Massachusetts General Hospital
Guide to Primary Care Psychiatry

Massachusetts General Hospital
Guide to Primary Care Psychiatry

SECOND EDITION

EDITORS

THEODORE A. STERN, M.D.

Chief, The Avery D. Weisman, M.D., Psychiatry Consultation Service
Massachusetts General Hospital
Professor of Psychiatry
Harvard Medical School
Boston, Massachusetts

JOHN B. HERMAN, M.D.

Director of Clinical Services
Director of Post-Graduate Education
Department of Psychiatry
Massachusetts General Hospital
Medical Director, EAP
Partners HealthCare, Inc.
Assistant Professor of Psychiatry
Harvard Medical School
Boston, Massachusetts

PETER L. SLAVIN, M.D.

President, Massachusetts General Hospital
Senior Lecturer
Department of Health Care Policy
Harvard Medical School
Boston, Massachusetts

McGraw-Hill
Medical Publishing Division

New York Chicago San Francisco Lisbon
London Madrid Mexico City Milan New Delhi San Juan
Seoul Singapore Sydney Toronto

Massachusetts General Hospital Guide to Primary Care Psychiatry, Second Edition

Copyright © 2004 by The **McGraw-Hill Companies**, Inc. All rights reserved. Printed in the United States of America. Except as permitted under the United States Copyright Act of 1976, no part of this publication may be reproduced or distributed in any form or by any means, or stored in a data base or retrieval system, without the prior written permission of the publisher.

Previous edition copyright © 1998 by The McGraw-Hill Companies, Inc.

1 2 3 4 5 6 7 8 9 0 DOC/DOC 0 9 8 7 6 5 4 3

ISBN 0-07-141001-5

This book was set in Times Roman by Pine Tree Composition.
The editors were Marc Strauss and Lisa Silverman.
The production supervisor was Catherine Saggese.
Project management was provided by Pine Tree Composition.
The index was prepared by Walsh Associates.
RR Donnelley was printer and binder.

This book is printed on acid-free paper.

Library of Congress Cataloging-in-Publication Data

Massachusetts General Hospital guide to primary care psychiatry / edited by
    Theodore A. Stern, John B. Herman, Peter L. Slavin.—2nd ed.
      p. ; cm.
    Rev. ed. of: MGH guide to psychiatry in primary care / editors, Theodore A. Stern, John
B. Herman, Peter L. Slavin. c1998.
    Includes bibliographical references and index.
    ISBN 0-07-141001-5
    1. Psychiatry—Handbooks, manuals, etc.   I. Title: Guide to primary care psychiatry.   II.
Stern, Theodore A.   III. Herman, John B.   IV. Slavin, Peter L.   V. MGH guide to psychiatry
in primary care.
    [DNLM: 1. Mental Disorders—diagnosis.   2. Mental Disorders—therapy.   3. Primary
Health Care. WM 140 M4139 2004]
    RC456.M368 2004
    686.89—dc21
                                                                    2003051018

To the former chiefs of The Massachusetts General Hospital's Psychiatry Consultation Service

Avery D. Weisman, M.D.	1959–1968
Thomas P. Hackett, M.D.	1968–1977
Ned H. Cassem, M.D.	1977–1990
George B. Murray, M.D.	1990–1995

and the MGH's extraordinary medical and surgical staff with whom we work and care for patients every day.

T.A.S.
J.B.H.
P.L.S.

. . . and to my first teacher of psychiatric medicine, my father, Marvin Stern, M.D., whose skill as a clinician and whose ability to teach with humor and intellect, has been a guiding force.

T.A.S.

Contents

Contributors   *xiii*
Foreword   *xxi*
Preface   *xxiii*

I: Introduction   1

CHAPTER 1
Collaborative Treatment by Primary Care Providers and Psychiatrists   3

CHAPTER 2
Overview of the Practice of Psychotherapy   13

CHAPTER 3
Effective Psychiatric Interviewing in Primary Care Medicine   19

CHAPTER 4
Making a Referral   27

CHAPTER 5
Approach to Informed Consent   35

II: Diagnostic Strategies   41

CHAPTER 6
How to Use the *DSM-IV-PC*   43

CHAPTER 7
Screening Tests for Detection of Psychiatric Disorders   51

CHAPTER 8
Use of Neuroimaging Techniques   61

III: Therapeutic Strategies   67

CHAPTER 9
Cognitive-Behavioral Therapy   69

CHAPTER 10
Cognitive-Behavioral Strategies for Specific Disorders   75

CHAPTER 11
Principles of Stress Management   85

IV: Approaches to Patients with Specific Conditions   95

Primary Psychiatric and Neurologic Illnesses

CHAPTER 12
Personality Disorders I: Approaches to Difficult Patients   97

CHAPTER 13
Personality Disorders II: Approaches to Specific Behavioral Presentations   105

CHAPTER 14
The Patient with Depression   111

CHAPTER 15
The Suicidal Patient   127

CHAPTER 16
The Anxious Patient   137

CHAPTER 17
The Patient with Acute Grief   153

CHAPTER 18
The Patient with Hallucinations and Delusions   157

CHAPTER 19
The Patient with Obsessions or Compulsions   165

CHAPTER 20
The Patient with Anorexia or Bulimia   171

CHAPTER 21
The Patient with Elevated, Expansive, or Irritable Mood   181

CHAPTER 22
The Patient with Memory Problems or Dementia   197

CHAPTER 23
The Patient with Neuropsychiatric Dysfunction   213

CHAPTER 24
The Patient with Seizures   225

CHAPTER 25
The Patient Following Closed Head Injury   237

CHAPTER 26
The Patient with Headache   243

CHAPTER 27
The Patient with Disordered Sleep   251

CHAPTER 28
The Patient with Dizziness   263

CHAPTER 29
The Patient with Multiple Physical Complaints   269

CHAPTER 30
Behavior Problems of Children and Adolescents   279

CHAPTER 31
The Patient with Attention-Deficit Hyperactivity Disorder   287

Medical-Related Illnesses

CHAPTER 32
The Patient with Chronic Medical Illness   301

CHAPTER 33
The Patient with Acute or Chronic Pain   311

CHAPTER 34
The Patient with Fatigue   329

CHAPTER 35
The Patient with Chronic Fatigue Syndrome   335

CHAPTER 36
**The Patient with Multiple Environmental Allergies/Idiopathic
Environmental Intolerance**   341

CHAPTER 37
The Patient with Irritable Bowel Syndrome   349

CHAPTER 38
The Patient with Cancer   359

CHAPTER 39
The Patient with HIV Infection   367

CHAPTER 40
The Patient Undergoing Organ Transplantation   385

CHAPTER 41
The Patient with Sexual Dysfunction   393

CHAPTER 42
The Patient with Impotence   405

CHAPTER 43
The Patient with Infertility   413

CHAPTER 44
The Patient with Premenstrual Syndrome   421

CHAPTER 45
The Patient Entering Menopause   429

CHAPTER 46
The Pregnant Patient   435

CHAPTER 47
The Patient with Post-partum Mood Disorders   443

CHAPTER 48
The Obese Patient   451

CHAPTER 49
The Geriatric Patient   469

CHAPTER 50
The Patient Requiring Rehabilitation   479

CHAPTER 51
The Patient Receiving Palliative Care   487

Other Patient Populations and Situations

CHAPTER 52
The Alcoholic Patient   499

CHAPTER 53
The Cocaine or Opiate-Abusing Patient   513

CHAPTER 54
The Patient Receiving Steroids   521

CHAPTER 55
The Patient Receiving Psychotropics   529

CHAPTER 56
The Patient Following a Traumatic Event   535

CHAPTER 57
The Patient Who Has Been Sexually Assaulted   545

CHAPTER 58
Approach to Domestic Violence   553

CHAPTER 59
The Family in Crisis   559

CHAPTER 60
The Violent Patient   567

CHAPTER 61
Civil Commitment and the Patient Refusing Treatment   577

CHAPTER 62
The Management of Denial   583

CHAPTER 63
The Patient Seeking Disability Benefits   589

CHAPTER 64
The Homeless Patient   595

CHAPTER 65
The Celebrity Patient   603

V: Therapeutic Complications and Considerations 611

CHAPTER 66
Management of Antidepressant-Induced Side Effects 613

CHAPTER 67
Cardiovascular Side Effects of Psychotropic Agents 629

CHAPTER 68
Drug-Drug Interactions: The Interface between Psychotropics and Other Agents 653

CHAPTER 69
Natural Medications in Psychiatry 671

CHAPTER 70
Treatment Decisions at the End of Life 687

VI: Quality-of-Life Enhancing Strategies 697

CHAPTER 71
Encouraging Your Patients to Live Healthier Lives 699

CHAPTER 72
Smoking Cessation Strategies 705

CHAPTER 73
Useful Exercise Programs and Strategies for Weight Loss 713

VII: Physician-Assistance Strategies 723

CHAPTER 74
Enhancing Patient Compliance with Treatment Recommendations 725

CHAPTER 75
Breaking Bad News 735

CHAPTER 76
Maintaining Boundaries in the Doctor-Patient Relationship 743

CHAPTER 77
Dealing with Psychiatric Issues in an Era of Managed/Capitated Care 749

CHAPTER 78
Coping with the Rigors of Medical Practice 757

Index 765

Contributors

Number in brackets refers to chapters of which contributor was author or co-author.

Susan Abbey, M.D., F.R.C.P. (C) [36]
Director
Program in Medical Psychiatry
Associate Professor
Department of Psychiatry
University of Toronto
Toronto, Ontario
Canada

Robert S. Abernethy III, M.D. [2]
Psychiatrist
Massachusetts General Hospital
Assistant Professor of Psychiatry
Harvard Medical School
Boston, Massachusetts

David Ahern, Ph.D. [11]
Chief Science Officer, The Abacus Group
Assistant Professor of Psychology
in the Department of Psychiatry
Harvard Medical School, Brigham
and Women's Hospital
Brigham and Women's Hospital
Boston, Massachusetts

Menekse Alpay, M.D. [33]
Clinical Assistant in Psychiatry
Massachusetts General Hospital
Instructor in Psychiatry
Harvard Medical School
Boston, Massachusetts

Jonathan Alpert, M.D., Ph.D. [68]
Assistant Psychiatrist and Associate Director
Depression Clinical and Research Program
Massachusetts General Hospital
Assistant Professor of Psychiatry
Harvard Medical School
Boston, Massachusetts

Claudia Baldassano, M.D. [26, 28]
Department of Psychiatry
University of Pennsylvania School of Medicine
Philadelphia, Pennsylvania

Anne E. Becker, M.D., Ph.D. [48]
Director, Adult Eating and Weight Disorders Program
Massachusetts General Hospital
Assistant Professor of Psychiatry
and Medical Anthropology
Departments of Psychiatry and Social Medicine
Harvard Medical School
Boston, Massachusetts

Eugene Beresin, M.D. [20]
Psychiatrist and Director, Child
and Adolescent Residency
Training Program in Psychiatry
Massachusetts General Hospital and
McLean Hospital
Associate Professor of Psychiatry
Harvard Medical School
Boston, Massachusetts

Joseph Biederman, M.D. **[31]**
Chief, Joint Program in Pediatric
Psychopharmacology
Massachusetts General and McLean Hospitals
Professor of Psychiatry
Harvard Medical School
Boston, Massachusetts

Michael F. Bierer, M.D. **[18, 52, 64]**
Assistant Physician
Massachusetts General Hospital
Director, Boston Health Care for the
Homeless Program
Massachusetts General Hospital
Instructor in Medicine
Harvard Medical School
Boston, Massachusetts

Stephen L. Boswell, M.D. **[39]**
Executive Director
Fenway Community Health Center
Assistant in Medicine
Massachusetts General Hospital
Assistant Professor of Medicine
Harvard Medical School
Boston, Massachusetts

Jennifer Bremer, M.D. **[20]**
Medical Director
Eating Disorders Program
University of Chicago
Chicago, Illinois

Lori Viscogliosi Calabrese, M.D. **[29]**
Assistant Clinical Professor of Psychiatry
Yale University School of Medicine
South Windsor, Connecticut

Barbara Cannon, M.D. **[26]**
Psychiatrist
Somerville Mental Health Clinic
Somerville, Massachusetts

Alexandra F.M. Cist, M.D. **[70]**
Internist
Massachusetts General Hospital
Instructor in Medicine
Harvard Medical School
Boston, Massachusetts

Lee S. Cohen, M.D. **[43, 44, 45, 46, 47]**
Director
Perinatal and Reproductive Psychiatry
Clinical Research Program
Clinical Psychopharmacology and
Behavior Therapy Unit
Massachusetts General Hospital
Associate Professor of Psychiatry
Harvard Medical School
Boston, Massachusetts

Andrew J. Cole, M.D., F.R.C.P. (C) **[24]**
Director
Epilepsy Service
Massachusetts General Hospital
Associate Professor of Neurology
Harvard Medical School
Boston, Massachusetts

Paul M. Copeland, M.D. **[73]**
Clinical Associate in Medicine
Massachusetts General Hospital
Assistant Clinical Professor of Medicine
Harvard Medical School
Boston, Massachusetts

M. Cornelia Cremens, M.D., M.P.H. **[49, 73]**
Assistant Psychiatrist and Geriatric Psychiatrist
Beacon Hill Senior Health Practice
Massachusetts General Hospital
Instructor in Psychiatry
Harvard Medical School
Boston, Massachusetts

Darin Dougherty, M.D. **[8, 19]**
Assistant Director, Psychiatric Neuroimaging Group
Massachusetts General Hospital
Assistant Professor of Psychiatry
Harvard Medical School
Boston, Massachusetts

Barbara A. Dunderdale, R.N., B.S.N., M.B.A. **[65]**
Senior Major Gifts Officer, Development Office
Massachusetts General Hospital
Formerly, Nurse Manager
Phillips House
Massachusetts General Hospital
Boston, Massachusetts

Steven A. Epstein, M.D. **[4]**
Chair, Department of Psychiatry
Georgetown University Medical Center
Washington, DC

William Falk, M.D. [22]
Psychiatrist and Co-director
Geriatric Neurobehavioral Clinic
Massachusetts General Hospital
Assistant Professor of Psychiatry
Harvard Medical School
Boston, Massachusetts

Maurizio Fava, M.D. [7, 14, 44]
Psychiatrist and Director
Depression Clinical and Research Program
Massachusetts General Hospital
Professor of Psychiatry
Harvard Medical School
Boston, Massachusetts

Anne K. Fishel, Ph.D. [59]
Assistant in Psychology
Massachusetts General Hospital
Assistant Clinical Professor of Psychology
Department of Psychiatry
Harvard Medical School
Boston, Massachusetts

Gregory L. Fricchione, M.D. [32]
Associate Chief and Director of the
Division of Psychiatry and Medicine
Massachusetts General Hospital
Associate Professor of Psychiatry
Harvard Medical School
Boston, Massachusetts

Melissa Frumin, M.D. [38]
Associate Physician in Medicine
Brigham and Women's Hospital
Instructor in Psychiatry
Harvard Medical School
Boston, Massachusetts

Christine Galardy, M.D., Ph.D. [74]
4th Year Resident in Psychiatry
Massachusetts General Hospital and
McLean Hospital
Clinical Fellow in Psychiatry
Harvard Medical School
Boston, Massachusetts

David R. Gastfriend, M.D. [53]
Psychiatrist and Director
Addiction Research Program
Massachusetts General Hospital
Director, Partners Healthcare Fellowship
in Addiction Psychiatry
Associate Professor of Psychiatry
Harvard Medical School
Boston, Massachusetts

Edith S. Geringer, M.D. [1]
Psychiatrist and Co-Director
Primary Care Psychiatry Unit
Massachusetts General Hospital
Instructor in Psychiatry
Harvard Medical School
Boston, Massachusetts

Christopher Gordon, M.D. [3]
Assistant Psychiatrist
Massachusetts General Hospital
Medical Director and Vice President
for Behavioral Health, Advocates, Inc.
Framingham, Massachusetts
Assistant Clinical Professor of Psychiatry
Harvard Medical School
Boston, Massachusetts

Allan H. Goroll, M.D. [3]
Physician
Massachusetts General Hospital
Associate Professor of Medicine
Harvard Medical School
Boston, Massachusetts

Donna B. Greenberg, M.D. [34, 35, 38]
Psychiatrist and Director
Medical Student Education
Department of Psychiatry
Massachusetts General Hospital
Associate Professor of Psychiatry
Harvard Medical School
Boston, Massachusetts

James E. Groves, M.D. [12, 13, 65]
Psychiatrist
Massachusetts General Hospital
Associate Clinical Professor of Psychiatry
Harvard Medical School
Boston, Massachusetts

Paul Hamburg, M.D. [75]
Associate Director
Eating Disorders Unit
Massachusetts General Hospital
Assistant Clinical Professor of Psychiatry
Harvard Medical School
Boston, Massachusetts

Joseph A. Harrington, M.D. [9, 10]
Charles River Medical Associates
Natick, Massachusetts

Stephan Heckers, M.D. [18, 23, 24]
Assistant Psychiatrist
Assistant Director of Psychiatric Neuroimaging
Research
Massachusetts General Hospital
Assistant Professor of Psychiatry
Harvard Medical School
Boston, Massachusetts

John B. Herman, M.D. [74]
Director of Clinical Services
Director of Post-Graduate Education
Department of Psychiatry
Massachusetts General Hospital
Medical Director, EAP
Partners HealthCare, Inc.
Assistant Professor of Psychiatry
Harvard Medical School
Boston, Massachusetts

David Herzog, M.D. [20]
Executive Director
Harvard Eating Disorders Center
Professor of Psychiatry (Pediatrics)
Harvard Medical School
Boston, Massachusetts

Jeff C. Huffman, M.D. [21, 62, 67]
Fellow in Consultation Psychiatry
Graduate Assistant in Psychiatry
Massachusetts General Hospital
Clinical Fellow in Psychiatry
Harvard Medical School
Boston, Massachusetts

Michael S. Jellinek, M.D. [30, 77]
Psychiatrist and Chief, Child Psychiatry Service
Senior Vice-President for Administration
Massachusetts General Hospital
President, Newton-Wellesley Hospital
Professor of Psychiatry and Pediatrics
Harvard Medical School
Boston, Massachusetts

Michael A. Jenike, M.D. [19]
Associate Chief of Psychiatry
Massachusetts General Hospital
Professor of Psychiatry
Harvard Medical School
Boston, Massachusetts

Gorman R. Jones III, M.D. [51]
Director
Medical Clinics
Baptist Princeton Hospital
Birmingham, Alabama

Lee M. Kaplan, M.D., Ph.D. [48]
Director
Obesity Center
Massachusetts General Hospital
Associate Chief
Gastrointestinal Unit
Massachusetts General Hospital
Associate Professor of Medicine
Harvard Medical School
Boston, Massachusetts

Helen G. Kim, M.D. [78]
Hennepin Women's Mental Health Program
Hennepin County Medical Center
Clinical Assistant Professor of Psychiatry
University of Minnesota Medical School
Minneapolis, Minnesota

Scott Kim, M.D., Ph.D. [70]
Assistant Professor of Psychiatry and
Medical Humanities
University of Rochester Medical Center
Rochester, New York

Andrea Kolsky, B.A. [55]
Clinical Research Coordinator
Depression and Clinical Research Program
Massachusetts General Hospital
Boston, Massachusetts

Jennifer M. Lafayette, M.D. [64]
*Assistant in Psychiatry and Associate Director of
the Acute Psychiatry Service
Massachusetts General Hospital
Instructor in Psychiatry
Harvard Medical School
Boston, Massachusetts*

Isabel T. Lagomasino, M.D. [15, 54]
*Assistant Professor of Psychiatry
Charles R. Drew University of Medicine
and Science
Clinical Instructor in Psychiatry
UCLA School of Medicine
Los Angeles, California*

Michael L. Langan, M.D. [49]
*Assistant in Medicine and Geriatrician,
Massachusetts General Senior Health and
Spaulding Rehabilitation Center
Massachusetts General Hospital
Instructor in Medicine
Harvard Medical School
Boston, Massachusetts*

Bandy X. Lee, M.D. [78]
*Former Resident in Psychiatry
Massachusetts General Hospital
Clinical Fellow in Psychiatry
Harvard Medical School
Boston, Massachusetts*

Dara K. Lee, M.D. [16, 66]
*Clinical Fellow in Cardiovascular
Medicine
Brigham and Women's Hospital
Instructor in Medicine
Harvard Medical School
Boston, Massachusetts*

Andrew B. Littman, M.D. [71, 72]
*Associate Psychiatrist
Massachusetts General Hospital
Instructor in Psychiatry
Harvard Medical School
Boston, Massachusetts*

Keith Luther, M.D. [8]
*Departments of Internal
Medicine and Pediatrics
Stevens Hospital
Edmonds, Washington*

Edward Marcantonio, M.D. [32]
*Associate Physician
Division of General Internal Medicine and Gerontology
Brigham and Women's Hospital
Instructor in Medicine
Harvard Medical School
Boston, Massachusetts*

Edward Messner, M.D. [78]
*Psychiatrist
Massachusetts General Hospital
Associate Clinical Professor of Psychiatry
Harvard Medical School
Boston, Massachusetts*

Patricia Mian, R.N., M.S., C.S. [57]
*Psychiatric Clinical Nurse Specialist
Emergency Department
Massachusetts General Hospital
Boston, Massachusetts*

David Mischoulon, M.D., Ph.D. [7, 69]
*Depression Clinical and Research Program
Massachusetts General Hospital
Assistant Professor of Psychiatry
Harvard Medical School
Boston, Massachusetts*

Andrew A. Nierenberg, M.D. [55, 69]
*Psychiatrist and Associate Director
Depression Clinical and Research Program
Massachusetts General Hospital
Associate Professor of Psychiatry
Harvard Medical School
Boston, Massachusetts*

Ruta Nonacs, M.D., Ph.D. [43]
*Clinical Assistant in Psychiatry
Massachusetts General Hospital
Instructor in Psychiatry
Harvard Medical School
Boston, Massachusetts*

James J. O'Connell III, M.D. [53]
*Director
Boston HealthCare for the Homeless
Program
Assistant in Medicine
Massachusetts General Hospital
Clinical Instructor in Medicine
Harvard Medical School
Boston, Massachusetts*

Kevin W. Olden, M.D. [37]
Departments of Gastroenterology and
Transplantation Medicine
Mayo Clinic Scottsdale
Scottsdale, Arizona

Rafael Ornstein, M.D. [56]
Assistant in Psychiatry
Massachusetts General Hospital
Instructor in Psychiatry
Harvard Medical School
Boston, Massachusetts

Michael W. Otto, Ph.D. [9, 10]
Psychologist and Director
Cognitive-Behavioral Therapy Program
Massachusetts General Hospital
Associate Professor of Psychology
Department of Psychiatry
Harvard Medical School
Boston, Massachusetts

Elyse R. Park, M.D. [11]
Psychiatrist
Massachusetts General Hospital
Instructor in Psychology
Harvard Medical School
Boston, Massachusetts

Roger C. Pasinski, M.D. [23]
Medical Director
MGH-Revere Health Care Center
Assistant Pediatrician and Physician
Massachusetts General Hospital
Instructor in Medicine
Harvard Medical School
Boston, Massachusetts

Mark H. Pollack, M.D. [16, 66]
Psychiatrist and Director
Anxiety Disorders Program
Clinical Psychopharmacology and
Behavior Therapy Unit
Massachusetts General Hospital
Associate Professor of Psychiatry
Harvard Medical School
Boston, Massachusetts

Alicia Powell, M.D. [18]
Clinical Associate in Psychiatry
Massachusetts General Hospital
Clinical Instructor in Psychiatry
Harvard Medical School
Boston, Massachusetts

Laura M. Prager, M.D. [40]
Psychiatrist
Massachusetts General Hospital
Clinical Instructor in Psychiatry
Harvard Medical School
Boston, Massachusetts

John Querques, M.D. [39]
Clinical Assistant in Psychiatry
Massachusetts General Hospital
Instructor in Psychiatry
Harvard Medical School
Boston, Massachusetts

Terry Rabinowitz, M.D., F.A.P.M. [50]
Director
Psychiatric Consultation Service
Fletcher Allen Health Care
Burlington, Vermont
Associate Professor of Psychiatry and
Family Practice
University of Vermont College of Medicine
Burlington, Vermont

Scott Rauch, M.D. [8]
Psychiatrist and Associate Chief
of Psychiatry for Neuroscience Research
Massachusetts General Hospital
Associate Professor of Psychiatry
Harvard Medical School
Boston, Massachusetts

Julia Reade, M.D. [58]
Clinical Assistant in Psychiatry
Massachusetts General Hospital
Clinical Instructor in Psychiatry
Harvard Medical School
Boston, Massachusetts

Noreen A. Reilly-Harrington, M.A. [9, 10]
Clinical Fellow in Psychology
Department of Psychiatry
Massachusetts General Hospital
Clinical Fellow in Psychology
Harvard Medical School
Boston, Massachusetts

John A. Renner, Jr., M.D. [52]
Associate Psychiatrist
Massachusetts General Hospital
Chief
Substance Abuse Treatment Program and
Associate Chief
Psychiatry Service
Veterans Administration Medical Center,
Boston, Massachusetts
Associate Professor of Psychiatry
Boston University School of Medicine
Clinical Instructor in Psychiatry
Harvard Medical School
Boston, Massachusetts

James M. Richter, M.D. [27]
Medical Director
Massachusetts General Hospital
Physicians Organization
Associate Professor of Medicine
Harvard Medical School
Boston, Massachusetts

Jerrold F. Rosenbaum, M.D. [14]
Chief, Department of Psychiatry
Massachusetts General Hospital
Professor of Psychiatry
Harvard Medical School
Boston, Massachusetts

Gary Sachs, M.D. [21]
Psychiatrist and Director
Harvard Bipolar Research Program
Massachusetts General Hospital
Associate Professor of Psychiatry
Harvard Medical School
Boston, Massachusetts

Kathy M. Sanders, M.D. [25, 60]
Psychiatrist and Director
Adult Residency Training Program in Psychiatry
Massachusetts General Hospital and
McLean Hospital
Assistant Professor of Psychiatry
Harvard Medical School
Boston, Massachusetts

Ronald Schouten, M.D., J.D. [5, 61, 63, 76]
Director
Law and Psychiatry Service
Massachusetts General Hospital
Associate Professor of Psychiatry
Harvard Medical School
Boston, Massachusetts

Linda Shafer, M.D. [41, 42]
Psychiatrist and Director
Human Sexuality/Sexual Dysfunction
Program
Massachusetts General Hospital
Instructor in Psychiatry
Harvard Medical School
Boston, Massachusetts

John L. Shuster, M.D. [51]
Medical Director
UAB Hospice
University of Alabama, Birmingham
Associate Professor of Psychiatry
University of Alabama, Birmingham

Peter L. Slavin, M.D., M.B.A.
President, Massachusetts General Hospital
Senior Lecturer
Department of Health Care Policy
Harvard Medical School

Felicia Smith, M.D. [25]
4th Year Resident in Psychiatry
Massachusetts General Hospital and
McLean Hospital
Clinical Fellow in Psychiatry
Harvard Medical School
Boston, Massachusetts

Jordan W. Smoller, M.D., S.M. [16, 66]
Assistant in Psychiatry
Massachusetts General Hospital
Assistant Professor of Psychiatry
Harvard Medical School
Boston, Massachusetts

Claudio N. Soares, M.D., Ph.D. [44, 45]
Assistant in Research
Massachusetts General Hospital
Instructor in Psychiatry
Harvard Medical School
Boston, Massachusetts

Thomas J. Spencer, M.D. [31]
Psychiatrist and Assistant Director of Pediatric
Psychopharmacology
Massachusetts General Hospital
Associate Professor of Psychiatry
Harvard Medical School
Boston, Massachusetts

Theodore A. Stern, M.D. [4, 6, 15, 17, 21, 26, 28, 29, 36, 50, 51, 54, 62, 65, 67]
Psychiatrist and Chief
The Avery D. Weisman, M.D., Psychiatry
Consultation Service
Massachusetts General Hospital
Professor of Psychiatry
Harvard Medical School
Boston, Massachusetts

Paul Summergrad, M.D. [77]
Psychiatrist and Director
Psychiatry Network
Partners HealthCare System, Inc.
Massachusetts General Hospital
Associate Professor of Psychiatry
Harvard Medical School
Boston, Massachusetts

Owen S. Surman, M.D. [40]
Psychiatrist and Psychiatric Consultant
for the Transplant Unit
Massachusetts General Hospital
Associate Professor of Psychiatry
Harvard Medical School
Boston, Massachusetts

George E. Tesar, M.D. [67]
Chairman
Department of Psychiatry & Psychology
Cleveland Clinic Foundation
Cleveland, Ohio

Adele C. Viguera, M.D. [45, 57]
Assistant in Psychiatry
Associate Director, Perinatal and Reproductive
Psychiatry
Clinical Research Program
Massachusetts General Hospital
Assistant Professor of Psychiatry
Harvard Medical School
Boston, Massachusetts

Jeffrey B. Weilburg, M.D. [27]
Director
Neuropsychiatry and Sleep Disorders
Section
Clinical Psychopharmacology and
Behavior Therapy Unit
Massachusetts General Hospital
Assistant Professor of Psychiatry
Harvard Medical School
Boston, Massachusetts

Avery Weisman, M.D. [17]
Senior Psychiatrist
Massachusetts General Hospital
Professor of Psychiatry, Emeritus
Harvard Medical School
Boston, Massachusetts

Timothy E. Wilens, M.D. [31]
Associate Psychiatrist
Pediatric and Adult Psychopharmacology Clinics
Massachusetts General Hospital
Associate Professor of Psychiatry
Harvard Medical School
Boston, Massachusetts

Thomas N. Wise, M.D. [6]
Professor and Vice Chairman
Department of Psychiatry
Georgetown University
Washington, D.C.
Associate Professor of Psychiatry
Johns Hopkins School of Medicine
Baltimore, Maryland

Jonathan L. Worth, M.D. [39]
Psychiatrist and Director
Robert B. Andrews (HIV Psychiatry) Unit and
Director, Outpatient Psychiatry
Massachusetts General Hospital
Instructor in Psychiatry
Harvard Medical School
Boston, Massachusetts

Foreword

Fifty percent of visits to primary care offices are for psychiatric rather than medical problems.

Pediatricians, family practitioners, internists, surgeons, and obstetricians have an increasing responsibility to keep abreast of the rapid advances in the diagnosis and treatment of these disorders. This timely and practical guide comes at a most important juncture in the practice of many busy practitioners.

In its 1811 charter, the Massachusetts General Hospital's founders declared

> *Among the unfortunate objects of this charitable*
> *project, particular provision is to be made for*
> *such as the wisdom of Providence may have seen*
> *fit to visit with the most terrible of all human*
> *maladies—a depravation of reason.*

In 1818, MGH's first patients, the mentally ill, were admitted to what would later be called McLean Hospital. In 1821, the General Hospital opened its doors to the medically ill. In 1934, endeavoring to bridge the gap between mind and body, the eminent neuropathologist Stanley Cobb established the nation's second general hospital department of psychiatry. Since then MGH has enjoyed its place at the frontier of modern medicine and modern psychiatry. The standard of care practiced on the surgical and medical wards by the psychiatric consultation service is characterized by practicality, efficiency, and interdisciplinary collegiality. This Guide expands the essence of that approach into the realm of the primary care clinician.

The editors of this book have created an accessible, practical reference source specifically intended for the busy practitioner. It recognizes common presenting problems and proposes straightforward treatment options. It does not assume training in psychiatry. Each chapter represents an interdisciplinary collaboration, either coauthored or reviewed and revised with a practicing primary care provider.

This book represents the best of MGH's tradition of patient care, teaching, and application of clinical research. Easily accessible, its design should find it a frequently used, effective reference tool on the desk and in the examining room of every busy practitioner.

Eugene Brauwald, M.D.
Distinguished Hershey Professor
  of the Theory and Practice of Medicine
Harvard Medical School
Boston, Massachusetts

Samuel O. Thier, M.D.
Professor of Medicine and Professor of
  Health Care Policy
Harvard Medical School
Boston, Massachusetts

Preface

Half of all mental illness goes untreated. Of those patients who do seek treatment, two-thirds receive their care from non-mental health clinicians. Therefore, this book was written for busy clinicians in general practice. It was designed to provide clear guidelines for the diagnosis and treatment of common emotional and behavioral problems. Since the publication of the first edition, we have been delighted to see this vision realized; dog-eared copies are frequently sighted on the desks of our physician colleagues at the MGH, across our country, and in translations around the globe. To ensure clarity and practicality each chapter was either co-authored or reviewed by a non-psychiatrist. One of us (P.L.S.) is an internist. For more than 25 years another of us (T.A.S.) has consulted to and answered the questions posed by this book's intended readers.

The odyssey of *MGH Guide to Primary Care Psychiatry* reflects the synergy of a good idea and great people. The blessings of fate played their mythic role. Steven Hyman, M.D., at the time a member of our staff and the Director of the National Institute of Mental Health and now the Provost of Harvard University, encouraged us to move forward on this journey. Our former Chief, Ned Cassem, M.D., and current Chief, Jerry Rosenbaum, M.D., endorsed the project as an essential feature of our department's mission and immediately set forth to enlist the support of our busy and talented faculty; their efforts were crucial to its completion and success.

Many individuals reviewed parts of this manuscript and were critical to its fate. The editors gratefully thank our medical colleagues.

Judi Greenberg of the MGH General Counsel's office navigated treacherous legal currents as we sailed past the Scylla of contractual jargon and the Charybdis of copyright law. John Morton, Sara Nadelman, and Judy Byford sculpted organization out of chaos and provided the essential administrative shape of this effort. Jim Groves, M.D., designed the cover logo of the Bulfinch Building. Our editors at McGraw-Hill, Marc Strauss and Lisa Silverman, intrepidly pushed through the e-mails, voice-mails, faxes, and express-mail packages associated with 78 chapters and nearly 100 authors, all the while maintaining good humor and a reassuring style.

T.A.S.
J.B.H.
P.L.S.

SECTION I

Introduction

CHAPTER 1

Collaborative Treatment by Primary Care Providers and Psychiatrists

EDITH S. GERINGER

I. Introduction

A. Psychiatric disorders are prevalent and often go untreated.
1. The prevalence of mental disorders, including addiction, in the United States is 28%.
2. Only 40% of those with a psychiatric disorder receive treatment during their lifetimes.

B. Psychiatric Illness in Primary Care Settings
1. **Depression**
   a. **The prevalence of depression in primary care settings ranges from 6–17%,** compared with a prevalence of 6% for hypertension.
   b. Unfortunately, **depression is diagnosed in only 50% of those with depression** who present to primary care providers (PCPs).
   c. **Adequate treatment ensues in only about 17% of depressed patients** in primary care settings.
2. **Anxiety**
   a. **Anxiety disorders have a lifetime prevalence of 11–25%.** In a 1-year period, only 33% of patients with anxiety disorders obtain treatment and only 15% obtain mental health services.
   b. **Lifetime prevalence for generalized anxiety disorder (GAD) is** 5% in the general population and **3–10% in the primary care medical population.** This makes GAD the most common anxiety disorder in primary care settings.
   c. Anxiety disorders are common in the medically ill, especially those with chest pain, pulmonary disease, cerebrovascular disease, irritable bowel syndrome, and diabetes. Anxiety disorders have been detected in 25–50% of patients in these groups.
3. **Suicide**
   a. **15% of patients with affective disorders commit suicide.**
   b. **Half the patients who commit suicide sought treatment in a primary care setting within 1 month of dying.**
4. **Medical utilization**
   a. **Two-thirds of patients with undiagnosed depression have six visits or more a year with PCPs for somatic complaints.**
   b. Patients with somatization disorder have a nine-fold increase in the use of PCP resources compared to general medical patients.
   c. Depressed patients have a two-fold increase in general health care costs compared to non-depressed patients.
   d. About two-thirds of high utilizers of medical care have undertreated psychiatric disorders.

II. Barriers to Diagnosis and Treatment of Psychiatric Disorders in Primary Care Settings

A. Patient Factors

1. **A patient may present with a somatic complaint and minimize the mood component** of the illness. An example of this would be a chronic pain patient who states, "I'm depressed because of my pain. Wouldn't you be?"

2. **Concurrent medical illness often obscures psychiatric symptoms.** It is important to sort out the effects of medical illness on the vegetative symptoms of psychiatric disorders. Examples include anorexia in a depressed cancer patient and anxiety in a patient with a cardiac arrhythmia.

3. **Denial of psychiatric issues** or their mood symptoms may occur. A patient may present with a full complement of depressive symptoms but deny feeling sad. In this case, the physician must determine whether the patient has no mood symptoms or is reluctant to disclose them.

4. **Stigma and shame** lead to fear of a mental health diagnosis or referral. A patient may refuse a psychiatric referral in the belief that only crazy people see psychiatrists.

5. **The belief that psychiatric referral will lead to abandonment** by the PCP is common. This is especially true if patients are told implicitly or explicitly that they are being referred to a psychiatrist because there is nothing physically wrong with them or if a referral occurs only after the physician has become thoroughly frustrated with his or her inability to calm and reassure these patients about their symptoms.

6. **The belief that psychiatric illness is untreatable** is held by many patients. This belief is most often expressed by patients who are hopeless and depressed.

7. **The belief that psychiatric drugs are mind-altering and/or addictive** is common. It is interesting that psychiatric medications are one of the few classes of medication that patients categorically refuse to take despite the fact that they want treatment for their suffering.

8. **The belief that treatment will be too expensive** is common. Patients often are unaware of pharmaceutical company programs that help cover the cost of medications for medically indigent patients.

B. Physician Factors

1. **Often there is a lack of time** to make an accurate diagnosis and/or referral during an appointment.

2. **Fear of being embarrassed** and inadvertently stigmatizing a patient, especially if that patient becomes emotional and upset, can be especially tricky if the patient has a clear-cut life situation that is triggering the difficulties.

3. There often is **uncertainty about when and how to make an appropriate referral** for psychiatric services.

4. There may be **fear that the patient will have an illness that is unresponsive to treatment.**

5. The physician may have had **prior negative experiences** in which psychiatric consultants were seen as unavailable, uncommunicative, or unresponsive.

6. There may be a **lack of knowledge** about the appropriate diagnosis, drugs, and duration of treatment.

C. Health System Factors
1. **Visits are too short** for a full evaluation.
2. **Fewer reimbursement incentives** exist for problems with a mental health focus.
3. **Psychiatric resources may be unavailable.**
4. **Carve-outs of mental health coverage** in managed care systems can make referral difficult.

III. Models of Outpatient Primary Care Psychiatry

A. **Comprehensive medical clinics** (Table 1-1) involve a psychiatrist as part of the team, providing consultation or joint care with internists.
1. **The staff** can consist of internists, psychiatrists, family practitioners, physician assistants, nurse practitioners, medical residents, psychiatric residents, psychologists, and/or social workers.
2. **The patients** seen are often complex and challenging and may have hypochondriasis, somatization disorder, or complex co-morbid medical and psychiatric disorders.
3. **The support staff** is shared by all the practitioners, and **medical charts** are kept within the clinic.
4. **The location** is most often within the outpatient medical, rather than the psychiatric, setting.
5. **Teaching conferences** can be a part of this clinic, especially if trainees are involved.
6. **Advantages for PCPs** of this type of clinic include minimal barriers to communication between disciplines, the chance to work side by side with psychiatrists, opportunities for education, and treatment continuity.

Table 1-1. Comparison of Primary Care Psychiatry Models

Type	Location	Staff	Shared Charts	Teaching	Follow-up
Comprehensive clinic	Medical clinics	PCP, mental health	Yes	Yes	Yes
Consultation-liaison	Medical clinics	Mental health	Yes	Yes	No
Psychiatric consultation clinic	Psychiatric clinics	Mental health	No	No	Yes
Collaborative management	Medical clinics	PCP, mental health	Yes	Yes	Yes
Hybrid	Medical clinics	Mental health	No	Yes	Yes
Teleconsultation	Non-clinic	Mental health	No	Yes (informal)	No

7. **Advantages for patients** treated in this setting include treatment in a familiar place and not being singled out for mental health treatment.

8. **Disadvantages for PCPs** can include being unable to provide ongoing treatment for psychiatric disorders in one setting, especially if the need for mental health resources overwhelms the available staff.

9. **Disadvantages for patients can include** fragmentation of care between too many treaters and subtle stigmatization if the clinic is seen as existing only for problem patients.

B. **Consultation and liaison services with other outpatient settings** are used when a psychiatrist accepts a referral and/or consultation and sees the patient in an outpatient medical setting (primary care or medical specialty).

1. **Staffing** is usually provided by a psychiatrist or psychiatric resident. The psychiatrist is often present on an as-needed basis and may see patients independently or as a "guest interviewer" at a patient's appointment with the PCP.

2. **Patients** can be varied and can include those with somatization disorder, those with difficulty adhering to medical regimens, and those having difficulty coping with physical illness.

3. **The support staff** includes those in the clinic with whom the psychiatrist consults, and the psychiatrist uses the clinic's medical chart for his or her notes.

4. **The location** is the medical outpatient clinic where the person requesting the consultation sees patients.

5. The psychiatric consultation may occur as part of a teaching program, or the psychiatrist may present his or her observations at a **teaching conference.**

6. **Advantages for practitioners** include the ability to develop ongoing relationships between the consultant and the consultee and informal teaching through liaison activities. **Advantages for patients** include being treated in a familiar setting and being seen with the medical practitioner present.

7. **Problems include** the need to refer patients for ongoing mental health treatment, and difficulties in maintaining availability on an *ad hoc* basis in a fee-for-service setting.

C. **Psychiatric consultation clinics** are separate psychiatric clinics.

1. **The staff** can include psychiatrists, psychologists, psychiatric trainees, and social workers.

2. **Patients** include those requesting the help of a psychiatrist as well as those whom medical practitioners refer for evaluation. **Comprehensive psychiatric treatment** is also provided.

3. The clinic has its own **support staff** and keeps its own **medical charts.**

4. The clinic is **not at the medical site;** usually it is situated wherever outpatient psychiatric treatment occurs.

5. **Teaching conferences** with medical practitioners are not routine.

6. **Advantages** include being able to match referrals to staff availability and being able to offer a variety of treatment modalities.

7. **Problems** include the potential for poor communication between medical and mental health practitioners and the greater possibility that patients will refuse a referral because of stigmatization and fear of abandonment by the medical practitioner.

IV. Alternative Models of Outpatient Primary Care Psychiatry

A. In collaboratve management models, patients pay alternate visits to primary care providers and psychiatrists within the same clinic.

1. **The staff** includes primary care medicine physicians, family practitioners, and psychiatrists.

2. **Patients** are identified by the PCP as having a psychiatric disorder that needs pharmacologic treatment. In a stepped collaborative care model, only those patients who have failed initial psychiatric treatment by the PCP are referred for collaborative care.

3. **The support staff** is shared by all the practitioners, and **medical charts** are shared by PCPs and psychiatrists.

4. Services are **located in the primary care medicine clinic.**

5. **Teaching conferences** are a routine part of the education provided by the psychiatrists. These conferences focus on pharmacologic and behavioral treatments for common psychiatric disorders. **Case-by-case consultation** is readily available.

6. **Advantages for PCPs** include enhanced communication between physicians, many opportunities for formal and informal physician education, and the ability to develop ongoing relationships between the disciplines. **Advantages for patients** include maintenance of continuity with the PCP, treatment in a familiar setting, easy access to specialists, and improved education. Studies have shown that patients have more depression-free days and greater adherence to medication with this approach.

7. Disadvantages include greater health care costs (mostly from filling antidepressant prescriptions).

B. Hybrid models combine the services of a psychiatric referral clinic, the availability of the consultation model, and familiarity with the staff in the comprehensive medical clinics.

1. **The staff** includes psychiatrists, psychologists, and psychiatric trainees. Patients are seen by scheduled appointment, with time set aside each week for urgent evaluations.

2. **Patients** include the full range of patients seen in a general outpatient psychiatry clinic plus those who have co-morbid medical and psychiatric disorders. Patients are seen only after referral by the PCP.

3. Some **support staff** is shared with the general medical clinic. The primary care psychiatry clinic keeps its own **medical records.** PCPs send a **written referral request** before a patient is scheduled to be seen, and patients give demographic and insurance information when an initial appointment is made by telephone with a person at the psychiatric clinic who has been trained in triage techniques.

4. The clinic is **situated within the outpatient internal medicine clinics.**

5. Some of the staff members participate in a regular **teaching conference** for primary care medical residents.

6. **Advantages for PCPs** include the ability to develop long-term relationships between consultants and consultees, to have frequent opportunities for informal consultation, and to have enough staff members to see patients in a timely fashion. **Advantages for patients** include increased medical legitimacy and decreased stigmatization

when being seen on site and being seen for evaluation and treatment by the same psychiatrist.

C. **The psychiatric teleconsultation unit can be provided as a full-time service with immediate telephone consultation to PCPs.**

1. The service is **staffed** by staff psychiatrists experienced in consultation and liaison psychiatry.

2. **Patients** do not have access to the service. **PCPs** use the service for consultation, triage, referral, psychopharmacologic management, behavioral management, and general psychiatry questions.

3. **Records** are kept in a computerized form. The record can be modified to generate a consultation letter to the PCP and a referral letter if one is needed.

4. **The support staff** is available to help facilitate referrals.

5. Although the service provides no formal teaching, by definition its function involves **teaching.**

6. **Advantages of the service include immediate responses by consultants** and regular staffing so that a PCP can establish an ongoing relationship with the teleconsultation staff.

7. **Disadvantages include a non-reimbursable service** in a fee-for-service setting. This may not apply to a setting with significant capitation.

8. Other telepsychiatry models use videoconferencing to allow patients at rural sites to be seen by psychiatrists at regional medical centers. This has been used for both evaluation and management.

V. Communication between PCPs and Psychiatrists

A. **Referrals** usually are initiated by the PCP, although occasionally they come from the patient. Referrals may be **communicated through notes, letters, phone calls, or face-to-face conversations.**

1. **Written referrals are the most effective method,** as they provide the consultant with an immediate reminder at the time of the consultation request. Written referrals should include the pertinent history and the specific reasons for the referral, including diagnostic or management issues. Even a one-sentence referral note or a copy of the patient's last visit note is preferable to nothing. Psychiatrists report that about one-half of PCPs send written information for a new referral, about one-third send no information at all. Especially confidential or sensitive material can be handled through an additional telephone call or a face-to-face meeting with the consultant, if that can be done in a timely manner.

2. Care must be taken to ensure that the referral reaches the consultant before the patient's visit. **Faxes and e-mail** can be very helpful if adequate confidentiality can be maintained through all phases of the communication.

3. **Phone referrals** ideally should be made to the consultant; however, if support staff members are adequately trained, they can gather pertinent screening information. A phone call to the support staff is always preferable to no information.

4. **Face-to-face conversations** between providers allow more detailed information to be given, and a brief conversation about the patient may bring out additional questions to be answered by the consultant. This is especially true with patients whose major difficulties include non-compliance or other behavioral problems.

An example of this is an initial referral to help assess and manage depression that is broadened to include assessment of a personality disorder when the patient's non-compliant and provocative behavior is discussed in a face-to-face conversation between the PCP and the consultant. The greatest disadvantage of this method of referral is the difficulty of arranging it. Phone calls have similar advantages and disadvantages.

B. Consultation notes can appear in a patient's clinic chart if the chart is shared, as in the collaborative management model, or in a separate chart, as in the hybrid or psychiatric consultation clinic model.

1. Consultation **notes should be dictated in a timely fashion** and sent to the PCP in the most efficient way possible that maintains confidentiality.
2. **A brief note should be sent to the PCP on the day of the consultation,** outlining the major findings of the consultation, any therapy that was initiated, and follow-up plans for the patient.
3. **Phone calls or electronic mail (e-mail) also can be used** to communicate consultation results quickly. Phone calls can be especially useful for communicating sensitive information or discussing ongoing patient management difficulties. E-mail is very timely, but one must be sure that the system is secure and does not compromise the confidentiality of psychiatric issues. Pertinent emails should be put in the patient's chart.

C. Follow-up visits by both the PCP and the mental health provider may provide new information or lead to changes in therapies. This information can be communicated by copies of visit notes, letters to update the other practitioner, phone calls, e-mails, or face-to-face conversation.

D. Confidentiality is a particularly important issue when a psychiatric disorder is the main focus of treatment. Notes should have enough detail to ensure medical safety but not so much that a patient's privacy is compromised. For example, a patient's history of intravenous drug abuse, which may not have been disclosed to the PCP, is medically pertinent to the patient's overall health status. The details of a patient's incest history, while potentially affecting the patient's overall ease in dealing with somatic complaints, remains a confidential issue unless the patient supports the disclosure. Sharing records within an institution or with a referring physician generally does not require written consent, although each state and institution may have their own standards.

VI. Successful Collaborations between PCPs and Psychiatrists

A. The characteristics of a successful referral clinic are listed in Table 1-2.

B. A successful referral can occur in any of the settings described above. The factors involved may include the following:

1. **Discussion of the referral** with the consultant before the patient is seen. This can be done in a verbal or written form and can be as brief as a possible diagnosis with a question mark.
2. **Knowledge of the consultants** and their strengths and weaknesses.
3. **Availability** of the consultant when the physician needs him or her. The less time a patient has to wait to be seen, the greater is the likelihood that the patient will

Table 1-2. Characteristics of a Model Primary Care Psychiatry Clinic
Availability Adequate staffing On-site consultation with PCPs Good communication among staff Adequate funding

follow through with the consultation. If a clinic is understaffed, good support staff members who maintain contact with the patient while waiting for the appointment can be an enormous help. Good relationships between the PCP's support staff and the consultant's support staff and between the patient and the PCP's support staff can help alleviate a patient's fears about a psychiatric referral and can minimize stigma.

4. **Minimization of stigma** can be achieved by seeing a patient in the medical setting.
5. **Anticipation of roadblocks** can help facilitate a referral. This includes discussion of a patient's fears about stigma, about fears of abandonment by the PCP, and about fears of psychotropic medications.

Suggested Readings

Carbone, L.A., Barsky, A.J., Orav, E.J., et al. (2000). Psychiatric symptoms and medical utilization in primary care patients. *Psychosomatics, 41,* 512–518.

Dolinar, L.J. (1993). A historical review of outpatient consultation-liaison psychiatry. *General Hospital Psychiatry, 15,* 363–368.

Epstein, S.A., & Gonzales, J.J. (1993). Outpatient consultation-liaison psychiatry: A valuable addition to the training of advanced psychiatric residents. *General Hospital Psychiatry, 15,* 369–374.

Katon, W., & Gonzales, J. (1994). A review of randomized trials of psychiatric consultation-liaison studies in primary care. *Psychosomatics, 35,* 268–278.

Katon, W., Von Korff, M., Lin, E., et al. (1999). Stepped collaborative care for primary care patients with persistent symptoms of depression: A randomized trial. *Archives of General Psychiatry, 56*(12), 1109–1115.

Montano, C.B. (1994). Recognition and treatment of depression in a primary care setting. *Journal of Clinical Psychiatry, 55*(suppl), 18–34.

Pincus, H.A., Vettorello, N.E., McQueen, L.E., et al. (1995). Bridging the gap between psychiatry and primary care: The DSM-IV-PC. *Psychosomatics, 36,* 328–335.

Simon, G.E., Katon, W.J., Von Korff, M., et al. (2001). Cost-effectiveness of a collaborative care program for primary care patients with persistent depression. *American Journal of Psychiatry, 158,* 1638–1644.

Smith, G.R. (1994). The course of somatization and its effects on utilization of health care resources. *Psychosomatics, 35,* 263–267.

Stoudemire, A. (1996). Epidemiology and psychopharmacology of anxiety in medical patients. *Journal of Clinical Psychiatry, 57*(suppl 7), 64–72.

Tanielian, T.L., Pincus, H.A., Dietrich, A.J., et al. (2000). Referral to psychiatrists: Assessing the communication interface between psychiatry and primary care. *Psychosomatics, 41,* 245–252.

Worth, J.L., & Stern, T.A. (2003). Benefits of an outpatient psychiatric teleconsultation unit: Results of a 1-year pilot. *Primary Care Companion Journal of Clinical Psychiatry, 5,* 80–84.

CHAPTER 2

Overview of the Practice of Psychotherapy

ROBERT S. ABERNETHY III

I. Introduction

This chapter describes the seven most common forms of psychotherapy and delineates which disorders or reactions to life situations should be referred to which types of therapy. The emphasis is on therapies that have been demonstrated to be effective and therapies that are good values. The chapter also discusses how one can evaluate the professional and personal credentials of a psychotherapist.

II. Types of Psychotherapy

A. **Psychoanalytic Psychotherapy** (Expressive Therapy or Psychodynamic Psychotherapy)
   1. **Principles.** Based on the Freudian tradition of uncovering unconscious aspects of a patient's mental life. **Unconscious conflicts, repressed feelings, family issues from early in a patient's life, and difficulty with current relationships are the themes commonly addressed in this therapy.**
   2. **Strategies.** The therapist is usually non-directive, allowing the patient to set his or her own pace. The therapist may interpret transference phenomena as a way to demonstrate unconscious factors in the patient's behavior.
   3. **Targets of treatment.** Severe and chronic personality disorders, as well as persistent problems in coping with life events. Anxiety disorders, depression, and eating disorders may also be treated with psychoanalytic psychotherapy.
   4. **Duration of treatment.** The length of therapy varies from a few months to a few years.
   5. **Comments.** Some research has supported the efficacy of this form of treatment, but cognitive and behavioral therapies (see below) are more efficient in terms of symptom-reduction and length of therapy and have more rigorous research evidence of effectiveness. **Although mood and anxiety disorders may respond to psychoanalytic psychotherapy, combinations of medication and cognitive or behavioral therapy tend to be more effective and efficient and to cost less.** Few if any insurance programs pay for this type of treatment, but many patients choose and pursue psychoanalytic psychotherapy, paying out-of-pocket because they find it emotionally and intellectually compelling.

B. **Behavior Therapy**
   1. **Principles. Behavior therapy is based on reducing symptoms by learning relaxation techniques, changing factors that reinforce symptoms, and giving the patient graduated exposure to distressing stimuli.**
   2. **Strategies of treatment. Behavior therapists usually are directive and encourage homework** experimentation that contributes to the efficiency of this therapy. **Homework may involve exposure to a feared situation,** such as speaking out during a committee meeting, to reduce the reinforcing expectation that catastrophe will occur

if one speaks out. Mental imaging allows the patient to learn how to relax while imagining the feared situation.

3. **Targets of treatment.** Research evidence shows that **behavior therapy works for a variety of anxiety disorders** as well as for some psychosomatic symptoms (e.g., pain). Behavior therapy equips the patient with concrete strategies that can be used after the termination of therapy.

4. **Duration of treatment.** Behavior therapy is **generally brief,** requiring 6 to 20 sessions.

5. **Comments.** Behavior therapy is effective, efficient, easy to understand, and focused on symptom-reduction.

C. **Cognitive Therapy**

1. **Principles. Cognitive therapy is based on the assumption that negative or distorted thoughts promote depression or anxiety.**

2. **Strategies.** Negative thoughts are documented by the patient during depressing or anxious experiences that occur between visits. During the therapy sessions, **the patient learns to challenge the negative thinking.**

3. **Targets of treatment.** Research evidence has demonstrated that cognitive therapy is an **effective treatment for depression and anxiety.** Cognitive therapy is indicated for depression, anxiety states, and problems related to substance abuse. Cognitive therapy is also being used to complement medication in the treatment of delusional thinking in schizophrenics. Cognitive-behavioral therapy (CBT) is the term used for the combination of cognitive and behavioral therapies. CBT is also effective for anxiety disorders and depression.

4. **Duration of treatment.** Cognitive therapy generally requires 10 to 20 sessions.

5. **Comments.** Cognitive therapy, like behavior therapy, is effective, efficient, easy to understand, and focused on symptom-reduction.

D. **Interpersonal Psychotherapy**

1. **Principles.** Interpersonal psychotherapy **assumes that depression is the result of problems in relationships in the here and now.**

2. **Strategies.** In the first few sessions, the therapist identifies one or two of four common interpersonal issues: grief, role transition, role dispute, and interpersonal deficits.

3. **Targets of treatment.** Interpersonal psychotherapy has most frequently been **used for the treatment of depression** but it may also be effective for anxiety disorders.

4. **Duration.** Interpersonal psychotherapy generally requires 12 to 20 sessions. Monthly sessions in follow-up have been used as a maintenance therapy for patients to prevent recurrence of depression.

5. **Comment.** Considerable research has demonstrated the effectiveness of interpersonal psychotherapy for depression. In spite of its demonstrated effectiveness, this therapy is not widely practiced.

E. **Psychoeducational Therapy**

1. **Principles. This form of therapy is used to educate patients about ways to manage and understand emotional or physical problems.**

2. **Strategies of treatment. Patients often meet with a therapist in groups,** and there is often family participation. The therapy involves both education and support as well as insight into psychological issues related to the problem.

3. **Targets of treatment.** This is **a here-and-now, problem-solving therapy** that is **effective for patients with schizophrenia.** It has also been used for a variety of other psychiatric and psychosocial problems. It can also be used for physical disorders, such as psychoeducational groups for women with breast cancer.
4. **Duration of treatment.** Psychoeducational therapy usually addresses chronic problems and, therefore, tends to be longer-term.

F. **Supportive Therapy**
1. **Principles. Supportive psychotherapy is based on the assumption that patients improve when there is someone to talk to who is validating.**
2. **Strategies of treatment.** Supportive therapy generally avoids interpreting the unconscious or addressing the transference. The therapist often gives advice and validates the patient's feelings and ideas.
3. **Targets of treatment.** Supportive psychotherapy can be helpful for **any emotional disorder or life problem.**
4. **Duration of treatment.** This therapy can vary in length from a few visits to a life-long endeavor. Many psychopharmacologists who see patients for maintenance medication will do 20-minutes of supportive psychotherapy as part of follow-up visits.
5. **Comment.** Although supportive psychotherapy is widely practiced, little formal research has focused on its effectiveness.

G. **Integrative Psychotherapy**
1. **Principles.** Integrative psychotherapy assumes that a patient could **benefit more from a combination of strategies** than a "pure form" of psychotherapy. Therefore, a therapist may use psychodynamic therapy but give behaviorally-focused homework assignments.
2. **Strategies of treatment.** The therapist tries to address the patient's problems using a custom-made amalgam of the six psychotherapies presented above.
3. **Targets of treatment.** Integrative psychotherapy can benefit any psychiatric diagnosis.
4. **Duration of psychotherapy.** Because this therapy is often not "manual driven" with a set protocol, its duration can vary greatly.
5. **Comment.** Integrative psychotherapy is probably widely practiced. A well-known example of a manual-driven integrative psychotherapy is dialectical behavior therapy for borderline personality disorder. This therapy involves dynamic, behavioral, cognitive, interpersonal, supportive, and psychoeducational features. Research has demonstrated its effectiveness.

III. Group Therapies

A. **Principles.** The principles of each of the therapies listed above can be applied to group therapy.

B. **Composition and membership.** Group therapy can be organized around psychiatric or medical diagnoses or life situations, such as panic disorder and breast cancer. Groups can also be heterogeneous, with a variety of diagnoses in one group. Groups can be open-ended and ongoing or can be brief experiences in which the patients begin and end the group together.

C. Value of groups. Group therapy is an excellent economic value and can be of significant benefit for many psychiatric, medical, and life situations.

D. Subsets of Treatment.
1. **Couples therapy** and family therapy are excellent modalities for dealing with marital tension or family crises and for families with a member who has a serious mental illness.
2. **Psychoeducational family therapy** is quite effective in the management of schizophrenia.
3. **Family therapy** also can be helpful for patients with eating disorders.

IV. What You Should Ask about a Psychotherapist before Referring

A. Ask about the therapist's training and experience. Ask for a resumé and about the therapist's experience in treating certain conditions. The therapist may have one or more degrees (e.g., M.D., Ph.D., Ed.D., Psy.D., M.S.W., or M.S.N.). Doctoral-level training is obviously more extensive, but many masters'-level psychotherapists are excellent. Conversely, many doctoral-level therapists can be narrow in their approach and, therefore, ineffective with many patients. An M.D. can both medicate and do psychotherapy, but many psychiatrists do only psychopharmacology and refer patients to other disciplines for psychotherapy.

B. Ask about the kinds of psychotherapies the therapist practices and the duration on average of these methods. Use the previous list of seven common psychotherapies to assess the breadth of the therapist's experience and expertise.

C. Ask about the therapist's availability to take new patients. How long does a patient have to wait for an appointment? How are emergencies handled under the therapist's care? What about a new patient in crisis?

D. Ask about the therapist's style of communication with the patient's family and with you, the primary care physician (PCP). The majority of patients will give the therapist permission to communicate discreetly with the PCP or with concerned family members, but some therapists choose not to communicate with anyone but the patient.

E. Ask about the psychotherapist's view of psychopharmacologic treatment. Unfortunately, some therapists believe that the use of medications can undermine personal growth and change. These therapists may overtly or covertly discourage a patient from continuing treatment with antidepressants or anxiolytics. These therapists also may have too high a threshold for referring an unmedicated patient for psychopharmacologic evaluation. This failure to refer can be harmful to the patient and be economically wasteful.

F. Determine whether the psychotherapist is someone you can work with. Try to get a gut reaction to this professional as a person. Is he or she warm? Does he or she maintain boundaries? Would you feel comfortable sending a loved one to this person? Would you feel comfortable calling this person to discuss a patient's lack of progress or to complain?

G. Ask if other patients whom you have referred have fared well. Patients are often the best judges of a therapist's competence.

V. Conclusion

Psychotherapies are definable entities with different goals and strategies for psychiatric or life problems. Understanding the varieties of treatment available and getting to know prospective psychotherapists for your patients will enhance the effectiveness of your referrals.

Suggested Readings

Abernethy, R.S. (1992). The integration of therapies. In S. Rutan (Ed.), *Psychotherapy for the 1990's*. New York: Guilford Press.

Basch, M.R. (1988). *Understanding psychotherapy: The science behind the art*. New York: Basic Books.

Beck, J.S. (1995). *Cognitive therapy*. New York: Guilford Press.

Eells, T.D. (2000). Psychotherapy of schizophrenia. *Journal of Psychotherapy, Practice, and Research, 9*(4), 250–254.

Klerman, G., Weissman, M., Rounsaville, B., & Chevron, E. (1984). *Interpersonal psychotherapy of depression*. New York: Basic Books.

Linehan, M.M. (1993). *Cognitive-behavioral treatment of borderline personality disorder*. New York: Guilford Press.

Mann, J. (1992). *Time-limited psychotherapy*. Cambridge, Mass.: Harvard University Press.

Misch, D.A. (2000). Basic strategies of dynamic supportive therapy. *Journal of Psychotherapy, Practice, and Research, 9*(4), 173–189.

O'Connor, R. (2001). Active treatment of depression. *American Journal of Psychotherapy, 55*(4), 507–530.

Rutan, J.S., & Stone, W.N. (2000). *Psychodynamic group psychotherapy*. New York: Guilford Press.

Swenson, C.R., Torrey, W.C., & Koerner, K. (2002). Implementing dialectical behavior therapy. *Psychiatric Services, 53*(2), 171–178.

Wachtel, P.L. (1977). *Psychoanalysis and behavior therapy: Toward an integration*. New York: Basic Books.

CHAPTER 3

Effective Psychiatric Interviewing in Primary Care Medicine

CHRISTOPHER GORDON AND ALLAN GOROLL

I. Overview

Encounters with patients in primary care medicine take place under considerable time pressure. However, patients often present in primary care settings with problems related to psychiatric or emotional issues that they are reluctant to reveal. In a brief period of time the primary care physician (PCP) needs to build a relationship with the patient that is conducive to self-revelation and treatment negotiation. **The goals of time-limited interviewing include the following:**

A. **Creation of an atmosphere in which the patient can convey information that may be shameful or frightening**

B. **Compilation of sufficient information to generate a differential diagnosis**

C. **Establishment of a relationship from which an effective treatment plan can be mutually designed and implemented**

II. Conceptualizing Psychiatric Conditions

In evaluating whether a person has a psychiatric problem, it is useful to listen to the history from three complementary perspectives: the biologic, the social and interpersonal, and the psychological.

A. **A discrete biologic illness** (e.g., hypothyroidism, panic disorder, obsessive-compulsive disorder) presenting as a psychiatric syndrome usually is recognized from constellations of discrete symptoms and signs, past similar episodes, a characteristic course, a positive family history of similar illness, and other features of the history. Biologic problems of this sort often are treatable entirely or in part by means of psychopharmacologic or other somatic treatments, sometimes in combination with psychotherapy.

B. **Social or interpersonal problems** (e.g., coming to terms with the recent death of a loved one, coping with an abusive relationship) arise in a setting of a current problematic relationship or social circumstance. These problems often improve after acknowledgment of the problem, ventilation, and catharsis; they sometimes require focused psychotherapy.

C. **Recurrent psychological problems** (e.g., repetitive problems dealing with authority or separation) are often more subtle and involve recurrent patterns of behavior and experience that undermine a person's optimal functioning. We all, of course, have such areas in our lives, but for some people the suffering or disability is more substantial, as in the case of a gifted person who repeatedly fails at work because of conflict with the boss or is self-defeatingly shy and non-assertive. Problems of this sort may respond to psychotherapy if the person is motivated to change.

1. These problems occur along a spectrum from mild/normal to progressively more severe.

2. In evaluating a psychological problem, the physician must consider whether there is a recurrent pattern of suffering or suboptimal functioning. If so, who are the key other people involved in this pattern? What are consequences of this pattern in the person's life? What is the person's interest and capacity to change this pattern? Clearer patterns of behavior with definable negative consequences for the individual or for people she or he cares about and a high desire for change are predictive of better outcomes with psychotherapy.

3. In extreme forms, these problems usually are associated with character disorders. In character disorders, there is a high degree of self-defeating behavior and distress either in the patient or in those around the patient, little appreciation for the perspective of others, and a low capacity to assume responsibility for one's difficulties. People with character disorders often react poorly to treaters and sometimes decompensate rather than improve with psychotherapy.

D. **The biologic, social and interpersonal, and psychological perspectives are not mutually exclusive.** Very often a single problem will involve biologic, social and interpersonal, and psychological aspects, as in the case of a middle-aged woman with major depression whose children are leaving home and who has long-standing poor self-esteem. As the physician conceptualizes the patient's problem, he or she may be able to use these three perspectives to collaborate with the patient about which seems most suitable to deal with the problem at hand.

III. Creating an Atmosphere Conducive to Self-Revelation and Mutual Treatment-Planning

Several strategies may facilitate self-revelation.

A. **Do not assume that the patient sees the problem in the same way you do.** Clarify the patient's main concerns and the main requests of the physician. These may be entirely different from the initially stated chief complaint, as it may take some time for the patient to express the real reason for his or her visit.

B. **Consider sharing what you may already know about the problem or situation and invite correction.** Sometimes the PCP receives information from a nurse, referrer, or other source. When such information is in the physician's possession, it is often efficient and facilitates communication for the physician to offer to share this information and invite correction: "Mr. Jones, the nurse practitioner, Ms. West, has told me a bit about the depression you've been experiencing. Would it be helpful if I told you what I have been told, and if I'm missing something you could straighten it out?" This going first by the doctor keeps the patient from having to repeat his or her story, shows that the physician is open to correction, and ideally gives the doctor a chance to build rapport by sensitively describing the person's situation in a way that feels accurate. Make sure, however, that the description of the problem is not inadvertently embarrassing or shaming (see below).

C. **Establish a mutual perspective** by making sure you understand how the patient sees the situation, using ordinary non-clinical language: "As you talk, Mr. Smith, I'm impressed that you sound like you've really been down over the past couple of months—

tired, sad, pessimistic. Do you see it the same way?" As you reflect your understanding of the problem, use the same words as the patient when possible. For example, if the patient says that she has been worrying a lot and dreading everyday things, use the words *worry* and *dread* rather than paraphrasing with words such as *concerned* and *frightened.* Otherwise, the disparity between your words and the patient's words will tend to accentuate differences rather than understanding.

D. Get permission to discuss the problem before jumping in to do so: "Shall we take a few minutes to discuss these feelings of worry and dread to see what we could do about it?"

E. Appreciate the patient's perspective.

1. **See the problem from the patient's eyes and try to appreciate the complexity of the problem as the patient experiences it.** When the psychiatric interviewer fails to do this, his or her proffered solutions seem facile to the patient, and the diagnosis, no matter how accurate or elegant, may seem from the patient's perspective to miss the point.

2. **Appreciate the patient's language, strengths, and problem-solving style.** As you approach the problem, consider what you know about this person: What kind of problems has the patient dealt with in the past, and how is she or he more comfortable talking about feelings or facts? Does the patient appreciate hearing the options or a clear recommendation? Is there someone the patient might like to confer with who could be brought in, such as a spouse? Is the patient especially sensitive to criticism and likely to experience a psychiatric problem as a fault? Knowing the person's strengths, weaknesses, and problem-solving style can help avert problems before they occur.

3. **Reflect and summarize.** Continually summarize what you hear from the patient and give the patient a chance to correct your impressions. Putting your summaries in ordinary language will tend to demystify the problem: "So let me summarize: You started feeling down about 3 months ago, roughly when you learned about the possibility of the new job, and since then you've been worrying almost constantly about it. You've been having a lot of trouble sleeping, eating, and concentrating, and lately it's gotten so bad that you feel filled with dread. Is that about right?" Getting something wrong and having the patient correct you is a good opportunity to welcome the patient's input and set a tone of receptivity.

4. **Get the "nod."** As you begin the interview and throughout it, look for the patient to give you non-verbal cues that you are in sync—ideally, a nodding affirmation that your summaries and reflections are on target. If you do not get "the nod," you must consider the possibility that something is interfering with your communication with the patient. Maybe you have said or done something inadvertently hurtful or are missing a critical point. Careful, thoughtful analysis and conferring with the patient about how she or he is experiencing the interview may be crucial.

F. Never underestimate the value of simple friendliness, warmth, kindness, appreciation, and demystification of the practice of medicine. In the long run these are probably the most important principles of successful interviewing in any setting. An apology when someone has been kept waiting, an acknowledgment of difficulty, and admiring a patient's attempts to deal with a problem may make all the difference in enabling the patient to confide in you.

IV. Data Gathering

A. Having established a tone of collaboration, identified the problem, and gotten "the nod," concentrate on the history of present illness.

1. **Let the patient tell his or her own story.** Listen actively by not interrupting and concentrate not on establishing the right diagnosis but on making sure you are "getting it right" from the patient's point of view. When you conceptualize the patient's problem as being more likely to be in the psychological or interpersonal realm, it is especially important to give the patient a chance to share what is troubling him or her in an atmosphere of acceptance and empathy. For many people it is a rare and healing experience to be listened to attentively, particularly about a subject that may have been a source of private suffering for some time.

2. **Do not rely immediately on symptom checklists to rule in or rule out a particular diagnosis.** Under the pressure of time, it is easy to slip quickly into asking a series of closed-ended questions to rule in or out a particular diagnosis, such as major depression. Doing this creates the risk of closing off prematurely important information that the patient might otherwise impart about the social or psychological aspects of the situation.

3. **Establish the last time the patient felt well with respect to this problem:** the earliest symptoms recollected; associated stresses, illnesses, and changes in medications; attempts to solve the problem and their effects; and how the person elected to get help for the problem now.

4. **Summarize, reflect, and invite correction.**

5. **As you move to different sections of the history, consider explaining what you are doing and why:** "I'd like to ask some questions about your past psychiatric history, if any, to see if anything like this has happened before." This guided interviewing tends to demystify what you are doing and elicits collaboration.

B. The patient's psychiatric history offers important clues to the nature of the present problem.

1. **Ascertain past episodes of similar or related suffering,** such as past episodes of depression or periods of anxiety, **how they were treated, and how the patient responded.**

2. **Ascertain past episodes of unrelated psychiatric illness,** such as problems with anxiety, phobias, fears, and obsessions. These episodes may point the way to a diathesis to affective or anxiety disorders that otherwise might be obscure.

3. **Ascertain past periods of emotional difficulty** as distinct from psychiatric illness *per se.*

C. Past medical history. The past medical history is a crucial element of the database for all patients who may have psychiatric or emotional complaints, as this history will point to possible organic causes of the presenting problem. The medical history can be obtained quickly and should include surgical procedures, hospitalizations, major illnesses, current medications, allergies, any history of substance abuse, and a review of systems, which may be limited to the question, "Are you having any physical symptoms or problems now that are concerning you that we haven't already discussed?"

D. The family history of psychiatric illness should be established, including treatment and the response to treatment.

E. The social and developmental history cannot be exhaustively developed in a time-limited format, but it is possible to get a general sense of the following:

1. **The patient's family experience** and whether there were major problems in the patient's childhood.

2. **The patient's education, marital status, and employment and professional status** and a general sense of the quality of the patient's current life.

3. **Whether there is a history of substantial physical or sexual abuse** in the past. When abuse has occurred, it is very likely to be contributing in some way to the current problem.

F. Mental Status

1. **Practically all of the patient's mental status can be inferred;** it is rarely necessary to do a formal mental status work-up, except when disturbances of reality testing are suspected, as in patients with psychosis, dementia, or delirium.

2. **For suspected mood disorders,** be sure to inquire about the characteristic neuro-vegetative symptoms of depression (*s*leep, *i*nterests, *g*uilt, *e*nergy, *c*oncentration, *a*ppetite, *p*sychomotor agitation/retardation, *s*uicide (**SIG E: CAPS).**

3. **Whenever a sign of impaired reality testing is suspected, be sure to inquire about hallucinations in all sensory modalities** and to perform a detailed cognitive evaluation.

4. **Whenever delirium or dementia is suspected,** perform a detailed evaluation of the person's cognition, including orientation, attention, concentration, and immediate and short-term memory. This topic is dealt with in detail in Chapters 22 and 23.

5. **Assessment of suicidal and homicidal risks** is dealt with in the following section and in Chapters 15 and 60.

V. Interviewing Difficulties

A. Approaching a sensitive subject. Some topics seem especially likely to shame or humiliate patients and therefore to drive the problem underground, making mutual treatment-planning difficult. Examples include sexual disorders, substance abuse problems, and even the presence of an anxiety disorder in people who are particularly prone to shame. (See as follows.)

1. **Be aware of the problem and plan for it.**

2. **Approach the problem indirectly at first,** giving the patient the opportunity to initiate the topic.

3. **If you must initiate, ask permission to bring up something that may be somewhat difficult to discuss.** This gives the patient a chance to brace himself or herself and affords the patient a greater sense of control. Moreover, the actual subject you then raise is almost always less threatening or difficult than the one the patient has braced for, and so the patient often feels relief rather than threat when you raise the topic.

4. **Having broached the subject, again establish permission to explore it; get the "nod."**

5. **In exploring the topic, use open-ended questions to deepen the discussion;** use close-ended questions to lighten or close the discussion.

B. Dealing with denial. In some circumstances it is clear that the patient either consciously (deliberately) or unconsciously is denying the existence of an important problem, such as serious substance abuse or severe depression. These situations are challenging and potentially dangerous and require special management.

1. **Acknowledge the problem of disagreement about the problem.** When it is impossible to address directly the problem that the physician sees as primary, the focus of discussion must shift. Try to get agreement that there is a serious disagreement and negotiate how to resolve it.

2. **Consider calling in a third party.** Try to determine whose judgment the patient most respects and suggest a conference with that person.

3. **Anticipate bad outcomes. Warn but do not threaten.** This is a crucial distinction, as threats often harden a patient's resistance. Consider the metaphor of a car stalled on railroad tracks, warning the patient of what you see coming and soliciting his or her help in avoiding the bad outcome.

4. **Know your limits and options.** Be clear about your legal and ethical limits and obligations, for example, that the patient as a competent adult has the right to refuse even reasonable options unless certain conditions exist. Be sure you understand what these conditions are, such as suicide threats or child or elder abuse, and have a clear plan for informing the patient of your obligation. Even when your behavior is mandated, you can use this eventuality to try to develop a mutually acceptable plan: "Mr. Jones, I am very sorry to say that these bruises on your child are so serious that I have to involve the Department of Social Services. I am mandated to do so, and I will. It will be better ultimately, though, if we can talk honestly about how this happened and what would be best. Shall we do that?"

5. **Keep the relationship alive.** No matter how much you may disagree, try to sustain the relationship. Set another time to meet or talk after further information has been gathered or after the patient has had time to confer with his or her family, for example.

C. **Uncovering an emergency situation.** In some circumstances it becomes clear that an emergency exists; for example, the person is actively suicidal or homicidal, the patient is acutely psychotic or delirious, or child abuse is ongoing. In these situations special management is required.

1. **Know your obligations and options.** Be clear about what you are mandated to act on. Plan ahead to be ready when these situations arise.

2. **Be ready before you intervene.** If you think that a person may need to be prevented from leaving the interview, if at all possible, excuse yourself and alert back-up resources, such as hospital security, other clinicians, or in extreme circumstances the police. Do not intervene unless and until you have adequate back-up to ensure your and others' safety.

3. **Once you have back-up, negotiate.** Again, warn but do not threaten; solicit advice and help from the patient about how best to resolve the problem safely.

VI. Negotiation and Treatment-Planning

A. **Establish agreement about the findings.**

1. **Take time to ensure that you and the patient agree about your findings** so that you can move on to explore the treatment options available.

2. **When disagreement exists, it is helpful to make it explicit and to revisit the data,** keeping your mind open to the patient's perspective.

B. **Use a psychoeducational approach to define the problem and pave the way to a solution.** As you discuss the problem, consider using the idea that most psychiatric problems can be thought of as being due to a chemical imbalance and/or to a problem in living that is hard to come to terms with (e.g., the death of a loved one that the person has not grieved). **The idea of a "chemical imbalance" is generally acceptable** and much less stigmatizing than the notion of a "mental illness." To illustrate an emotional cause of a problem, most people find the example of **unresolved grief** familiar and demystifying. Recurrent psychological problems, such as problems with authority and problems dealing with separations, are often harder for patients to see and accept, and special care must be taken not to make the patient feel criticized or "put down" by the suggestion that there is a recurrent problem of this sort. Gently pointing out clear examples of the pattern and inviting the patient's comments are ways of beginning a dialogue about whether such a problem exists. Sorting out with the patient whether the problem is more like a problem in living, more like a chemical imbalance, more like a recurrent psychological problem, or some combination sets the stage for deciding about treatment together.

C. **Try to present treatment options** rather than a single recommendation unless one is compellingly better, as this permits the patient to participate fully in designing the treatment plan.

VII. Common Errors in Interviewing

A. **Inadvertently shaming, embarrassing, or humiliating the patient,** for example, by calling the patient by his or her first name when the physician has been introduced as "Dr."; using terms that the person may feel demeaned by, such as "Does anyone else in the family have a mental illness?"; conducting the interview while the patient is unclothed; or plunging into a sensitive area without the patient's permission.

B. **Jumping to conclusions about the nature of the problem,** for example, not permitting the patient to tell his or her story; prematurely using a symptom checklist; over-medicalizing a psychological or interpersonal problem, such as attributing a painful marital problem or unresolved grief to a "chemical imbalance"; overly psychologizing a medical-psychiatric condition, such as suggesting that a major depression occurs because a person has not worked out a problem from childhood or with his or her spouse.

C. **Prematurely offering solutions or advice.** Usually when people confide in a physician about a problem, they have been worrying about it for some time and have tried to solve the problem. When caregivers offer quick solutions or advice, no matter how sagacious, that can have the unintended effect of alienating the patient, who may feel insulted or demeaned by a ready answer. "After all, if the answer is so obvious, I must really be a mess," may be the patient's inner experience, or "If she thinks that is all it takes to fix this, then she really doesn't get it." It is vital to acknowledge the complexity of the problem as well as the possible obstacles to a solution to maximize your alliance with the patient: "It sounds like you have been in a lot of distress for a long time. I appreciate your confiding in me. I hope we can work together to find a solution."

Suggested Readings

Gordon, C.D. (1994). Crisis intervention: A general approach. In S.E. Hyman, & G.E. Tesar (Eds.), *Manual of psychiatric emergencies* (3rd ed.). Boston: Little, Brown, pp. 12–18.

Lazare, A. (1973). Hidden conceptual models in clinical psychiatry. *New England Journal of Medicine, 288*(7), 345–351.

Lazare, A. (1979). A negotiated approach to the clinical encounter. In A. Lazare (Ed.), *Outpatient psychiatry.* Baltimore: Williams & Wilkins, pp. 141–156.

Lazare, A. (1987). Shame and humiliation in the medical encounter. *Archives of Internal Medicine, 147*(9), 1653–1658.

Lipkin, M., Putanam, S.M., & Lazare, A. (Eds.). (1995). *The medical interview: Clinical care, education and research.* New York: Springer-Verlag.

Levinson, W. (2001). Generalist's approach to the medical interview. In J. Noble (Ed.), *Textbook of primary care medicine.* St. Louis: Mosby, pp. 9–17.

CHAPTER 4

Making a Referral

STEVEN A. EPSTEIN AND THEODORE A. STERN

I. Introduction

Recent health care reforms have led to the expectation that primary care clinicians will diagnose and treat many psychiatric disorders themselves, minimizing referrals to mental health clinicians. To aid in this task, experts have developed diagnostic and treatment guides such as *PRIME-MD, DSM-IV-PC,* and the *AHCPR Guideline on Depression in Primary Care.* Nonetheless, the primary care clinician's ability to diagnose and treat psychiatric disorders may be hindered by time constraints and by a lack of comfort with, or expertise in, some mental health problems. Thus, as is true regarding referral to other specialists, a primary care clinician needs to have a systematic approach to making a referral to a mental health clinician.

II. Consultation or Referral

The primary care provider (PCP) should attempt to be as clear as possible with the patient and with the mental health practitioner (MHP) about whether a referral or consultation is being requested. The MHP will want to be clear with the patient about the goals of the initial visit.

A. Consultation. A consultation is a situation in which the MHP gives an opinion about diagnosis and treatment but the ongoing treatment is implemented by the PCP. Situations in which a consultation is needed include a diagnostic dilemma (e.g., depression or dysthymia; Is this patient psychotic? Are medications or medical problems causing mood symptoms?) and uncertainty about appropriate medication management (Which antidepressant should be started? How can the sexual side effects of an antidepressant be managed?). Most practicing MHPs should be available within 1 to 2 weeks for a consultation. However, some may be unavailable for ongoing treatment, particularly when treatment will be intensive (e.g., twice-weekly sessions with a severely depressed patient). In such situations it is often useful to discuss the case briefly by phone with the MHP so that if he or she is unavailable, an appointment can be scheduled with another clinician for evaluation and treatment.

B. Referral. A referral implies that ongoing care will be implemented by the MHP.

C. Rationale for distinguishing between a Consultation and a Referral
1. Some patients are more likely to accept a consultation than a referral.
2. Some patients prefer that all mental health care be confidential and thus they do not want the results of a mental health consultation communicated to others or will not agree to ongoing collaborative care. For such patients, a referral without ongoing PCP-MHP communication (unless essential) is more appropriate.

III. Psychiatric Diagnoses That Warrant a Referral

A. Common psychiatric problems. The most common psychiatric problems seen in primary care are depression and anxiety. Depending on the PCP's level of expertise and comfort, patients with uncomplicated depression and anxiety do not necessarily have to be referred to a mental health professional. However, the circumstances outlined in Table 4-1 warrant a referral.

B. Less common psychiatric problems. The PCP may want to refer a patient with less common problems because he or she neither feels comfortable with, nor skilled in, the treatment of those problems. Even if the PCC would feel comfortable treating such a problem, medicolegal concerns may warrant that the problem be treated by a specialist. Table 4-2 gives examples of psychiatric problems that usually warrant a referral.

Table 4-1. When to Refer a Depressed or Anxious Patient

1. When there are severe symptoms of depression or anxiety (e.g., psychosis or suicidal ideation)
2. When there are features suggestive of less common anxiety or depressive disorders (e.g., obsessive-compulsive disorder, post-traumatic stress disorder, seasonal affective disorder, depression in a person with a history of mania, dysthymia)
3. When symptoms may be due to a medical condition, medication, or drug abuse
4. When there are concomitant cognitive deficits (e.g., dementia)
5. When there are significant co-existing psychiatric conditions (e.g., alcohol dependence, or a personality disorder)
6. When the diagnosis is unclear (e.g., depression vs. bereavement, or "normal" worry vs. an anxiety disorder)
7. When depression or anxiety is not responding to usual treatment

---

Table 4-2. Examples of Psychiatric Disorders That Usually Warrant a Referral

1. Psychotic disorders (e.g., schizophrenia, schizoaffective disorder, and delusional disorders)
2. Substance-related disorders (e.g., alcoholism and cocaine abuse)
3. Sexual and gender identity disorders (e.g., premature ejaculation, female orgasmic disorder, and paraphilias)
4. Eating disorders (e.g., anorexia nervosa and bulimia nervosa)
5. Severe personality disorders (e.g., borderline and antisocial personality disorders)
6. Adult attention deficit disorder

IV. Clinical Situations or Treatments That Warrant a Referral

A. Patient's request for a referral. In some circumstances the patient may request that a psychiatric history not be taken by the PCP. Within the constraints of managed care, it may be appropriate to refer such a patient directly to a mental health professional.

B. The patient may need a treatment that the PCP has neither the time nor the expertise to provide (Table 4-3).

C. The patient may be treated initially by a PCP but during treatment a referral becomes appropriate (e.g., when treatment-refractory depression develops).

V. To Whom Should One Refer?

PCPs should refer to practitioners with whom they have had good experiences in the past, and to those known to have specialty expertise in the area of a patient's problem. Although referrals may be made to any mental health professional, increasingly PCPs will be forced to make referrals to members of a designated provider panel. Referrals should be made to colleagues who have had good results, who are well liked by prior patients, who communicate clearly with the PCP by letter or phone, and who use treatment plans that make sense. Table 4-4 shows how to decide which type of MHP is appropriate for a particular referral.

VI. How to Present the Recommendation for a Referral to a Patient

A. The goal of a referral is to help the patient. The patient should be made aware that a referral to a MHP indicates that the PCP wants to help him or her; it is not an indication of abandonment. A referral made for a patient the PCP knows well often goes smoothly, but it may be made during an initial visit if history reveals that a referral is warranted. It is often helpful, especially with a reluctant patient, to say that a referral is being made for a consultation only and that the PCP will continue to care for the patient. It is particularly important to take this approach in the treatment of somatizing patients. One would not want to tell such a patient that the referral is being made because "it looks

---

Table 4-3. Diagnostic Tests and Treatments Usually Provided Only by MHPs

1. Complex pharmacotherapy, especially for disorders such as those in Table 4-2
2. Insight-oriented psychotherapy, especially when sessions are frequent (e.g., weekly) and/or long-term (e.g., 6 months to years)
3. Cognitive-behavioral treatments (e.g., relaxation training, biofeedback-assisted relaxation, and cognitive psychotherapy)
4. Light therapy (for seasonal affective disorder)
5. Electroconvulsive therapy
6. Psychiatric hospitalization or partial hospitalization
7. Psychological or neuropsychological testing

Table 4-4. Type of Mental Health Practitioner to Refer to, Based on the Reason for Referral

Reason for Referral	To Whom to Refer
Diagnostic dilemma	Psychiatrist or clinical psychologist
Medication management or consultation	Psychiatrist
Cognitive-behavioral psychotherapy	Psychologist generally, but some psychiatrists may be skilled in this approach
Biofeedback-assisted relaxation	Psychologist who has a biofeedback program
Electroconvulsive therapy	Psychiatrist with experience with this treatment
Light therapy	Psychiatrist with experience with this treatment
Psychiatric disorders requiring specialized treatment	MHP with experience and resources to treat the disorder (e.g., eating disorder requiring a multidisciplinary program)
Psychotherapy (general)	Psychiatrist, psychologist, or psychiatric social worker
Psychiatric hospitalization or partial hospitalization (day treatment)	Psychiatrist with admitting privileges (ideally at a facility where the PCP also has admitting privileges)
Psychological or neuro-psychological testing	Clinical psychologist

like the problem is all in your head." A straightforward and less caustic explanation is usually more successful: "I will continue to treat your migraines with sumatriptan, but a psychologist may be able to augment this approach with stress management and biofeedback."

B. **Mention early in treatment that there is a possibility of referral.** The PCP might tell a patient that he or she would be happy to prescribe an antidepressant, but if there is not full recovery in 6 weeks, a consultation will be requested. Raising this possibility early may lead to easier acceptance of the referral if it is ultimately needed.

C. **Engage family members.** It may be helpful to engage family members in the recommendation for referral. Every PCP recalls a situation in which he or she was called aside by a patient's family member, who then requested a mental health referral for the patient. In such a situation, a meeting with the patient and family members may help a reluctant patient accept a referral.

D. **Refer to a known colleague when possible.** It is helpful to make a referral to someone known to the PCP, as the patient is likely to find this reassuring. If it is necessary to make a referral to a panel, the PCP can offer to obtain a recommendation from a mental health colleague for a specific member of the panel.

E. **Suggest a therapeutic trial.** For a patient who appears convinced that a mental health referral will not help, suggest that he or she meet with the MHP once or twice before deciding against ongoing treatment.

F. **Offer ongoing collaboration whenever possible.** The PCP may tell a patient that if he or she wishes, there will be ongoing collaboration with the MHP, particularly with regard to medically important areas, such as drug–drug interactions. Conversely, the PCP may tell a patient that if the patient wishes, mental health treatment will be confidential (except for pharmacotherapy).

G. **Educate the patient.** Provide the patient with an explanation of and literature about the nature of the psychiatric problem and the effectiveness of treatment.

VII. How to Make a Referral

A. **Write a letter or phone.** A referral to a MHP can be made just as one would make a referral to any specialist. A brief referral letter is often helpful, as is a transmittal of a recent medical summary. A referral should not be made merely by giving the patient a single MHP's phone number; the numbers for a few MHPs should be given, since the first choice may not be available. If the PCP wants to know whether a particular practitioner is available and appropriate for the patient, the PCP should call that practitioner first. Some academic medical centers offer telephone consultations for primary care providers, which also facilitates referrals.

B. **Make direct contact for a difficult patient.** When one is referring a difficult patient, it may be helpful to phone the MHP first, since important information, such as personality traits and non-compliance, may not be readily discernible from a review of the medical record. The PCP should be honest about what it feels like to take care of the patient. For example, the information that the PCP finds the patient to be frustrating may provide a clue for the MHP regarding the patient's interpersonal style.

C. **Call directly for urgent referrals.** MHPs may not always be able to take urgent referrals. If it is important that a patient be seen within one week, it is wise to call the MHP first. Emergency evaluations and referrals (e.g., for acute psychosis, suicidality, or homicidality) should be performed at a nearby emergency room or at an urgent care mental health clinic; referrals should not be handled in a casual manner.

D. **Be honest with the patient about the reason for the referral.** It is never wise to avoid telling a patient the true reason for a referral because of concerns about the patient's potential reaction. For example, if the PCP believes that a patient has a problem with alcohol, the patient should not be told that the referral is for anxiety. MHPs are put at an immediate disadvantage if the patient being referred has not explicitly made the appointment for reasons with which he or she agrees. (The exception is involuntary hospitalization, for reasons of imminent danger to oneself or others.)

E. **Do not promise that a specific MHP will treat the patient.** For example, a psychiatrist often performs the initial evaluation and refers the patient to another practitioner for psychotherapy.

F. **Clearly articulate the reason for referral.** When making a referral by letter or by phone, it is important for the referring physician to articulate clearly the specific reason for the referral, i.e., the referral question. For example, a referral of a patient with chronic pain should specify whether the referral is being made for depression, to rule out somatization, or both. It is not necessary to use *DSM-IV* diagnoses when making a referral ("Please evaluate for a major depressive episode versus generalized anxiety disorder.").

VIII. How to Evaluate a Referral

A. **Communication of the results of the evaluation.** The PCP should expect to hear from the MHP by phone or by letter within a few days (if semiurgent) or within 2 weeks (if not). If the PCP has not heard anything by this time, a call should be made directly to the MHP. A MHP will indicate whether the patient did not allow further discussion (i.e., did not sign a release of information) or whether administrative problems arose.

B. **Clarity of the opinion.** The PCP should expect the MHP to communicate clearly without overuse of psychiatric jargon. A *DSM-IV* diagnosis may be used, but the MHP should be able to explain clearly why a particular diagnosis was chosen. A tentative formulation should be made, for example, from a biopsychosocial perspective. The treatment plan should be clear and should consider all aspects of treatment, including the medical causes of the symptoms, medications that could be responsible, stressors, and social supports. Medication options should be outlined clearly. Finally, a good evaluation should specifically answer the referral question.

C. **The patient's opinion.** The PCP should ask the patient for his or her assessment of the mental health visit. If the patient has reservations about a particular practitioner whom the PCP knows is skilled, the PCP should encourage the patient to return for one or two more visits. If after that point the patient is still dissatisfied, the PCP should call the MHP to discuss the case. A good MHP will be aware of the patient's dissatisfaction, and he or she will be able to shed some light on why this has occurred.

D. **Clinical improvement.** The PCP should not rely solely on the MHP to monitor mental health symptoms. If the patient is not improving within a reasonable period, such as 6 weeks for a major depressive episode, the PCP should feel free to discuss this situation with the MHP. A good MHP will convey an understanding of why the patient has not improved and will have prepared an alternative plan. A good MHP, like any good clinician, is flexible, resourceful, and open to suggestions.

IX. What Should Be Done if a Patient Will Not Accept a Referral?

A. **If the problem is not urgent or serious.** If a patient with a mild problem does not want to see a MHP, **the PCP should not insist on a referral.**

B. **If the problem is urgent or serious.** In this situation, it is appropriate to urge the patient to see a MHP. If a patient refuses, the PCP should attempt to involve family members or even work colleagues. For example, an intervention for an alcoholic may involve a coordinated effort including family members, friends, colleagues, the PCP, and an alcohol treatment specialist. If the patient appears to be acutely suicidal, homicidal, or unable to care for himself or herself because of mental illness, the PCP is responsible for arranging an immediate mental health evaluation. Ideally, such an evaluation should occur in an emergency room or in another setting in which the safety of the patient can be assured and from which elopement can be prevented.

1. Is it permissible for the PCP to refuse to prescribe a psychotropic agent and insist on a psychiatric referral? If the PCP feels comfortable treating the problem, it is certainly appropriate for the PCP to be the treating practitioner. However, if the PCP does not feel qualified to treat a specialized problem, he or she is under no obligation to do so. The PCP may tell the patient that he or she will continue to treat primary care medical problems but that a MHP must treat the psychiatric problem. Consultation with a colleague, attorney, or medical ethicist should be considered in such circumstances.

2. If a patient's untreated psychiatric condition makes medical treatment impossible, the PCP may insist on a psychiatric referral. For example, if a patient is so severely depressed that he or she has refused to take insulin and becomes ketoacidotic on multiple occasions, it is appropriate for the PCP to insist that the patient seek psychiatric help. The justification for insisting on a referral is that not doing so may constitute tacit acceptance of the patient's dangerous behavior. Another example of this situation occurs in transplantation settings. Many transplant programs require psychosocial evaluations of potential transplant recipients to determine suitability for transplantation. For example, a candidate for a liver transplant who is an active alcoholic would need to participate in a treatment program before being permitted a transplant. Refusal to do so would result in ineligibility for transplantation. Consultation with a colleague, attorney, or medical ethicist should be considered in such circumstances.

X. Referral or Collaborative Care

After the referral has been made, the PCP should discuss with the MHP whether the treatment plan should be instituted by the PCP or by the MHP. Possible treatment arrangements are outlined in Table 4-5. Which of these arrangements is implemented depends on a number of factors, including the following:

A. Availability of practitioners. In some rural areas it is logistically easier for a patient to receive medications from a PCP instead of traveling to see a psychiatrist.

B. Managed care requirements. Some managed care plans insist that psychotherapy not proceed without an initial medication evaluation by a psychiatrist.

Table 4-5. Possible Ongoing Treatment Arrangements	
Medication Management	*Psychotherapy/Behavioral Medicine*
Psychiatrist	Psychiatrist
Primary care clinician	Psychiatrist, psychologist, or psychiatric social worker
Psychiatrist	Psychologist or psychiatric social worker
Primary care practitioner or psychiatrist	None
None	Psychiatrist, psychologist, or psychiatric social worker

C. Comfort level and expertise of the practitioners

D. Ability of the practitioners to work together effectively

E. Timing. An initial arrangement need not be permanent. For example, psychotherapy may be time-limited, but medication management may continue indefinitely. Or a psychiatrist may initiate medication treatment and treat the patient until the patient is in remission, at which point the PCP may feel comfortable taking over the treatment. A consultant who is available at the beginning of treatment should be happy to see the patient again for a follow-up consultation.

Suggested Readings

Agency for Health Care Policy and Research. (1993). Clinical Practice Guideline Number 5, *Depression in primary care,* vols 1 and 2. AHCPR Publication No. 93–0551. Rockville, Md.: U.S. Department of Health and Human Services.

Diagnostic and statistical manual of mental disorders, primary care version (DSM-IV, PC). (1996). Washington, DC: American Psychiatric Press.

Kates, N., Craven, M.A., & Crustolo, A. (1997). Sharing care: The psychiatrist in the family physician's office. *Canadian Journal of Psychiatry, 42,* 960–965.

Katon, W., Von Korff, M., Lin, E., et al. (1995). Collaborative management to achieve treatment guidelines: Impact on depression in primary care. *Journal of the American Medical Association, 273*(13), 1026–1031.

Olfson, M. (1991). Primary care patients who refuse specialized mental health services. *Archives of Internal Medicine, 151,* 129–132.

Smith, G.R., Rost, K., & Kashner, T.M. (1995). A trial of the effect of a standardized psychiatric consultation on health outcomes and costs in somatizing patients. *Archives of General Psychiatry, 52*(3), 238–243.

Spitzer, R.L., Williams, J.B., Kroenke, K., et al. (1994). Utility of a new procedure for diagnosing mental disorders in primary care: The PRIME-MD 1000 study. *Journal of the American Medical Association, 272*(22), 1749–1756.

Worth, J.L., & Stern, T.A. (2003). Benefits of an outpatient teleconsultation unit: Results of a one-year pilot. *Primary Care Companion Journal of Clinical Psychiatry, 5,* 80–84.

CHAPTER 5

Approach to Informed Consent

RONALD SCHOUTEN

I. Introduction

Informed consent is a process through which a physician gets the permission of a patient or a substitute decision-maker to provide treatment to that patient. The decision-maker must be **competent** (have the capacity to make the decision), must be given enough **information** to make an informed decision, and must make the decision **voluntarily.** Informed consent is an effective means of improving the clinical outcome, reducing the risk of malpractice, fulfilling an ethical obligation, and meeting a legal requirement.

A. Process versus Event

1. To the extent that the clinical circumstances allow, **informed consent should be obtained over a period of time,** with an interval elapsing between the time when the information is provided and the time when the patient is asked to make a decision. During this period the patient has an opportunity to consider the information provided and to ask more questions. This is the **process model.**

2. The **event model,** in which **the physician makes the treatment recommendation, reviews the risks and benefits, and asks the patient to make a decision in one sitting,** increases the risk that the patient or family will have unanswered questions, feel pressured, or fail to comply with the recommended treatment. **The signing of a form titled "Informed Consent" does not constitute informed consent. It is the process leading up to the signing that constitutes informed consent; the form is only a piece of evidence that the process occurred.**

B. Role of Informed Consent

1. **Informed consent is a means of improving the clinical outcome.**

   a. Patients who understand the purpose of the treatment and the importance of following directions (e.g., the length of a course of antibiotic therapy) and participate in the decision-making process are more likely to comply with the prescribed treatment.

   b. Patients who are informed about potential side effects in advance are less likely to discontinue treatment when those side effects occur.

2. **Informed consent is a risk management tool.**

   a. Unpleasant feelings in the doctor–patient relationship can increase the likelihood of a malpractice suit being filed after an adverse event.

      i. The informed consent process allows for person-to-person contact in which the patient and his or her family see the physician as a real person who is attempting to help them.

      ii. A physician who obtains informed consent in a reasonable way is less likely to be perceived as arrogant and deserving of a lawsuit by distressed patients if there is an adverse outcome.

    b. Explanation of the lack of certainty in regard to the outcome can help patients and their families develop reasonable expectations about the results, decreasing their degree of upset if there is a less than perfect outcome.

    c. Appropriate documentation of the informed consent process is extremely helpful if a lawsuit is filed alleging that treatment was conducted without appropriate consent.

3. **Informed consent is an ethical obligation.**

    a. Patient autonomy is an essential ethical construct and lies at the heart of the doctor-patient relationship.

       i. **Autonomy**—the patient's right to make his or her own decisions regardless of what the physician or society believes is the best choice—has become the controlling principle in medical ethics.

       ii. **Beneficence**—the physician's obligation to do what is in the best interests of the patient is secondary to autonomy.

    b. Physicians have an obligation to promote patient autonomy.

       i. This is true even when the patient's wishes are at odds with the wishes of the patient's family or the physician.

       ii. When a competent patient wishes to pass the right to make a decision to a family member or to the physician, the patient may do so.

4. **Informed consent is a legal obligation.**

    a. The legal concept of informed consent started to develop in the 1960s.

    b. Liability may arise in several ways.

       i. Civil liability (**malpractice**)

- **Malpractice is based on the concept of battery** (touching another person without consent or justification).
- This is rarely the sole basis for a suit, because the plaintiff must prove that he or she would have rejected the treatment if informed consent had been obtained.

       ii. Liability for fraud, for example, when a patient is deceived into accepting care

       iii. Civil rights violations, such as violations of liberty interests when treatments are imposed without the patient's informed consent

       iv. Liability or administrative penalties for violation of regulations

II. Elements of Informed Consent

A. Competency

1. For a patient to give adequate informed consent, **that patient must have the physical and mental capacity to make informed treatment decisions. The degree of capacity required depends on the nature of the condition and the risks of the proposed treatment.** Less capacity is required for low-risk treatments with a high likelihood of a good result, such as intravenous fluids for dehydration. A higher level of capacity is required when the treatment has a higher level of risk or is more invasive and the results are less likely to be favorable, such as amputation in an elderly diabetic patient with renal failure.

    a. Keep in mind that **competency is a legal term, not a clinical term,** although physicians tend to overlook this distinction. **A legal declaration of incompetence** strips a person of certain rights and privileges normally accorded to adults, such as making treatment decisions, making contracts, voting, and executing a will.

      i. All adults are presumed to be competent to make their own treatment decisions in the eyes of the law.

     ii. **Only a judge can declare a person incompetent.**

   iii. **Clinical assessments of capacity,** which are often referred to as competency evaluations, **have no effect on a patient's legal status,** although they can serve as an indication of the likely outcome of legal proceedings.

- Competency evaluations are used as evidence in judicial proceedings.
- A competency evaluation that concludes that a patient has the capacity to make treatment decisions can allow treatment to proceed if there are doubts about the patient's mental status.
- The conclusion that a patient lacks the capacity to give informed consent requires the choice of an alternative decision-maker except in an emergency or when the patient has a valid advance directive.

2. **Competence (capacity) can be global or task-specific.**

  a. **Global capacity refers to a person's ability to undertake and carry out all the normal responsibilities and rights of an adult.** A declaration of global incapacity strips an individual of his or her rights as **a legal person.**

  b. **Specific capacities** include the following:

      i. **Testamentary capacity** is the capacity to execute a will. Specific legal standards for testamentary capacity apply in all jurisdictions. Be aware of the legal standard in your jurisdiction before agreeing to render an opinion that you may have to defend in court if the will is challenged.

     ii. **Testimonial capacity** is the capacity to serve as a witness in court.

   iii. There is also the **capacity to make treatment decisions.**

3. **The physician must evaluate the patient's capacity to make treatment decisions.**

  a. **Does the patient express a preference?**

      i. Patients who are unable to express a preference are presumed to lack decision-making capacity.

     ii. Capacity should be questioned further in individuals who shift their expressed preferences back and forth.

  b. **Is the patient able to attain a factual understanding of the information provided?**

      i. The patient need not be a medical expert to give informed consent but must be able to understand the basic information.

     ii. The ability to understand and retain information regarding the diagnosis, proposed treatment, and risks and benefits of the treatment satisfies this requirement.

  c. **Is the patient able to appreciate the seriousness of the condition and the consequences of accepting or rejecting treatment?**

      i. Appreciation represents more than an understanding of the basic facts.

     ii. The patient should be able to appreciate the significance and impact of the various options available and make decisions accordingly.

  d. **Can the patient manipulate the information provided in a rational fashion and come to a decision that follows logically from that information in the context of the individual's personal beliefs, experience, and circumstances?**

      i. The process of reaching a decision, not the decision itself, must be rational. Competent people have a right to make decisions that may seem irrational to the rest of the world.

     ii. Disagreement with the treating clinician's recommendations is in and of itself not a basis for judging that a patient is irrational.

B. Information

1. The amount and type of information which must be given to the patient to meet the requirements of informed consent vary among jurisdictions. Check with your hospital attorney or medical society to determine the standard in your state. There are three basic standards.
   a. **The professional standard** is the amount of information a reasonable professional would provide in similar circumstances.
   b. **The materiality standard** is what the average patient would need to make a decision under the same circumstances.
      i. It is also referred to as a **patient-oriented standard.**
      ii. In some jurisdictions, such as Massachusetts, the concept is extended to require provision of the information that would be material to the particular patient's decision.
   c. **The combined standard** requires the information that a reasonable medical practitioner would provide but also examines whether it was "sufficient to ensure informed consent."
2. **Providing the following information to patients will fulfill the information requirements in most jurisdictions.**
   a. The nature of the condition to be treated and the treatment proposed.
   b. The nature and probability of the risks associated with the treatment. Minor risks or side effects that occur frequently, such as dry mouth, and significant risks that occur infrequently, such as hepatic failure secondary to sodium valproate, should be reviewed with the patient.
   c. Inability to predict the results of the treatment.
   d. The irreversibility of the procedure, if applicable.
   e. The alternative treatments available, including no treatment. This should include a discussion of the risks and benefits associated with these options.

C. Voluntary

1. This simply means **free of coercion** by those proposing the treatment.
2. Persuasion by family members does not invalidate informed consent as long as the circumstances do not put the physician on notice that the treatment is being imposed against the patient's will or indicate that the patient is incompetent.

III. Obtaining Informed Consent

A. Informed consent must be obtained for all medical treatment. The question here is whether the informed consent must be written.
   1. Consult the informed consent policies of your hospital, clinic, or health maintenance organization to determine which treatments or procedures require written informed consent. Organizations usually have specific informed consent forms which must be used.
   2. If written consent is not required, a verbal discussion with the patient or decision-maker covering the issues outlined above is sufficient.

B. Informed consent need not be obtained in some situations.
   1. **In an emergency**, treatment can be provided to stabilize a patient and prevent deterioration of the patient's condition even if appropriate informed consent cannot be obtained.
   2. **There may be a waiver** of informed consent by the patient: "You do what you think is necessary, Doctor, and spare me the details." The patient must be **competent** to waive informed consent, however.

3. Informed consent need not be obtained from a patient **if the patient is incompetent.** Reasonable treatment can be provided until a substitute decision maker is appointed.

4. **If a patient's physical or mental condition would deteriorate as a direct result of the process of providing information,** informed consent may be deferred under the doctrine of therapeutic privilege. This exception should be invoked rarely and is open to challenge.

C. **The patient or decision-maker should be given an opportunity to ask questions** and should be informed of the right to withdraw consent at any point during the course of treatment.

D. **The consent process should be documented in the patient's record** even if a separate informed consent form is used. The note can be brief but should include the fact that the patient was informed of the risks and benefits associated with the treatment. It also should indicate that side effects and risks of specific relevance to the patient were mentioned, such as hand tremor during lithium treatment for those who use fine motor skills in their work. It is useful to **document the questions** asked by the patient to indicate that the patient was truly involved in the decision-making process.

Suggested Readings

Appelbaum, P.S., & Gutheil, T.G. (2000). *Clinical handbook of psychiatry and the law* (3rd ed.). Baltimore: Williams & Wilkins.

Berg, J.W., Appelbaum, P.S., Parker, L.S., & Lidz, C.W. (2001). *Informed consent: Legal theory and clinical practice.* New York: Oxford University Press.

Harnish v. Children's Hospital Medical Center, 439 NE2d 240 (Mass 1982).

Schouten, R. (1989). Informed consent: Resistance and reappraisal. *Critical Care Medicine, 17,* 1359–1361.

Sprung, C.L., & Winick, B.J. (1989). Informed consent in theory and practice: Legal and medical perspectives in the informed consent doctrine and a proposed reconciliation. *Critical Care Medicine, 17,* 1346–1354.

Winick, B.J. (1991). Competency to consent to treatment: The distinction between assent and objection. *Houston Law Review, 28,* 15–61.

Diagnostic Strategies

CHAPTER 6

How to Use the *DSM-IV-PC*

Thomas N. Wise and Theodore A. Stern

I. Why Should One Use a Primary Care Version of the *Diagnostic and Statistical Manual of Mental Disorders-Fourth Edition (DSM-IV)?*

A. **The *DSM-IV* Text-Revision (TR) is not widely used in training or in practice by primary care physicians.**
1. *DSM* iterations are organized according to major subclasses of disorders that assume the user knows to which section to refer.
2. The *DSM* system includes detailed and complex information for many disorders that are rarely diagnosed in primary care settings.
3. A more user-friendly guide for diagnosis according to *DSM-IV* criteria may help physicians in primary care to recognize better the psychiatrically-disordered patients in their practices. Thus, the American Psychiatric Association collaborated with organizations of primary care specialties to develop a diagnostic manual better suited for primary care settings.

B. **Only half of individuals with psychiatric and/or substance abuse disorders seek treatment. When they do, it is generally in primary care settings.**
1. These disorders are often underdiagnosed; detection rates range from 20–80% in primary care settings.
2. Many patients diagnosed with psychiatric disorders in primary care settings do not actually meet formal diagnostic criteria and may represent subthreshold mental disorders or psychosocial distress that is not clearly defined in the *DSM-IV.*
3. Proper recognition of psychiatric disorders is essential in providing effective treatment, which costs approximately $67 billion annually in the United States.

C. **Patients with psychiatric, addictive and substance abuse disorders have an increased mortality rate, an increased risk for general medical co-morbidity, and a reduction in work productivity.** Psychiatric patients with co-morbid general medical conditions have longer hospital stays, more medical procedures, and higher global health care costs.

II. Elements that Inhibit the Recognition and Treatment of Psychiatric Conditions

A. **Patient Factors**
1. Shame and embarrassment inhibit patients from discussing psychiatric issues and substance abuse problems with their physician.
2. Patients diagnosed with a psychiatric disorder may refuse referral to a psychiatrist owing to fears of stigmatization attached to such treatment.

3. Financial concerns, such as lack of insurance, may prevent patients from seeking proper treatment.

B. Health System Variables

1. Inadequate time may be allocated for a proper psychosocial and drug use evaluation in busy primary care settings.
2. Reimbursement policies for primary care providers (PCPs) provide little incentive for them to diagnose and to treat mental disorders.
3. Mental health carve-outs effectively partition the PCP from freely referring mental health practitioners and misalign incentives.
   a. The mental health panel of carve-outs is often a free-standing entity with no financial or organizational relationship to the larger general medical panel.
4. Psychiatric physicians, particularly in rural areas, may not be readily available.

C. Physician-Related Areas

1. Some PCPs have had prior negative experiences with psychiatrists.
2. Inadequate interview techniques may preclude a full psychosocial history (e.g., one marked by closed-ended and rapid questions that ignore psychosocial factors).
3. Limited training regarding diagnosis and treatment of alcoholism and psychiatric disorders interferes with timely and appropriate treatment.
4. An inadequate understanding of psychiatric taxonomy may lead to improper diagnosis.

D. The nature of psychiatric disorders may also inhibit proper recognition and treatment.

1. Psychiatric disorders may be incorrectly viewed as an "understandable" reaction to a life stressor or medical illness.
2. An inadequate understanding of current psychiatric nosology impedes diagnosis and treatment.
3. Diagnosis depends on a psychiatric history rather than on specific laboratory tests.

III. The Genesis of the *DSM-IV-PC*

A. Primary care organizations were invited to participate in the organization and production of the *DSM-IV-Primary Care Version.*

B. Representatives from internal medicine, family practice, obstetrics and gynecology, pediatrics, and psychiatry produced this version of psychiatric nosology for PCPs.

IV. Guiding Principles

A. The *DSM-IV-PC* is organized around symptoms and is user-friendly.

B. The manual facilitates creation of differential diagnoses and provides essential clinical facts in an educationally useful format.

C. Appropriate research criteria (using *DSM-IV*'s Appendix B) for disorders commonly seen in primary care, such as a minor depressive disorder, were included. These criteria are found in Appendix B of the *DSM-IV.*

D. The manual was made compatible with the *DSM-IV* and the ICD10-CM to facilitate communication and proper medical record notation.

V. The Four Sections of the *DSM-IV-PC*

A. Nine common symptoms were deemed present in primary care.
   1. An algorithm was included for each symptom to facilitate a differential diagnosis.
   2. Psychosocial problems commonly seen, but not formally considered mental disorders, were also included.
   3. Disorders rarely found in primary care were listed with their common presenting symptoms.
   4. Symptoms seen in infancy, adolescence, and childhood were also included.

B. Symptom presentation was the organizing basis for the manual, with algorithms provided for common symptoms.
   1. The order of each algorithm is based on frequency, salience, or severity of symptoms.
   2. Consistency across algorithms allows the physician to first consider whether a general medical condition, substance abuse, or organic disorder is the likely syndromal cause of a symptom.
   3. **Within each algorithmic step, a code and definition of the condition was emphasized** to allow additional information.
   4. **An introductory text accompanied each algorithm.**
      a. Epidemiology of the various disorders within the general population or primary care was presented.
      b. Common primary care presentations were described.
      c. The differential diagnosis and common associated conditions were listed.
      d. An explanation of how the algorithm was organized was included.

VI. How Should One Use the Manual? (See Table 6-1)

A. Interview carefully, gather corollary information from other sources, and identify the specific symptoms.

B. Select the appropriate sections of the *DSM-IV-PC* that focus on the symptoms elicited.

C. Determine whether the symptoms are caused by a medical disorder, by a medication that causes such symptoms, or by substance abuse.

D. If organic etiologies do not seem to explain the symptoms, follow the algorithm to define the specific disorder.

Table 6-1. An Example of How to Use the DSM-IV-PC; the Algorithm for Depressed Mood

Presenting symptoms might also include

   Decreased energy

   Insomnia

   Weight loss

   Unexplained general medical complaint (e.g., chronic pain, gastrointestinal distress, dizziness)

(continued)

Table 6-1. (*Continued*)

Step 1: Consider the etiological role of a general medical condition or substance use, and whether the depressed mood is better accounted for by another mental disorder:

    A. 293.83 Mood Disorder Due to a General Medical Condition

    B. ---.-- Substance-Induced (including medication) Mood Disorder

    C. ---:-- Other Mental Disorders

Step 2: If depressed mood or loss of interest or pleasure persists over a 2-week period, consider:

    296.2x   Major Depressive Disorder, Single Episode

    296.3x   Major Depressive Disorder, Recurrent

NOTE: If individual has ever had a major depressive episode (but current symptoms do not meet full criteria), consider: 296.x5 Major Depressive Disorder, in Partial Remission

NOTE: If criteria for a major depressive episode are met, and there is a history of elevated, expansive, or euphoric mood, consider: 296:-- Bipolar I Disorder or 296.89 Bipolar II Disorder

Step 3: If depressed mood has been present for most of the past 2 years (in adults; or 1 year in children), consider:

    300.4   Dysthymic Disorder

Step 4: If depressed mood occurs within 2 months of the death of a loved one, consider:

    V62.82   Bereavement

Step 5: If depressed mood occurs in response to an identifiable psychosocial stressor and does not meet criteria for any of the preceding disorders, consider:

    309.0   Adjustment Disorder, With Depressed Mood, or

    309.28   Adjustment Disorder, With Depressed Mood and Anxiety

Step 6: If criteria are not met for any of the previously described disorders, consider:

    311   Depressive Disorder Not Otherwise Specified

Step 7: If the clinician has determined that a disorder is not present but wishes to note the presence of symptoms, consider:

    780.9   Sadness

    780.7   Decreased energy

    780.52   Insomnia

VII. Disorders Defined in *DSM-IV-PC* via Algorithms That Are Based on Presenting Symptoms

A. Depressed Mood
1. Mood disorder caused by a general medical condition
2. Major depressive disorder
3. Bipolar I disorder
4. Bipolar II disorder
5. Dysthymic disorder
6. Bereavement—not a formal psychiatric disorder, but a V-coded phenomenon (V-coded phenomena refer to conditions that may be a focus of clinical attention but are not defined as an Axis I, II, or III disorder; academic problems or relationship issues exemplify this)
7. Adjustment disorder with either depressed mood or mixed anxiety and depression

B. Anxiety Symptoms
1. Caused by a general medical condition, by alcohol, or by another substance
2. Panic disorders
3. Phobias
4. Separation anxiety disorder
5. Obsessive-compulsive disorder
6. Post-traumatic stress disorder
7. Acute general stress disorder
8. Generalized anxiety disorder
9. Adjustment disorder with anxiety

C. Unexplained Physical Symptoms
1. Conversion disorder
2. Pain disorder
3. Hypochondriasis
4. Body dysmorphic disorder
5. Somatization disorder
6. Malingering (this is also a V code)
7. Factitious disorder

D. Cognitive Disturbance (e.g., delirium, dementia)

E. Problematic Substance Abuse
1. Dependence
2. Abuse
3. Alcohol-induced disorders
4. Other substance-induced disorders

F. Sleep Disturbance

G. Sexual Dysfunction—erectile and orgasmic disorders

H. Weight Change or abnormal eating

I. Psychotic Symptoms (including hallucinations, delusions, disorganized speech, or catatonia)

VIII. Psychosocial Problems That Are Not Formal Diagnoses but That Are Coded under the V Codes

A. Psychological and behavioral factors that affect health, such as non-compliance with treatment or other psychological factors, may affect a medical condition

B. Relational or family problems

C. Problems related to abuse or to neglect

D. Problems related to personal roles, such as religious or spiritual problems, or to occupational difficulties

E. Social problems, such as housing or economic difficulties, or problems with access to healthcare services, legal representation, or acculturation to our society

F. Other problems previously listed, such as bereavement, borderline intellectual functioning, or malingering

IX. Other Mental Conditions or Symptoms

A. Symptoms of mania

B. Symptoms of impulse dyscontrol, such as kleptomania, or intermittent explosive disorder

C. Deviant sexual arousal (this is in contradistinction to the sexual disorder section, which includes difficulties in sexual functioning in the phases of arousal or orgasm)

D. Symptoms related to dissociation, such as fugue and amnestic states

E. Abnormal movements and/or vocalizations, such as seen in Tourette's disorder or tic disorders

F. Traits of a dysfunctional personality, such as those found in Clusters A, B, and C of *DSM-IV*

X. Disorders Usually First Diagnosed in Infancy, Childhood, or Adulthood

A. Disorders of intellectual functioning, such as mental retardation

B. Disorders of academic skill, such as learning disorders

C. Disorders of motor skills

D. Disorders of disruptive behavior and inattention, such as attention-deficit/hyperactivity disorder

E. Negativistic or antisocial behaviors, such as conduct disorder

F. Disorders of feeding, eating, or elimination, such as enuresis or encopresis

G. Disorders of communication, such as stuttering

H. Conditions with impaired social interaction, such as autistic disorder or Asperger's disorder

I. Disorders of gender identity in children, adolescents, or adults

XI. Conclusion

Once the specific disorder is defined, treatment should be carried out in an appropriate manner. If more information is needed, the clinician should refer to the full

DSM-IV manual or to appropriate texts. At present there are no plans to revise the *DSM-IV-PC*. The *DSM-V* is expected to be published in 2008.

Suggested Readings

Borus, J.F., Howes, M.J., Devins, N.P., et al. (1989). Primary health care providers' recognition and diagnosis of mental disorders in their patients. *General Hospital Psychiatry, 10,* 317–321.

Branch, W.T., & Malik, T.K. (1993). Using "windows of opportunities" in brief interviews to understand patients' concerns. *Journal of the American Medical Association, 269,* 1667–1668.

Diagnostic and statistical manual of mental disorders (4th ed., primary care version). (1995). Washington, DC: American Psychiatric Press.

Diagnostic and statistical manual of mental disorders (4th ed.). (1994). Washington, DC: American Psychiatric Press.

Kirmayer, L.J., Robbins, J.M., Dworkind, M., et al. (1993). Somatization and the recognition of depression and anxiety in primary care. *American Journal of Psychiatry, 150,* 734–741.

Pincus, H.A., Vettorello, N.E., McQueen, L.E., et al. (1995). Bridging the gap between psychiatry and primary care: The *DSM-IV-PC. Psychosomatics, 36,* 328–335.

Reiger, D.A., Narrow, W.E., Rae, D.S., et al. (1993). The de facto U.S. mental and addictive disorders service system. *Archives of General Psychiatry, 50,* 85–94.

CHAPTER 7
Screening Tests for Detection of Psychiatric Disorders

David Mischoulon and Maurizio Fava

I. Introduction

A. **Overview**

When screening for psychiatric disorders, physicians typically rely on information obtained from the clinical interview, from review of medical records, and from other ancillary sources. Although diagnostic instruments are used primarily in clinical research studies, some of these instruments may serve as useful adjuncts to the clinical interview, particularly in cases where the diagnosis is in doubt, or when the efficacy of a treatment is unclear. Psychiatric rating scales attempt to translate clinical observations into objective and (sometimes) quantifiable information, and may help ensure the accuracy of a diagnosis, quantify the severity of symptoms, and assess the degree of effectiveness of a given treatment. We will review general concepts to clarify the usefulness of diagnostic instruments, review some commonly used instruments, and provide suggestions for the implementation of some of these instruments in the primary care setting.

B. **Reliability and Validity**

1. **Reliability refers to a scale's ability to convey consistent, reproducible information.** Diagnostic instruments are usually tested for their reliability by having more than one person administer, or rate, them, and then compare the results. This is called **inter-rater reliability.** If the instrument is designed to measure phenomena that are consistent over time, **test-retest reliability** becomes the relevant measure.

2. **Validity refers to the scale's ability to measure what it intends to measure.** For a diagnostic instrument to be valid, it must be reliable, although a reliable instrument may not necessarily be valid.

C. **Types of Diagnostic Instruments: Clinician-Rated vs. Self-Rated**

1. **Clinician-Rated Instruments, as their name implies, are diagnostic instruments administered by the clinician.** These instruments are advantageous in that they are generally valid and reliable. Most diagnostic instruments are of this kind.

2. **Self-Rated Instruments, on the other hand, are instruments that the patient must complete independently.** Self-rating scales have the advantage that they require less clinician time. This makes them especially useful for screening purposes. However, the reliability of self-rated scales is often difficult to assess, and some patients may be too impaired to complete them. The concordance rate between self-rating and observer scales is not well established.

D. **Diagnostic Interviews**

Structured clinical interviews were developed because of a perceived unreliability of psychiatric diagnoses. This problem was especially serious with regard to international studies, as psychiatrists from different countries or cultural backgrounds often had diverging views of what constituted mental disorders. Several scales were developed in the hope of improving the reliability and validity of diagnosis. In the following section, we will review the Structured Clinical Interview for *DSM-IV* (SCID), which is the most commonly used psychiatric diagnostic instrument.

II. The Structured Clinical Interview For *DSM-IV* (SCID)

A. Overview of the SCID

The SCID is essentially a semi-structured interview that applies the *DSM-IV* criteria to a patient. It is organized into modules that cover most of the major Axis I disorders (Mood Disorders, Psychotic Disorders, Anxiety Disorders, Substance Use Disorders, Somatoform Disorders, Post-Traumatic Stress Disorder, Adjustment Disorders, and Eating Disorders).

B. Administration of the SCID

The SCID is administered by a clinician, sometimes as an exclusive diagnostic tool, often after the patient has already screened positive for a given disorder (e.g., depression) through a shorter, self-administered questionnaire (such as the Beck Depression Inventory). **The SCID begins with a general introductory section on demographics, general medical and psychiatric history, and use of medications.** Questions here tend to be open-ended, and similar to those asked during general medical history-taking.

The SCID then proceeds by modules to the different Axis I psychiatric disorders. Questions here cover the specific *DSM-IV* symptoms of the different disorders, and are asked exactly as written. Answers are generally rated on a scale of 1–3 (1 = doubtful, 2 = probable, 3 = definite). Based on the number of positive answers, a diagnosis is determined. **A SCID-based interview may take between 1–3 hours to complete,** depending on how complicated a patient's history is, and on the patient's ability to provide a good history.

C. Value of the SCID

Although the SCID is probably the most reliable means of diagnosing psychiatric disorders, it is time-consuming to administer, and may require up to three hours to administer fully. For this reason, **it is used almost exclusively in the research setting.** Nonetheless, each individual SCID module is relatively quick to administer (some require no more than a few minutes), so in some instances (e.g., in the primary care setting), clinicians may use an individual module—such as the mood disorder module—if they suspect the presence of a particular psychiatric disorder.

III. Depression Scales

A. Hamilton Rating Scale for Depression (HAM-D)

1. Overview of the HAM-D

The HAM-D was designed to quantify the severity of depression in patients who already have a diagnosis of major depression. Questions focus on symptoms experienced only over the past week. It is administered by the clinician, and generally does not require more than 20 minutes to complete. **The HAM-D is a useful tool for measuring the progress of a patient during the course of treatment,** either in the research or clinical setting.

2. **Description of the HAM-D**

There are several different versions of the HAM-D, differing only in the number of questions included. The longest version includes 31 items; the shortest includes only six items. The longer versions include questions about atypical depression symptoms, psychotic symptoms, psychosomatic symptoms, and symptoms associated with obsessive-compulsive disorder (OCD). **The standard form, which is most often used in research studies, is the 17-item Hamilton D (HAM-D-17).**

3. **Scoring of the HAM-D**

There is a structured version of this instrument, in which questions are asked exactly as written, and are rated on a scale of 0–4 or 0–2, depending on the answers given by the patient. This version is typically used in research studies. Other versions allow more open-ended questioning, and may be useful in a clinical setting. Scores on the HAM-D-17 measure severity of depression as follows:

a. Not depressed: 0–7

b. Mildly depressed: 7–15

c. Moderately depressed: 15–25

d. Severely depressed: over 25

4. **The HAM-D as a Research Tool**

Clinical trials rely on the Hamilton-D to quantify responses to a given treatment over time. Studies will often cite a change in HAM-D score as a criterion for response. For example, a decrease of 50% or more in the HAM-D score is considered to be a positive response to antidepressant treatment, while a final score of 7 or less is considered typical of remission. The HAM-D is the most widely studied instrument for depression, and its reliability and validity are high. **In a primary care setting, the six-item HAM-D may prove a useful diagnostic adjunct, as it may be administered in less than three minutes,** and has been shown to be of comparable reliability and validity to the longer versions.

B. **Clinical Global Improvement (CGI) Scale**

The CGI scale is a three-item instrument used as an adjunct in the treatment of psychiatric disorders. It is administered by the clinician after a history has been obtained, and after the HAM-D or other instruments have been completed and reviewed by the clinician. Based on history and scores on other instruments, **it measures the following:**

a. **CGI-S (severity): the current condition of the patient on a scale of 1–7** (1 being normal, and 7 being among the most severely ill patients)

b. **CGI-I (improvement): the degree of improvement (as perceived by the clinician) since the start of treatment on a scale of 1–7** (1 being very much improved, and 7 being very much worse). Improvement in CGI ratings is also used in research to determine the degree of improvement over time with a given treatment.

C. **Beck Depression Inventory (BDI)**

1. **Overview of the BDI**

This 21-item questionnaire for assessment of degree of depression is probably the most widely used self-rating scale; it is self-administered by the patient, and can be completed in a few minutes. It is often used as a screening tool for determining the likelihood of a patient meeting criteria for major depression. A clinician may also use it to determine the degree of improvement over time. Questions are different from those found on the HAM-D, in that they **focus more on cognitive symptoms of depression.**

2. **Scoring of the BDI**

Patients generally must choose between four answers on each item (numbered 0–3 for degree of severity of depression). **Scores correlate with severity of depression as follows:**

a. Not depressed: 0–7

b. Mildly depressed: 7–15

c. Moderately depressed: 15–25

d. Severely depressed: over 25

The BDI has been shown to correlate well with the HAM-D and CGI, and because of its sensitivity to change over time, it is often used in medication trials. **It is also a popular screening tool in some primary care settings.**

D. **Zung Self-Rating Depression Scale (SDS)**

1. **Overview of the Zung SDS**

This is a 20-item self-administered rating scale. Items are rated based on frequency rather than intensity.

2. **Scoring of the SDS**

The raw score is converted into an index score as follows:

$$\text{Index} = \frac{\text{Raw Score Total}}{\text{Maximum Score of 80}} \times 100$$

SDS Index correlates with severity of depression as follows:

a. Not depressed: Below 50

b. Minimal to mild depression: 50–59

c. Moderate to marked depression: 60–69

d. Severe to extreme depression: over 70

The SDS is not thought to be sensitive to change over time, so it is not widely used in clinical trials. However, **it is popular for screening purposes, given its ease of administration,** and it has been widely used on National Depression Screening Day.

E. **The Harvard Department of Psychiatry National Depression Screening Day Scale (HANDS)**

1. **Overview of the HANDS**

The HANDS questionnaire is a brief self-rating scale that patients can self-administer in the office setting. It can be completed by the patient in a few minutes, and is scored by the clinician. It is typically used as part of National Depression Screening Day, and by primary care physicians (PCPs) as an indicator for further evaluation of the patient, when depression is suspected.

2. **Scoring of the HANDS**

The screening form includes 10 questions about symptoms of depression; for each item, the patient must answer whether he or she feels this way "none or little of the time" (0 points), "some of the time" (1 point), "most of the time" (2 points), or "all of the time" (3 points). **Scores correlate with likelihood of depression as follows:**

a. Unlikely depression: below 8

b. Likely depression: 9–16

c. Very likely depression: 17–30

The HANDS questionnaire has been shown to be valid and reliable, but has not yet achieved widespread use in psychiatric research settings. It may prove very useful in the primary care setting, given its ease of administration.

IV. Anxiety Scales

A. Anxiety Disorder Interview Scale, Revised (ADIS-R)
The ADIS-R is a semi-structured interview used for arriving at *DSM-III-R* diagnoses of anxiety disorders. It provides information on panic, generalized anxiety, and phobic avoidance, and also measures one's degree of disability. The scale includes the Hamilton-A and Hamilton-D scales for anxiety and depression, respectively. Its inter-rater reliability is high for most of the anxiety disorders, except generalized anxiety disorder (GAD).

B. Hamilton Rating Scale for Anxiety (HAM-A)
This is the most widely used scale for measurement of anxiety. It is used for patients with diagnosed anxiety disorders. It is similar to the HAM-D in that **it emphasizes somatic symptoms and experiences.** It has reasonable validity and reliability. This scale is easy and quick to administer in a primary care setting.

C. Yale-Brown Obsessive-Compulsive Scale (Y-BOCS)
The Y-BOCS is the most widely used scale for assessment of severity of obsessive-compulsive disorder (OCD) symptoms. It includes 10 items, and a symptom checklist. Inter-rater reliability is excellent. This scale has been used extensively in medication trials for measuring changes in severity of OCD symptoms.

V. Mania Scales

A. Manic State Rating Scale (MSRS)
The MSRS is a 26-item scale; it is rated on a 0–5 scale, and is based on the frequency and intensity of symptoms, particularly elation-grandiosity, and paranoid-destructiveness. The MSRS is designed primarily for use on inpatient units, and has been found to be reliable and valid.

B. Young Mania Rating Scale (Y-MRS)
This scale has 11 items, and is scored following a clinical interview. Four items (irritability, speech, thought content, and aggressive behavior) are given extra weight and scored on a 0–8 scale, while the other items are scored from 0–4. The scale has a high inter-rater reliability; scores on the Y-MRS correlate well with length of hospital stay.

VI. Schizophrenia Scales

A. Overview
The complexity of schizophrenia requires that clinicians use several different instruments to assess and study this illness. **Scales have been designed to assess positive and negative symptoms, social and vocational adjustment, and medication side effects.** Virtually all schizophrenia scales must be administered by a clinician, as many patients would not be able to complete a self-rated form. These scales are less likely to be used in a primary care setting. We will cover two of the more commonly used scales.

B. Description of Scales
1. Brief Psychiatric Rating Scale (BPRS)
The BPRS includes between 16 and 24 items, each rated on a scale of 1–7. **Items primarily cover symptoms of psychosis, but also address depression, and anxiety symptoms.** Ratings are expressed as a sum total of all items. **The scale is brief and may be administered in 15 to 30 minutes.** One limitation of the BPRS is that some

definitions of items tend to be vague, and are subject to interpretation. However, the scale has shown high inter-rater reliability.

2. **Positive and Negative Symptoms Scale (PANSS)**

As its name implies, the PANSS, similar to the BPRS, **focuses more on the positive symptoms** (such as hallucinations and delusions) **and negative symptoms** (such as alogia, affective flattening, avolition-apathy, anhedonia-asociality, and inattention). This scale is frequently used in clinical trials of antipsychotic drugs, largely because of its inclusion of negative symptoms. However, it requires more time to complete than does the BPRS. It has excellent inter-rater reliability and has been validated against other instruments.

VII. Cognitive Impairment Scales

A. Overview

Cognitive scales are useful as an initial screen for organic psychopathology; results of these scales can help the clinician decide whether or not to request formal neuropsychological testing or imaging studies. **These scales, however, may be influenced by the patient's intelligence, level of education, and literacy;** consequently, clinicians need to be careful not to make erroneous conclusions based on scores of these scales.

B. Description of Scales

1. **Mini-Mental State Examination (MMSE)**

The MMSE is **the most widely used instrument for measuring cognitive impairment.** It is a highly structured instrument, which may be administered by non-clinicians. **It includes questions about orientation, memory, attention, naming, as well as ability to follow commands, write a sentence, and copy intersecting polygons.** The MMSE may be **administered in less than 10 minutes;** it has established reliability and validity. It is an excellent tool for PCPs who may suspect dementia in elderly patients.

2. **Blessed Dementia Scale (BDS)**

This instrument **includes 50 items which assess orientation, recent and remote memory, and the ability to carry out activities of daily living.** It is used primarily to diagnose Alzheimer's dementia.

VIII. Personality Disorder Scales

A. Overview

The accurate diagnosis of personality disorders is difficult under most circumstances. **Most diagnostic scales have demonstrated poor reliability,** largely due to the subjective quality of the criteria, patient unreliability, and the tendency for many patients to meet criteria for more than one disorder at a time. Diagnostic reliability of these scales needs to be improved.

B. Description of Scales

1. **Structured Clinical Interview for *DSM-III-R* Personality Disorders (SCID-II)**

The SCID-II instrument is **used for the diagnosis of personality disorders.** As with the SCID-I, the SCID-II is organized around different personality disorders; questions are based on the criteria for each personality disorder, and are answered "yes" or "no." This instrument is **time-consuming to administer,** and is used almost exclusively for research purposes. It is not of practical use in the primary care setting.

2. **Personality Disorder Examination (PDE)**

   The PDE is a lengthy and semi-structured interview consisting of 359 items; it is rated on a 3-point scale (absent, clinically significant, or doubtful). It requires 1 to 2 hours to complete, and provides fairly rich information that places less burden on the assessor's judgment. As with the SCID-II, it is too lengthy for practical use in the primary care setting.

IX. Substance Abuse Scales

A. CAGE Questionnaire

This brief instrument is **widely used as a screening tool.** The name of the scale is an acronym for:

1. Have you ever felt a need to **cut down** on drinking?
2. Have people **annoyed** you by criticizing your drinking?
3. Have you ever felt **guilty** about drinking?
4. Have you ever had an **eye-opener**?

Answering "yes" to two or more of these questions strongly suggests an alcohol-related problem, particularly in a male population. It is an excellent instrument for use in the primary care setting.

B. Michigan Alcoholism Screening Test (MAST)

The MAST consists of 25 true-false questions that may be self-rated or administered by the clinician. Briefer versions have been developed, with comparable validity to the original. The Drug Abuse Screening Test (DAST) is similar to the MAST, and may discriminate between alcohol and drug abusers.

C. Addiction Severity Index (ASI)

The ASI assesses severity of problems with drug and alcohol abuse, with medical illness, with the legal system, with the family system, as well as with one's system of support (social and employment). **It appears to be a valid instrument,** that is useful in research as well as in treatment-planning. It may be administered in less than an hour. It may be useful in primary care clinics where there are large numbers of patients with substance-related problems.

X. Social Functioning Scales

A. Overview

These scales are often used to **assess the outcome of an illness** or its overall effect on the patient.

B. Description of Scales

1. **Global Assessment of Functioning Scale (GAF)**

   The GAF is used on Axis V of the *DSM-IV;* **it is based on collected information on psychological, social, and occupational function.** It rates the patient on a scale of 1–100, with a higher score indicating higher function. Usually there are two ratings made, one for current function, and one for highest function in the past year. A PCP may refer to this scale in order to assess the patient's overall function and the need for psychiatric or supportive services (e.g. visiting nurse or home health aide) or placement.

2. **Social Adjustment Scale (SAS)**

The SAS measures social functioning during the past month. Subjects answer questions about work role, household role, parental role, extended family role, sexual roles, social and leisure activities, and overall well-being. This scale covers the widest domain of social function, but may be less useful for severely dysfunctional patients, who may be unable to work and/or who have very limited social contacts.

XI. Drug Side Effect Scales

A. Abnormal Involuntary Movement Scale (AIMS)

The AIMS is widely used to measure neuroleptic-induced, late-onset movement disorders, such as tardive dyskinesia. Movements of the head, trunk, and extremities are observed, and rated on a scale of 1–5. **It is typically administered every 3 to 6 months to patients receiving antipsychotic medication.** PCPs who work in conjunction with psychiatric practitioners may benefit from familiarity with this scale, particularly if they see their patients with more frequency than their psychiatric counterparts.

XII. Conclusion

Diagnostic and psychiatric instruments can be useful diagnostic tools, both in research as well as in the clinical setting. These tools may be used independently or in conjunction with a thorough clinical interview. They may help the clinician ascertain the degree and type of illness and the response to treatment over time. **Many of these tools can be used effectively in the busy primary care medical setting, as a means of helping physicians ascertain the presence of psychiatric disorders, and the need for treatment and/or referral to a psychiatrist.**

Suggested Readings

Andreasen, N.C. (1982). Negative symptoms in schizophrenia: Definition and reliability. *Archives of General Psychiatry, 39,* 784–788.

Baer, L., Jacobs, D.J., Meszler-Reizes, J., et al. (2000). Development of a brief screening instrument: The HANDS. *Psychotherapy and Psychosomatics, 69,* 35–41.

Beck, A.T., Ward, C.H., Mendelson, M., et al. (1961). An inventory for measuring depression. *Archives of General Psychiatry, 4,* 561.

Beigel, A., Murphy, D., & Bunney, W. (1971). The manic state rating scale: Scale construction, reliability, and validity. *Archives of General Psychiatry, 25,* 256.

Blessed, G., Black, S.E., Butler, T., & Kay, D.W. (1991). The diagnosis of dementia in the elderly. A comparison of CAMCOG (the cognitive section of CAMDEX), the AGECAT program, DSM-III, the Mini-Mental State Examination and some short rating scales. *British Journal of Psychiatry, 159,* 193–198.

Blessed, G., Tomlinson, B.E., & Roth, M. (1968). The association between quantitative measures of dementia and of senile change in the cerebral grey matter of elderly subjects. *British Journal of Psychiatry, 114,* 797–811.

Di Nardo, P., Moras, K., Barlow, D.H., Rapee, R.M., & Brown, T.A. (1993). Reliability of DSM-III-R anxiety disorder categories. Using the Anxiety Disorders Interview Schedule-Revised (ADIS-R). *Archives of General Psychiatry, 50,* 251–256.

Endicott, J., Spitzer, R.L., Fleiss, J.L., & Cohen, J. (1976). The global assessment scale. A procedure for measuring overall severity of psychiatric disturbance. *Archives of General Psychiatry, 33,* 766–771.

Fenton, W.S., & McGlashan, T.H. (1992). Testing systems for assessment of negative symptoms in schizophrenia. *Archives of General Psychiatry, 49,* 179–184.

Folstein, M.F., Folstein, S.E., & McHugh, P.R. (1975). "Mini-mental state." A practical method for grading the cognitive state of patients for the clinician. *Journal of Psychiatric Research, 12,* 189–198.

Frank, E., Prien, R.F., Jarrett, R.B., et al. (1991). Conceptualization and rationale for consensus definitions of terms in major depressive disorder. Remission, recovery, relapse, and recurrence. *Archives of General Psychiatry, 48,* 851–855.

Goodman, W.K., Price, L.H., Rasmussen, S.A., et al. (1989). The Yale-Brown Obsessive Compulsive Scale. II. Validity. *Archives of General Psychiatry, 48,* 1012–1016.

Goodman, W.K., Price, L.H., Rasmussen, S.A., et al. (1989). The Yale-Brown Obsessive Compulsive Scale. I. Development, use, and reliability. *Archives of General Psychiatry, 46,* 1006–1011.

Gur, R.E., Mozley, P.D., Resnick, S.M., et al. (1991). Relations among clinical scales in schizophrenia. *American Journal of Psychiatry, 148,* 472–478.

Hamilton, M. (1959). The assessment of anxiety states by rating. *British Journal of Psychology, 32,* 50.

Hamilton, M. (1960). A rating scale for depression. *Journal of Neurology Neurosurgery and Psychiatry, 23,* 56–62.

Kay, S.R., Fiszbein, A., & Opler, L.A. (1987). The Positive and Negative Syndrome Scale (PANSS) for schizophrenia. *Schizophrenia Bulletin, 13,* 261–276.

Lewis, S.J., & Harder, D.W. (1991). A comparison of four measures to diagnose DSM-III-R borderline personality disorder in outpatients. *Journal of Nervous and Mental Disease, 179,* 329–337.

Loranger, A.W., Sartorius, N., Andreoli, A., et al. (1994). The International Personality Disorder Examination. The World Health Organization/Alcohol, Drug Abuse, and Mental Health Administration international pilot study of personality disorders. *Archives of General Psychiatry, 51,* 215–224.

Marder, S.R. (1995). Psychiatric rating scales. In H.I. Kaplan, & B.J. Saddock (Eds.), *Comprehensive textbook of psychiatry* (6th ed., pp. 619–635). Baltimore, MD: Williams & Wilkins.

Mischoulon, D., & Fava, M. (2000). Diagnostic rating scales and psychiatric instruments. In T.A. Stern, & J.B. Herman (Eds.), *Psychiatry update and board preparation.* New York: McGraw-Hill, pp. 233–238.

Oldham, J.M., Skodol, A.E., Kellman, H.D., et al. (1992). Diagnosis of DSM-III-R personality disorders by two structured interviews: Patterns of comorbidity. *American Journal of Psychiatry, 149*(2), 213–220.

Overall, J.E., & Gorham, D.R. (1962). The brief psychiatric rating scale. *Psychology Reports, 10,* 799.

Shear, M.K., & Maser, J.D. (1994). Standardized assessment for panic disorder research. A conference report. *Archives of General Psychiatry, 51,* 346–354.

Spitzer, R.L., Williams, J.B., Gibbon, M., & First, M.B. (1992). The Structured Clinical Interview for DSM-III-R (SCID). I: History, rationale, and description. *Archives of General Psychiatry, 49,* 624–629.

Williams, J.B., Gibbon, M., First, M.B., et al. (1992). The Structured Clinical Interview for DSM-III-R (SCID). II. Multisite test-retest reliability. *Archives of General Psychiatry, 49,* 630–636.

Williams, J.B. (1990). Structured interview guides for the Hamilton Rating Scales. *Psychopharmacology Series, 9,* 48–63.

Williams, J.B. (1988). A structured interview guide for the Hamilton Depression Rating Scale. *Archives of General Psychiatry, 45,* 742–747.

Young, R.C., Biggs, J.T., Ziegler, V.E., & Meyer, D.A. (1978). A rating scale for mania: Reliability, validity and sensitivity. *British Journal of Psychiatry, 133,* 429–435.

Zimmerman, M. (1994). Diagnosing personality disorders. A review of issues and research methods. *Archives of General Psychiatry, 51*(3), 225–245.

Zung, W.W.K. (1965). A self-rating depression scale. *Archives of General Psychiatry, 12,* 63.

CHAPTER 8

Use of Neuroimaging Techniques

DARIN DOUGHERTY, SCOTT RAUCH, AND KEITH LUTHER

I. Introduction

In general, neuroimaging is used as an aid in the differential diagnosis of neuropsychiatric conditions; rarely does neuroimaging alone establish the diagnosis. When one is contemplating the use of neuroimaging, a variety of factors must be considered, including the indications, risks, cost, advantages, and limitations. This chapter reviews these factors and provides general guidelines for the use of neuroimaging in neuropsychiatric syndromes.

II. Modalities

A. Structural

1. **Computed tomography (CT)**
   a. Technology
      i. Uses x-rays which are differentially attenuated, depending on the material through which they pass (higher attenuation in dense material, such as bone, and lower attenuation in less dense material, such as air and fluid).
      ii. CT uses serial x-rays acquired in an axial slabwise (i.e., tomographic) manner.
   b. CT with contrast
      i. Radiopaque iodine-based contrast material introduced intravenously allows visualization of lesions that compromise the integrity of the blood-brain barrier (e.g., cerebrovascular accident [CVA], tumor, inflammation).
      ii. Contrast media which enhance the visibility of pathology by CT are either ionic or non-ionic. Non-ionic contrast is more expensive than is ionic contrast; however, ionic contrast has a greater risk of the side effects.

      - Idiosyncratic reactions occur in 5% of cases and include hypotension, nausea, flushing, urticaria, and sometimes frank anaphylaxis. Risk factors include age less than 1 year or above 60 years and a history of asthma, allergies, cerebrovascular disease, or prior contrast reactions.
      - Chemotoxic reactions can occur in the brain and kidneys. Chemotoxicity may present as impaired renal function or even renal failure, with the main risk factor being pre-existing renal insufficiency. In the brain, chemotoxic reactions manifest as seizures. Such reactions occur in approximately 1 in every 10,000 cases but develop in up to 10% of cases in which gross disruption of the blood–brain barrier is present.

   c. Newer CT methods
      i. Spiral CT
      ii. CT angiography

    d. Advantages and limitations

        i. CT offers excellent spatial resolution (< 1 mm).

        ii. **CT is useful for the detection of acute bleeding** (less than 48 to 72 hours old) but less helpful in subacute bleeding (more than 72 hours old) and in severely anemic patients (hemoglobin below 10 g/dL).

        iii. CT is not helpful in visualizing subtle white matter lesions.

        iv. CT uses ionizing radiation and so is strongly contraindicated in pregnancy.

2. **Magnetic resonance imaging (MRI)**

    a. Technology

        i. MRI exploits the magnetic properties of hydrogen atoms in water molecules to construct a representation of tissue. Nuclei are excited; as they relax, they give off energy that is used to construct the images. Different components of the relaxation process exist and occur at different rates (called T1 and T2) in different tissues. Specific imaging parameters (T1-weighted versus T2-weighted) are selected according to the clinical circumstances.

          • **T1-weighted images are used for optimal visualization of normal anatomy.**

          • **T2-weighted images are used to detect areas of pathology.**

    b. MRI with contrast

        i. **Gadolinium** is used as the contrast medium because of its paramagnetic properties. Like CT contrast, it is introduced intravascularly. The use of **MRI contrast highlights vascular structures and aids in the detection of pathology in areas where blood vessel walls or the blood–brain barrier is compromised**. Gadolinium causes fewer and less severe side effects than does CT contrast, with one reported death in over 5 million dosings.

    c. Diffusion-weighted imaging (DWI)

        i. DWI utilizes magnetic resonance (MR) acquisition parameters that allow for the detection of water molecule movement in tissue. The rate of movement (or diffusion) may be expressed as an apparent diffusion coefficient (ADC). Soon after the onset of an ischemic stroke, the ADC of the affected brain tissue is reduced. DWI may soon become the modality of choice for clinical situations where acute ischemia is suspected.

    d. Advantages and limitations

        i. MRI provides excellent spatial resolution and **superior soft-tissue contrast** in comparison to CT (e.g., more useful for visualization of white matter).

        ii. MRI is **superior for surveying the posterior fossa and brainstem.**

        iii. MRI does not use ionizing radiation, and so it is **preferable to CT in pregnancy** but still is relatively contraindicated.

        iv. MRI is **contraindicated in patients with metallic implants** for the following reasons:

          • Metal can cause artifacts in MR images.

          • Metal can shift position or absorb heat within the magnetic field, causing burn injuries.

          • Mechanical devices, such as pacemakers, can malfunction within the magnetic field.

3. **CT versus MRI (Table 8-1)**

    a. CT is more economical than MRI and is available at more centers.

    b. CT is the modality of choice in patients with acute bleeds or acute trauma, although diffusion-weighted MRI may soon supercede CT in this regard.

Table 8-1. Summary Comparisons of CT and MRI	
Consideration	*CT versus MRI*
Economy	CT ≥ MRI
Availability	CT ≥ MRI
Speed	CT ≥ MRI
Comfort	CT > MRI
Quality of visualization	
Bleeding	
Acute (< 48–72 hours)	CT > MRI
Subacute (> 48–72 hours)	MRI > CT
Ischemia	
Acute	DWI > MRI ≈ CT
Chronic	DWI ≈ MRI > CT
Bone	CT > MRI
Gray matter	MRI > CT
White matter	MRI > CT
Posterior fossa	MRI > CT
Spatial resolution	CT ≥ MRI

    c. MRI is superior to CT for the differentiation of white from gray matter and the identification of white matter lesions.

    d. MRI is superior to CT for the detection of posterior fossa and brainstem pathology.

B. Functional

  1. Positron emission tomography (PET)

    a. Technology

      i. **PET uses positron emission from administered radionuclides to measure cerebral blood flow or cerebral glucose metabolism, both of which correspond to neuronal activity.**

      ii. With PET one can use inhaled or intravenous (IV) radionuclides to look at the brain in the resting state or when activated by specific tasks.

      iii. One can also use radioactive ligands to perform receptor characterization studies.

    b. Advantages and limitations

      i. **PET is the gold standard of functional neurolmaging modalities.**

      ii. **PET offers excellent spatial resolution (4 to 8 mm).**

      iii. **PET is very expensive and requires immediate access to the cyclotron,** which produces positron-emitting radionuclides.

  2. Single photon emission computed tomography (SPECT)

    a. Technology

      i. **SPECT also uses radionuclides** for functional imaging but measures single photon emission rather than positron emission.

      ii. As with PET, both inhaled and IV radionuclides are available, as are radioligands for measuring indexes of gross brain activity and performing receptor characterization.

Table 8-2. Summary Comparisons of PET and SPECT	
Consideration	*PET versus SPECT*
Economy	
Institutional	SPECT >> PET
Per scan	SPECT > PET
Availability	SPECT > PET
Spatial resolution	PET > SPECT
Temporal resolution	PET ≥ SPECT
Sensitivity	PET > SPECT
Signal: noise ratio	PET > SPECT
Variety of ligands	PET > SPECT

   b. Advantages and disadvantages
      i. **SPECT is more affordable than PET** and does not require a cyclotron for the production of nucleotides.
      ii. **SPECT provides inferior spatial resolution (≥ 8 mm)** compared with PET.
      iii. **SPECT resolution worsens as one attempts to image deeper brain structures.**
   3. **PET versus SPECT (Table 8-2)**
      a. PET provides superior spatial resolution, especially for deeper brain structures.
      b. PET offers a broader array of radioligands for use in receptor studies and is the only modality that allows for the measurement of metabolism.
      c. SPECT is less expensive than PET and is more widely available.

III. Indications

   A. **Structural**
      1. **Computed tomography**
         a. There have been numerous studies of the results of CT imaging in psychiatric populations. These studies have culminated in **Weinberger's criteria (1984) for CT imaging for psychiatric symptomatology:**
            i. **Confusion or dementia**
            ii. **New-onset psychosis**
            iii. **Movement disorder**
            iv. **Anorexia nervosa**
            v. **Prolonged catatonia**
            vi. **New-onset major affective disorder or personality change after the age of 50 years**
      2. **MRI**
         a. When MRI became available in the 1980s, the neuroimaging literature reflected a shift toward the use of MRI in psychiatric populations.
         b. Many studies found an increased incidence of white matter lesions in psychiatric populations. However, studies also revealed that 30% of normal persons over age 60 have white matter abnormalities of no apparent clinical significance.

c. The largest study was done at McLean Hospital over a 5-year period and included all patients who received an MRI during that time (Table 8-3).

d. Finding a structural abnormality on neuroimaging is of questionable value if it does not alter the treatment or outcome.

3. **Pre-electroconvulsive therapy neuroimaging**

a. Patients who require electroconvulsive therapy (ECT) often have a more treatment-refractory affective illness and may warrant a more thorough organic work-up.

b. Pre-ECT neuroimaging may be helpful in identifying lesions that may lead to an adverse outcome with ECT (aneurysms, tumors, arteriovenous malformations, hydrocephalus, and basal ganglia infarction).

4. **General guidelines for structural neuroimaging**

a. Criteria

   i. **Patients with acute changes in mental status** (including changes in affect, behavior, or personality) **plus one of three additional criteria:**

   * **Age greater than 50 years**
   * **Abnormal neurologic exam (especially focal abnormalities)**
   * **History of significant head trauma (i.e., with extended loss of consciousness, neurologic sequelae, or temporally related to mental status change in question)**

   ii. New-onset psychosis

   iii. New-onset delirium or dementia of unknown course

   iv. Prior to an initial course of ECT

b. Considerations

   i. Adherence to the criteria listed above should yield positive findings in 10–45% of cases. However, only 1–5% will produce findings that lead to specific medical intervention.

   ii. If structural neuroimaging is indicated, one should use MRI unless the problem is an acute trauma, or an acute bleed is suspected.

Table 8-3. Brain MRI Results in 6,200 Psychiatric Inpatients: Unexpected and Potentially Treatable Findings

MRI Findings	No. Cases	%
Multiple sclerosis	26	0.4
Hemorrhage	26	0.4
Temporal lobe cyst	22	0.4
Tumor	15	0.2
Vascular malformations	6	0.1
Hydrocephalus	4	0.1
Total	99	1.6

NOTE: Results from 6,200 consecutive MR scans performed at McLean Hospital over a 5-year period. Patients receiving MR scans represent approximately 40% of the total number of patients seen during that period.

SOURCE: Adapted from Rauch, S.L., & Renshaw, P.R. (1995). Clinical neuroimaging in psychiatry. *Harvard Review of Psychiatry, 2,* 297–312.

B. Functional. Most applications of functional neuroimaging in psychiatry occur in the field of research. However, a clinical role for functional neuroimaging in dementia and seizures is evolving and shows promise.

1. Dementia
   a. Characteristic neuroimaging profiles of various forms of dementia are emerging. Some studies have indicated that functional neuroimaging can offer better than 90% sensitivity and specificity in distinguishing Alzheimer's disease from other kinds of dementia.
   b. However, most forms of dementia are irreversible, and specific diagnoses may not affect the treatment. Furthermore, an adequate clinical examination often is the only thing necessary to reach a diagnosis of dementia.

2. **Seizures**
   a. Some seizures, especially complex partial seizures, are not always detected by an electroencephalogram (EEG). EEG measures cortical surface electrical activity but is less efficacious if the seizure focus is deep.
   b. PET and SPECT images demonstrate ictal hypermetabolism and interictal hypometabolism. This allows for the detection of seizure foci during the predominant inter-ictal period.
   c. To evaluate a possible seizure disorder, functional neuroimaging is performed in conjunction with EEG. PET also is useful for more precise localization of seizure foci in a patient with a known seizure disorder if neurosurgical intervention is indicated.

Suggested Readings

Dougherty, D.D., & Rauch, S.L. (Eds.). (2001). *Psychiatric neuroimaging research: Contemporary strategies.* Washington DC: American Psychiatric Publishing Inc.

Osborn, A.G. (1994). *Diagnostic neuroradiology.* St. Louis: Mosby-Year Book.

Rauch, S.L., & Renshaw, P.R. (1995). Clinical neuroimaging in psychiatry. *Harvard Review of Psychiatry, 2,* 297–312.

Renshaw, P.F., & Rauch, S.L. (1999). Neuroimaging in clinical psychiatry. In A.M. Nicholi (Ed.), *The Harvard guide to psychiatry* (3rd ed.). Cambridge, Mass.: Belknap Press, pp. 84–97.

Toga, A.W., & Mazziotta, J.C. (Eds.). (1996). *Brain mapping: The methods.* Boston: Academic Press.

Weinberger, D.R. (1984). Brain disease and psychiatric illness: When should a psychiatrist order a CAT scan? *American Journal of Psychiatry, 141,* 1521–1527.

SECTION III

Therapeutic Strategies

CHAPTER 9

Cognitive-Behavioral Therapy

Michael W. Otto, Noreen A. Reilly-Harrington, and Joseph A. Harrington

I. Cognitive-Behavioral Therapy

A. **Definition.** Cognitive-behavioral therapy (CBT) is a form of psychotherapy that is rooted in learning theory and relies on empiric investigation to obtain information about the nature of disorders, guide the development of new interventions, and document the effectiveness of existing treatments. CBT is not limited to overt behaviors and intellectual life. Instead, **it is concerned with a patient's emotional functioning and emphasizes modification of the maladaptive behavioral, emotional, and cognitive responses that characterize individual disorders.**

B. **Differences between CBT and insight-oriented therapy.** CBT is characterized by the following factors:
1. **CBT is short-term.** The length of therapy is dependent on the time needed to help a patient develop alternative patterns of behavioral and emotional responses.
2. **CBT is active.** Therapy provides a context for learning, and **it is the therapist's role to provide the patient with the information, skills, and opportunity to develop alternative patterns.**
3. **CBT is structured.** Portions of sessions are devoted to specific interventions. In many cases, **specific homework** (i.e., assignments to employ alternative responses) **is assigned for the patient to practice between sessions.** Each session may strike a balance between novel material introduced by the patient and a set of ordered interventions designed to eliminate the disorder that is being treated.
4. **CBT is collaborative.** The therapist and the patient act as collaborators to eliminate disorders and solve life issues by developing alternative skills or patterns.
5. **CBT is focused on the modification of emotions and behaviors.** Although the historic roots of current behavior may be examined, the greatest focus is on the modification of current patterns of behavior and emotion rather than on achieving historic insight.

C. **Effectiveness of CBT.** Empiric studies provide clinicians with information to inform, guide, and improve clinical practice. **To date, the best studied and most efficacious treatments for a wide range of mental disorders include CBT and pharmacotherapy. At present, the efficacy of CBT tends to approximate or surpass that of medication for the treatment of anxiety disorders, eating disorders, and non-psychotic major depression,** particularly when the longer-term outcome is considered.

II. Basis of Cognitive-Behavioral Therapy

A. **CBT has as its roots principles of learning derived from empiric study.** The application of those principles takes into account the individual's ability to rapidly generalize experiences from one situation to another and people's reliance on verbal behavior and symbolic information processing. The over-reliance on thoughts about the world rather than actual experiences has been implicated as a potential cause of psychopathology. Accordingly, cognitive-behavioral interventions frequently target the content, quality, and style of thoughts, images, beliefs, and rules regarding the nature of the world.

B. **Attention to distortions and inaccuracies in thoughts and beliefs** creates a perspective on the "unconscious" that is very different from traditional approaches to psychotherapy. Rather than being thought of as a unique structure, the unconscious is viewed as the default program. Consciousness rather than the absence of consciousness is seen as the most important, although frequently distorted, cognitive achievement.

C. **Conceptualizations of normal and pathologic patterns rely on the analysis of inter-related chains of thoughts, feelings, and behavior as well as the identification of behavioral excesses and deficits.** Cognitive-behavioral principles are easily exportable to a range of behavioral issues from the analysis and modification of interactions between physician and the patient to the modification of the marked anxiety, avoidance, or depression that characterizes anxiety and affective disorders.

D. **Specific models of the nature of pathology have been developed for various disorders,** and treatment programs thus are becoming increasingly specialized for each disorder.

E. **Attention to patterns of pathology** and the behavioral and emotional responses that maintain them **does not exclude a biologic contribution to disorders.** Biologic risk factors are assumed for a number of disorders and are implicated in the temperamental factors that may provide the context for the development of a disorder.

F. **CBT** attends to the complex interaction between biology and environment and focuses on **changes in cognition, behavior, and emotion to achieve changes in pathology.** These changes undoubtedly have an impact on the central nervous system and underscore the absence of a clear distinction between the somatic and the psychosocial effects of an intervention. For example, research has shown that CBT results in some of the same changes in brain activation that occur when patients respond successfully to pharmacotherapy for obsessive-compulsive disorder.

III. Clinical Rapport: Motivation and Compliance

A. **Interpersonal interactions are a rich target for behavioral analysis. Attention from a high-status individual frequently serves as a powerful reinforcer; thus, the clinician should be aware of her or his own behavior.** Changes in eye contact, body posture, and verbal tone can play an important role in encouraging or discouraging behaviors, including verbal behaviors. Similarly, extra attention devoted to on-task behaviors (e.g., the completion of recommended physical therapy) can be a powerful force in helping patients enhance adaptive rather than maladaptive patterns.

B. **In CBT, motivation is seen** not as a static variable that is personality-dependent but **as a behavioral state that is modifiable and a focus of treatment. Poor motivation can result from information deficits, skill deficits, or fear.** Consequently, informational interventions, including descriptions of the disorder and its associated symptoms, options for treatment, the change process, likely outcomes, and the step-by-step approach to achieving this outcome, can provide patients with a supportive framework that enhances motivation.

C. **Collaborative goal-setting and participation in decision-making** (e.g., selection of one of several treatment options) **can help increase motivation and compliance.** Similarly, discussion of a patient's conceptualization of the problem can provide an opportunity to deliver corrective information and enhance the patient's motivation for change.

D. Because motivation is influenced by the success of initial attempts, **feedback on initial performance can be a crucial factor during the early stages of the change process** or treatment regimen. Occasional follow-up can help remind patients of adaptive changes and maintain change over the long term.

IV. Common Elements of Clinical Treatment

A. **Informational Interventions. Part of the role of the behavioral clinician is to teach patients about the nature of their disorders, including common patterns that maintain a disorder and strategies for returning to normal functioning.**
   1. Information about the symptoms that define a disorder helps reduce self-blame and/or catastrophic misinterpretations of symptoms.
   2. Information about symptoms sets the stage for active collaboration between the clinician and the patient.
   3. Information about the nature of the disorder enhances the patient's motivation for therapeutic change. This is particularly important because initial interventions may require a great effort.

B. **Definition and Monitoring of Outcome**
   1. Treatment motivation and goal achievement are aided by clear specification and monitoring of goals and goal-directed activity by both the patient and the therapist.
   2. Regular assessment of outcome provides the therapist with a means to judge progress and can alert the clinician to update her or his case formulation or consider alternative interventions if the expected treatment gains are not achieved.

C. **Self-monitoring. Monitoring helps individuals become aware of the timing and occurrence of target behaviors, providing additional awareness and opportunities for change.**
   1. Smoking cessation. Smokers who wish to quit may use monitoring cards (i.e., a folded 3 by 5 card that is carried inside the cellophane wrapper of a cigarette pack). Before lighting a cigarette, the smoker is asked to note the situation, emotional context, and desire for a cigarette. Monitoring provides not only a record of the number of cigarettes smoked per day but also the situational and emotional cues for lighting up. The use of the monitoring card before lighting up can help some individuals reconsider their need for a cigarette by slowing the progression from desiring a cigarette to automatically lighting up.
   2. Treatment of work inhibition. Monitoring of work and non-work behavior can help individuals learn about problems of time management, motivation, and procrastination. Monitoring then can be extended to include behavioral change interventions, such as the scheduling of specific work topics, the inclusion of breaks, and the use of rewards.

D. **Cognitive Interventions**
   1. Cognitive interventions target systematic negative biases in thinking and help patients recognize how these thinking patterns affect moods and behaviors. By treating distorted thoughts as hypotheses (guesses) rather than statements of fact, patients begin to entertain and ultimately adopt more adaptive patterns of thought.

2. Examples of cognitive distortions include all-or-nothing thinking (e.g., "If I'm not respected by everyone, I'm a total failure"), overgeneralization (e.g., "Because I was not invited to speak at the upcoming conference, my research will never be well received"), and personalization (e.g., "My colleague acted distantly because I must have done something wrong"). In anxiety disorders, distortions frequently target the probability of negative outcomes or one's ability to cope if such outcomes occur.

3. Distorted thoughts often occur automatically, and patients are taught to monitor their thoughts and respond to them with alternative, more adaptive explanations. Patients record thoughts verbatim, using changes in emotion, difficult interactions, and avoidance behavior as cues for formal (often written) monitoring.

4. In addition to examining automatic thoughts that are situation-specific, cognitive interventions examine more pervasive core beliefs by assessing the themes that lie behind recurrent thought patterns. Those themes may be evaluated in regard to a patient's learning history to assess the genesis of such beliefs, but greater emphasis is placed on the logical evaluation and alteration of maladaptive beliefs.

E. Exposure Interventions

1. **Exposure is designed to help patients develop alternative emotional (and behavioral) responses to a variety of situations (usually feared situations) by allowing maladaptive emotional responses to dissipate (habituate and eventually be extinguished) upon continued successful exposure to a situation or event.**

2. **Exposure treatments may include direct exposure to feared situations (*in vivo* exposure), imaginal exposure to feared situations or events, exposure to feared feelings** (this is termed interoceptive exposure because the exposure involves the elicitation of feared somatic sensations, typically sensations similar to anxiety and panic), and exposure to feared cognitions (exposure to feared scenarios using imaginal techniques).

3. **Exposure can be conducted in a gradual, stepwise fashion or as an extended exposure to strong cues (flooding).** The preference of most therapists (and patients) is for more gradual exposure.

4. **It is preferable to terminate an individual exposure session only after anxiety has started to dissipate.** Prolonged exposure and massed practice (several sessions close together) aid in fear reduction.

F. Skill Rehearsal

1. Intellectual knowledge or intent is not the same as behavior change. Skill rehearsal helps ensure that individuals can utilize new skills when they are needed.

2. Skill rehearsal may involve modeling new behaviors and then role-played rehearsal of those behaviors in sessions.

3. Rehearsal allows for the evaluation of cognitive and emotional reactions to new behaviors and for the provision of constructive feedback.

4. Rehearsal in session is frequently followed by home behavioral assignments.

G. Behavioral Assignments

1. Behavioral assignments may be used to reinstate normal patterns of behavior (e.g., activity assignments for a depressed individual), to provide an opportunity for learning (in the case of exposure or cognitive interventions), or to ensure the acquisition of new behaviors (after instruction and rehearsal in sessions).

2. When used in the context of exposure and cognitive interventions, behavioral assignments provide individuals with opportunities to examine the veracity of their cognitions and expectations about the outcomes of events and behaviors. In this way, behavioral assignments provide "behavioral tests" of hypotheses about the outcomes of events.

3. Behavioral assignments also ensure that new behaviors are practiced independently of the therapist, and provide for a rehearsal for independent functioning over the long term.

H. **Contingency management** refers to **the management of a target behavior by modifying events after that behavior.** Contingency management usually involves the following:

1. An initial analysis of the target behavior with attention to the events that reliably appear to elicit and follow it

2. Clear specification of the behavior to be changed and the alternative behaviors desired

3. Rehearsal of alternative behaviors (never take away a behavior without providing an adaptive alternative)

4. Application of alternative consequences (e.g., the use of reasonable rewards or punishments)

I. **Relapse prevention skills** often are included as part of the treatment. **Patients are trained to recognize early warning signs of relapse and taught to "be their own therapists"** (e.g., to analyze difficulties and apply skills on their own) or, with some disorders, to schedule booster sessions when needed.

CHAPTER 10

Cognitive-Behavioral Strategies for Specific Disorders

MICHAEL W. OTTO, NOREEN A. REILLY-HARRINGTON, AND JOSEPH A. HARRINGTON

I. Treatment Approaches for Specific Disorders

Basic and applied research has advanced the understanding of the nature of individual psychiatric disorders, and cognitive-behavioral therapy (CBT) accordingly has become increasingly specialized, seeking to modify the core patterns that underlie each disorder. **Outlined below are examples of the common elements of such CBT treatment packages as they are applied to specific Axis I and Axis II disorders.** In addition to these examples, CBT has been applied successfully to a variety of difficulties and disorders ranging from marital conflict and child management problems to chronic pain, hypochondriasis, sexual dysfunction, and substance abuse disorders.

II. Depression

A. **CBT for depression is a structured, active approach that emphasizes modification of the patterns of negative evaluations and dysfunctional behaviors that characterize the disorder.**
   1. **The thought patterns of depressed patients are characterized by cognitive distortions and logical errors.** These distorted cognitions or thoughts are often automatic and may precede negative shifts in mood.
   2. **A CBT therapist helps patients examine the evidence for and against such thoughts and generate alternative, more adaptive responses.** Assigned monitoring of thoughts is helpful in identifying, evaluating, and changing these dysfunctional cognitions.
   3. **Goal-setting, activity assignments, and careful monitoring of cognitions are used to address the behavioral inaction that frequently characterizes depression.**
B. **Informational interventions** represent the first stage of cognitive interventions.
   1. **Information is provided on the nature of the disorder, common symptoms, and the interventions that will follow.** These interventions can help a patient view depression as something external to the self and help prepare the patient for adaptive change.
   2. Informational interventions also can help inhibit the downward spiral of depressogenic responses to symptoms (negative self-evaluation in response to symptoms of depression, which is referred to as depression about depression).
C. **Activity Assignments**
   1. **Active behavioral techniques,** such as scheduling weekly activities (e.g., exercise, social interactions, and shopping) **are particularly useful for severely depressed patients.**

2. In addition to activating behavior and decreasing avoidance, such techniques help provide a context for challenging the maladaptive cognitions associated with problematic behaviors.

D. Training in problem-solving skills may be required to help patients return to adaptive patterns of functioning in social and work situations.

E. Core Belief Work
1. **The long-term goal of CBT for depression is to identify underlying, long-standing maladaptive beliefs which may predispose patients to depression.**
2. Patients are taught to identify and evaluate these beliefs as they are discovered during monitoring assignments. Modification of these beliefs may be especially important in reducing the risk of relapse.

F. Suicide Risk
1. In working with depressed patients, **it is crucial to assess suicide risk** and the need for protective hospitalization.
2. Assessment and modification of the dysfunctional cognitions that underlie feelings of hopelessness and helplessness provide a strategy for reducing suicide risk.

G. Other Treatment Considerations
1. A basic course of CBT commonly ranges from 16 to 20 sessions, with many patients showing benefit after 8 to 10 sessions.
2. CBT provides an effective alternative to antidepressant medications for patients with non-psychotic depression.
3. In severe cases of depression, combined pharmacotherapy and CBT should be considered.
4. In addition, CBT is useful in preventing relapse in patients and should be considered for patients who wish to discontinue antidepressant medication (e.g., as part of a planned pregnancy).

III. Bipolar Disorder

A. The goal of CBT for bipolar disorder is to decrease the frequency and severity of episodes of mania and depression.
1. The interventions listed below are designed to be an adjunct to ongoing medication treatment and focus on the elimination of risk factors for additional episodes (e.g., psychosocial or biologic stressors), early detection of episodes, compliance with medication, and modulation of manic symptoms.
2. Interventions for major depression are applied in patients with a bipolar disorder.

B. Regularity of the circadian rhythm. Interventions targeting the maintenance of a regular circadian rhythm include monitoring and/or scheduling of regular patterns of sleep, eating, and exercise.

C. Stress management. Risk reduction for future episodes also is achieved by targeting the occurrence and impact of interpersonal conflicts and other external stressors with instruction in problem-solving and stress management skills (see Chapter 11).

D. Early detection. Mood charts are used to graph changes in mood and watch for early warning signs of mania or depression.

E. Cognitive restructuring. Modification of negative (depressogenic) or hyperpositive thinking utilizes cognitive restructuring strategies.

F. Compliance

1. Training in active problem-solving targets the consistent use of medications and the minimization of side effects.
2. Cognitive interventions also can be used to identify and modify maladaptive beliefs about medication or a disorder.

G. Empiric evidence

1. Studies published to date have provided consistent evidence for reductions in numbers and severity of episodes when CBT is combined with pharmacotherapy.
2. This promising evidence from, primarily, smaller studies needs to be confirmed in larger trials. Nonetheless, the evidence to date is particularly encouraging.

IV. Panic Disorder with or without Agoraphobia

A. Nature of the Disorder

1. Panic disorder is characterized by the fear of panic attacks and the sensations of arousal that herald such attacks.
2. **Catastrophic interpretations of anxiety sensations** (e.g., a rapid heart rate or parasthesias interpreted as an impending heart attack or stroke) **intensify and maintain anxious responses to arousal.**
3. **Avoidance of situations in which panic attacks occurred** (or in which an attack is feared) **helps maintain and extend fears and prevents more adaptive emotional processing.**

B. Informational Interventions

1. Informational interventions target self-perpetuating cycles of fearful interpretations of and anxiogenic reactions to the somatic sensations of anxiety.
2. Patients are provided with a model of panic disorder, including information on the body's response to danger, the role of catastrophic thoughts in providing a "danger" interpretation of symptoms, and the role of CBT in eliminating the "fear of fear" cycle that maintains the disorder.

C. Cognitive restructuring targets the catastrophic fears and misinterpretations of panic sensations. Common interventions include the provision of corrective information and logical analysis of the actual outcome of panic attacks.

D. Interoceptive Exposure

1. **Cognitive interventions are combined with exposure to the feared sensations of anxiety.**
2. This exposure, which is termed interoceptive exposure, includes procedures (such as running in place, hyperventilating, and spinning) to re-create feared sensations (e.g., tachycardia, numbness and tingling, dizziness) in a controlled fashion so that the patient can eliminate fears and anxiogenic responses to these sensations.

E. Stepwise situational exposure is commonly used to eliminate the agoraphobic avoidance that frequently accompanies panic disorder.

F. Somatic management skills, such as breathing retraining and progressive deep muscle relaxation, are used to help patients minimize their responses to symptoms (e.g., hyperventilating as a response to anticipatory anxiety) that can produce additional panic sensations.

G. Course and Efficacy

1. **CBT programs** are widely used, commonly consist of 12 to 15 structured sessions, and **provide an effective alternative to medication treatment of panic disorder.**

2. CBT also has been found to be effective for partial responders or non-responders to medications and it offers long-term maintenance of treatment gains.

3. CBT is an effective strategy to aid patients who wish to discontinue medication, particularly benzodiazepine treatment.

4. Patients need to be informed that effective non-medication treatment is available.

V. Social Phobia

A. Nature of Treatment

1. **Whereas patients with a panic disorder fear having a panic attack, patients with social phobia are concerned about humiliation, embarrassment, and negative evaluations by others.**

2. Those fears motivate avoidance of social situations, and this avoidance helps prevent the acquisition of the social confidence and skills that typify non-phobic patterns.

3. **CBT for social phobia usually emphasizes two core treatment components: cognitive restructuring to alter anxiogenic social expectations and exposure to help patients develop skills and decrease anxiety as part of regular social rehearsal.**

4. Although the majority of patients with social phobia can be typified as having adequate social skills but impaired social performance (i.e., anxiety prevents them from utilizing and displaying their skills), some social phobics may require additional training in specific social-interactional skills.

B. Informational interventions are designed to alert patients to the anxiogenic nature of their thoughts and the role of avoidance in heightening socially phobic patterns.

C. Cognitive Restructuring

1. Cognitive restructuring interventions are designed to modify maladaptive cognitions that detract from competent social performance.

2. **Typical cognitive distortions include negative expectations of social performance** ("I will not know what to say"), **distorted evaluations of the self** ("Everyone can do it but me"), **and distorted expectations and interpretations of the reactions of others** ("She will think I am a jerk"), combined with underestimates of one's ability to cope with a suboptimal performance and an overfocus on and attentional search for signs of social failure.

3. **Self-monitoring interventions, instruction, and rational evaluation of the accuracy of thoughts are combined with exposure interventions to help patients develop more accurate thought patterns.**

D. Exposure Interventions

1. Exposure interventions provide patients with the ability to practice, examine cognitions in, and habituate to, social situations.

2. Recently developed treatment protocols utilize a group format to allow the efficient construction of exposure situations.

3. After adequate preparation, including the preliminary identification of likely cognitive distortions as well as the desired outcome of the exposure practice, patients rehearse feared interactions in the group and in homework assignments.

E. Social Skills Training

1. **Training in social skills utilizes instruction and programmed practice to help patients develop skills in a role-playing (exposure) format.**

2. Videotapes may be used to provide specific feedback on performance.

F. Additional considerations. Because the symptoms of social phobia may resemble those of panic disorder (e.g., shaking, trembling, shortness of breath, and increased heart rate), newer treatment packages sometimes include exposure to feared internal bodily sensations, with the goal of decreasing performance-related worries about those symptoms.

G. Effectiveness. Recent research trials have indicated that CBT is a treatment for social phobia that approximates the effectiveness of the most successful pharmacologic alternatives (e.g., phenelzine and clonazepam) but appears to offer maintenance and even extension of treatment gains over follow-up periods.

VI. Generalized Anxiety Disorder

A. Targets for Treatment
1. Generalized anxiety disorder (GAD) is characterized by unrealistic or excessive worry about several life circumstances and is accompanied by chronic symptoms of anxious arousal.
2. **Typical cognitive-behavioral interventions target the worry process with cognitive restructuring of anxiety, using a variety of symptom management techniques (frequently emphasizing relaxation procedures).**

B. Informational interventions identify maladaptive cognitions and the worry process as a primary cause of anxiety and set the stage for the interventions that will follow.

C. Cognitive Interventions
1. **Self-monitoring of cognitions is used to help patients identify maladaptive cognitions** as they occur in high-anxiety situations.
2. Patients then **learn to evaluate those cognitions logically,** examining the evidence and probability for anticipated negative events, and generate alternative explanations of events to challenge catastrophic thoughts.
3. As patients learn to better identify and evaluate the content of their thoughts, **specific "worry times" may be assigned to help them gain control** over a constant tendency to worry.
4. **A problem-solving approach to worries can then be introduced** around the specific worry time topics.
5. In some cases, **imaginal exposure to core worries can help patients decrease their anxiety** responses to specific concerns.

D. Relaxation training, such as training in progressive muscle relaxation and biofeedback-assisted procedures, is used to decrease the arousal that accompanies worry and provide patients with a coping tool to use in high-anxiety situations.

E. Effectiveness
1. CBT tends to be as effective as medication (benzodiazepine or antidepressant treatment).
2. There is a consensus that more effective treatments need to be developed for GAD.

VII. Obsessive-Compulsive Disorder

A. Targets for Treatment
1. Obsessive-compulsive disorder (OCD) is characterized by cycles of intrusive thoughts or concerns followed by ritualistic attempts to reduce the anxiety or discomfort caused by these concerns.

2. When the concerns are recurring unwanted thoughts, they are termed **obsessions.**

3. The ritualistic behaviors—**compulsions**—range from repeated hand washing in response to fears of contamination to the inability to discard trash because of catastrophic concerns about the potential meaning of discarding an item.

B. Exposure and Response Prevention

1. Treatment for OCD emphasizes exposure and response prevention to break the chronic cycles of intrusive concerns that are ameliorated by compulsive rituals.

2. **Exposure involves the programmed confrontation of a situation that triggers intrusive or obsessive thoughts and/or compulsive rituals.**

3. **Response prevention requires patients to resist performing compulsive rituals (that reduce the anxiety and discomfort) to break the link between the trigger and the compulsive response.**

4. As patients repeatedly expose themselves to previously avoided cues without performing compulsions, anxiety decreases over time.

C. Cognitive interventions. Recently developed cognitive strategies may complement exposure and response prevention by providing patients with additional skills for breaking the link between intrusive thoughts and compulsive responses.

D. Effectiveness

1. Evaluation of the treatment outcome literature indicates that **CBT is at least as effective as medication for OCD,** but for severe patients a combination of CBT and medication (particularly a serotonin selective antidepressant) typically is recommended.

2. CBT should be considered for every patient with this disorder.

VIII. Post-traumatic Stress Disorder

A. Nature of the Disorder

1. Severe trauma can disrupt an individual's sense of safety in the world to the extent that chronic vigilance, arousal, and attempts to avoid perceived danger characterize functioning.

2. When trauma results in chronic patterns characterized by re-experiencing symptoms (feeling or responding as if the trauma were recurring), arousal, and avoidance (typically avoidance of the emotional, cognitive, or situational cues of the trauma), a diagnosis of post-traumatic stress disorder (PTSD) should be considered.

3. This severe disorder can be underdiagnosed because of the frequent presentation of prominent depression or panic that may draw therapeutic attention away from the underlying PTSD.

B. Nature of Treatment

1. CBT interventions are designed to break the link between trauma-related cues and the severe anxiety responses (chronic vigilance) and avoidance that characterize PTSD.

2. In treatment, patients learn to identify the symptoms that characterize PTSD, identify what was learned at the time of the trauma, distinguish trauma memories and trauma-related emotions from current reality, and re-establish a sense of safety in the world.

C. Informational Interventions

1. Informational interventions serve a crucial function in helping patients understand their symptoms.

2. In particular, careful discussion of dissociation and flashback phenomena can help decrease the marked fear of these symptoms that characterizes many individuals with this disorder.

3. Review and discussion of each symptom as described in *DSM-IV* constitute a way to organize the experience of PTSD for patients.

4. Informational intervention also may need to focus on the quality of trauma-related memories. It is not unusual for these memories to be experienced as abnormal and frightening; they often consist of flashes of sensory experience that are devoid of the verbal narration that characterizes non-trauma memories.

5. Review of the nature of these memories provides an important prelude to cognitive and exposure-based interventions.

D. **Cognitive interventions.** Cognitive interventions are designed to help patients identify distortions in their thoughts that may have arisen as a consequence of trauma (e.g., "The world is dangerous and unpredictable," "I cannot trust anyone," "It is not safe to relax," "I do not have any power") and develop a broader cognitive organization that places the trauma in the proper context of a patient's life and future. Recent evidence supports the strength of cognitive interventions in this disorder.

E. **Exposure Interventions**

1. Exposure interventions are used to help patients eliminate emotional reactions tied to trauma cues. That is, while it may be adaptive to retain aspects of a fear reaction to a dark alley at night when a stranger is following, exposure may be used to eliminate the broad-based fears (e.g., fears of the dark, all streets, or all strangers) that characterize PTSD.

2. With repeated exposure and appropriate instruction, patients learn to discriminate between exaggerated fear reactions left over from the trauma and the safety of current situations; the result is an elimination of exaggerated fear (or other emotional) reactions.

F. **Symptom management skills.** As with many of the anxiety disorders, additional symptom management or symptom exposure strategies may be used to help patients cope with their symptoms during the early stages of treatment.

G. **Other Interventions**

1. Empiric examination of treatment outcome for PTSD tends to lag behind that for other disorders (i.e., depression and panic disorder), but evaluation of the well-controlled trials that have been completed to date supports the efficacy of exposure-based interventions.

2. At present, the benefit offered by CBT appears to be far greater than that achieved in medication trials, but additional evidence is needed, particularly for the efficacy of the combination of CBT and pharmacotherapy.

IX. Specific Phobias

A. **Exposure Interventions**

1. Fears of specific events that lead to clinically significant distress or disability and are not better accounted for by other conditions are termed specific phobias.

2. **Exposure-based interventions remain the mainstay of interventions for specific phobias** (e.g., fear of dogs, storms, heights, or snakes), although benzodiazepine treatment may be preferred to help an individual cope with a feared event that is rarely encountered (e.g., trips to the dentist).

3. Exposure can be conducted according to a wide variety of procedures.

4. Systematic desensitization refers to a procedure of relaxation training accompanied by gradual exposure (frequently imaginal) to a feared stimulus.

5. **To aid in exposure, the feared stimulus may be broken into logical components, with independent exposure to each feared element occurring before exposure to the full phobic cue.** As was noted above, exposure can be imaginal or *in vivo* and can be to internal sensations or thoughts, external situations, or both.

B. **Participant-Modeling**

1. **Participant-modeling, a procedure in which a therapist enacts (models) a behavior and then encourages the patient to repeat that behavior, is also used in the treatment of phobias.**

2. For example, participant-modeling of the handling of snakes can be used to help snake phobics.

3. As with all exposure-like procedures, modeling of progressively more fear-provoking behaviors is done in a stepwise fashion.

X. Eating Disorders

A. **Interventions for Bulimia Nervosa**

1. **CBT for bulimia nervosa seeks to control binge eating and identify and challenge distorted beliefs regarding food, body shape, and weight.** Standardized CBT programs of treatment consist of approximately 20 sessions.

2. **Self-monitoring of food intake, binge episodes, and purging** is helpful in identifying the precipitants and consequences of binge eating.

3. Stimulus-control procedures are aimed at **manipulating the cues for inappropriate eating** (e.g., these interventions may change the rate or place of eating). Scheduling of meals is used to normalize eating patterns and decrease dietary restraint.

4. **Training in problem solving** may help patients develop alternative strategies to use when confronted by the urge to binge. Scheduling of pleasurable activities may be used to increase non-food pleasurable activities.

5. **Cognitive restructuring** is used to help identify and modify distorted beliefs regarding shape and weight. Informational interventions are designed to educate patients about body weight, nutrition, the deleterious consequences of the binge–purge cycle, and the effects of dieting on mood.

6. Behavioral experiments also provide a context that helps patients alter distorted beliefs regarding shape and weight and gain evidence incompatible with those beliefs.

B. **Interventions for Anorexia Nervosa**

1. The first goal of treatment for anorexia nervosa is to restore weight and normal eating.

2. **Contingency management (positive and negative reinforcement) frequently is used to directly manipulate maladaptive eating and weight control patterns,** especially in the acute phase of treatment.

3. Cognitive restructuring is useful in challenging distorted thoughts and beliefs about the relationship between weight, self-esteem, body shape, and eating.

4. Additional interventions, similar to those for bulimia, also can be applied.

XI. Psychotic Disorders

A. Cognitive-behavioral interventions for psychotic disorders can be used as an important adjunct to antipsychotic medications.

B. CBT has been used successfully to increase **social and daily living skills** in schizophrenics.

C. Cognitive-behavioral techniques also can be used to assist patients in dealing with the side effects of medication and **to help identify and modify irrational beliefs about medication.**

D. **Stress management and problem-solving skills** assist patients in dealing with stressors which may act as **precipitants to relapse.**

E. **Cognitive techniques** aimed at reducing the frequency and distress associated with hallucinations are in development; there is early support for the efficacy of these interventions.

XII. Personality Disorders

A. Personality disorders are characterized by long-standing and pervasive maladaptive patterns of behavior which lead to distress or impairment in functioning.

B. Early empiric support has been found for the use of CBT in the treatment of personality disorders. Such work typically places additional emphasis on the clinical relationship and may devote a great deal of attention to maladaptive behaviors that interrupt the flow of treatment.

C. **Because many personality disorders involve emotional dysregulation, training may be provided to help patients learn basic skills for labeling, tolerating, and modifying emotions.** Patients may have pervasive problem-solving and social skills deficits that require repeated rehearsal of new ways of dealing with interpersonal conflicts or other life issues.

D. Treatment typically requires a much longer course because the targets of treatment are long-standing and pervasive patterns.

XIII. Referral for Cognitive-Behavioral Therapy

A. Both the referring clinician and the patient must be careful consumers of mental health services. Discussion of a clinician's specialty area and the type of interventions frequently employed can help the referring physician identify an appropriate CBT clinician.

B. **Lists of CBT providers can be acquired** from the following sources:
    1. Association for the Advancement of Behavior Therapy, (www.aabt.org)
    2. Anxiety Disorders Association of America, (www.adaa.org).

C. **Therapist and patient manuals.** A variety of therapist manuals and patient workbooks are available for the treatment of anxiety disorders and affective disorders and the discontinuation of anxiolytic medication.

D. A variety of **self-help books** emphasizing CBT interventions are also available.
    1. Depression
        a. Burns, D.D. (1981). *Feeling good: The new mood therapy.* Chicago: Signet.

2. Panic Disorder
   a. Clum, G.A. (1990). *Coping with panic: A drug-free approach to dealing with anxiety attacks.* Pacific Grove, Calif: Brooks/Cole.
   b. Hecker, J.E., & Thorpe, G.L. (1992). *Agoraphobia and panic: A guide to psychological treatment.* Needham Heights, Mass.: Allyn and Bacon.
3. Social Phobia
   a. Markway, B.G., Carmin, C.N., Pollard, C.A., & Flynn, T. (1992). *Dying of embarrassment: Help for social anxiety and phobias.* Oakland, Calif.: New Harbinger.
4. Obsessive-Compulsive Disorder
   a. Baer, L. (1991). *Getting control: Overcoming your obsessions and compulsions.* Boston: Little, Brown.
   b. Steketee, G., & White, K. (1990). *When once is not enough: Help for obsessive compulsives.* Oakland, Calif.: New Harbinger.

Suggested Readings

Barlow, D.H. (Ed.). (1993). *Clinical handbook of psychological disorders.* New York: Guilford.

Beck, A.T., Freeman, A., and associates. (1990). *Cognitive therapy of personality disorders.* New York: Guilford.

Hawton, K., Salkovskis, P.M., Kirk, J., & Clark, D.M. (1989). *Cognitive behaviour therapy for psychiatric problems: A practical guide.* Oxford: Oxford University Press.

Hofmann, S.G., & Tompson, M. (Eds.). (2002). *Handbook of psychosocial treatments for severe mental disorders.* New York: Guilford.

Pollack, M.H., Otto, M.W., & Rosenbaum, J.F. (Eds.). (1996). *Challenges in clinical practice: Pharmacologic and psychosocial strategies.* New York: Guilford.

CHAPTER 11

Principles of Stress Management

DAVID AHERN AND ELYSE PARK

I. Overview

Stress is defined as a state of extreme difficulty, pressure, or strain with negative effects on physical and emotional health and well-being. Stressors are the circumstances that induce the stress response. A stress response occurs when internal or external demands exceed a patient's ability to adapt or cope. It is the patient's cognitive and psychophysiologic responses in the context of certain life circumstances that determine the experience of stress. Coping responses are attempts to do something about, or adjust to, the stressor. Individuals may use problem-focused or emotion-focused coping skills (Table 11-1).

Situations become stressors for an individual only if they are perceived as threatening or dangerous to that individual (cognitive appraisal). Primary appraisal is the process by which individuals assess and evaluate an event and determine its impact. Secondary appraisal is the process by which individuals evaluate their coping resources. (Lazarus & Folkman, 1984).

Table 11-1. Examples of Stressors, Stress Responses, and Coping Strategies

Examples of Stressors	*Examples of Stress Responses*	*Examples of Coping Strategies*
Frustration (a goal's being blocked)	**Mental and emotional signs** (lack of concentration, memory lapses, anxiety, fear, panic, anger, hostilily, aggression)	**Cognitive strategies** (developing awareness, detachment, self-esteem, and compassion; learning anger management)
Conflict (uncertainty, making choices)	**Behavioral signs** (smoking, drinking, overeating, Type A behavior, social withdrawal)	**Behavioral strategies** (assertiveness, social support, resilient behavior)
Pressure (time pressure, emotional pressure)	**Physiological signs** (erratic breathing, tense muscles, aches and pain, fatigue, palpitations, sweating, dry mouth, indigestion, allergies, hypertension, depression)	**Physiological strategies** (breathing exercises, relaxation, visualization, meditation, biofeedback)

SOURCE: Adapted from Lehrer, P.M., & Woolfolk, R. (1993). *Principles and practice of stress management* (2nd ed.). New York: Guilford Press, p. 116. Reprinted by permission of the Guilford Press.

Coping strategies can be combative and preventive. **Combative coping** is a provoked reaction to a stressor in an attempt to suppress or end an existent stressor. **Preventive coping** is an attempt to actively prevent the stressor from appearing. Types of combative strategies include: monitoring stressors and symptoms, organizing personal and social resources, tolerating or attacking stressors, and lowering arousal. Types of preventive strategies include: avoiding stressors, adjusting demand levels, altering stress-inducing behavior patterns, and developing coping resources.

A stress reaction is an individual's response to a given stressor, which can be physical, behavioral, emotional, or cognitive. Examples of stress reactions include:

Physical: Increasing heart rate, elevated blood pressure, headache, fatigue, shortness of breath, and sweating.
Emotional: Irritability, depression, anxiety, impatience, restlessness, and hostility.
Cognitive: Forgetfulness, lack of concentration, distraction, and disorganization of thought.
Behavioral: Increased smoking and alcohol use, nervous laughter, carelessness, and aggressive behavior.

Two types of stress are distinguishable and each has a different strategy for medical management.

A. **Acute stress is intense but time-limited, with a clear starting and stopping point and individualized physiologic reactions** (including increased heart rate and blood pressure, muscular tension, and lowered peripheral skin temperature). Reactivity is the change in response to stress that may occur in autonomic, neuroendocrine, and or immune responses.
   1. Often referred to as the **"fight or flight" response,** acute stress is the body's natural reaction to threatening situations.

B. **Chronic stress is present for extended periods of time with sustained physiologic changes in muscle tension, skin temperature, and negative emotional states** (including irritability, nervousness, and depressed mood).
   1. Chronic stress often is associated with physical symptoms or complaints in the absence of detectable pathophysiology.
   2. **Chronic stress may exacerbate existing medical conditions, reduce adherence to medical recommendations, and complicate medical care.** Hence, the evaluation and treatment of chronic stress is paramount for the primary care clinician.

II. Primary Sources of Stress

A. **Personal sources of stress** relate to characteristics of the patient that predispose him or her to stress responses.
   1. **Daily hassles**
      Daily events are experienced as hassles; for example, being stuck in traffic or waiting in long lines.
   2. **Self-doubt**
      Lack of confidence in decision-making or poor self-esteem leads to self-doubt.
   3. **Physical ailments**
      Acute, recurrent, or chronic medical conditions are associated with stress.

4. **Psychiatric disorders**

Anxiety disorders, depression, and substance abuse disorders are both a source of and a result of chronic stress.

B. **Personality and Stress**

Each individual's personality influences how he or she will appraise and cope with an event. Some personality characteristics make stressful situations worse or better. Negative affectivity is a pervasive negative mood marked by anxiety, depression, and hostility. A pessimistic explanatory style is one in which an individual attributes the negative events in their life in terms of internal, stable, and global qualities. **Negativity and pessimism are related to poor health.** An optimistic nature can lead one to cope more effectively with stress.

Hardiness is a personality trait that may protect a person from stressful effects. Hardiness consists of three characteristics: **Commitment** (a tendency to involve oneself in whatever one encounters); **control** (the sense that one causes the events that happen in one's life and one can influence one's environment); and **challenge** (a willingness to undertake change and to confront new activities that represent opportunities for growth).

C. **Social relationships** are important determinants of overall health status. When relationships are conflicted or dysfunctional they are a source of chronic stress in one of the following ways.

1. **Lack of social support**

The patient does not receive necessary encouragement or assistance from family or friends. Four types of social support that are needed include appraisal, tangible, informational, and emotional. Social support can help a person cope with stressors. People with high levels of social support may confront a stressful experience more successfully. The quantity of support is not as important as the quality of support.

2. **Marital/family conflict**

Marital discord, separation, and divorce are prevalent and constitute a major source of recurrent and chronic stress.

3. **Co-worker and supervisor conflict**

Dissatisfaction in the workplace is a known risk factor for musculoskeletal injury, pain, and other bodily complaints.

D. **Organizational changes** are common as businesses seek to respond to economic and market pressures. Stress responses may result from one or more of the following sources.

1. **Down-sizing**

Job loss, increased job duties for remaining employees, and "survivor syndrome" (i.e., a sense of guilt and remorse associated with co-worker job loss).

2. **Job insecurity**

Uncertainty, anxiety, and fear about job stability.

3. **Overload of responsibilities**

"Working twice as hard for half as much," and excessive time pressure.

4. **Role transitions.** Increase or decrease in position status, being moved to a different position, or being moved to a different area of work.

E. Economic difficulties can affect many aspects of one's life.

    1. **Living conditions.** Living in an overcrowded setting or in one that does not feel safe.

    2. **Health care costs.** Being unable to afford adequate health care.

    3. **Educational opportunities.** Lack of ability to obtain needed education.

F. Environmental Stress

    1. **Pollution**

    2. **Overcrowding.** Lack of space in work environment or in one's outside environment.

    3. **Commuting.** Enduring long travel routes between work and home.

III. Evaluation

A. General Approach

    1. The evaluation of chronic stress in the primary care setting should include a determination of the following factors:

        a. Bodily complaints that do not follow an anatomic distribution or for which no plausible underlying pathophysiology can be found.

        b. Personal, social, and work-related factors as mentioned previously that might be potential sources of chronic stress for the patient.

        c. The degree to which the patient possesses coping resources and skills.

        d. The identified stressful life circumstances that exceed the patient's coping resources.

    2. Patients may not necessarily be aware of the nature of their stress levels or the fact that stress can contribute to somatic complaints. A non-judgmental and "normalizing" approach is likely to facilitate the patient's report of life circumstances perceived as stressful. For example, it is helpful to say, "Stress can make us more aware of bodily sensations and can produce negative changes in our health" or "Tell me more about your [personal, family, work] situation so we can better understand if chronic stress is playing a role here."

    3. It is important to emphasize that stress *per se* is not the single cause of symptoms, but rather a contributor. On one hand, patients may fear that their symptoms are "all in the head" if the clinician inadvertently curtails attention to possible physical causes in the examination or diagnostic evaluation. On the other hand, the earlier the clinician introduces stress as a legitimate and appropriate concern and focus of inquiry the greater the likelihood that the patient will be receptive to recommendations for managing stress more effectively.

    4. Stress may also inhibit immune functioning. When patients are under stress they are more vulnerable to infectious diseases, including the common cold, the flu, herpes, chicken pox, mononucleosis and Epstein-Barr virus.

B. History

    1. Physicians receive more complaints about stress than they do about symptoms of the common cold. Because stress is a common experience for many patients it is challenging to discern whether a given patient's symptoms, either without clear medical explanation or in the context of a medical or psychiatric diagnosis, are associated with recurrent or chronic stress

    2. **New-onset complaints necessitate an examination of recent or current life circumstances** that are perceived as stressful to the patient. Occasionally, a major life event (e.g., death of a loved one or close friend, loss of a job, unexpected job change or demotion, or onset of a medical illness) is identified as a triggering stressful life event. However, stressors are frequently more subtle and recurrent and may be mini-

mized by the patient. Hence, the clinician may need to probe further into personal, social, and job history if there is a strong suspicion of recurrent or chronic stressors that are salient to the presenting complaints.

3. A history of unexplained vague or diffuse symptoms that spontaneously resolved or responded to reassurance from the clinician should be sought. Patients who experience recurrent stress may present with episodic somatic complaints, such as headache, gastrointestinal distress, or fatigue.

C. **The medical history may elicit information helpful in determining a patient's stress responsivity and coping strategies.**

1. For many patients the medical history may be unremarkable, lacking any established medical conditions or clear diagnoses (especially if the symptoms or complaints are of recent onset).

2. For patients with chronic medical conditions, the medical history is important for evaluation of the extent of exposure to stressful medical experiences and the patient's successes and failures in coping.

3. Psychophysiological recording (e.g., peripheral skin temperature) or surface electromyography (EMG) may be useful in determining autonomic nervous system reactivity to stressful life circumstances. High EMG activity of the frontalis muscle or low digital skin temperature are indicators of stress responsivity.

D. **The interview requires a balance between an appropriate focus on plausible medical causes for symptoms and a thorough personal, social, and work history** as they relate to stress. Fortunately, many patients view stress as a "normal" experience and even will acknowledge it as a cause of their symptoms.

1. In some cases, however, **there is a stigma associated with stress-related symptoms** or conditions. The clinician should alleviate any concerns on the patient's part that his or her symptoms are real and not imagined.

2. **Behavioral analysis** (i.e., determination of the antecedents, behavioral responses, and consequences to challenging and potential stressful life circumstances) **is useful** to pinpoint the sources of stress and the patient's coping abilities (see Chapter 9).

IV. Chronic Stress and Psychiatric Disorders

The most common psychiatric disorders associated with chronic stress are the anxiety disorders: panic disorder, agoraphobia, social phobia, simple phobia, generalized anxiety disorder, obsessive-compulsive disorder, and post-traumatic stress disorder.

Adjustment disorders with anxious and/or depressed mood, depression, and substance abuse disorders are also associated with chronic stress.

A. **Differential diagnosis** is an important first step to rule out any existing psychiatric disorder that may account for the presenting symptoms and complaints. If an anxiety disorder or other psychiatric disorder is found, then treatment should commence according to appropriate psychopharmacologic and non-psychopharmacologic guidelines (see Chapters 14 and 16).

B. The *Diagnostic and Statistical Manual of Mental Disorders, Fourth Edition (DSM-IV)* permits coding of conditions, that is, **the "V" codes,** which are a focus of clinical attention but are not due to a mental disorder. These codes are appropriate to use when there is no psychiatric disorder to account for the anxiety or distress associated with chronic stress, but rather a phase-of-life problem or other life circumstance problem.

C. Given that **chronic stress is not a diagnosis but rather a behavioral and psychophysiological problem,** the most critical step is to **identify the primary stressors, recognize the associated individualized psychophysiologic stress reactions, and gauge the adequacy of coping skills** and resources available to the patient. This process provides a framework for organizing the evaluation data and leads to treatment formulation and implementation.

V. Treatment Strategies

A. Pharmacologic interventions

1. **Acute stress and associated anxiety may require pharmacologic intervention.** The benzodiazepines are the treatment of choice for emergency situations and short-term use (see Chapter 16). Even with chronic stress conditions, occasional use of anxiolytics is beneficial for breakthrough episodes of acute distress.

2. However, **patients should not use medication as the sole intervention for chronic stress** conditions when alternative non-pharmacologic strategies are available. Reliance on medication alone precludes the patient's learning more long-term and adaptive coping skills.

B. Non-pharmacologic interventions

1. **Self-control skills are behavioral coping strategies** that patients can learn; these include diaphragmatic breathing, relaxation training, cognitive restructuring, and exercise.

   a. **Diaphragmatic breathing** is a relatively simple technique that patients can learn to evoke a relaxation response. Patients are instructed to take a deep, cleansing breath, bringing the air in through the nose, using the diaphragmatic rather than the intercostal muscles, holding for a moment, and then exhaling slowly through the mouth with lips pursed. Each inspiration/expiration cycle should be 5 to 7 seconds in duration. Patients are also instructed to note any sensations while performing the technique. Patients are also instructed to practice at home a series of five breaths followed by a short break and then five more breaths twice a day.

   b. **Relaxation training** is the most effective technique available for reducing the effects of chronic stress. A variety of techniques exist including autogenic training, progressive muscle relaxation training, hypnosis, and mindfulness meditation. Evidence suggests that certain techniques are more effective for particular psychophysiologic disorders, but any one of them can elicit a relaxation response. An abbreviated progressive muscle relaxation training approach is efficient and useful in furthering a patient's sense of self-control and producing a stress-reduction effect. The technique involves progressively tensing and releasing large muscle groups throughout the body: hands and fingers; forearms, upper arms, and shoulders; facial muscles (forehead and scalp, eyes, nose, lips and mouth, chin and jaw); neck; chest, shoulders, and back; stomach and abdomen; hips and buttocks; and legs and feet. Patients are instructed to tense the muscles for a few seconds, just long enough to feel the tension, then relax the muscles and notice the difference between tension and relaxation (Table 11-2). This is done systematically from the hands and fingers to the legs and feet for approximately 10 to 15 minutes. Diaphragmatic breathing is interspersed throughout the training to maximize the relaxation response.

   c. **Guided imagery** is a technique that involves closing one's eyes, taking easy breaths, and envisioning a peaceful and relaxing place. Imagine being at that place and concentrating on sights, sounds, and smells.

Table 11-2. Optimal Tension-Release Procedures for 16 Major Muscle Groups

Muscle Group	*Method of Tensing*
1. Dominant hand and forearm	Make a tight fist while allowing upper arm to remain relaxed
2. Dominant upper arm	Press elbow downward against chair without involving lower arm
3. Non-dominant hand and forearm	Same as dominant
4. Non-dominant upper arm	Same as dominant
5. Forehead	Raise eyebrows as high as possible
6. Upper cheeks and nose	Squint eyes and wrinkle nose
7. Lower face	Clench teeth and pull back corners of the mouth
8. Neck	Counterpose muscles by trying to raise and lower chin simultaneously
9. Chest, shoulders, and upper back	Take a deep breath; hold it and pull shoulder blades together
10. Abdomen	Counterpose muscles by trying to push stomach out and pull in simultaneously
11. Dominant upper leg	Counterpose large muscle on top of leg against two smaller ones underneath (specific strategy will vary considerably)
12. Dominant calf	Point toes upward
13. Dominant foot	Point toes downward, turn foot in, and curl toes gently
14. Non-dominant upper leg	Same as dominant
15. Non-dominant calf	Same as dominant
16. Non-dominant foot	Same as dominant

Once a patient has mastered this technique, this exercise should be condensed by combining sets of muscles into four groups.

SOURCE: Lehrer, P.M., & Woolfolk, R.L. (Eds.). (1993). *Principles and practice of stress management* (2nd ed.). New York: Guilford Press, p. 71.

d. **Meditation.** Meditation involves being still and concentrating on a single stimulus, such as a word or image. This technique slows the breathing rate, increases oxygen consumption, and increases blood flow.

e. **Autogenic training** is a technique that involves focusing on internal stimulations, such as warmth and heaviness, and repeating verbal thoughts about that stimulus.

f. **Biofeedback and biofeedback-assisted relaxation** are methods employing physiologic recording equipment and feedback systems, typically auditory or visual, that permit patients to receive direct feedback regarding changes in certain physiological parameters. For example, patients with Raynaud's disease often benefit from biofeedback proportional to alterations in peripheral skin temperature. Similarly, muscular contraction headache sufferers benefit from surface EMG feedback from the frontalis muscle. Biofeedback-assisted relaxation uses biofeedback to augment the acquisition of the relaxation response.

g. **Cognitive restructuring** involves assisting patients to determine any maladaptive thoughts associated with the identified stressful life circumstances and encouraging them to evaluate these beliefs and develop alternative, adaptive, countering statements. For example, patients may make self-referential statements such as, "I'm always making mistakes in response to external demands." Examples of countering statements would be "I can prepare and do a good job" and "I have dealt with this situation before so I'm prepared."

h. **Exercise,** especially aerobic exercise, reduces anxiety and can serve as a buffer to chronic stress. Unfortunately, patients may find it difficult to exercise consistently when they become overwhelmed by stressful life circumstances. Instructing patients to start walking short distances, perhaps with a friend or neighbor, can be helpful. Joining a health club is a good way to combine exercise with social activity, which serves to promote and maintain adherence.

2. **Instrumental coping** refers to behavioral skills that can alleviate chronic stress and prevent the occurrence of adverse stress reactions.

a. **Effective time management** is essential to prevent stress reactions. Patients can be encouraged to set priorities and break down goals into small, achievable pieces. Goal-setting and pacing activities toward goals serve to minimize feeling overwhelmed.

b. **Assertiveness training** involves teaching patients to learn appropriate assertiveness skills to better manage external demands. Often an assertive response can help a patient avoid an adverse stress response and improve self-esteem. Assertiveness is necessary for delegating responsibilities and reducing workload.

3. **Cognitive-behavioral approaches** involve looking at how cognitions (beliefs and appraisals) and behaviors are interrelated.

a. Meichenbaum's Stress Inoculation Training (SIT). Involves evaluating one's stress and learning and practicing coping strategies.

b. Ellis's Rational-Emotive Therapy (RET). Involves identifying and ridding oneself of irrational beliefs that are causing emotional distress.

c. Beck's Cognitive Therapy. Involves identifying faulty ideas or automatic thoughts that are associated with stress.

Suggested Readings

American Psychiatric Association Task Force on *DSM-IV.* (1995). *Diagnostic and statistical manual of mental disorders-fourth edition.* Washington, DC: American Psychiatric Association.

Auerbach, S.M., & Gramling, S.E. (1998). *Stress management: Psychological foundations.* Upper Saddle River, NJ: Prentice Hall.

Barlow, D.H. (1988). *Anxiety and its disorders.* New York: Guilford Press.

Barsky, A.J., Delamater, B., Clancy, S.A., et al. (1996). Somatized psychiatric disorder presenting as palpitations. *Archives of Internal Medicine, 156,* 1102–1108.

Basmajian, J.V. (Ed.). (1989). *Biofeedback: Principles and practice for clinicians* (3rd ed.). Baltimore: Williams & Wilkins.

Benson, H. (1975). *The relaxation response.* New York: William Morrow and Co.

Bernstein, D.A., & Borkovec, T.D. (1973). *Progressive relaxation training: A manual for the helping professions.* Champaign, IL: Research Press.

Blumenthal, J.A., Williams, R.S., Needels, T.L., & Wallace, A.G. (1982). Psychological changes accompany aerobic exercise in healthy middle-aged adults. *Psychosomatic Medicine, 44,* 29–36.

Kobasa, S.C. (1979). Stressful life events and health. *Journal of Personality and Social Psychology, 37,* 1–11.

Lazarus, R.S., & Folkman, S. (1984). *Stress, appraisal, and coping.* New York: Springer.

Lehrer, P.M., & Woolfolk, R. (1993). *Principles and practice of stress management* (2nd ed.). New York: Guilford Press.

Lovallo, W.R. (1997). *Stress and health: Biological and psychological interactions.* Thousand Oaks, CA: Sage Publications.

Matheny, K.B., Aycock, D.W., Pugh, J.L., et al. (1986). Stress coping: A qualitative and quantitative synthesis with implications for treatment. *Counseling Psychologist, 14,* 499–549.

Meichenbaum, D. (1985). *Stress inoculation training.* Elmsford, NY: Pergamon Press.

Rice, P.L. (1999). *Stress and health* (3rd ed.). Thousand Oaks, CA: Brooks/Cole Publishing Company.

Sapolsky, R.M. (1998). *Why zebras don't get ulcers: An updated guide to stress, stress-related diseases, and coping.* New York: W.H. Freeman and Company.

Seligman, M.E., Castellon, C., Cacciola, J., et al. (1988). Explanatory style change during cognitive therapy for unipolar depression. *Journal of Abnormal Psychology, 97*(1), 13–18.

Watson, D., & Clark, L.A. (1984). Negative affectivity: The disposition to experience aversive emotional states. *Psychological Bulletin, 96,* 465–490.

SECTION IV

Approaches to Patients with Specific Conditions

CHAPTER 12

Personality Disorders I: Approaches to Difficult Patients

JAMES E. GROVES

I. Introduction

The primary care physician can cultivate one of two approaches to difficult patients: (1) lump them together conceptually and over time develop a number of management strategies that tend to work with any difficult patient; or (2) divide them into various categories and tailor a management strategy to each type. If the physician leans toward being a lumper, this chapter is the relevant one; if the physician is a splitter, Chapter 13 will be of greater interest. In either case, the same material, arranged differently, is presented in both chapters.

II. Scope of the Problem

A. **What a personality disorder is. In psychiatric diagnosis, a difficult patient is almost always an individual with a personality disorder. In practical terms, a personality-disordered patient is one who gives the physician that "uh-oh" feeling in the gut** on hearing, reading, or thinking of the patient's name. In other words, the type of patient most caregivers want to avoid. There are patients who almost produce this feeling—psychotic individuals, patients with organic brain syndromes, very sick and pitiable individuals—but these tough cases do not consistently (and over the years) make the physician dread them.

B. **Abnormalities of affect and cognition.** Patients with personality disorders have abnormally intense affects, are poorer-than-average neutralizers of affect, or both. In any case, raw rage, naked dependency, and primitive shame are present and frequently on the surface. The cognitive structures that ordinarily modulate intense affects are distorted and primitive. The "ego weakness" of this type of patient is seen in the absence of higher level defenses and in the primitive nature of the ones that are present. In *DSM-IV,* the **Axis II diagnoses** (personality disorders) **apply to individuals with exaggerations of normal personality traits.** In psychiatry, *personality* means basically what it means elsewhere: the **style** of an individual's dealings with the world. Personality traits are **stylistic peculiarities all people bring to social relations,** traits such as shyness and seductiveness, rigidity and suspiciousness. When these traits are exaggerated to the point where they cause emotional pain or dysfunction in the social sphere, psychiatry refers to them as *personality disorders.*

III. The Etiology of Personality Disorders

A. **Biologic and Social Determinants**
1. **Innate origins.** Personality disorders used to be called *character disorders* because they seem to reside in the deepest layers of the personality, which sometimes are called *character.* Personality traits and their exaggerations probably are largely innate

and on some level biologic and may be present from infancy, although they do not usually start to look like disorders until adolescence. Although personality and its disorders have a large innate or inborn component, psychiatry distinguishes a personality disorder from other diagnostic categories, the Axis I disorders. By contrast, the Axis I disorders are more "medical" in a sense, look more like diseases, tend to appear to be less related to development and environment, and tend to be affected less by acts of will on the part of the individual. These diagnoses include schizophrenia, manic-depressive illness, and obsessive-compulsive disorder.

2. **Social interactions.** Although personality disorders are to some extent outside the individual's control, people as social beings still expect an individual to exert a degree of free will. Social intuition dictates that one not excuse a criminal's behavior just because he or she has an antisocial personality disorder; without a demand for self-control, social intuition dictates that individuals with personality disorders would act worse than they already do.

3. **Primitive defenses.** Figure 12-1 schematizes how the outrageous and troublesome behaviors of these individuals are thought to arise from intense affect, distorted cognitions, and inadequate or primitive defenses. These behaviors are complicated by dissociation; many patients with personality disorders are less in contact with the real world than they appear to be and often are in a dreamlike state without appearing to be so or without realizing it. Under the pressure of intense affect (a fusion of rage, terror, and shame), such a patient uses dissociation to an even greater extent and enters this dream-like state, which normal individuals ordinarily enter only in extreme emergencies. Such patients are hard to reach in this dissociated state, which probably is present much of the time to some degree, especially at times when the individual is under stress, such as during a medical illness.

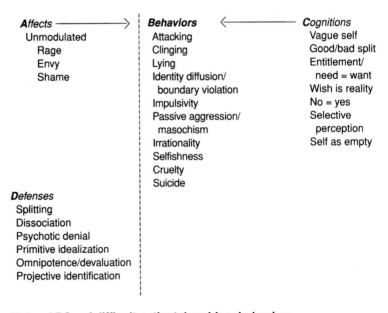

Affects ────────→ | *Behaviors* ←──────── *Cognitions*
Unmodulated | Attacking | Vague self
Rage | Clinging | Good/bad split
Envy | Lying | Entitlement/
Shame | Identity diffusion/ | need = want
 | boundary violation | Wish is reality
 | Impulsivity | No = yes
 | Passive aggression/ | Selective
 | masochism | perception
 | Irrationality | Self as empty
 | Selfishness |
 | Cruelty |
 | Suicide |

Defenses
Splitting
Dissociation
Psychotic denial
Primitive idealization
Omnipotence/devaluation
Projective identification

Figure 12-1.   ABCs of difficult patients' problem behaviors.

4. **Vague self-definition.** To complicate matters, in most personality disorders the boundaries between the self and others are blurred so that closeness seems to lead to fusion. As a relationship intensifies, such individuals have difficulty telling whether an emotion or idea comes from themselves or from the other person. Sexuality and dependency are confused with aggression. Needs are experienced as rage. Long-term relationships disintegrate because of an inability to find the optimal interpersonal distance. Because of inadequate ego mechanisms of defense, there is little ability to master painful feelings and channel needs or aggression into creative outlets. Ambivalence is poorly tolerated; impulse control is dismal. The patient has a fragmented mental picture of the self and others as all bad and simultaneously all potent, a chaotic mixture of shameful and grandiose images.

IV. Clinical Presentations

A. Dependency: The Common Thread
1. **Troublesome Behavior**
   a. When personality disorders show up in the medical setting, they typically are characterized by troublesome behavior. To some extent the leading edge of these patients' problems has to do with severe dependency in interpersonal relationships, including the relationship with the physician.
   b. One of the most difficult tasks in life is to find ways to get close to others without getting too close. Schopenhauer likened this universal human dilemma of emotional closeness to the predicament of two porcupines in the cold: If they get close enough for warmth, they prick each other with their quills. If they get distant enough to avoid each other's quills, they become too cold. For every person the trick in friendship, love, and parenting is to get close enough for warmth without being too close for comfort. In practice this always involves compromise and a constant dynamic tension. What is close enough for one party is too close or not close enough for the other.
   c. **Individuals with personality disorders have trouble tolerating distance and closeness** and often do not know the difference. If they complain about too much distance, the caregiver's stance probably is about right. It is when they get "close enough" that the caregiver should worry.
   d. Most of these persons have **deep feelings of shame** which they cover and hide even from themselves by means of rage and contempt.
   e. Everyone knows that it is easier to be mad than sad; nothing is a better antidepressant than a case of righteous indignation.

B. Patients' Projections onto the Doctor
1. **Problems with Interpersonal Closeness**
   a. Difficult patients' problems with interpersonal closeness always involve the physician, because doctors also have needs. Most doctors go into medicine in the hope of being useful to their suffering fellows. Most doctors want to help people and get paid in both coin and gratitude, a particular case of the universal wish to nurture and teach the young and receive love and respect in return. However, as every parent knows, ingratitude and trouble are inevitable.
   b. A complicating factor in the caregiver's wish to help is the normal tendency of the patient to put a caregiver in the parental role. **This is universal: People idealize their doctors** and in fact any other helper to some extent. This tendency to form **transferences** to doctors, as Freud called this normal but inappropriate displacement, has some social value by occasionally creating receptivity to medical advice and help.

      c. However, when this transference is too strong and inappropriate, trouble arises. When doctors are seen as the too-beloved or too-hated parent, they react.

      d. Dependent patients sometimes make doctors happy at first, but after a while physicians get tired of their constant neediness and avoid them.

      e. **The difficult patient's sense of entitlement, especially when backed up by a hostile, devaluing attitude, makes doctors defensive and sometimes hostile,** counterattacking and devaluing back.

      f. The difficult patient's manipulativeness depresses doctors, making them feel deskilled and devalued because they can never satisfy the patient's wish to be close and distant at the same time.

      g. The difficult patient's excessive denial makes physicians fearful.

C. The "Maladaptive" Defenses of Difficult Patients

  1. **Interaction between Environment and Heredity**

      a. Figure 12-1 is a schematic that shows how both environment and heredity play a role. The affects—or feelings—of those with personality disorders, which are innately exaggerated, interact with cognitions—thoughts—which are learned at an early age and produce the outrageous and unfair behaviors seen in difficult patients.

      b. The defenses of difficult patients are inadequate to keep their affects damped down and to prevent their toxic resonance with the odd ideas personality-disordered individuals learn in childhood.

      c. What stands out about patients with personality disorders who enter the medical system is their great use of **entitlement** and **manipulativeness** as defenses and their increased use of the psychological defenses psychiatrists call **splitting** and **projective identification.** In the phenomenology of personality disorders, entitlement, manipulativeness, defensive splitting, and projective identification have a devastating impact on the treating physician's self-esteem.

  2. **Splitting**

      a. Personality-disordered patients utilize splitting as a defense. Some do this dramatically in the medical context. For instance, **they frequently see one caregiver as omnipotent and omniscient while devaluing and denigrating another.**

      b. They utilize an "idealizing transference," not only to protect themselves from the illness but also to protect themselves from their own projected envy and rage, qualities they project onto anyone they get close to.

      c. Because of their intense dependency, they use the physician as a "transitional object," a Linus' blanket. However, as physicians know or soon find out, a primitive patient's adoration is not really love: It is like getting a letter in the mail which says, "I love you, I love you, I *love* you!" and then realizing that the letter is addressed to "Occupant."

      d. A doctor who does not recognize that the adulation is marked "occupant" is prone to reciprocate as if it were the real thing and thus to overstimulate the patient. It is no good to tear away the patient's idealization altogether, since it serves a good adaptive function, but for patients with unfillable emptiness, there is no such thing as enough.

      e. A caregiver who attempts to supply "enough" will end up giving too much, overstimulating the patient, exhausting his or her capacity to care, and eventually abandoning the patient.

  3. **Projective Identification**

      a. The half of the splitting mechanism that is opposite to idealization is seen when the patient uses something called **projective identification** to dump pathology, particularly envy and rage, onto the physician.

    b. Projective identification differs from simple projection in several respects. In projection, a disowned feeling or impulse is conferred on another person; in projective identification, it is not only the feeling or impulse that is conferred but also a whole personality trait or disposition.

    c. In projective identification, the person projecting "holds on to" part of the feeling and simultaneously reacts to that which is projected.

    d. In projective identification, there is an almost uncanny tendency for the victim of the projection to begin to act out the negative role which is projected and end up validating the projection. In other words, such individuals get just what they expect, and that is nothing good.

    e. The clinical implication of projective identification for a difficult patient in the medical setting is that patient's tendency to see certain caregivers as being as "bad" as the patient feels. This gets translated into behavior based on the following kind of logic: "I'm bad and you take care of me, which means you're as rotten as I am, or you wouldn't care for me." This perception is so powerfully held that the individual receiving it tends to act it out unconsciously.

4. **Entitlement**

    a. **Entitlement** is an emotionally deprived individual's attempt to collect now what he or she should have gotten "back then." Babies really are entitled to be babied; otherwise they would not survive. Adults who wish to collect on the same promises of caregiving are referred to as **entitled.**

    b. In the hospital or doctor's office, the dependent individual attempts to wrest from the medical relationship that which he or she did not get from the mother-child relationship. Of course, this does not work.

    c. If one tries to tell an entitled individual the realities of life, that individual usually becomes more entitled or, worse, regresses to an even more primitive and helpless level.

    d. Thus, entitlement may act as a psychological defense. Like the other defensive actions of personality-disordered patients, it is inefficient.

    e. **Thus, with an entitled patient, the doctor eventually gets tired and drained and then frightened and finally counterattacks the patient's entitlement head-on.**

    f. In essence this represents the physician's attempt to get across to the patient the fact that the doctor-patient relationship is not the mother-child relationship.

    g. Entitlement is like a personality-disordered patient's religion, and to attack it is blasphemy, a stripping away of something felt to give life its meaning and adversity its cure: the primitive, intense belief that one *deserves*. This attitude may enrage the physician, especially if his or her own defenses are shaky and there is regression on the doctor's part toward his or her own entitlement as a defense. It is best in this situation not to attack the patient's defensive entitlement but instead to attempt to substitute the medical relationship as a defense against the patient's fear of abandonment.

5. **Manipulativeness**

    a. **Manipulativeness** has a defensive function for the patient similar to that of entitlement.

    b. These difficult patients manipulate the relationship by staying symptomatic but reject whatever help is offered.

    c. This paradox is a maladaptive "solution" to the **need-fear dilemma** and illustrates the fact that these patients crave close relationships—intimacy—yet have a terrible fear of that intimacy.

    d. To resolve this dilemma, the physician may have to resort to a countermaneuver that consists of finding a middle ground between the patient's wish to be cared for and the patient's fear of being gobbled up.

    e. The physician should begin by recognizing his or her own feelings of pessimism and then state honestly that the treatment is not a panacea.

    f. Thus, even if improvement in the condition occurs, the medical relationship will have to be maintained over time. This should occur at regular intervals determined by the physician, not by the patient's manipulation of symptoms.

    g. Such patients need to learn that losing the symptom does not mean losing the doctor.

    h. In dealing with manipulation, the physician should try not to attack the defense but instead attempt to substitute for it the medical relationship to ease the patient's fear of abandonment.

    i. By sharing a kind of pessimism with the patient—"This is a chronic condition we'll never entirely cure."—and by scheduling regularly spaced appointments, the doctor can substitute the relationship for the defensive manipulativeness.

    j. **In limit-setting confrontations with manipulative, entitled patients the physician practices repetition and an appeal to the patient's sense of entitlement rather than an assault on it:** "You *deserve* the best medical care we can give, and that's why we're recommending X, Y, and Z."

    k. The doctor has to keep uppermost in mind the appeal to the entitlement and not get drawn into logical or illogical arguments.

    l. **Repetition is crucial.** Encounters to engage compliance often have to be repeated two or three times at varying intervals before the patient agrees, if in fact the patient does agree.

6. **Denial**

    a. **Denial** is like distance and closeness; it is hard to get the right mixture. Without healthy denial, people could not get through daily life. Without some degree of denial, people could not get on a plane or see their children off to school.

    b. To survive, people have to ignore selectively the fact that bad things happen to good people. Without healthy denial everyone would run around waving his or her arms and screaming, "How can God let such things happen?"

    c. Individuals with personality disorders, however, deny too much. They ignore dangers most people take seriously. They drink heavily or smoke, disobey laws, have unsafe sex, drive too fast without seat belts, and ignore the counsel of their physicians, which in turn makes doctors crazy.

    d. **The doctor's tendency is to take too much responsibility for deniers,** attempting to overcontrol them on the one hand or ignoring the denial on the other.

    e. A balance is important. The caregiver should **confront the most dangerous aspects of the denial without feeling responsible for it.**

    f. Patients in denial need constant repetitions of a single theme.

    g. They also need for physicians to cope with their own feelings of hate and aversion in an honest way. Moral behavior in the medical relationship has nothing to do with what doctors think and feel and everything to do with how they behave. It is not important how doctors feel, but it is important that they treat patients fairly, respectfully, and with all the skills they hire doctors for.

V. Summary

Individuals who dislike finely divided categories generally prefer word pictures to long summaries. For them, the following mnemonic is offered:

Neutralize	**a**ffects with structure,
contain destructive	**b**ehaviors with distancing and/or limits,
repair distorted	**c**ognitions with accurate information,
do not challenge needed	**d**efenses such as entitlement and manipulation,
and "lend	**e**go" to defects by reasoning.

For physicians who like to categorize various types of patients by working from their symptomatic presentations toward a "diagnosis," Chapter 13 will be more relevant.

Suggested Readings

American Psychiatric Association. (1995). *Diagnostic and statistical manual of mental disorders* (4th ed., primary care version). Washington, D.C.: American Psychiatric Association, pp. 169–174.

American Psychiatric Association. (2001). Practice guidelines for the treatment of patients with borderline personality disorder. *American Journal of Psychiatry, 158*(Suppl), 4–24.

Groves, J.E. (1981). Borderline personality disorder. *New England Journal of Medicine, 305,* 259–262.

Groves, J.E. (1997). Difficult patients and their management. In N.H. Cassem, T.A. Stern, J.F. Rosenbaum, & M.S. Jellinek (Eds.), *MGH handbook of general hospital psychiatry* (4th ed.). Chicago: Mosby Year Book.

Gunderson, J.G. (2002). Ire fighters: Physicians can learn to respond effectively when patients lose their patience. *Harvard Medical School Alumni Bulletin, 75,* 26–31.

Reich, P., & Kelly, M.J. (1976). Suicide attempts by hospitalized medical and surgical patients. *New England Journal of Medicine, 294,* 298–301.

CHAPTER 13
Personality Disorders II: Approaches to Specific Behavioral Presentations

JAMES E. GROVES

I. Introduction

Chapter 12 dealt with individuals with personality disorders and their interactions in the medical setting. Those phenomena, however, can be viewed not only through the lens of psychology but also through the lens of behavior. **For doctors who are less interested in theory and more interested in practice, this chapter describes specific troublesome behavioral presentations that are frequently encountered by physicians who treat individuals with moderate to severe personality disorders.** By focusing on behavior, a doctor can ignore the issue of whether a patient has a personality disorder diagnostically, yet be effective in establishing behavioral management. **The problematic patient behaviors considered here include anger and demandingness; seductive, clinging, or dramatic behavior; suspiciousness and paranoia; remoteness and detachment; and long-suffering behaviors and help-rejecting attitudes.** Manipulation and manipulative behaviors are often found in a list such as this, but manipulativeness in personality disorders is so pervasive and is associated with so many of the difficult behaviors in the list above that it should lead off the discussion.

II. Manipulativeness

A. **Clinical manifestations. Manipulativeness is a by-product of dependency and a usually angry reaction against it. These individuals are terribly dependent but have trouble turning their care over to a doctor.** They are very passive but extremely uncomfortable with their own passivity. They continually say that they want help but seem to do everything in their power to defeat the helper's attempts.

   In Chapter 12 the metaphor of the two cold porcupines showed how individuals with personality disorders can never find the optimal interpersonal distance from important people in their lives; they are always too close and too distant at the same time. Manipulativeness is their maladaptive "solution" to this dilemma. The demand for help satisfies the need for closeness, and the self-defeating behavior satisfies the need for distance because the distance keeps them from feeling that those they depend on will exploit them or gobble them up. (Also, the messes these people make of their lives seem to provide perverse "atonement" for deep feelings of shame.)

B. **Practical Approaches**

   1. When a patient says, "Well, if you don't give me the Valium, I'll just buy it on the street," this is a typical manipulation. On the surface it seems like a simple search for medication to use or abuse, but the interaction is more complex: It is an attempt to **control** the source of nurture—the doctor.

2. To deal with this behavior, the clinician needs to address both the **wish** for supplies and the patient's **fear** of becoming dependent (ironic as that may seem in the case of a drug-seeking patient). The doctor might say, "Well you could buy it on the street, but before you do that, why don't you let me give you a prescription for Paxil. [I'll provide your drug.] It's an antidepressant. Some of your anxiety may come from a depression that will respond to this medication. Give it a try for 2 weeks if you can. After all, I can't stop you from buying drugs on the street. I can't even make you fill this prescription. [See, I won't gobble you up.] Give it a shot."

III. The Angry or Demanding Patient

A. Clinical Manifestations

1. **Panicky obsessionals** and injured narcissists can present as angry demanders, but despite the initial surface presentation, there is a world of difference between the two. Obsessionals may be sticky, but **they are easy to deal with once the physician provides them with information and shares control of their care with them.**

2. **Injured Narcissists**

   a. Injured narcissists, who also are called **entitled demanders,** are a different story. They have serious underlying character pathology despite the fact that many of them have made a "success" of their lives, usually in the sphere of work.

   b. They have a deep sense of profound defectiveness and ugliness despite their outward bluster.

   c. They bully anyone and everyone in an attempt to avoid the feelings of vulnerability and helplessness that inevitably cast them into the pit of despair over their basic badness.

   d. They feel so terrible about themselves that they will do almost anything to keep from feeling vulnerable and thus slipping into profound self-contempt. Most of these individuals are, at the moment of demanding and bullying, completely unaware of their profound self-hatred, and so it is useless to suggest that their behavior is not based on what they think it is based on.

   e. **Entitlement represents an emotionally deprived individual's attempt to collect now what he or she should have gotten back then.** In the hospital or doctor's office a dependent individual attempts to wrest from the medical relationship that which he or she did not get from the mother-child relationship. Of course this does not work, but if one tries to tell an entitled individual the realities of life, that individual usually becomes more entitled or, worse, regresses to an even more primitive and helpless level.

   f. It is best in this situation not to attack the patient's defensive entitlement but instead to attempt to use the medical relationship as a defense against the patient's fear of abandonment.

3. **Entitled Demanders**

   a. **Demanders can be identified as being entitled by the doctor's impulse to devalue them.**

   b. The entitlement discussed in Chapter 12 is the behavior they lead with, and it is obnoxious. If the physician can catch it quickly enough, the desire to counterattack or become defensive can tell the physician about the patient and provide a behavioral remedy for the patient's potentially injured narcissism. These patients need to have their feelings of total deservedness rechanneled into a partnership that acknowledges their entitlement not to unrealistic demands but to good medical care. While the doctor should not attack the patient's wish for a restoration of what is essentially a parent-child relationship rather than a doctor-patient relationship, **the doctor can explicitly reassure the pa-**

tient that there is a real relationship—a medical relationship, a doctor-patient relationship—and that the patient does have rights, especially the right to the best possible medical care that can be provided.

c. **In limit-setting confrontations** with manipulative, entitled patients **the physician should use repetition and an appeal to the patient's sense of entitlement** rather than an assault on it: "You *deserve* the best medical care we can give, and that's why we're recommending this course of action." **The doctor has to keep uppermost in mind the appeal to the entitlement and not get drawn into logical or illogical arguments.**

d. **Repetition is crucial** in this maneuver, which is called **channeling entitlement.**

e. Demanders want too much, a lot of it unearned and undeserved. You should not, however, say this in a way that personally challenges them. You should instead follow a very conservative and orthodox plan of treatment and never say anything to them you would not want to read on the front page of the newspaper. You should contain them but not challenge them. You should not let them bully you. You again and again point out the realities of the illness and its treatment and state that you will try to get them part of what they deserve. When they feel entitled to something extra, you should pull their attention back to what they are medically entitled to and emphasize that.

IV. The Seductive or Dramatic Patient

A. Clinical Manifestations

1. **Patient characteristics.** Anxious clingers and angry and anxious trauma victims present as seductive or dramatic patients. Although their surface presentation is compliant or even sticky-sweet, they bear a remarkable resemblance to entitled demanders. They want the same things and fear the same dependency but use the carrot rather than the stick. Often, when they are frustrated or disappointed by the doctor, they suddenly turn into angry, entitled demanders.

2. **Physician Reactions**

   a. **The doctor's reaction to seductive patients is usually a feeling of aversion,** but that is a good signal that tells the doctor how to manage their care.

   b. **Clingers need to be identified early by means of the feelings of aversion they create and to be told gently but firmly and explicitly that the doctor is going to set limits** on the duration and number of visits and therefore on the depth of intimacy in the relationship. These **limits on clingers' expectations for an intense doctor-patient relationship are set so that clingers do not collapse in despair and feel rejected when disappointments occur,** as they inevitably do.

B. Theoretical models. Such individuals are said to be utilizing an **idealizing transference** not only to protect themselves from the illness but also to protect themselves from their own projected envy and rage, qualities they project onto anyone they get close to. They unconsciously want to use the physician as a "transitional object," like Linus' blanket. However, **a clinger's adoration is not really love; it is generic dependency.**

C. Practical Approaches

1. **Clingers**

   a. **Clingers need a good deal of factual information and education about your work situation (nothing about you personally).**

   b. **They need to know explicitly that you may not return their phone calls immediately.** You are busy working for them and others, and they should write down their concerns and keep a list to use your time and their money efficiently when you meet.

    c. They need to know that you will never call them by the first name or inquire about their personal lives except when these issues are directly related to their health.

    d. It is important with clingers, especially seductive ones, never to be alone in the office with them and never to answer personal questions about yourself.

  2. **Victims of Abuse**

    a. Related to seductive and dramatic patients are victims of abuse. Over the last 10 years psychiatry has recognized that the abuse of children and others with little or no power—especially sexual abuse—is far more common than had been thought. The newsstands and bookstores are full of stories reflecting this epidemic, and one cannot turn on the television without seeing a story about or an interview with an abuse victim. One of the most useful things to know about psychology is that in both normal development and abnormal circumstances all people display something psychiatry terms **identification with the aggressor.** In normal development, such imitations of the power of the parent promote healthy assertiveness and self-esteem. In pathologic situations, it means that people take on the traits of those who abuse them. One hears about hostages, for instance, who come to love and identify with their kidnappers. It is the same with abuse victims. In order to survive, they to some extent become like their abusers.

    b. Primary care physicians may encounter a lot of abuse victims, and these people display two important characteristics related to identification with the aggressor. First, they are on some level **abusive toward the doctor.** Second, they **disown responsibility for their actions.** Victims of child abuse are notorious for abusing their own children (and others) and almost universally feel diminished responsibility for their actions. It is as if they were locked in a time warp when they were abused.

    c. The implication for dealing with abuse victims is to know that they are abusive at times and are stuck in the role of victim, two traits that can interfere with attempts to help them. Helping them depends on being prepared for their abusiveness and not letting it happen. It also depends on understanding how limited they are in taking responsibility.

    d. Above all with abuse victims, one needs to maintain the strictest possible boundaries in the doctor-patient relationship. Never, regardless of their gender or age, let yourself be long in their presence without some sort of chaperonage nearby.

V. The Withdrawn, Unsociable, or Remote Patient

A. Clinical manifestations. Compared with some of the patient behaviors listed above, withdrawal is easy to deal with. Patients who seem withdrawn may behave that way because of their culture of origin. They also may be depressed, in which case you should proceed through the usual work-up for depressed patients in the primary care setting. However, there are people who characterologically want to keep a great distance from others, a stance they make obvious by their speech and even body language.

B. Practical approaches. This sort of person is relatively easy to deal with. **First, give yourself permission not to engage the patient too much; second, convey a respectful distance by your manner and the way you talk about the patient's medical care.** In an emotional sense, you have to let them come to you.

VI. The Fearful or Paranoid Patient

A. Clinical Manifestations

  1. Fearful individuals are almost identical to the withdrawn, unsociable, or remote patients described above.

2. In addition to such behaviors, however, they have subtle (or not so subtle) cognitive distortions.

3. They have no ability to trust and display exaggerated suspiciousness.

B. Practical Approaches

1. **To work with a paranoid individual, listen carefully and try to see what the patient is afraid of.** Often there are real things bothering such a patient as well as the myriad imagined ones, and a focus on the realities of the situation helps diminish their paranoia.

2. **Also, do not ask the patient to trust you. Your stance should be, "You don't know me. Why should you trust me?"** This they find respectful of them as individuals, allowing you to convey a further reassuring idea: "Your medical care doesn't depend on your trusting me. Just listen to what I have to say and see if the advice makes sense. Then you decide if you can trust that."

VII. The Long-Suffering, Depressed, Help-Rejecting Patient

A. Clinical Manifestations

1. These individuals are trying unsuccessfully to cope with chronic depression by using manipulation to get care. You might think of them as clingers with a different style or as demanders whose demandingness is converted into passive-aggressive behavior.

B. Practical Approaches

1. Help-rejecters need what clingers and demanders need but also need a kind of countermanipulation. For instance, **it is best to schedule visits on a regular basis to diminish the patient's need to generate new symptoms in order to assume the cared-for role.**

2. **Help-rejecters need to be allowed to have some of their symptoms within the context of regular visits determined by the calendar, not by generating an illness to maintain the relationship.**

3. The type of negative emotion the doctor experiences in response to these patients is like a laboratory test. If the doctor feels depressed and deskilled by the patient's continued and seemingly deliberate failure to comply with and respond to treatment, the patient needs the kind of structured, "pessimistic" treatment outlined above. **Never tell a long-suffering help-rejecter that everything is going to be fine;** such a statement is in their world untrue and will drag you into an enormous time sink.

VIII. Summary

A. The type of negative emotion a doctor experiences in response to certain patient behaviors is like a laboratory test.

B. If the doctor experiences suffocation and a feeling of aversion toward the patient, the patient is likely to be a clinger.

C. If the doctor is at first wary of the patient and then begins to want to counterattack that repulsive sense of innate deservedness, the patient is probably an entitled demander.

D. If the doctor feels depressed and deskilled by the patient's continued and seemingly deliberate failure to comply with and respond to treatment, the patient is probably a manipulative help-rejecter.

E. From the outset, clingers need to have gentle but firm limits set on their dependent behaviors and attempts at seduction. This is done by conveying great respect for formal boundaries.

F. Demanders need to have their entitlement channeled away from the destructive things they seek and into what they actually are entitled to: good medical care, not a mother-child relationship. This is accomplished by repetition and the projection of a reasonable attitude.

G. Help-rejecters need to be allowed to have some of their symptoms within the context of regular visits determined by the calendar, not by generating an illness to maintain the relationship. The physician's stance here is one of shared pessimism.

H. Paranoid and withdrawn individuals need to be allowed to keep their distance.

Suggested Readings

American Psychiatric Association. (2001). Practice guidelines for the treatment of patients with borderline personality disorder. *American Journal of Psychiatry, 158*(Suppl), 25–45.

Groves, J.E. (1978). Taking care of the hateful patient. *New England Journal of Medicine, 298,* 883–887.

Groves, J.E., & Newman, E. (1992). Terminating psychotherapy: Calling it quits. In J.S. Rutan (Ed.), *Psychotherapy for the 1990s.* New York: Guilford Press, pp. 339–358.

Hackett, T.P. (1969). Which patients turn you off? It's worth analyzing. *Medical Economics, 46*(15), 94–99.

Messner, E., Groves, J.E., & Schwartz, J.H. (Eds.). (1994). *What therapists learn about themselves and how they learn it.* Northvale, N.J.: Jason Aronson.

Millon, T., & Davis, R. (2000). *Personality disorders in modern life.* New York: John Wiley & Sons.

Perry, J.C., Banon, E., & Ianni, F. (1999). Effectiveness of psychotherapy for personality disorders. *American Journal of Psychiatry, 156,* 1312–1321.

Winnicott, D.W. (1949). Hate in the countertransference. *Interntional Journal of Psychoanalysis, 30,* 69–74.

CHAPTER 14
The Patient with Depression

JERROLD F. ROSENBAUM and MAURIZIO FAVA

I. Introduction

A. Definition

Unipolar depressive disorders are characterized by a constellation of physical, behavioral, and psychological symptoms (see Table 14-1) that cause significant distress and impairment in psychosocial functioning and occur in the absence of a history of mania or hypomania. The *DSM-IV* has established specific criteria for classification of these disorders, whose severity and course can vary greatly (see Table 14-2). **The most severe form of unipolar depression is major depressive disorder (MDD),** which consists of a history of one or more **major depressive episodes** (see Table 14-3 for specific criteria). **Dysthymic disorder is a milder but chronic form of depression** (see Table 14-4) and **minor depressive disorder** is probably the most common form of **depressive disorder not otherwise specified, and is characterized by fewer than five symptoms of MDD, with the duration of the illness being at least two weeks.**

Table 14-1. Physical, Behavioral, and Psychological Symptoms of Unipolar Depressive Disorders

• Depressed mood	• Irritable mood
• Anxiety, excessive worrying	• Nervousness
• Panic attacks	• Anger attacks
• Crying spells	• Hypochondriacal concerns
• Loss of interest or pleasure	• Lack of motivation
• Weight loss, decreased appetite	• Weight gain, increased appetite
• Carbohydrate craving	• Dizziness, lightheadedness
• Insomnia	• Hypersomnia
• Headaches	• Muscle tension
• Backaches	• Heart palpitations
• Psychomotor agitation	• Psychomotor retardation
• Fatigue	• Heaviness in arms or legs
• Feelings of worthlessness	• Excessive guilt
• Diminished concentration	• Forgetfulness
• Indecisiveness	• Distractability
• Recurrent thoughts of death	• Suicidal ideation, attempt, or plan

---

Table 14-2. The *DSM-IV* Unipolar Depressive Disorders

1. Major depressive disorder (MDD)
   - Single major depressive episode
   - Two or more major depressive episodes (recurrent)
2. Dysthymic disorder
3. Depressive disorder not otherwise specified
   - Minor depressive disorder
   - Recurrent brief depressive disorder

Table 14-3. *DSM-IV* Criteria for Major Depressive Disorder

- Depressed mood (in children and adolescents, can be irritable mood) or markedly diminished interest or pleasure in almost all activities
- Duration ≥ two weeks
- At least five of the following symptoms:
  - depressed mood most of the day, nearly every day (in children and adolescents, can be irritable mood)
  - loss of interest or pleasure in almost all activities most of the day, nearly every day
  - significant weight loss or gain or decreased or increased appetite nearly every day
  - insomnia or hypersomnia nearly every day
  - psychomotor agitation or retardation nearly every day
  - loss of energy or fatigue nearly every day
  - feelings of worthlessness or excessive or inappropriate guilt nearly every day
  - diminished ability to think or concentrate, or indecisiveness, nearly every day
  - recurrent thoughts of death or suicidal ideation, or a suicide attempt or plan
- The symptoms cause clinically significant distress or psychosocial impairment.
- Symptoms are not better accounted for by bereavement or are not due to a general medical condition or psychotropic substance.
- Presence of a single or multiple major depressive episodes
- There has never been a manic or hypomanic episode.
- The major depressive episode is not superimposed upon psychotic disorders and is not better accounted for by schizoaffective disorder.

II. Epidemiology

A. **Major depressive disorder (MDD) is quite prevalent** in the general population and has been reported in men and women of all ages. **The lifetime risk of MDD ranges from 7–12% in men, and from 20–25% in women.** It appears that the chances of suffering from this disorder are increasing in younger age groups. **Between 5 and 10% of primary care patients typically meet criteria for MDD,** although in many patients

---

Table 14-4. *DSM-IV* Criteria for Dysthymic Disorder

- Depressed mood (or can be irritable mood in children and adolescents for at least one year) for most of the day, for more days than not, for at least two years
- Presence, when depressed, of at least two of the following symptoms:
  - poor appetite or overeating
  - insomnia or hypersomnia
  - low energy or fatigue
  - low self-esteem
  - poor concentration or difficulty making decisions
  - feelings of hopelessness
- During a two-year period (one year for children or adolescents), never without depressed mood (or irritable mood in children and adolescents) for more than two months at a time
- No evidence of major depressive episode during the first two years of the disturbance
- No history of mania, hypomania, or cyclothymia
- Symptoms are not caused by a general medical condition or by psychotropic substance.
- The symptoms cause clinically significant distress or by psychosocial impairment.
- The disturbance does not occur exclusively during the course of psychotic disorders.

---

this disorder goes unrecognized and untreated. **Less than 50% of MDD patients receive treatment for their condition.** Of those patients treated for MDD, 57% received all care from non-psychiatric physicians. **MDD is a disabling condition, associated with high levels of impairment in work, social, and physical activities.** Compared to patients with chronic medical disorders, depressed patients have generally **worse physical and social functioning and perceived current health.** The **total costs** related to MDD in the United States are estimated to be **greater than $70 billion** per year. In addition, this disorder is a well-known **risk factor for suicide,** with 15% of severely depressed patients eventually committing suicide. Finally, failure to diagnose and treat MDD can lead to chronicity and poor outcome.

B. Dysthymic disorder has a **prevalence** rate of approximately **4%** among primary care patients, with a **lifetime risk** up to **6.4%** in the general population, and a female-to-male **ratio of 7:1.**

C. The prevalence of minor depressive disorder is less well known. Among primary care outpatients, a prevalence rate of 9.8% has been noted.

D. The etiology of unipolar depressive disorders is unknown; many believe that these disorders are the result of interactions of **genetic, biological, developmental, and psychosocial factors.** In particular, great attention has been paid to the central nervous system activities (e.g., neurotransmitters, neuromodulators, and neuronal gene expression) affecting mood, behavior, and cognition. The studies on the etiology of unipolar depressive disorders have been complicated by the great heterogeneity of these disorders. It is possible that a greater knowledge of the different subtypes of depression may lead to a better understanding of the pathophysiology of depression.

III. Evaluation of the Problem

A. General Recommendations

1. The **evaluation** of the depressed patient should include a determination of the following:
   a. **Physical, behavioral, and psychological symptoms** occurring during the month before the visit.
   b. **Onset, duration, and course** of these symptoms (e.g., depressive symptoms starting six months before the visit and continuing unremittingly until the present).
   c. **Current and past psychiatric history,** in particular the presence of possible anxiety disorders and substance abuse, which are quite common among patients with unipolar depressive disorders.
2. Clinicians must **be aware** that many patients who abuse **drugs or alcohol** may experience **depression** as a result of their psychotropic substance use; however, when they stop, their depression may remit or improve significantly. Before making the definite diagnosis of depressive disorder, it is imperative to make sure that the symptoms of depression are not the result of **recent bereavement** (i.e., the patient has not experienced the loss of a loved one in the past month).
3. The **use of self-rating scales** (e.g., the Beck Depression Inventory or the HANDS) may help the clinician in making the diagnosis of unipolar depressive disorders. In fact, the use of these scales has been found to increase primary care physicians' ability to recognize MDD by 2.5-fold to 25-fold.
4. When **evaluating** a patient with unipolar depressive disorders, the clinician must address the following questions:
   a. **What are the depressive physical, behavioral, and psychological symptoms reported by the patient?** How severe and frequent are these symptoms? For how long have they been present?
   b. **Are these symptoms new or have they occurred before?**
   c. **What is the impact of these symptoms?**
      i. Does the patient have difficulties in functioning at work and at home?
      ii. Are interpersonal relationships affected by these symptoms (i.e., is there social impairment as result of these symptoms)?
5. The **communication** with the depressed patient should include the following:
   a. **Frame the depressive disorder as a medical illness,** with specific signs and symptoms.
   b. **Refer to a neurochemical dysregulation** in the brain.
   c. **Emphasize that having depression is not indicative of a personal weakness or fault.**
6. **When proposing the treatment** to the patient, it is important to explain that:
   a. **Depression will not just go away.**
   b. **It takes three to five weeks for antidepressants to work.**
   c. **Adhering to treatment is very important** and treatment itself should have a **minimum duration** (e.g., six months).
   d. **Antidepressants are not "happy pills."**

B. Medical History

1. The **evaluation** of the patient with a depressive disorder should also include a determination of the following:
   a. **Medical history and medications** currently being used. Several medical conditions (e.g., hypothyroidism, folate deficiency, hypoadrenalism, rheumatoid arthritis, and Parkinson's disease) may be associated with the emergence of depressive symptoms,

and the use of certain medications (e.g., reserpine, and metoclopramide) may trigger symptoms of depression.

    b. **Assess the patient's use of psychotropic drugs, alcohol, and other dietary habits** (in particular, carbohydrate intake). **Psychoactive substances may mimic some of the symptoms of depressive disorders.** In addition, the **use of these substances may increase during worsenings of depressive disorders,** perhaps as an attempt to obtain relief from the psychological distress. Whereas depressed patients of the melancholic subtype may report a significant **decrease in appetite with subsequent weight loss,** patients with depressive **disorders of the atypical subtype may report carbohydrate craving and increased appetite, with subsequent weight gain.**

C. Examination of the Patient

    1. In addition to obtaining psychiatric and medical history, the examination of the patient should include a mental status examination, possibly a physical examination, and laboratory tests, when indicated.

        a. **The mental status examination** of the patient with unipolar depressive disorders is often unremarkable. Patients typically present with **depressed mood,** accompanied by **diminished interest/motivation** and, in some inviduals, **irritability and/or nervousness. Decreased concentration and attention** may affect the patient's performance in the Mini-Mental State Examination (MMSE), although the scores on the MMSE tend to be in the normal range. **Suicidal ideation** has been reported **in up to 40%** of depressed populations. The concomitant presence of **psychotic symptoms** suggests a diagnosis of MDD with psychotic features.

        b. **The physical examination** of the patient with unipolar depressive disorders is typically either unremarkable or non-specific.

        c. **Laboratory tests** should be obtained only when there is a specific concern about an underlying medical condition associated with depression. **Many studies have failed to document significantly higher rates of medical conditions associated with depression (e.g., hypothyroidism)** among outpatients with unipolar depressive disorders. For this reason, there is no need to obtain both standard and specific (e.g., thyroid function) laboratory tests in the evaluation of a depressed patient. However, **laboratory tests can be helpful when assessing patients who do not respond to standard treatments.** In particular, **thyroid function tests and B_{12} and folate levels** should be checked in these populations, as these abnormalities are known to be associated with depression and they can be easily corrected.

IV. Psychiatric Differential Diagnosis

A. Patients with dementia complain of symptoms (e.g., apathy, diminished concentration, and reduced memory) that may be hard to distinguish from the cognitive symptoms of unipolar depressive disorders. It is rare to see depressed outpatients with MMSE scores of less than 23. Therefore, very low scores on this test suggest the presence of dementia, although the term "pseudodementia" has been used in the past to describe non-demented depressed individuals with significant cognitive impairment.

B. Patients with **bipolar depression** may present with depressive symptoms that mimic unipolar depressive disorders. However, patients with bipolar disorder typically have a history of periods of mood elevation or irritability (mania or hypomania) that will help clinicians recognize that these patients are bipolar.

C. Many psychotic disorders may be accompanied by depressive symptoms. In particular, schizophrenic disorders of the catatonic subtype may be difficult to distinguish from MDD.

D. Premenstrual dysphoric disorder may present with symptoms that mimic unipolar depressive disorders in women. A clear distinction may be difficult at times, as **many depressive disorders fluctuate in severity,** with some of these fluctuations being the result of premenstrual worsening among cycling women. It is therefore important to **distinguish between premenstrual worsening** of unipolar depressive disorders and **true premenstrual dysphoric disorder.** This can be determined by ensuring that the female patient is symptomatic, perhaps to a lesser degree, during the follicular and midcycle phases as well.

E. Anxiety disorders can be accompanied by symptoms such as irritability, nervousness, insomnia, and diminished concentration. In particular, there is substantial overlap in symptoms between depressive disorders and generalized anxiety disorder. When patients describe the onset of depressive symptoms accompanied by generalized anxiety symptoms, only the diagnosis of unipolar depressive disorders (e.g., MDD or dysthymic disorder) is typically made. **Somatoform disorders, bulimia nervosa, substance use disorders, and personality disorders** may also present with symptoms of depression. When appropriate, the diagnosis of co-morbid unipolar depressive disorders can be made.

F. Patients with general medical conditions may also present with depressive symptoms. When appropriate, certain medical conditions (e.g., thyroid and other endocrine disorders that can mimic symptoms of depression) should be distinguished from unipolar depressive disorders by laboratory testing or physical examination.

V. Treatment Strategies

A. Pharmacotherapy with Antidepressants

1. **Selective Serotonin Reuptake Inhibitors (SSRIs)** have been widely used over the past few years as a treatment for depressive disorders. The rationale for their use as a **first-line treatment** is based on their **excellent safety record** and their **safety during overdose.** Table 14-5 lists all the available **SSRIs** in the United States, the usual

Table 14-5. Selective Serotonin Reuptake Inhibitors (SSRIs)

Generic Name	Brand Name	Tablets	Customary Initial Dose	Titrate Dose Up To
Citalopram	Celexa	10, 20, 40 mg	10–20 mg/day	20–60 mg/day
Escitalopram	Lexapro	10, 20 mg	10 mg/day	10–40 mg/day
Fluoxetine	Prozac/ Prozac Weekly	10, 20, or 90 mg	10–20 mg/day	20–60 mg qd or 90–180 mg weekly
Fluvoxamine	Luvox	25, 50, 100 mg	50–100 mg/day	100–250 mg/day
Paroxetine	Paxil/ Paxil CR	10, 20, 30, 40, 12.5, and 25 mg	10–20 mg/day or 12.5–25 mg CR	25–60 mg/day
Sertraline	Zoloft	50, 100 mg	50 mg/day	50–250 mg/day

starting dose, and the customary **target doses.** SSRIs are structurally unrelated to tricyclic or tetracyclic antidepressants and **lack associated anticholinergic, antihistaminic, and anti-α_1-adrenergic effects,** so that certain side effects (e.g., dry mouth, constipation, urinary retention, increased appetite, and orthostatic hypotension) are relatively infrequent with these antidepressants. **The most common side effects of the SSRIs are nausea, lack of appetite, weight loss, excessive sweating, nervousness, insomnia, sexual dysfunction, sedation, fatigue, headache, and dizziness. SSRIs do not have cardiac toxicity or blood pressure effects. Uncommon side effects** reported with SSRIs **are dry mouth, constipation, bleeding difficulties, nocturnal bruxism, hair loss, and reduced short-term memory. Most side effects tend to subside after a few weeks,** particularly if dosage escalation has been slow and gradual.

2. **Serotonin Norepinephrine Reuptake Inhibitors (SNRIs)** are efficacious, **safe during overdose,** and appear to be particularly **effective for the treatment of physical/somatic symptoms of depression.** Table 14-6 lists the only two available **SNRIs** in the United States (venlafaxine and duloxetine), the usual **starting doses,** and the customary **target doses.** SNRIs, like the SSRIs, are structurally unrelated to tricyclic or tetracyclic antidepressants and **lack associated anticholinergic, antihistaminic, and anti-α_1-adrenergic effects,** so that certain side effects (e.g., dry mouth, constipation, urinary retention, increased appetite, and orthostatic hypotension) are relatively infrequent with these antidepressants. The **most common side effects of the SNRIs are nausea, lack of appetite, weight loss, excessive sweating, nervousness, insomnia, sexual dysfunction, sedation, fatigue, headache, and dizziness. SNRIs do not have cardiac toxicity. At higher doses, venlafaxine treatment has been associated with blood pressure elevations in some patients.**

3. **Tricyclic Antidepressants (TCAs)** are agents structurally related to each other that have been used for decades in the treatment of depressed patients. **Table 14-7** lists all the available **TCAs** in the United States, the usual **starting doses,** and the customary **target doses.** By **blocking cholinergic muscarinic receptors,** TCAs can cause **dry mouth, constipation, urinary retention, sinus tachycardia, blurred vision, and memory dysfunction. Through a blockade of histamine H_1-receptors,** TCAs can also produce **sedation, increased appetite, weight gain, and potentiation of central depressant drugs.** Finally, **by blocking α_1-adrenergic receptors,** TCAs can cause **postural hypotension, dizziness, reflex tachycardia, and potentiation of the antihypertensive effect of drugs,** such as prazosin, terazosin, doxazosin, and labetalol.

Table 14-6. Serotonin Norepinephrine Reuptake Inhibitors (SNRIs)

Generic Name	Brand Name	Tablets	Customary Initial Dose	Titrate Dose Up To
Venlafaxine	Effexor/ Effexor XR	25, 37.5, 50, 75, 100 mg	37.5 mg b.i.d. or 75 mg XR qd	150–300 mg q.d.(XR) or 75–150 mg b.i.d.
Duloxetine	Cymbalta	30, 60 mg	30–60 mg qd	60–120 q.d.

Table 14-7. Tricyclic Antidepressants (TCAs)

Generic Name	Brand Name	Tablets	Customary Initial Dose	Titrate Dose Up To
Amitriptyline	Elavil or Endep	10, 25, 50, 75, 100, 150 mg	25 mg qhs	150–300 mg qhs
Amoxapine	Asendin	50, 100, 150 mg	50 mg b.i.d.	100–200 mg b.i.d.
Clomipramine	Anafranil	25, 50, 75 mg	25 mg qhs	150–200 mg qhs
Desipramine	Norpramin	10, 25, 50, 75, 100, 150 mg	25–50 mg qhs or qam	150–300 mg qhs or in divided doses
Doxepin	Adapin	10, 25, 50, 75, 100, 150 mg	25–50 mg qhs	150–300 mg qhs
Imipramine	Tofranil	10, 25, 50, 75, 100, 150 mg	25 mg qhs	150–300 mg qhs or in divided doses
Nortriptyline	Pamelor	10, 25, 50, 75 mg	10–25 mg qhs	50–150 mg qhs
Protriptyline	Vivactil	5, 10 mg	10 mg qam	30–60 mg qam
Trimipramine	Surmontil	25, 50, 100 mg	25 mg qhs	150–250 mg qhs
Tetracyclic Antidepressant				
Maprotiline	Ludiomil	25, 50, 75 mg	50 mg qhs	150–200 mg qhs or in divided doses

Sexual dysfunction can occur during treatment with TCAs, which can also have **significant effects on cardiac conduction,** through a quinidine-like effect. TCAs are contraindicated in the treatment of patients with narrow-angle glaucoma and prostatic hypertrophy. **Most side effects** tend to **subside** after a few weeks, particularly if dosage escalation has been slow and gradual. **Persistence of** bothersome **anticholinergic side effects** is usually **handled by decreasing the dose or by adding cholinergic smooth-muscle stimulants** (e.g., bethanecol). An important caution in the use of TCAs is their **lethality in overdose.** It is useful to **obtain an EKG before treatment and after four weeks of TCA treatment, with plasma levels** of TCAs being a rough guide to dosing adequacy. The side-effect profile of TCAs may be advantageous in the treatment of depressed patients who complain of insomnia and weight loss, as these symptoms can be helped quite rapidly by these drugs. On the other hand, side effects such as **weight gain and sedation** may **create difficulties with atypical depressed patients** who complain of hypersomnia and hyperphagia. For these reasons, and because of the required dose titration, **adherence to TCA treatment can be poor** at times, in spite of the relatively low cost of these drugs.

4. A number of **atypical antidepressants** (bupropion, mirtazapine, nefazodone, and trazodone) have been used in the treatment of depression. These agents have chemical structures different from those of TCAs and SSRIs, and their **side-effect profile is variable** depending on the agent. They are **all relatively safe in overdose,** as they lack significant cardiac effects. **Table 14-8** lists all the available **atypical anti-**

Table 14-8. Atypical Antidepressants

Generic Name	Brand Name	Tablets	Customary Initial Dose	Titrate Dose Up To
Bupropion	Wellbutrin/ Wellbutrin XL	75, 100, 150, or 300 mg	150 XL q.d. or 75–100 mg b.i.d.	150–300 mg XL q.d. or 150 mg t.i.d.
Mirtazapine	Remeron/ Remeron Sol Tab	15, 30, and 45 mg	15 mg qhs	30–45 mg qhs
Nefazodone	Serzone	50, 100, 150, 200, 250 mg	100 mg b.i.d.	150–300 mg b.i.d.
Trazodone	Desyrel	50, 100, 150, 300 mg	50–100 mg qhs	200–600 mg/day

depressants in the United States, the usual **starting doses,** and their customary **target doses.**

The most common **side effects of bupropion** are **anxiety/nervousness, agitation, dry mouth, insomnia, headache, nausea, constipation, and tremor.** Bupropion lacks significant anticholinergic, antihistaminic, and anti-α_1-adrenergic effects, so that side effects, such as blurred vision, urinary retention, increased appetite, weight gain, sedation, and orthostatic hypotension, are relatively infrequent with this antidepressant. **Bupropion is contraindicated in the treatment of patients with a seizure disorder or bulimia,** as the incidence of seizures is about 0.4% at doses up to 450 mg/day of bupropion, increasing almost 10-fold at higher doses, so that **450 mg with t.i.d. dosing is the maximum recommended daily dose of the immediate-release formulation and 150 mg is the maximum single dose to avoid high peak plasma concentrations.** A sustained release (XL) formulation is now available, allowing for once-a-day administration.

Mirtazapine lacks significant anticholinergic and anti-α_1-adrenergic effects. Mirtazapine does have significant antihistamine H_1-receptor blocking activity, which accounts for the **sedation, drowsiness, increased appetite, and weight gain** observed with this drug. **Other side effects** of mirtazapine are **dry mouth, constipation, and dizziness.** The relative **lack of significant drug–drug interactions** with other antidepressants makes mirtazapine a good candidate for **combination strategies** (i.e., combining two antidepressants together at full doses).

Nefazodone lacks significant anticholinergic and antihistaminic effects, so that side effects, such as blurred vision, urinary retention, and weight gain, are relatively infrequent with this antidepressant. **The most common side effects of nefazodone are headache, fatigue, orthostatic hypotension (caused by the blockade of α_1-adrenergic receptors), dry mouth, nausea, constipation, sedation, and blurred vision. In view of reported cases of severe hepatotoxicity associated with nefazodone, caution has been suggested** when nefazodone is prescribed with other drugs, especially those metabolized by CYP 450 3A4, or is prescribed to **patients with pre-existing liver disease.** It has also been recommended that **baseline and regular liver**

function tests should be obtained in all patients on nefazodone therapy in the first 6 months, and the drug should be discontinued if abnormalities are found.

Trazodone is an agent somewhat related to nefazodone, although the former is much more sedating than the latter. **The most common side effects of trazodone are drowsiness, dizziness, headache, nausea, and orthostatic hypotension, with priapism being an extremely rare but potentially serious side effect in men.**

5. **Monoamine Oxidase Inhibitors (MAOIs)** have been used primarily in the **treatment of certain depressive subtypes (e.g., atypical)** or as a **third or fourth line** of treatment of depression, mostly in **treatment-resistant patients. MAOIs inhibit the MAO enzymes (type A and B)** located in monoamine-containing nerve terminals, and in the liver and other tissues that metabolize such monoamines as norepinephrine, serotonin, and dopamine. Three of the four currently marketed MAO inhibitors **(phenelzine, tranylcypromine, and isocarboxazid) are non-selective** and inhibit both isozymes, while ʟ-deprenyl preferentially inactivates MAO-B within a dosage range of 5 to 10 mg/day, and is therefore used at higher doses to obtain non-selective inhibition. **Table 14-9** lists all the MAOIs available in the United States and Canada, the usual starting doses, and the customary target doses.

These four *MAOIs* have a **prolonged biological half-life** and are considered relatively **irreversible inhibitors of MAO,** in that they exert a persistent inhibitory effect on these isoenzymes, with **normal function** of these enzymes being **restored only after several drug-free days** to allow regeneration of new stores of enzymes. MAOIs are relatively devoid of any post-synaptic receptor affinity. Since MAO enzymes are crucial in inactivating exogenous monoamines arising from foods or the action of bacteria in the gut, including the sympathomimetic pressor amine tyramine, the use of MAOIs is associated with **a RISK OF LETHAL HYPERTENSIVE CRISIS** related to *interactions with foods containing tyramine, and with sympathomimetic drugs.* They can also be associated with **severe** drug–drug **interactions** with *meperidine.* **Moclobemide,** a newer antidepressant with **reversible effects of inhibition of MAO** and greatly **diminished risk** of dietary or other interactions, has been available in Europe and Canada for several years.

Serotonergic syndromes, characterized by heat stroke, vascular collapse, fever, tachycardia, or even death, have been reported **when MAOIs have been combined with potent serotonergic agents** (e.g., the SSRIs). The most common side effects of

Table 14-9. Monoamine Oxidase Inhibitors (MAOIs)

Generic Name	Brand Name	Tablets	Customary Initial Dose	Titrate Dose Up To
Isocarboxazid	Marplan	10 mg	10 mg b.i.d.	30–60 mg/day
Phenelzine	Nardil	15 mg	15 mg b.i.d.	45–90 mg/day
Tranylcypromine	Parnate	10 mg	10 mg b.i.d.	40–80 mg/day
ʟ-Deprenyl	Eldepryl	10 mg	10 mg b.i.d.	30–40 mg/day
Moclobemide	Available only in Canada	150 mg	150 mg b.i.d.	450–900 mg/day

MAOIs are **insomnia, sedation, orthostatic hypotension, weight gain, and sexual dysfunction,** with less common side effects being **tremor, blurred vision, dry mouth, constipation, and urinary retention.** It is usually best to administer the last MAOI dose in the early afternoon, as insomnia is a potential side effect. To avoid the risk of severe (and possibly lethal) drug–drug interactions, one must **wait two weeks after discontinuing antidepressants and five weeks after discontinuing fluoxetine or protriptyline before starting treatment with MAOIs.** It is also recommended to **wait two weeks before starting another antidepressant following discontinuation of an MAOI.**

B. Psychotherapy

1. **Cognitive therapy and interpersonal psychotherapy** are probably the **most efficacious forms of psychotherapy** in the treatment of patients with depressive disorders. Both therapies are **short-term** and focused on the "here and now."
2. **Behavioral therapy and short-term dynamic psychotherapy** have also been studied in the treatment of major depression, but their **efficacy is less well established.**
3. Many other forms of therapy are currently used in the treatment of depressed patients, but more studies are needed to establish their usefulness.

C. Combined Psychotherapy and Pharmacotherapy with Antidepressants

1. It is **common practice** to treat patients with depressive disorders with a **combination of psychotherapy and pharmacotherapy with antidepressants.** This combination is **often prescribed from the beginning** when the depressive disorder emerges **in the context of severe psychosocial stressors or in the absence of social support.** More typically, **psychotherapy is added to pharmacotherapy** once the patient has reported a significant **clinical improvement,** in order to **consolidate** the progress, address **residual symptoms,** and **prevent relapses.** The usefulness of this combination, particularly when antidepressants are combined with cognitive therapy, has been demonstrated in research studies.

D. Electroconvulsive Therapy (ECT)

1. **Electroconvulsive therapy (ECT)** was first introduced in 1938 and involves a safe **application of an electrical current to the skull to induce a generalized seizure.** It is usually administered by placing on the head either **bilateral or unilateral** nondominant electrodes and by delivering either sine-wave or brief-pulse current to induce seizures of adequate intensity and duration in patients under anesthesia. **ECT should primarily be used only after several adequate antidepressant trials have failed** or with patients with **depression marked by delusions or other psychotic symptoms.** The most common side effect of ECT is **retrograde and anterograde amnesia;** patients very frequently experience difficulty retaining new information during the course of ECT and up to several months after the last treatment, followed by gradual normalization of memory functions. **Heart arrhythmias or hypertension** can also occur during the course of ECT, and **death,** mostly caused by cardiovascular complications, is an **extremely rare** complication of ECT. Although there are no absolute contraindications to ECT, **relative contraindications** are the presence of **coronary artery disease, digitalis toxicity, increased intracranial pressure, and intracranial lesions** (e.g., arteriovenous malformation, arterial aneurysm, hemorrhagic stroke). Specific modifications in anesthetic technique are necessary to safely treat patients with recent myocardial infarction, congestive heart failure, conduction abnormalities, coronary artery disease, hypertension, and impaired pulmonary function.

E. Light Therapy

1. **Light therapy** involves the **exposure** of the **eyes** to **light containing very little ultraviolet light.** Its **primary indication** for use is **seasonal affective disorder** (SAD), characterized by **recurrent fall and winter depressions** alternating with non-depressed periods in spring and summer. There is no clear evidence yet for the efficacy of light therapy in non-seasonal depressives. Most frequent side effects observed during the course of phototherapy are **insomnia, headaches, eyestrain, and irritability.**

F. Other Treatments

1. Many drug treatments have shown some efficacy in the treatment of depressive disorders either in small studies or case reports. Their efficacy, however, has not been established yet. These agents include **s-adenosyl-l-methionine (SAMe), St. John's wort (hypericum), psychostimulants** (e.g., dextroamphetamine and methylphenidate), certain **anticonvulsants** (e.g., gabapentin, lamotrigine, carbamazepine, and valproic acid), **steroid suppressing agents, dehydroepiandrosterone (DHEA), methylfolate, inositol,** and **dopaminergic agonists.** Many of these agents are used **as adjuncts** to standard antidepressants in the event of **non-response.**

VI. Frequent Misconceptions in the Use of Antidepressants

A. **Most depressed patients (70–80%) recover acutely after antidepressant treatment.** In reality, **less than 50%** of the patients typically **show a very robust response, with a substantial proportion of patients showing only a partial but significant improvement.**

B. **Two to four weeks of antidepressant treatment is an adequate period of time.** Many patients will actually take **five to eight weeks to show a significant improvement.** Therefore, patients should be treated for at least six weeks with an antidepressant at adequate doses.

C. **One should use antidepressants alone.** In clinical practice, however, **polypharmacy is quite common.** For example, many patients receive treatment with a combination of antidepressants and antianxiety drugs to address symptoms of nervousness and agitation, which are relatively common in depression.

D. **All antidepressants are the same.** In reality, however, when patients have no history of antidepressant treatment, **experienced clinicians tend to choose a drug with the lowest predictable side-effect burden.** Similarly, the likelihood of continuing antidepressant treatment is greater if the first treatment is provided with drugs with a relatively well-tolerated side effect profile (e.g., the **SSRIs) as opposed to tertiary-amine TCAs** (e.g., amitriptyline or doxepin).

VII. Factors Limiting Adequate Dose, Duration, and Compliance

A. Prescriber-Related Factors

- **Prescribers may lack sophistication with dose requirements** (52% of primary care physicians versus 17% of psychiatrists use lower-than-recommended doses).
- **There may be variable comfort with side effects and risks** of the specific drug treatments.

- The degree of **education and preparation of the patient** is likely to affect treatment adherence.

B. Patient-Related Factors

- **Patients' attitudes toward drug treatment** may influence their ability to adhere to treatment.
- **Patients' level of education and knowledge** is also an important factor in increasing motivation.
- **The tolerability of the agent prescribed** affects the patients' ability to continue taking it.

VIII. Change in Drug Treatment: When and How Should One Do It?

A. Circumstances in which prescribers should change pharmacologic strategy:

- **Patients who do not experience significant improvement** with continuing current medication **at full dose** for an additional **four weeks;** in such cases, an **increase in dose** may be tried first, then **augmentation or combination** strategies, unless a **switch** to a different antidepressant may seem appropriate.
- Patients may experience a **relapse within a few months** of treatment initiation; in such cases, a **dose increase** can be the first option, then a **switch** to a different antidepressant is quite reasonable.

B. Augmentation strategies are typically carried out by adding:

- **Lithium** (e.g., 600 to 900 mg/day, often at bedtime)
- **Thyroid** (e.g., 50 to 75 µg/day of T$_3$)
- **Psychostimulants** (e.g., 20 to 40 mg/day of methylphenidate, or dextroamphetamine 10 to 20 mg/day)
- **Dopaminergic agents** (e.g., 0.125–0.25 mg t.i.d. of pramipexole)
- **Atypical antipsychotic agents** (e.g., 5–15 mg qhs of olanzapine, 40–160 mg/day of ziprasidone, or 1–4 mg/day of risperidone)
- **Anticonvulsant agents** (e.g., 600–1,800 mg/day of gabapentin, or 100–200 mg of lamotrigine)
- **Antianxiety drugs** (e.g., 10–30 mg b.i.d. of buspirone, or benzodiazepines)

C. Combination strategies are usually obtained by combining the following drugs:

- an **SSRI** at full dose and a **low-dose TCA** (e.g., 25 to 50 mg/day)
- an **SSRI** at full dose and **mirtazapine** at full dose (e.g., 15 to 30 mg/day)
- an **SSRI** at full dose and **bupropion** at full dose (e.g., 100 to 200 mg b.i.d. of a sustained release formulation)

D. Switching antidepressants is usually carried out by the following means:

- **Switching** to an **agent** of the **same class** (e.g., from an SSRI to another SSRI)
- **Switching** to an **agent** of a **different class** (e.g., from an SSRI to an SNRI or a TCA)
- **Switching** to an **atypical agent** (e.g., bupropion, mirtazapine)
- **Switching** to an **MAOI**

IX. Continuation and Maintenance Therapies

A. Continuation Therapy

There are **three phases** in the treatment of depressive disorders with antidepressant drugs: **acute therapy** (the first 8 to 12 weeks), **continuation therapy,** and **maintenance therapy.** Whereas **continuation** therapy is the continued administration of the drug for **four to six months following the disappearance** of acute symptoms in order to maintain control over the episode, **maintenance** therapy refers to pharmacological treatment extending beyond the continuation phase and being administered for **long periods of time (months or years) to prevent recurrences.** The risk of **relapse** is **significantly higher** when recently improved patients **discontinue their antidepressant,** as compared to patients **receiving continuation treatment** with antidepressants. The **risk of relapse** after antidepressant withdrawal only **abates after at least four months** of sustained response. Therefore, it is **best to continue** the antidepressant treatment **for at least four to six months** after obtaining a clinical response.

B. Maintenance Therapy

Since **most of the patients** who have had at least one episode of major depression are **likely to suffer a recurrence, maintenance antidepressant treatment is important,** particularly for patients with a **high probability of having recurrences.** The main **risk factors** for recurrent depression are a history of **frequent or multiple episodes of depression,** a history of **double-depression** (i.e., major depression superimposed upon dysthymic disorder), and a **long duration of the index episode** (i.e., more than two years). **Antidepressants,** in dosages comparable to those used during the acute phase, have been found to be **effective in preventing recurrent depressive episodes** in populations at risk. The **combination of maintenance pharmacotherapy with psychotherapies** appears to be a promising strategy as well.

X. When Should One Refer a Patient to a Psychiatrist?

A. Primary care physicians should consider referring a patient to a psychiatrist when:

- The patient presents a significant **suicidal risk.**
- The patient is **pregnant** or **plans to become pregnant.**
- There is **very little or no social support.**
- The patient is **disabled** by the depression.
- The patient has certain **co-morbid conditions** (i.e., substance abuse, panic disorder, obsessive-compulsive disorder).
- The patient **fails to respond** to one or two **adequate trials** of antidepressants.
- The patient has symptoms of **psychosis.**

XI. Conclusion

To effectively treat the patient who suffers from symptoms of depression, it is crucial for the clinician to assess physical, behavioral, and psychological symptoms and establish a diagnosis. There are many pharmacological treatment strategies available for patients suffering from depressive disorders. Pharmacological treatment with antidepressants is clearly a cost-effective approach. Psychotherapy, in particular with cognitive and interpersonal strategies, represents an alternative approach that can be considered, particularly when a patient is reluctant to take medications.

Suggested Readings

Alpert, J.E., Mischoulon, D., Nierenberg, A.A., & Fava, M. (2000). Nutrition and depression: Focus on folate. *Nutrition, 16*(7–8), 544–546.

Chan, C.H., Janicak, P.G., Davis, J.M., et al. (1987). Response to psychotic and nonpsychotic depressed patients to tricyclic antidepressants. *Journal of Clinical Psychiatry, 48,* 197–200.

Fava, M., Rosenbaum, J.F., Pava, J., et al. (1993b). Anger attacks in unipolar depression, Part I: Clinical correlates and response to fluoxetine treatment. *American Journal of Psychiatry, 150,* 1158–1163.

Fava, M., & Kendler, K.S. (2000). Major depressive disorder. *Neuron, 28*(2), 335–341.

Fava, M. (2001). Augmentation and combination strategies in treatment-resistant depression. *Journal of Clinical Psychiatry, 62*(Suppl 18), 4–11.

Fawcett, J., & Kravitz, H.M. (1988). Anxiety syndromes and their relationship to depressive illness. *Journal of Clinical Psychiatry, 44,* 8–11.

Keitner, G.I., Ryan, C.E., Miller, I.W., et al. (1992). Recovery and major depression: Factors associated with twelve-month outcome. *American Journal of Psychiatry, 149,* 93–99.

Keller, M., Lavori, P., Endicott, J., et al. (1983). "Double depression": Two year follow-up. *American Journal of Psychiatry, 140,* 689–694.

Nierenberg, A.A., Farabaugh, A.H., Alpert, J.E., et al. (2000). Timing of onset of antidepressant response with fluoxetine treatment. *American Journal of Psychiatry, 157*(9), 1423–1428.

Parker, G., Hadzi-Pavlovic, D., & Pedic, F. (1992). Psychotic (delusional) depression: A meta-analysis of physical treatments. *Journal of Affective Disorders, 24,* 17–24.

Quitkin, F.M., Stewart, J.W., McGrath, P.J., et al. (1993). Columbia atypical depression: A subgroup of depressives with better response to MAOI than to tricyclic antidepressants or placebo. *British Journal of Psychiatry, 163*(suppl 21), 30–34.

Rush, A.J., & Weissenburger, J.E. (1994). Melancholic symptom features and *DSM-IV. American Journal of Psychiatry, 151,* 489–498.

Stewart, J.W., McGrath, P.J., Quitkin, F.M. (1992). Can mildly depressed outpatients with atypical depression benefit from antidepressants? *American Journal of Psychiatry, 149,* 615–619.

Winter, P., Philipp, M., Buller, R., et al. (1991). Identification of minor affective disorders and implications for psychopharmacotherapy. *Journal of Affective Disorders, 22,* 125–133.

CHAPTER 15

The Suicidal Patient

ISABEL T. LAGOMASINO AND THEODORE A. STERN

I. Introduction

Suicide is the eighth leading cause of death in the United States, accounting for more than 30,000 deaths each year (1–2% of the total number of deaths each year). For every person who completes suicide, 8 to 10 people attempt suicide, and for every completed suicide, 18 to 20 attempts are made (some individuals make more than one attempt). As many as 1–2% of emergency department visits, 5% of intensive care unit admissions, and 10% of general medical admissions result from failed suicide attempts.

II. The Evaluation of Current Suicidal Tendencies (Table 15-1)

The evaluation of suicide risk relies on a detailed clinical examination of the patient who has contemplated, threatened, or attempted suicide. **The thoughts and feelings of the individual must be elicited and placed in the context of known risk factors for suicide.**

A. Patients Requiring Evaluation

Keep a low threshold when considering whether to evaluate a patient for suicidal tendencies. Certainly, **all patients who have made a suicide attempt, voiced suicidal ideation or intent, admitted suicidal ideation or intent upon questioning, or whose actions have suggested suicidal intent despite their protests to the contrary should undergo an evaluation.** Patients with psychiatric disorders or those who express a sense of hopelessness about the future should undergo an evaluation as well.

Table 15-1. Components of the Suicide Evaluation

Evaluate suicidal ideation and intent.

Examine details of the suicidal plan.

    Risk–rescue ratio

    Level of planning

Evaluate the degree of hopelessness.

Identify possible precipitants.

Consider available social supports.

Examine the mental status.

Corroborate the history with family and friends.

B. The General Approach

The patient at potential risk for suicide must be approached in **a non-judgmental, supportive, and empathic manner.** Initial rapport may be established by creating some degree of privacy, attempting to maximize the physical comfort of the patient, and proceeding from general questions to more specific ones. The patient who senses interest, concern, and compassion is more likely to trust the examiner and provide a detailed and accurate history.

C. Evaluation of Suicidal Ideation and Intent

Questions regarding suicidal ideation and intent must be made in an open and direct manner. Patients with suicidal thoughts and plans are often relieved and not offended when they find someone with whom they can speak about the unspeakable. Those without suicidal ideation will not have suicidal thoughts planted in their mind and will not be at greater risk for suicide. General questions concerning any suicidal thoughts can be introduced in a gradual manner while obtaining the history of present illness:

1. "Has it ever seemed that things just aren't worth it?" or "Have you had thoughts that life is not worth living?" may lead to a further discussion of depression and hopelessness.

2. "Have you gotten so depressed that you've considered killing yourself?" or "Have you had thoughts of killing yourself?" may allow a further evaluation of suicidal thoughts and plans.

D. Evaluation of Suicide Plans

Specific questions concerning potential suicide plans and preparations must follow any admission of suicidal ideation or intent. The patient must be asked when, where, and how an attempt would be made and any potential means should be evaluated for both feasibility and lethality. An organized and detailed plan involving an accessible and lethal method may place the patient at greater risk for suicide.

1. The "risk–rescue ratio" is a concept that may be used to examine the intent and lethality of a planned attempt. The greater the relative risk or lethality and the lesser the likelihood of rescue, the more serious the potential for completed suicide. For example, a man who makes detailed plans to kill himself by traveling to an isolated wooded area where he will not be seen or heard and then shooting himself in the head has a high risk–rescue ratio and should be considered at serious risk for suicide. The woman who acts impulsively and takes a few extra fluoxetine capsules directly in front of her spouse has a low risk–rescue ratio and may not be of high risk for suicide. Although helpful, the risk–rescue ratio must always be examined from the perspective and beliefs of the particular patient.

    a. A patient who makes an attempt with a low risk of potential harm but who sincerely wants to die and believes that the plan will be fatal has a relatively high risk–rescue ratio and is at risk for suicide.

    b. A patient who survives an attempt that carries a high probability of death, such as an acetaminophen overdose, but who has very little desire to die and very little understanding of the severity of the attempt has a relatively low risk-rescue ratio and is less at risk for suicide.

2. The patient who survives a premeditated attempt may be at greater risk for a repeat attempt than the patient who survives an impulsive attempt, or an attempt made while intoxicated.

E. Evaluation of Hopelessness

The patient who has no hopes or plans for the future is at greater risk for suicide. Potential questions that address hopelessness include the following:

1. "What do you see yourself doing five years from now?"
2. "What things are you still looking forward to doing or seeing?"

F. Identification of Possible Precipitants

The identification of possible precipitants for an ongoing crisis will help in the effort to understand why the patient is suicidal. The patient who must face the same problems or stressors following the evaluation, or who cannot or will not discuss potential precipitants, may be at greater risk.

G. Consideration of Social Supports

A lack of outpatient care providers, family, or friends, may elevate the potential risk for suicide.

H. Examination of Mental Status

A careful mental status examination will detect psychiatric difficulties and assess cognitive capacities. Relevant aspects of the examination include the level of consciousness, appearance, behavior, attention, mood, affect, language, orientation, memory, thought form, thought content, perception, insight, and judgment.

I. Corroboration with Family and Friends

Family and friends can be interviewed to corroborate gathered information and to obtain new and pertinent data. Families may provide information that patients are hesitant to provide and that may be essential to care. The evaluation of suicidal risk is an emergency procedure that takes precedence over the desire of the patient for privacy and over the maintenance of confidentiality in the doctor-patient relationship.

III. Examination of Risk Factors for Suicide (Table 15-2)

A thorough psychiatric, medical, social, and family history of the patient at risk for suicide will allow the clinician to consider the presence and significance of potential risk factors. The existence of more than one significant risk factor may confer an additive risk.

A. Demographic Factors

1. **Age.** People over the age of 65 are more likely to suicide than are younger individuals; the elderly account for 20% of all completed suicides although they comprise only 13% of the population. Young adults, however, have recently experienced a dramatic increase in the rate of suicide; among individuals between the ages of 15 and 24, suicide has become the third leading cause of death.
2. **Gender.** Four times more men than women complete suicide, although three to four times more women than men attempt suicide.
3. **Race.** Whites are twice as likely to attempt and to complete suicide than are blacks and Hispanics, although American Indians and Alaskan natives have the highest suicide rates of any ethnic groups.

B. Psychiatric Disorders

Psychiatric disorders are associated with more than 90% of completed suicides and with the vast majority of attempted suicides.

1. **Major depressive disorder accounts for roughly 50% of suicides,** and 15% of patients with depression eventually die by suicide. The risk appears to be greater in

---

Table 15-2. Risk Factors for Suicide

Elderly, male, white

Psychiatric disorders

Medical illnesses

Widowed, divorced, or separated

Living alone

Recent personal loss

Unemployment

Financial/legal difficulties

Firearm possession

Family history of suicide or psychiatric illness

Tumultuous early family environment

Prior suicide attempts

Suicidal ideation or intent

Hopelessness

---

the early stages of a depressive episode and during the initial phases of treatment and recovery.

2. **Alcohol and drug dependence is responsible for 25% of suicides.** The majority suffer from both alcohol and drug dependence as well as from co-morbid depressive disorders. In addition, acute alcohol or drug intoxication may impair judgment and foster impulsivity, resulting in more attempted and completed suicides.

3. **Psychosis is present in 10% of suicides.** As many as 10% of patients with schizophrenia eventually complete suicide, mostly during periods of improvement from a relapse or during episodes of depression. Among patients with psychotic or affective illness, the presence of command hallucinations that urge self-harm may increase the risk of suicide.

4. **Personality disorders account for roughly 5% of suicides.** Impulsive suicide gestures or attempts must be taken seriously; even manipulative gestures may become fatal.

5. **Anxiety disorders** (especially panic disorder) are being increasingly recognized among suicides.

C. **Medical Illnesses**

Medical illnesses are associated with as many as 35–40% of suicides and with as many as 70% of suicides occurring in those over the age of 60. The increased risk observed among patients with certain medical conditions may be partly owing to the presence of influential demographic factors, co-morbid psychiatric conditions, or use of medications that induce psychiatric symptomatology. Individuals with the following severe or chronic illnesses have been reported to be at greater risk for suicide:

1. Acquired immune deficiency syndrome and cancer

2. Head trauma and organic brain syndromes

3. Epilepsy, multiple sclerosis, and Huntington's chorea
4. Spinal cord injuries
5. Cardiopulmonary disease
6. Peptic ulcer disease
7. Chronic renal failure
8. Cushing's disease
9. Rheumatoid arthritis
10. Porphyria

D. **Social Influences**

1. **Marital status.** Widowed, divorced, or separated adults are at greater risk for suicide than are single adults, who are at greater risk than are married adults. Married adults with young children carry the least risk.

2. **Living situation.** Living alone substantially increases the risk for suicide, especially among widowed, divorced, or separated adults.

3. **Personal loss.** Significant loss, from the death of a loved one, or to a diminution of self-esteem or status, may place individuals (especially young adults and adolescents) at greater risk for suicide.

4. **Occupational status.** Unemployment accounts for as many as one-third to one-half of completed suicides and may be a particularly strong risk factor for men.

5. **Financial and legal difficulties.** Financial troubles, legal involvement, and imprisonment confer an added risk for suicide.

6. **Firearm possession.** The presence of firearms in the home appears to independently increase the risk of suicide among all age groups and both genders.

E. **Familial Factors**

1. **A family history of suicide or psychiatric illness** is an important risk factor for suicide.

2. **A tumultuous early family environment,** characterized by early parental death, parental separation, frequent moves, emotional abuse, physical abuse, or sexual abuse, increases the risk for suicide.

F. **Past and Present Suicidal Tendencies**

1. **Patients with a history of suicide attempts account for 50% of completed suicides,** and as many as 10–20% of them will eventually die from suicide. They carry a markedly elevated risk during the year after their failed attempt, although the risk remains high for almost 10 years.

2. **The severity of prior suicide attempts** increases the risk for completed suicide.

3. **Present suicidal ideation and intent** are communicated by as many as 80% of people who complete suicide. The communication may be direct or indirect; death or suicide may be discussed, new wills or life insurance policies may be written, valued possessions may be given away, or uncharacteristic and destructive behaviors may arise. Patients may be more likely to discuss their intent with family and friends than with health care providers. Although 50% of people who commit suicide see a physician in the month before their death, only 60% communicate some degree of suicidal ideation or intent to the physician.

4. **Hopelessness,** or negative expectations about the future, appears to be one of the strongest predictors of suicide risk.

IV. The Treatment of Suicide Risk

Following a thorough exploration of current suicidality and an examination of potential risk factors, the clinician must make a clinical judgment regarding the immediate risk for suicide. Initial steps need to be taken in the treatment of patients at risk.

A. **Stabilization of Medical Conditions**

Patients who are at risk for suicide must have prompt attention and complete treatment for all current or potential medical conditions. The severity of the psychiatric presentation must not distract the clinician from the provision of good medical care.

B. **Protection from Self-harm**

Patient safety must be ensured throughout the evaluation and treatment of suicide risk.

1. **Patients who are at potential risk for suicide and who threaten to leave before an adequate evaluation is completed must be detained,** even against their will, in accordance with state statutes that allow for the detention of individuals deemed dangerous to themselves or others. Those patients who insist on leaving must be contained by locked environments or restraints.

2. **Potential means for self-harm must be removed from the reach of patients at risk.** Sharp objects, including scissors, sutures, needles, glass bottles, and eating utensils, must be removed from the immediate area. Open windows, stairwells, or potential hanging areas must be locked. Substances or medications that patients may have in their possession must be confiscated.

3. **Appropriate supervision and restraint must be provided** at all times for patients at risk for suicide:

   a. **Frequent supervision** may be provided for patients who are neither psychotic nor delirious and who can reliably "contract" not to hurt themselves and to alert staff if they are feeling out of control.

   b. **Constant one-to-one supervision** may be used for patients who cannot reliably "contract," who are of a relatively small size and have little strength, and who have lesser intent and impulsivity.

   c. **Physical restraint** may be necessary for patients who cannot reliably "contract," who are of a relatively large size and have significant strength, and who have greater intent and impulsivity. Physical restraint may also be indicated when staff are not available for supervision.

   d. **Medication** is indicated for patients who remain out of control even while in physical restraints. Actions that include spitting at staff, attempting to bite staff, or jerking wildly at restraints, endanger both the staff and the patient, and require the prompt use of medication.

C. **Serial Assessments of Mental Status**

Patients who are thought to be at significant risk for suicide and who are admitted to medical floors should be reassessed on at least a daily basis. The need for supervision and restraint should be readdressed continually.

D. **Initiation of Treatment**

Treatment may be initiated for patients at risk for suicide who are admitted to medical floors. Pharmacotherapy for any underlying diagnoses and brief psychotherapy that emphasizes a sense of control by the patient may both be indicated and helpful.

E. Choice of Disposition

A choice of disposition will follow the careful evaluation of suicidal tendencies, consideration of risk factors for suicide, and initial stabilization of psychiatric and medical conditions. A conservative approach should be employed, and errors, if necessary, should be made on the side of excess restraint or hospitalization. Acting in concordance with good clinical judgment is in the best interest of the patient and will bring little danger of liability. Possible dispositions include the following:

1. **Discharge home with an outpatient referral.** Patients may be allowed to return home if they are not currently suicidal; are able to contract to call or to return if suicidal thoughts or impulses recur; are medically stable; and are not delirious, demented, psychotic, significantly depressed, or intoxicated. Firearms need to be removed from the home; acute precipitants must be identified and addressed; social supports need to be in place; and outpatient treatment must be arranged and agreed upon.

2. **Admission to a medical floor with psychiatric consultation.** Patients may require medical hospitalization if they have any current or potential unstable medical illness. Psychiatric consultation should provide recommendations regarding supervision and restraint, reassessments of mental status, suggestions for potential treatments, and determination of subsequent disposition options.

3. **Voluntary admission to a psychiatric unit.** Patients should be hospitalized for further evaluation and treatment when a clinician cannot be reasonably certain that they are not at imminent risk for suicide. Those who agree to a voluntary hospitalization and who cooperate with their caregivers have the highest likelihood of effective treatment.

4. **Involuntary commitment to a psychiatric unit.** Patients who are at a high risk for suicide, who cannot control their suicidal urges, or who are at high risk for suicide but refuse hospitalization, must be committed involuntarily. They must be detained, by security personnel in the emergency room if necessary, until a transfer to a locked inpatient psychiatric facility can take place. Psychiatric consultation can help to confirm the need for commitment, arrange for an appropriate transfer, and complete necessary commitment papers. Patients should be informed of the disposition decision in a clear and direct manner. Transfers should proceed quickly and efficiently; patients should travel in restraints, by ambulance. Patients who are deemed to be at high risk for suicide and who elope before a transfer to a psychiatric facility can take place should be reported to their local police, who have the authority to bring them back to the hospital against their will.

V. Difficulties In the Assessment of Suicidal Risk

A. Patient Factors

Certain patients may present added difficulties in the evaluation of suicide risk.

1. Patients who are **intoxicated** may voice suicidal ideation or intent that they frequently retract when sober. A brief initial evaluation while they are intoxicated and their psychological defenses are impaired may reveal the depth of suicidal ideation and possible precipitants. A more thorough final evaluation when they are sober must also be completed.

2. Patients who are **threatening** should be evaluated in the presence of security officers and should be placed in restraints, if necessary, to protect both them and staff.

3. Patients who are **uncooperative** may refuse to answer questions despite all attempts to establish rapport and to create a supportive and empathic connection. Stating "I'd like to figure out how to be of help, but I can't do that without some information from you" in a calm but firm manner might be helpful. Patients should be informed that safety precautions will not be discontinued until the evaluation can be completed and that they will not be allowed to leave against medical advice. Their competency to refuse medical treatment should be carefully questioned.

B. Clinician Factors

Clinicians may experience personal feelings and attitudes toward patients at risk for suicide that must be recognized and that must not be allowed to interfere with appropriate patient care.

1. Clinicians may feel **anxious** because of the awareness that an error in judgment might have fatal consequences.

2. Clinicians may feel **angry** at patients with histories of multiple gestures or at patients who plan to use trivial methods, often resulting in poor evaluations and punitive interventions. Angry examiners may inappropriately transfer a patient with a low risk for suicide to a psychiatric facility or may discharge a patient with a high risk to home.

3. **Some clinicians may be prone to deny the seriousness of the risk** and may conspire with the patient or family in the stance that voiced suicidal ideation was "just talk" and that an attempt was "just an accident."

4. Some clinicians may **intellectualize** and choose to believe that suicide is "an act of free will" and that patients should have the personal and legal right to kill themselves.

5. Clinicians may **overidentify** with patients with whom they share personal characteristics. The thought "I would never commit suicide" may become translated into the thought "This patient would never commit suicide," and serious risk may be missed. The examiner may try to assure patients that they will be fine or may try to convince them that they do not feel suicidal. Patients may thus be unable to express themselves fully and may not receive proper evaluation and treatment.

C. The Evaluation Itself

Although helpful in guiding the evaluation, the epidemiological risk factors for suicide are neither sensitive nor specific in the prediction of suicide; they identify potential groups, but not individuals, at risk and have high false-positive and false-negative rates. **The clinician ultimately must rely on a detailed examination and clinical judgment.** While eliciting the thoughts and feelings of the patient, the clinician must assess the degree of suicidal intent in the present and attempt to predict what it might be in the immediate future. The prediction becomes increasingly unreliable with the passage of time.

Suggested Readings

Adamek, M.E., & Kaplan, M.S. (2000). Caring for depressed and suicidal older patients: A survey of physicians and nurse practitioners. *International Journal of Psychiatry and Medicine, 30*(2), 111–125.

Bartels, J.J., Conkley, E., Uxman, T.E., et al. (2002). Suicidal and death identification in older primary care patients with depression, anxiety, and at-risk alcohol use. *American Journal of Geriatric Psychiatry, 10*(4), 417–427.

Buzan, R.D., & Weissberg, M.P. (1992). Suicide: Risk factors and prevention in medical practice. *Annual Review of Medicine, 43,* 37–46.

Buzan, R.D., & Weissberg, M.P. (1992). Suicide: Risk factors and therapeutic considerations in the emergency department. *Journal of Emergency Medicine, 10,* 335–343.

Frierson, R.C., Melikien, M., & Wadman, P.C. (2002). Principles of suicide risk assessment: How to interview depressed patients and tailor treatment. *Postgraduate Medicine, 112*(3), 65–66, 69–71.

Hirschfeld, R.M.A., & Russell, J.M. (1997). Assessment and treatment of suicidal patients. *New England Journal of Medicine, 337,* 910–915.

Hofmann, D.P., & Dubovsky, S.L. (1991). Depression and suicide assessment. *Emergency Medical Clinics of North America, 9*(1), 107–121.

Hyman, S.E., & Tesar, G.E. (1994). The emergency psychiatric evaluation, including the mental status evaluation. In S.E. Hyman, G.E. Tesar (Eds.), *Manual of psychiatric emergencies* (3rd ed.). Boston: Little Brown, pp. 3–11.

MacKenzie, T.B., & Popkin, M.K. (1987). Suicide in the medical patient. *International Journal of Psychiatry and Medicine, 17*(1), 3–22.

Maris, R.W. (2002). Suicide. *Lancet,* 27;360(9329), 319–326.

Moscick, E.K. (1995). Epidemiology of suicidal behavior. *Suicide and Life-Threatening Behavior, 25*(1), 22–35.

Roy, A. (1995). Suicide. In H.I. Kaplan, & B.J. Sadock (Eds.), *Comprehensive textbook of psychiatry* (6th ed.). Baltimore: Williams & Wilkins, pp. 1739–1752.

Shuster, J.L., Lagomasino, I.T., & Stern, T.A. (1999). Suicide. In R.S. Irwin, F.B. Cerra, and J.M. Rippe (Eds.), *Intensive care medicine* (4th ed.). Philadelphia, PA: Lippincott-Raven, pp. 2415–2419.

Simon, R.L. (2002). Suicide risk assessment: What is the standard of care? *Journal of the American Academy of Psychiatry and the Law, 30*(3), 340–344.

Stern, T.A., Lagomasino, I.T., & Hackett, T.P. (1997). Suicidal patients. In N.H. Cassem, T.A. Stern, J.F. Rosenbaum, et al, (Eds.), *Massachusetts General Hospital handbook of general hospital psychiatry* (4th ed.). St. Louis: Mosby, pp. 69–88.

CHAPTER 16

The Anxious Patient

MARK H. POLLACK, JORDAN W. SMOLLER, AND DARA K. LEE

I. Introduction

Anxiety in the medical setting may be expected as a transient response to the stress of medical illness. However, excessive or pathological anxiety has a negative impact on patient morbidity and compliance with treatment. It should be diagnosed when present and treated in a timely fashion.

II. Definition of Anxiety

A. Anxiety vs. Fear

Anxiety and fear may be difficult to distinguish in the clinical setting. However, fear refers to the sense of dread and foreboding that occurs in response to an external threatening event, whereas anxiety derives from an unknown internal stimulus inappropriate or excessive to the reality of the external stimulus.

B. Manifestations of Anxiety

1. **Physical symptoms:** Generally those of autonomic arousal (e.g., tachycardia, tachypnea, diaphoresis, and lightheadedness)
2. **Affective symptoms:** Ranging from mild edginess to terror and panic
3. **Behavior:** Characterized by avoidance (e.g., including non-compliance with medical procedures) or compulsions
4. **Cognitions:** Include worry, apprehension, obsession, and thoughts about emotional or bodily damage

C. Pathological vs. "Normal" Anxiety

Anxiety in the medical setting is ubiquitous. The non-specific symptoms of anxiety may lead to underdiagnosis of pathologic anxiety, incorrect attribution to other physical causes, or its dismissal as minor, insignificant, or appropriate to the setting. **Pathological anxiety warrants evaluation and may be distinguished from "normal" anxiety by four criteria:**

1. **Autonomy:** Distress with a minimal relation to an external cause
2. **Intensity:** A high level of discomfort and severity of symptoms
3. **Duration:** Persistence of symptoms over time
4. **Behavior:** Development of disabling behavioral strategies (e.g., avoidance or compulsive behaviors). Pathologic anxiety is autonomous, persistent, and distressing, and results in impaired function owing to abnormal behavior.

III. Etiology

The biological underpinnings of anxiety likely include dysregulation in a number of pertinent neurobiologic systems (Johnson & Lydiard, 1995; Charney & Deutsch, 1996):

A. **Central Noradrenergic Systems**

Stimulation of the locus coeruleus (LC), the major source of the brain's noradrenergic innervation, generates panic attacks; **agents that block LC firing (e.g., antidepressants, high-potency benzodiazepines) decrease panic-anxiety.**

B. **The limbic system, including the septohippocampal areas, mediates general anxiety,** worry, and vigilance. High concentrations of benzodiazepine receptors in these areas modulate anxiety by increasing binding of the inhibitory neurotransmitter gamma-amino butyric acid (GABA).

C. **Serotonergic systems and neuropeptides** also appear important in the regulation of anxiety. The interconnections among all pertinent brain systems may help explain the apparent efficacy of interventions with diverse mechanisms of action (e.g., antidepressants affecting norepinephrine and serotonin; benzodiazepines; and cognitive-behavioral therapy) on pathologic anxiety.

IV. Epidemiology

A. **Anxiety disorders are among the most prevalent psychiatric disorders in the general population, with approximately a quarter of the individuals in the United States experiencing pathologic anxiety over the course of their lifetime** (Kessler et al., 1994).

B. **Anxiety is particularly common in the general medical setting.** The National Ambulatory Medical Care Survey (1980-1991) documented that anxiety is one of the most common chief complaints for people seeking care from a primary care doctor, **occurring in 11% of patients** (Schurman et al., 1985). Anxiety is the most common psychiatric problem seen by primary care doctors, with one study demonstrating that up to 20% of patients in this setting received benzodiazepines during a 6-month period (Wells et al., 1986).

C. **Most anxiety-disordered patients first seek care in the primary care setting** including the emergency room. **The majority of heavy users of primary care services have significant mood or anxiety difficulties** including panic disorder, generalized anxiety disorder (GAD), or depression (Katon et al., 1990). Patients with chronic illness and those who make frequent medical visits have higher rates of anxiety and depressive disorders (Leon et al., 1995).

V. Impact of Anxiety Disorders on Quality of Life

Anxiety disorders are associated with marked impairment in physical and psychosocial function as well as quality of life. For instance, panic disorder leads to a perceived deterioration of physical and emotional health, and it increases alcohol abuse, marital problems, and suicide attempts (Klerman et al., 1991). Panic and phobic anxiety may be associated with increased rates of premature cardiovascular mortality in men (Coryell et al., 1982; Kawachi et al., 1994). Panic disorder is associated with excessive use of medical resources including hospitalizations. Panic patients lose workdays twice as often as the general population, with 25% of panic patients chronically unemployed and up to one-third receiving public assistance or disability (Markowitz et al., 1989).

VI. Course of Anxiety Disorders

Systematic studies suggest that most patients are improved with treatment for panic and other anxiety disorders, but relatively few are "cured" (Pollack & Smoller, 1995). High rates of relapse after discontinuation of pharmacotherapy for anxiety disorders support the need for maintenance therapy for many patients.

VII. Problems with the Diagnosis of Panic in Primary Care

Most anxious and depressed patients in the medical setting present with somatic complaints rather than affective symptoms. The range and intensity of somatic symptoms may obscure the underlying psychiatric disorder and lead to extensive work-ups and misdirected treatment.

VIII. Populations of Particular Interest

A. Cardiac Patients

Chest pain is common among patients with panic; panic disorder occurs in 10–20% of patients who present to emergency rooms with chest pain. Up to 40–60% of patients with atypical chest pain and normal findings on cardiac catheterization have panic disorder (Katon et al., 1988). The concurrence of panic and chest pain results in increased use of emergency and intensive care facilities, and extensive cardiac work-ups; early treatment targeted at anxiety disorders, particularly in those with minimal risk factors for cardiac disease (i.e., younger and with normal physical examinations, electrocardiograms, and serum lipid profile), results in decreased patient morbidity and more rational use of medical resources.

B. Patients with Dizziness

In some studies, **15–20% of patients who are referred for evaluation of dizziness have panic disorder** (Stein et al., 1994). Studies examining vestibular function in panic disorder report mixed results, but patients not responding to standard antivertigo agents may benefit from treatments aimed at panic disorder.

C. Gastroenterology Patients

Twenty to 40% of patients with irritable bowel syndrome have panic disorder, and irritable bowel symptoms are frequently found among patients with panic disorder (Walker et al., 1995).

D. Dyspneic Patients

Many patients with COPD and asthma may have panic disorder or significant levels of anxiety (Smoller et al., 1996). In such patients, treatments aimed at reducing anxiety symptoms have positive effects on perceived dyspnea and functional capacity.

IX. Differential Diagnosis

The diagnostic approach to the anxious patient in the medical setting involves consideration of at least three overlapping areas. The clinician needs to assess whether the anxiety is secondary to the following conditions:

1. An **organic factor** (a medical illness or its treatment)
2. A **primary psychiatric disorder** (e.g., panic disorder or depression)
3. **Reactive or situationally related distress**

A. Organic Causes of Anxiety

Assessment of anxiety in the medical setting includes an evaluation of the patient's known medical illness (e.g., COPD), its complications (e.g., hypoxia), and its treatment (e.g., bronchodilators). Anxiety associated with organic etiologies is more likely to present with physical symptoms and less likely to be associated with avoidance behavior or onset with emotional trauma. **Diagnostic evaluation should be directed toward the somatic system most closely related to the anxiety symptoms** (e.g., the respiratory system in patients with shortness of breath).

The following **six factors are associated with an organic anxiety syndrome** and help distinguish it from a primary anxiety disorder (Rosenbaum et al., 1996):

1. **Onset of anxiety symptoms after the age of 35**
2. **Lack of personal or family history of an anxiety disorder**
3. **Lack of childhood history of significant anxiety, phobias, or separation anxiety**
4. **Absence of significant life events generating or exacerbating the anxiety symptoms**
5. **Lack of avoidance behavior**
6. **Poor response to antipanic agents**

B. General Medical Evaluation of the Anxious Patient

1. The extent of a medical work-up indicated for the patient with significant anxiety will vary depending on the age of the patient, the nature of the anxiety, the range and severity of associated symptoms, and the concomitant health status of the patient. The list of medical illnesses, medications, and substances that can produce anxiety is extensive, but in most cases only a small subset requires consideration.

2. The medical evaluation ideally includes the following:
   a. A history and physical examination, including a screening neurologic exam
   b. Consideration of the anxiogenic effects of medications, including beta-adrenergic agonists, theophylline, corticosteroids, thyroid hormone, and sympathomimetics
   c. Consideration and treatment of potentially contributory medical illness (e.g., thyroid dysfunction, hypoglycemic episodes in diabetes, hyperparathyroidism, arrhythmias, COPD, and seizure disorder)
   d. Consideration of the possible effects of substance use (e.g., caffeine, amphetamines, cocaine) or withdrawal (e.g., alcohol, sedative-hypnotics)
   e. Laboratory or other medical tests as indicated by clinical suspicion (e.g., thyroid function tests, serum calcium, and EEG)

X. Primary Psychiatric Disorders

A. Panic Disorder

1. **Definition**

   Panic disorder is a syndrome characterized by recurrent panic attacks (i.e., discrete episodes of intense anxiety associated with at least four other symptoms of autonomic arousal and anxiety that develop rapidly and typically peak within 10 minutes) (American Psychiatric Association, 1994). Associated symptoms include cardiopulmonary, gastrointestinal, and neurologic symptoms, autonomic arousal, and psychological symptoms (including derealization or depersonalization and fears of losing control, going crazy, or dying; see Table 16-1).

   The initial attack is usually spontaneous. Patients typically develop apprehension about attacks (i.e., **anticipatory anxiety).** Panic disorder may be complicated by **agoraphobia,** in which patients associate panic attacks with situations where escape

Table 16-1. Panic Attack Symptoms

- Palpitations, tachycardia
- Shortness of breath
- Chest pain or discomfort
- Nausea or abdominal distress
- Sweating
- Trembling and shaking
- Feeling of choking
- Dizziness, lightheadedness, or faintness
- Paresthesias
- Chills or hot flashes
- Derealization and depersonalization
- Fear of losing control or going crazy
- Fear of dying

may be difficult or embarrassing, or in which help may not be readily available (e.g., in a crowd or on a highway). Agoraphobia may result in significant avoidance behavior and restriction of patients' daily activities to the point at which they become dependent on companions to enter many situations or become housebound.

2. **Demographics and Course**

   Panic disorder typically begins in the second or third decade of life, though many patients first experience anxiety difficulties in childhood. Its course is often chronic or recurrent, and relapse rates after discontinuation of treatment are high. Panic disorder is more typically diagnosed in women than in men. This finding may reflect unknown biological or psychological gender differences, or the fact that men may be more likely to self-medicate with alcohol and be less likely to seek attention for their symptoms.

3. **Limited-Symptom Attacks**

   Although the diagnosis of full panic attacks requires four associated symptoms, many patients experience limited-symptom attacks, characterized by one or two symptoms (e.g., lightheadedness, dyspnea, or tachycardia). The symptomatic overlap with other medical illnesses may represent a source of diagnostic confusion. Limited-symptom attacks, like full attacks, cause distress and disability and respond to treatment with antipanic interventions.

4. **Treatments**

   Patients with untreated panic disorder develop significant morbidity, social dysfunction, increased medical use, and increased risk of mortality (from cardiovascular complications and suicide). **Established treatments include antidepressants, high-potency benzodiazepines, and cognitive-behavioral therapy.**

B. **Generalized Anxiety Disorder**

   GAD is defined as excessive anxiety or worry, in the absence of, or out of proportion to, situational factors; in most cases it lasts for longer than six months

(American Psychiatric Association, 1994). Patients are often called "nervous" or "worriers" by those who know them, and the anxiety is typically associated with symptoms of muscle tension, restlessness, insomnia, difficulty concentrating, easy fatigability, and irritability. The disorder may be differentiated from panic disorder by the presence of persistent anxiety rather than discrete panic attacks. GAD frequently presents co-morbidly with panic disorder, social phobia, depression, or alcohol abuse. The anxiety is often chronic and may worsen during periods of stress. **Treatment includes antidepressants, benzodiazepines, buspirone, and cognitive-behavioral therapies.**

C. Social Phobia

1. **Definition**

   Patients with social phobia experience marked anxiety in situations where they are exposed to possible scrutiny by others and fear they will behave in a way that will be humiliating or embarrassing (American Psychiatric Association, 1994). Social, occupational, or other situations may cause marked distress and avoidance, resulting in significant impairment. The social anxiety may be limited to circumscribed performance situations, that is, "performance anxiety" (e.g., speaking, writing, or eating in public), or more globally affect social interactions (e.g., maintaining conversations, participating in small group activities, or speaking to authority figures). Although fears of public speaking are not unusual in the general population, the intensity of the distress or resulting impairment must be significant to warrant a diagnosis of social phobia.

2. **Onset and Course**

   Social phobia typically has onset in the teens though it is often associated with childhood anxiety difficulties. **It tends to be chronic, although it may fluctuate** in intensity in response to stress.

3. **Treatments**

   Treatments **include antidepressants, particularly the serotonin selective reuptake inhibitors (SSRIs) and monoamine oxidase inhibitors (MAOIs), high-potency benzodiazepines, β-blockers, and cognitive-behavioral therapies.** Tricyclic antidepressants (TCAs) are generally less effective than other antidepressants for social phobia.

D. Specific Phobias

1. **Definition**

   Patients with a specific phobia have a marked and persistent fear of circumscribed situations or objects (e.g., heights, closed spaces, small animals, or blood) (American Psychiatric Association, 1994). Exposure to the stimulus causes marked anxiety and avoidance that interferes with the patient's life. Although phobias are not unusual in the general population, the intensity of the distress or resulting impairment must be significant to warrant a diagnosis of a specific phobia.

2. **Onset**

   Onset of phobias is often in childhood or the mid-20s and may be associated with traumatic events (e.g., being attacked by an animal), cued by observing others undergoing trauma, or result from frightening information transmission (e.g., media coverage). Feared objects tend to include things that may actually represent a threat or may have done so during our evolutionary past (e.g., snakes).

3. **Treatments**
   Benzodiazepine administration may be helpful in an acute situation, but comprehensive treatment usually includes behavior therapy (e.g., exposure and desensitization to the feared object or situation).

E. **Post-traumatic Stress Disorder**

1. **Definition**
   Patients with PTSD have been exposed to an event that involved the threat of death, injury, or severe harm to themselves or others (e.g., experiencing an assault or witnessing a serious accident or act of violence) (American Psychiatric Association, 1994). **Affected patients persistently re-experience the traumatic event in the form of nightmares, flashbacks, or marked arousal when exposed to situations reminiscent of the event.** The patient may develop avoidance of situations or cues related to the trauma and may become emotionally numb or detached from others. Associated symptoms also include sleep disturbance, irritability, and hypervigilance. PTSD may occur both in combat veterans and in civilians who suffer life-threatening situations.

2. **Onset and Course**
   Symptoms usually begin within the first three months after the trauma, although they may be delayed for months or years. The course is varied: complete recovery occurs within three months in half of the patients; many others experience symptoms for longer than a year after the trauma.

3. **Treatment**
   Clinical experience and systematic assessment suggest **SSRIs are generally effective for the treatment of PTSD. Cognitive-behavioral therapy (CBT) and other pharmacologic agents, including atypical antipsychotics and anticonvulsants, can also be effective.**

E. **Obsessive-Compulsive Disorder**

1. **Definition**
   Obsessive-compulsive disorder (OCD) is characterized by recurrent, intrusive, unwanted thoughts (obsessions) (e.g., fears of contamination) and compulsive behaviors or rituals (compulsions) (e.g., handwashing or checking) (American Psychiatric Association, 1994). The behaviors are excessive and are performed to decrease anxiety or are connected unrealistically to avoidance of a dreaded event or outcome. The obsessions and compulsions are time consuming (i.e., take more than an hour a day), cause significant distress, and interfere with a patient's normal functioning.

2. **Onset and Course**
   OCD typically develops during adolescence, but may occur earlier; in general it has a chronic course.

3. **Treatments**
   Treatments involve **serotonergic antidepressants, including the SSRIs and the TCA, clomipramine, and CBT** aimed at extinguishing intrusive thoughts and compulsive behavior.

XI. Co-morbid Depression

More than half of anxious patients also experience significant depression (Gorman & Coplan, 1996). Patients with anxiety symptoms in the medical setting should be evaluated for the presence of depression to avoid the scenario of targeting monotherapy with benzodiazepines for anxiety and leaving the depression un-treated. In cases of confirmed or suspected co-morbidity, treatment with an antide-pressant is recommended. Overlapping anxiety and depressive symptoms may be responsive to monotherapy with an antidepressant or to combined treatment with antidepressants and benzodiazepines.

XII. Reactive or Situational Anxiety

Patients may develop anxiety in reaction to a stressful situation (e.g., the onset of serious medical illness). The criteria for **an adjustment disorder with anxiety** in-clude the development of nervousness or anxiety in response to an identifiable stres-sor within three months of the onset of the stressor (American Psychiatric Associa-tion, 1994). The symptoms are clinically significant and cause marked distress or impairment in social functioning. This should only be diagnosed if the symptoms do not meet criteria for another disorder and last no longer than six months following cessation of the stressor. This disorder may be considered chronic if the stressor is persistent or its effects enduring, and the anxiety continues for six months or longer.

   Treatment may include general support, therapy aimed at exploring the meaning of the situation with the patient, environmental manipulations to re-duce the impact of the stressor (e.g., job change, financial assistance) **or sympto-matic relief of anxiety and depressive symptoms with an anxiolytic or antide-pressant.** Despite the fact that the anxiety may be "understandable" given the nature of the stressor, the provision of symptomatic relief can markedly improve the patient's quality of life and prevent more intense symptoms and complications from developing.

XIII. Treatment of Anxiety Disorders: General Considerations

A. **A supportive, reassuring approach is important** in treating the patient with significant anxiety. Patients with panic disorder, for instance, may be quite frightened about the medical significance of their symptoms or, alternatively, may be worried that the physi-cian will dismiss them as "crazy." Patients with social phobia may be anxious about the encounter itself and may be embarrassed by their anxiety. Patients with PTSD and histo-ries of abuse may have difficulty trusting the physician or may be apprehensive about the physical examination. The physician's awareness and anticipation of these issues along with a readiness to listen to the patient's concerns can in themselves be therapeutic.

B. Once a diagnosis of an anxiety disorder has been made, **educating the patient about the disorder and the availability of effective therapies is an important prelude to treatment.** Although some PCPs may not feel equipped to provide focused therapy, simple interventions (such as encouraging phobic patients to gradually expose them-selves to feared situations) can be quite helpful.

C. **When pharmacotherapy is initiated, the patient should be monitored closely (e.g., every two to three weeks depending on the complexity of the presentation) until a stable dosage and relief of symptoms are achieved.** If this is not feasible, referral to a psychiatrist may be indicated. In general, patients with PTSD and OCD have complex presentations with co-morbid psychiatric conditions, and expedient referral to a psychi-atrist is often appropriate (Figure 16-1).

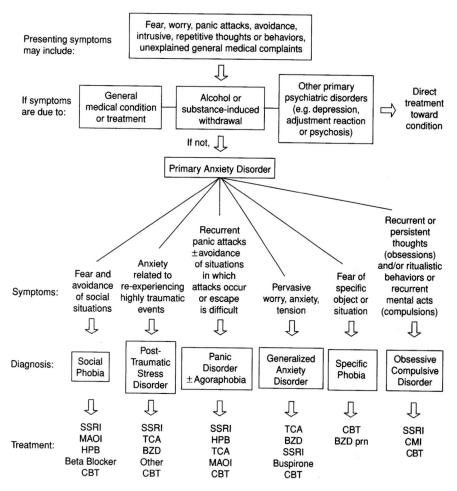

Figure 16-1. Approach to the anxious patient in the primary care setting.
NOTE: BZD, benzodiazepine; CBT, cognitive-behavioral therapy; CMI, clomipramine; HPB, high-potency benzodiazepine; MAOI, monoamine oxidase inhibitors; prn, as needed; SSRI, selective serotonin reuptake inhibitor; TCA, tricyclic antidepressant; other, e.g., anticonvulsant, neuroleptic, lithium.

XIV. Pharmacotherapy of Anxiety

A. Antidepressants

1. **Serotonin selective reuptake inhibitors (SSRIs), serotonin norepinepherine reuptake inhibitors (SNRIs) and newer agents**

   a. **The SSRIs and SNRIs have become first-line treatment for most of the anxiety disorders** (including panic disorder with or without agoraphobia, PTSD, social phobia, OCD, and GAD) because of their broad spectrum of efficacy for anxiety and depressive conditions, greater tolerability and safety compared with older classes of antidepressants, and lower potential for physical dependence as compared with the benzodi-azepines (see Table 16-2).

   b. These agents include the following drugs:

       i. fluoxetine (Prozac) 20 to 80 mg/day

       ii. sertraline (Zoloft) 50 to 200 mg/day

       iii. paroxetine (Paxil) 20 to 50 mg/day

       iv. paroxetine controlled-release (Paxil-CR 25–62.5 mg/day)

       v. fluvoxamine (Luvox) 50 to 300 mg/day

       vi. citalopram (Celexa) 20 to 50 mg/day

       vii. escitalopram (Lexapro) 10–20 mg/day

       viii. venlafaxine (SNRI: Effexor-XR) 75–225 mg/day)

   c. **Treatment of anxious patients is typically started with half the usual starting dose** (e.g., 10 mg for fluoxetine, 25 mg sertraline, 10 mg paroxetine, 12.5 mg paroxetine-CR, 25 mg fluvoxamine, 10 mg citalopram, 5 mg escitalopram, 37.5 mg/d venlafaxine) used for depression in order to minimize anxiety often associated with antidepressant initiation. Doses can usually be raised, after a week of acclimation, to typical therapeutic levels. Patients with OCD and PTSD may require higher doses (e.g., fluoxetine 60 to 80 mg/day) to receive maximum benefit.

   d. **Onset of benefit with SSRIs/SNRIs and other antidepressants usually occurs within two to three weeks of treatment.** SSRIs/SNRIs are better tolerated than older classes of antidepressants (e.g., TCAs), yet may be associated with transient or persistent adverse effects, including nausea, headaches, sexual dysfunction or apathy, sleep disturbance, and increased anxiety. SSRIs/SNRIs are usually administered in the morning to minimize associated sleep disturbance, although they may be sedating (particularly paroxetine) for some patients.

   e. Other newer agents, including nefazodone (Serzone), and mirtazapine (Remeron) appear to be effective for anxious patients in clinical practice though there is relatively little systematic data for these indications. Nefazodone may cause increased stimulation

Table 16-2. Pharmacotherapy of Anxiety Disorders

	SSRIs/SNRIs	TCAs	MAOIs	BZDs	Buspirone	CBT
Panic Disorder	+	+	+	+	+/_ [b]	+
GAD	+	+	+	+	+	+
Social Phobia	+	–	+	+	+/_ [b]	+
Specific Phobia	–	–	–	+/_	–	+
PTSD	+	+	+	+/_	–	+
OCD	+	– [a]	+	+/– [b]	+/– [b]	+

[a]Clomipramine is effective.
[b]Used adjunctively with serotonergic antidepressants.

NOTE: BZDs, Benzodiazepines; CBT, cognitive-behavioral therapy; GAD, generalized anxiety disorder; MAOIs, monoamine oxidase inhibitors; OCD, obsessive-compulsive disorder; PTSD, post-traumatic stress disorder; SSRIs, selective serotonin reuptake inhibitors; SNRIs, serotonin-norepinephrine reuptake inhibitors; TCAs, tricyclic antidepressants.

early in the treatment of anxious patients, and so should be initiated at low doses (e.g., 50 mg/day) with doses titrated up to therapeutic levels as tolerated; concerns about hepatotoxicity have also limited use of this agent. Limited data suggest that trazodone may be less effective for panic disorder than other available agents; data addressing the efficacy of bupropion for panic disorder is mixed.

2. **Tricyclic Antidepressants**
   a. **The TCAs are effective for panic disorder and generalized anxiety disorder, but less so for social phobia, and are, with the exception of clomipramine, largely ineffective for OCD.** The TCAs are also effective for depressive and anxiety symptoms associated with PTSD. The TCAs have largely been supplanted by the SSRIs as first-line interventions for the treatment of anxiety and depressive disorders because of their greater side-effect burden and more narrow spectrum of efficacy, but they remain potentially useful medications for patients who fail to respond to the newer agents.
   b. The TCAs include the following drugs:
      i. Imipramine (Tofranil)
      ii. Nortriptyline (Pamelor)
      iii. Desipramine (Norpramin)
      iv. Amitriptyline (Elavil)
      v. Doxepin (Sinequan)
   c. **Initiation of treatment with the TCAs may be associated with worsening of anxiety, so treatment is started with a "test dose" (e.g., 10 mg of imipramine or desipramine). Doses are titrated up as tolerated over the first few weeks of treatment.**
   d. The target dose of imipramine (or its equivalent) for panic disorder is approximately 2.25 mg/kg/day (100 to 200 mg/day for most patients) with a total 12-hour plasma level of imipramine plus desipramine of 110 to 140 ng/ml (Mavissakalian & Perel, 1995). Doses of nortriptyline are generally half those of imipramine.
   e. **Side effects of the TCAs include anticholinergic effects (e.g., dry mouth, constipation), cardiac conduction disturbance, orthostatic hypotension, weight gain, and sexual dysfunction. In addition, the TCAs, unlike the SSRIs, may be fatal in overdose.**

3. **Monoamine Oxidase Inhibitors (MAOIs)**
   a. **The MAOIs are broadly effective agents for the treatment of panic disorder, social phobia, agoraphobia, OCD, PTSD, GAD, and depression.**
   b. These agents include phenelzine (Nardil 45 to 90 mg/day) and tranylcypromine (Parnate 30 to 60 mg/day). The MAOIs are less likely to cause increased anxiety at treatment initiation than are the other antidepressants, but over time they may be associated with a variety of side effects, including weight gain, insomnia, edema, sexual dysfunction, and myoclonus.
   c. **In addition, patients on MAOIs are vulnerable to hypertensive reactions if they ingest tyramine (contained in certain foods and beverages) or sympathomimetic agents (e.g., pseudoephedrine),** so patients need to monitor their diet carefully and avoid a number of prescribed substances. Because of the potential adverse effects associated with their use, the MAOIs are generally reserved for patients who fail to improve with safer and more "user-friendly" interventions, and are typically prescribed by psychiatrists or others experienced in their use. All physicians should be aware that MAOI-treated patients should not receive meperidine (Demerol) because of a potentially fatal toxic interaction.
   d. Although supplanted by the SSRIs, which have a generally shared spectrum of efficacy but superior safety and side-effect profile, MAOIs may be useful to patients refractory to other interventions.

B. Benzodiazepines

1. **General Considerations**

   a. **All benzodiazepines are effective for generalized anxiety and insomnia; however, high-potency benzodiazepines (e.g., alprazolam, clonazepam) are generally preferred for panic disorder, although all agents may be effective at equipotent doses.**

   b. **Drug selection includes consideration of pharmacokinetic properties** (see Table 16-3). For single or acute dosing, the onset of effect is determined by the rate of absorption from the stomach and the lipophilicity of the benzodiazepine. The half-life of a drug predicts its accumulation in plasma with multiple dosing and the rapidity of washout during drug discontinuation. Rapid washout contributes to inter-dose rebound anxiety and withdrawal-related symptoms. Drug selection may depend on the desired clinical effect.

      i. A long-acting agent (e.g., clonazepam) can minimize inter-dose rebound anxiety and permit less frequent dosing.

      ii. A rapid-onset agent (e.g., alprazolam or diazepam) can provide acute anxiolysis.

      iii. A short-acting agent (e.g., alprazolam or lorazepam) can minimize drug accumulation and oversedation.

Table 16-3. Characteristics of Commonly Used Benzodiazopines

Drug (Trade Name)	Half-life (hours)	Dose (Mg Equivalent)	Onset	Significant Metabolites	Route of Administration
Alprazolam (Xanax; Xanax-XR)	12–15	0.5	Intermediate–Fast	No	PO
Chlordiazepoxide (Librium)	5–30	10	Intermediate	Yes	PO; IV
Clonazepam[a] (Klonopin)	15–50	0.25	Intermediate	No	PO
Clorazepate (Tranxene)	30–200	7.5	Fast	Yes	PO
Diazepam (Valium)	20–100	5.0	Fast	Yes	PO; IV
Flurazepam (Dalmane)	40	5.0	Fast	Yes	PO
Lorazepam (Ativan)	10–20	1.0	Intermediate	No	IV, IM, PO
Oxazepam (Serax)	5–15	15	Slow	No	PO

[a]Commonly used to treat panic disorder

c. **Side effects of benzodiazepines include sedation, ataxia, psychomotor impairment, and behavioral disinhibition.** Tolerance to these effects often develops with continued treatment. Respiratory depression is generally only a concern in patients with COPD or sleep apnea, or in overdose. Elderly patients generally require lower doses and are at higher risk for adverse psychomotor effects (e.g., confusion, amnesia, oversedation, falls). Prolonged use of benzodiazepines in the elderly should be avoided when possible.

d. **Patients with a history of alcohol or drug abuse are at increased risk for benzodiazepine abuse;** studies suggest that anxiety patients without a substance abuse predisposition do not misuse benzodiazepines. Rapid-onset agents (e.g., diazepam or alprazolam) have higher abuse potential than do slower-onset agents (e.g., oxazepam). The potential for benzodiazepine abuse can be minimized by avoiding repeated phone prescribing, by monitoring refills, and by encouraging regular follow-up. Although patients do not seem to develop tolerance to the anxiolytic effects of benzodiazepines, they do develop physical dependence and may experience rebound or withdrawal symptoms during drug discontinuation.

e. **Benzodiazepines should be initiated at low doses (e.g., 0.5 mg b.i.d. to t.i.d. alprazolam, 0.25 to 0.5 mg qhs clonazepam) to minimize initial sedation and increased every three to four days as tolerated until therapeutic.** Although some panic disorder patients respond to relatively low doses, **typical therapeutic doses are 2 to 8 mg/day for alprazolam and 1 to 4 mg/day for clonazepam.** Treatment of GAD may be initiated with benzodiazepines (e.g., lorazepam 1 to 2 mg/day or its equivalent and titrated up with a general dose range on the order of 2 to 8 mg/day). Inadequate dosing with benzodiazepines may be associated with continued symptoms, distress, and disability and contribute to patient non-compliance. Because of its relatively short half-life, alprazolam is generally administered on a q.i.d. dosing basis; patients may notice inter-dose rebound and morning rebound anxiety as plasma levels of the drug drop between doses. The longer-acting agent, clonazepam, can be administered on a b.i.d. basis with less interdose rebound symptomatology. An extended release formulation of alprazolam (Xanax-XR) was recently introduced. It permits once-a-day dosing though it does not significantly change the elimination half-life and need for gradual taper with discontinuation.

f. Given that both antidepressants and benzodiazepines are effective for many anxiety conditions, drug selection involves consideration of the risks and benefits of each class of agents. **The advantages of the benzodiazepines include a rapid onset of effect and relatively favorable side-effect profile. Potential drawbacks include their propensity to cause sedation, disinhibition (particularly in organically-impaired individuals), and physical dependence.** Depression, frequently co-morbid with anxiety disorders, does not generally respond as well to benzodiazepines as to antidepressants, and mood symptoms may be worsened by the benzodiazepine.

C. Buspirone

Buspirone is an azapirone anxiolytic with effects on serotonin and dopamine receptors; it is indicated for treatment of GAD. As a non-benzodiazepine, it lacks sedative or anticonvulsant properties or abuse potential. It is not effective alone for the treatment of panic disorder. At higher doses (60 to 90 mg/day) buspirone may have some weak antidepressant properties, although this is uncertain. Treatment is generally initiated with 10 mg b.i.d. and titrated up if necessary to 30 mg b.i.d. Perhaps in part because of a therapeutic lag to efficacy of several weeks and the need for dose titration, buspirone has had variable and often disappointing results in clinical practice, particularly when used in patients with prior exposure to benzodiazepines.

D. Alternative Agents

1. **Gabapentin (Neurontin)**

   The anticonvulsant gabapentin is being increasingly used in psychiatry for a variety of indications, including anxiety (panic as well as generalized anxiety), mood instability, sleep disturbance, and pain. It tends to show its anxiolytic effect within a few days to weeks of treatment-onset. Dosing is usually initiated at 300 mg qhs and titrated up in b.i.d. to t.i.d. fashion against therapeutic effects and side effects, such as sedation and dizziness, to a typical range of 900–3600 mg/day.

2. **Trazodone**

   The atypical antidepressant trazodone is sedating and has been effective for relief of generalized anxiety and anxiety-related sleep disturbance in some patients. Low doses (e.g., 50 to 100 mg qhs) may be an effective sleep aid, and doses of up to 400 mg/day may be tried for generalized anxiety. Besides sedation, potential side effects include orthostatic hypotension, GI distress, and a risk of priapism in men (approximately 1 in 6000). Its propensity to induce orthostasis may be particularly problematic in the elderly or medically compromised in whom it may result in falls and attendent morbidity.

3. **Beta-Blockers**

   Beta-blockers (e.g., propranolol, 10 to 40 mg/day prn 1 to 2 hours before a performance situation) may reduce peripheral autonomic symptoms of anxiety, such as tremor or tachycardia, but are less effective in blocking cognitive and emotional symptoms, such as worry or fear. Thus, with the exception of performance anxiety, they are generally not first-line agents for the treatment of anxiety, although they may be useful adjunctively to reduce the physical symptoms of arousal. Atenolol (25 to 100 mg) is also effective, and because it is less lipophilic may be less likely to cause fatigue or dysphoria.

E. Combining Antidepressants and Benzodiazepines

Antidepressants and benzodiazepines can be combined at the initiation of treatment to obtain the rapid anxiolysis associated with benzodiazepines, decrease the activation associated with antidepressant initiation, and provide antidepressant coverage of co-morbid depression. For many patients, benzodiazepines may be tapered after a few weeks when the antidepressant exerts its therapeutic effect, but some patients remain on combined treatment indefinitely with generally good results.

F. Discontinuation of Treatment for Anxiety Disorders

1. **Long-term use of antidepressants and benzodiazepines for anxious patients is often required to maintain ongoing benefit and prevent relapse.** For patients who do attempt discontinuation, withdrawal and rebound symptoms are more common with discontinuation of benzodiazepines than with other antianxiety treatments. Withdrawal symptoms can occur, however, even with discontinuation of antidepressants (e.g., a flu-like syndrome with the SSRIs or so-called cholinergic rebound with the TCAs), and these agents should be tapered when possible. Abrupt discontinuation of prolonged benzodiazepine treatment can be associated with rebound anxiety and insomnia, irritability, tremulousness, and even seizures. Short-half-life agents are more often associated with discontinuation difficulties.

2. **Strategies for Discontinuation**

   a. **The critical strategy in discontinuing benzodiazepines or other antianxiety medication is a slow taper,** particularly with the benzodiazepines or shorter-acting antidepressants (e.g., TCAs, sertraline, paroxetine, or venlafaxine). For instance, alprazolam should generally be tapered at rates of no greater than 0.5 to 1 mg/week, clonazepam 0.25 to 0.5 mg/week, paroxetine 10mg/week, or venlafaxine 75 mg/week. Many patients may benefit from even more gradual rates of discontinuation. Rapid rates of taper are associated with increased withdrawal symptomatology and patient distress and should thus be avoided when possible.

b. **For some patients, switching from a shorter-acting agent (e.g., alprazolam) to a longer-acting agent (e.g., clonazepam) can be helpful before initiating a taper;** a longer half-life may be associated with more gradual decreases in plasma levels during discontinuation and thus attenuate emergent symptomatology. The switch from alprazolam to clonazepam can be accomplished by substituting an equivalent amount of clonazepam for alprazolam (generally a 1:2 ratio) with use of alprazolam prn up to the former standing dose for the first seven days (Herman et al., 1987). After the first week, residual anxiety can be managed by adjusting the dose of clonazepam. Cognitive-behavioral interventions during the discontinuation process can also be useful; they are discussed in greater detail in Chapters 9 and 10.

XV. Non-pharmacologic Interventions for Anxiety Disorders

A. Cognitive-Behavioral Therapy (CBT)

CBT is predicated on the theory that the distress and impairment associated with anxiety and panic are mediated by maladaptive cognitive responses that promote anxiety and avoidance. **The core components of CBT for panic disorder include correction of cognitive misperceptions and overreactions to anxiety symptoms, breathing retraining, and muscle relaxation as well as exposure and desensitization to phobic situations.** Behavior therapy for OCD emphasizes "exposure" (to feared situations or objects) and "response prevention" (preventing compulsive behavior in response to the exposure). CBT and behavior therapy can produce results comparable to pharmacotherapy and can be used in combination with medications. Cognitive behavioral interventions are discussed in greater detail in Chapters 9 and 10.

B. Psychotherapies

An individual's psychological make-up, coping style, interpersonal dynamics, and situational stressors may contribute to the genesis and maintenance of pathologic anxiety in the clinical setting. Supportive, insight-oriented, family, and other types of therapy may be helpful when these factors appear prominently in the patient's presentation (see Chapter 2).

Suggested Readings

American Psychiatric Association. (1994). *Diagnostic and statistical manual of mental disorders* (4th ed., primary care version). Washington, DC: American Psychiatric Association, pp. 47–63.

Charney, D.S., & Deutsch, A. (1996). A functional neuroanatomy of anxiety and fear: Implications for the pathophysiology and treatment of anxiety disorders. *Critical Reviews in Neurobiology, 10*(3–4), 419–446.

Coryell, W., Noyes, R., & Clancy, J. (1992). Excess mortality in panic disorder. *Archives of General Psychiatry, 39,* 701–703.

Gorman, J.M., & Coplan, J.D. (1996). Comorbidity of depression and panic disorder. *Journal of Clinical Psychiatry, 57*(suppl 10), 34–41.

Herman, J., Rosenbaum, J., & Brotman, A. (1987). The alprazolam to clonazepam switch for the treatment of panic disorder. *Journal of Clinical Psychiatry, 7,* 175–178.

Johnson, M.R., & Lydiard, R.B. (1995). The neurobiology of anxiety disorders. *Psychiatric Clinics of North America, 18,* 681–725.

Katon, W., Hall, M.L., Russo, J., et al. (1988). Chest pain: The relationship of psychiatric illness to coronary arteriography results. *American Journal of Medicine, 84,* 1–9.

Katon, W., Von Korff, M., Lin, E., et al. (1990). Distressed high utilizers of medical care: *DSM III-R* diagnoses and treatment needs. *General Hospital Psychiatry, 12,* 355–362.

Kawachi, I., Colditz, G.A., Ascherio, A., et al. (1994). Prospective study of phobic anxiety and risk of coronary heart disease in men. *Circulation, 89,* 1992–1997.

Kessler, R.C., McGonagle, K.A., Zhao, S., et al. (1994). Lifetime and twelve-month prevalence of *DSM III-R* psychiatric disorders in the United States: Results from the National Comorbidity survey. *Archives of General Psychiatry, 51,* 8–19.

Klerman, G.L., Weissman, M.M., Ouellette, R., et al. (1991). Panic attacks in the community: Social morbidity and health care utilization. *Journal of the American Medical Association, 265,* 742–746.

Leon, A.C., Olfson, M., Broadhead, W.E., et al. (1995). Prevalence of mental disorders in primary care: Implications for screening. *Archives of Family Medicine, 4*(10), 857–861.

Markowitz, J.S., Weissman, M.M., Ouellette, R., et al. (1989). Quality of life in panic disorder. *Archives of General Psychiatry, 46,* 984–992.

Mavissakalian, M.R., & Parel, J.M. (1995). Imipramine treatment of panic disorder with agoraphobia: Dose ranging in plasma level response relationships. *American Journal of Psychiatry, 152,* 673–682.

Pollack, H.M., & Smoller, J.W. (1995). The longitudinal course and outcome of panic disorder. *Psychiatric Clinics of North America, 18,* 789–801.

Rosenbaum, J.F., Pollack, M.H., Otto, M.W., et al. (1996). Anxiety. In N.H. Cassem, T.A. Stern, J.F. Rosenbaum, & M.S. Jellinek (Eds.), *Massachusetts General Hospital handbook of general hospital psychiatry* (4th ed.). St. Louis, MO: Mosby-Year Book Inc., pp. 173–210.

Schurman, R.A., Kramer, P.D., Mitchell, J.B. (1985). The hidden mental health network: Treatment of mental illness by nonpsychiatric physicians. *Archives of General Psychiatry, 42,* 89–94.

Smoller, J.W., Pollack, M.H., Rosenbaum, J.F., et al. (1997). Panic, anxiety, and pulmonary disease: Theoretical and clinical considerations. *American Journal of Respiratory and Critical Care Medicine, 154,* 6–17.

Stein, M.B., Asinundson, J.G., Ireland, D., et al. (1994). Panic disorder in patients attending a clinic for vestibular disorders. *American Journal of Psychiatry, 151,* 1697–1700.

Van der Kolk, B., Dreyfuss, D., Michaels, M., et al. (1994). Fluoxetine in posttraumatic stress disorder. *Journal of Clinical Psychiatry, 55*(12), 517–522.

Walker, E.A., Gelfand, A.N., Gelfand, M.D., et al. (1995). Psychiatric diagnoses, sexual and physical victimization, and disability in patients with irritable bowel syndrome or inflammatory bowel disease. *Psychological Medicine, 25,* 1259–1267.

Wells, K.B., Goldberg, G., Brook, R.H., et al. (1986). Quality of care for psychotropic drug use in internal medicine group practices. *Western Journal of Medicine, 145,* 710–714.

CHAPTER 17

The Patient with Acute Grief

AVERY D. WEISMAN AND THEODORE A. STERN

I. Introduction

A. Definition

Grief is a variable but normal response, the price of having loved and needed, and now of being lost and bereaved. **Acute grief, along with its characteristic signs, is the first phase of the bereavement process.** It typically starts with the recent death of a person who was significant to the well-being and effective functioning of the bereaved. However, grief is not limited to loss via death; it can follow any recent or sudden loss, deprivation, injury, insult, illness, or disenfranchisement.

B. Severity of Grief

Grief is usually proportionate to the disruption caused by loss. Seldom does acute grief cause a medical or psychiatric emergency, but the clinician may be called upon for a compassionate intervention.

II. Who Suffers from Acute Grief?

A. Primary Mourners

Be aware that a mourner has the right to mourn, because of the love held for the deceased. **The primary mourner is the person who stands to lose the most by a recent death.** The primary mourner may suffer silently, appear under control, and be able to cope, without frightening family or friends. Such mourners may relapse later, when no one is around to listen and help them voice grief. Sometimes, another death, even of someone relatively distant, evokes the acute signs missing from the earlier bereavement.

B. Secondary Mourners

Secondary mourners, for whom the death causes less disruption and far less withdrawal, also suffer.

III. Signs of Acute Grief

A. Characterization of Grief

Acute grief is not an illness, but a normal part of life. It is an existential response that sooner or later normalizes, regardless of how extreme it seems at first. Designating the mourner as a "patient" or the signs of acute grief as "symptoms" is not helpful.

B. Typical Signs of Acute Grief

Symptoms include agitation, weeping, wailing, as well as feelings of aimlessness, hopelessness, helplessness, and a devaluation of the empty world. Idealization of the person now dead or the status of the prior situation now gone also arise. Signs of grief are typical, but do vary.

C. Stages of Mourning

The mourner should not be stereotyped as undergoing an expectable series of responses. **Not everyone mourns in the same way, for the same reasons, and in a given sequence.** Mourning is influenced by age, culture, community pressure, religious beliefs, and personal factors. Some feelings of grief cannot be voiced, others are mixed with relief at change, such as happens sometimes following a divorce.

IV. What Should or Can Be Done about Acute Grief?

A. Psychological Interventions for Acute Grief

Once the clinician realizes that acute grief is normal despite upsetting signs, and recognizes that pressure to treat often comes from secondary mourners, management is neither medical nor psychiatric. It becomes a question of how best to intervene and how to encourage the next phase of the mourning process, which is called bereavement.

1. **The right to mourn. Do not discourage open emotional expression (or catharsis) by urging total control.** As a rule, statements made by well-meaning friends and family unwittingly attempt to abort the mourning process.

2. **What shall I say? Presence is most important, avoiding the pressure to provide directives about control, or instructions about the philosophy or theology of death and loss.** There are a multitude of sayings, bromides, and faulty expressions of sympathy that are ineffective and counterproductive. "Try to control yourself. . . . Think of the children." "I understand exactly how you're feeling." Talking about your own past sorrows and triumphs is definitely out of place.

3. **What about grief that is hidden or unacceptable? As a rule, whenever someone intervenes and makes explicit what has been hidden heretofore, that grief becomes legitimate and acceptable.** Death of a mistress or a homosexual lover, loss of a pet, and many other deep attachments that society may not approve of also deserve informed intervention (sometimes more so because there are no established rules or ceremonies for a lost love that conventional society looks away from).

4. **Catharsis versus control. Appropriate intervention in acute grief strives for a balance between acknowledging a loss, legitimizing it, expressing sorrow, and starting to cope with the implications (including impairment of social function) of the loss.**

5. **Character of a good intervention. Not every practitioner is equally capable of intervening effectively in situations of acute loss accompanied by grief.** This is because clinicians have different abilities to preserve an equidistant stance between empathy (which amounts to making the clinician a professional mourner) and clinical objectivity (which may be devoid of sympathy). **Frequently, intervention depends on a balance between acceptance of a loss and denial of it.**

   Although anyone with a medical license can prescribe an antidepressant or a tranquilizer, **not everyone has credibility** (true sincerity), **compassion** (which respects a loss and does not expect it to vanish immediately), and **the capacity to collaborate** (without being overly directive). These qualities are like any other skill: they can be learned if a practitioner is earnest enough, willing to listen, and can refrain from uttering platitudes about loss and compensation, or giving gratuitous advice based on opinion. Be aware that help for a mourner is limited, and that acute grief gradually transforms itself. Signs of helplessness must change in time to dealing with tasks of adaptation, living without the significant other, and re-entering the newly-defined world. Significant family members among friends and family can assist with longer-term support, especially when decisions are to be made and practical matters are concerned. These people are particularly important and should be carefully alerted when there is risk of self-harm.

6. **Other guidelines.** In the presence of helplessness and hopelessness, there is always a tendency to give pep talks, exhorting the victim to do something other than what he or she is doing. Sometimes this is like blaming the victim and putting pressure on the person to conform to the way society finds comfortable and acceptable.

B. **Pharmacological Therapy of Grief**

Pharmacological agents, which help mute the more overt and disturbing signs of recent loss, **should be used judiciously, for a brief time, and with specific aims in mind.** Frequently, the secondary mourners become agitated by the seeming intractable symptoms of the primary mourner and call upon the physician to do something about it. Despair, to the level of self-harm or potential suicide, deserves a psychiatric evaluation, but temporary insomnia and loss of appetite do not. Without a history of depression, suicide is unlikely, but might be mentioned if the affected person talks about worthlessness, being better off dead, having unusual guilt, wanting to join the deceased, and so on. Other symptoms are treated "symptomatically," but not by psychotherapeutic interpretations, which are usually irrelevant and unhelpful. Lorazepam, 0.5 mg for sleep, is mild enough and effective enough.

1. **Tranquility versus sedation. A small dose of tranquility through medication (e.g., lorazepam) may be helpful,** provided that it stops short of sedation and does not interfere with the right to mourn. "Here, this will help you to sleep tonight. You'll need some sleep, to feel a little better than you do right now." Sedation can be painful, because a groggy mourner may also feel guilty, without clear thought and feeling, and unable to cope with what is expected.

V. How Long Should Grief Last?

A. **Duration of Grief**

In some respects this is like asking, "How high is up?" However, when asked in the light of acute grief, it usually means that other people, sometimes the practitioner, are becoming impatient. **Acute grief, in general, lasts months beyond the standard expectations or ceremonies that observe grief.** There are pangs of remembrance, semi-hallucinatory flashbacks, and loneliness. The tasks of mourning are acceptance of loss and re-entry into a transformed world. Practitioners can offer check-ups during the first nine months, depending on the mourner's inclination. How often one sees the grief-stricken varies; the process is one of normalization. The message is "I care."

Caution: **Do not promise more than can be delivered.** As a rule, patients do not ask for immediate resolution. **Put no time limit on recovery, and don't talk too much.**

VI. Principles of Managing Acute Grief

A. **There is not only one way to grieve;** not everyone expects one type of treatment.

B. **There is not only one reason for acute grief** (i.e., a recent death of a loved one). Other acute and chronic losses precipitate grief. Mourning is measured by the social and emotional disruption caused by a loss.

C. **There is no sole reason to intervene with patients suffering from acute grief.** The goal is not just to get rid of it as quickly as possible. Remember, instead, that grief is normal; the wound needs to be talked about, but not by the professional, who is more effective when listening.

D. **Psychopharmacological treatment is not the primary treatment for grief.** Despite urgings by bystanders made uncomfortable by grief, medication is usually secondary to the grief work put in motion. Medication may soothe, promote sleep, and relieve anxiety and depression, but must do no harm.

E. **Acute grief tends to become less painful over time. However, do not count on bereavement ever to disappear entirely.** Memories are precious; many subsequent situations reactivate grief. Social and emotional support are, perhaps, the most important and least expensive interventions. Gratuitous advice or inspirational exhortation is either useless or harmful.

F. **The practitioner makes a mistake when believing that grief is for the other person,** usually a patient. We are all prospective patients, and the sorrowing human currently suffering grief, might one day be you. Consequently, composure and compassion are important virtues to cultivate and practice.

G. **Not every person wants to talk, especially during the early hours and days of acute grief.** This must be respected; **the practitioner must not try to force a patient to talk.** A few quiet moments away from the emotional and social hubbub may be rewarding. Formal interviews should be conducted by professionals with enough time and skill, and should be held in a proper place.

Suggested References

Casaret, D., Kutner, J.S., & Abrahm, J. (2001). End-of-life care consensus panel. Life after death: A practical approach to grief and bereavement. *Annals of Internal Medicine, 134*(3), 208–215.

Fuller, R.L., & Geis, S. (1985). Communicating with the grieving family. *Journal of Family Practice, 21*(2), 139–144.

Kaunonem, M., Tarkka, M.T., Laippala, P., & Paunonen-Ilmonen, M. (2000). The impact of supportive telephone call intervention on grief after the death of a family member. *Cancer Nursing, 23*(6), 483–491.

Pasnau, R.D., Fawsy, F.I., & Fawsy, N. (1987). Role of the physician in bereavement. *Psychiatric Clinics of North America, 10*(1), 109–120.

Prigerson, H.G., & Jacobs, S.C. (2001). Perspectives on care of the close of life. Caring for bereaved patients: "All the doctors just suddenly go." *Journal of the American Medical Association, 286*(11), 1369–1376.

Shapiro, E.R. (1996). Family bereavement and cultural diversity: A social developmental perspective. *Family Process, 35*(3), 313–332.

Zeitlin, S.V. (2001). Grief and bereavement. *Primary Care, 28*(2), 415–425.

Zerbe, K.J., & Steinberg, D.L. (2000). Coming to terms with grief and loss. Can skills for dealing with bereavement be learned? *Postgraduate Medicine, 108*(6), 97–98, 101–104, 106.

Zisook, S., & DeVaul, R. (1985). Unresolved grief. *American Journal of Psychoanalysis, 45*(4), 370–379.

CHAPTER 18

The Patient with Hallucinations and Delusions

ALICIA POWELL, STEPHAN HECKERS, AND MICHAEL BIERER

I. Introduction

Hallucinations and delusions often are considered pathognomonic for psychotic disorders, especially schizophrenia. However, they can occur in many medical and neurologic conditions and also are found in other psychiatric disorders. They may be symptoms of reversible or life-threatening medical conditions; an erroneous diagnosis of schizophrenia can lead to ineffective or potentially harmful treatment of psychotic symptoms, whereas a thorough differential diagnosis can lead to specific, effective, and potentially curative interventions.

A. Definitions
1. **Hallucinations** are perceptions that occur in the absence of a corresponding sensory stimulus, have the full force or impact of real perceptions, and are not under the voluntary control of the experiencer. **Pseudohallucinations** either do not have the full force of real perceptions or are considered by the experiencer not to be true. **Hallucinosis** is an ongoing series of hallucinatory experiences, for example, during alcohol withdrawal or after a traumatic brain injury. **Illusions** are perceptions of external stimuli that are misinterpreted.
2. **Delusions** are persistent and unshakeable acceptances of false beliefs. **Preoccupation** refers to the recurrence of a thought that is neither unshakeable or necessarily false.

B. Classification. Hallucinations and delusions can be classified according to etiology and pathophysiology or according to the sensory domain and thought themes involved (Tables 18-1 and 18-2).

Table 18-1. Types of Hallucinations

Sensory Domain	Conditions	Examples
Visual	Decreased visual acuity	Cataract, choroidal disorders, Charles Bonnet syndrome, hemianopia, macular abnormalities, recent eye surgery
	Delirium	Delirium tremens
	Drug-induced	Hallucinogens, alcohol
	Migraine	Photism, bright lights
	Narcolepsy	Hypnagogic
	Peduncular hallucinations	Brainstem, thalamic lesion

(continued)

Table 18-1. Types of Hallucinations *(Continued)*

Sensory Domain	Conditions	Examples
Visual *(cont'd)*	Cerebrovascular	Occipital and/or temporal lesions
	Seizures	Micropsia, macropsia
Auditory	Seizures	Complex partial seizures
	Drug withdrawal states	Alcohol
	Psychiatric disorders	Schizophrenia
Olfactory and/or gustatory	Seizures	Especially complex partial seizures: foul smell, metallic taste
	Olfactory reference syndrome	
	Tumors	Meningioma
Tactile and/or pain	Formication	Drug-induced, psychosis
	Phantom limb	
Others	Autonomic	Complex partial seizures
	Somatosensory	Complex partial seizures
	Vestibular	
	Synesthesia	Sound-induced photism

Table 18-2. Types of Delusions

Thought Content	Phenomenology and Conditions
Persecution	Loss of property, poisoning, infection, influence (radio waves, x-rays, radar)
Somatic	Body dysmorphic disorder, hypochondriasis, parasitosis, somatization
Grandeur	Mania
Love/jealousy	Erotomania (de Clerambault's syndrome), phantom lover
Reduplication	Capgras' syndrome (person is replaced by an imposter), delusion of de Fregoli (person changes into many different people), doppelganger (self-double)

II. Evaluation

A. General Recommendations

1. Make the patient as comfortable as possible to facilitate the description of abnormal experiences. Allow the patient to talk freely and do not take a dismissive stance.
2. Assess the risk for self-harm or harm of others. If auditory hallucinations are suspected, ask about command hallucinations.
3. Rule out life-threatening medical causes of delusions or hallucinations and consider other medical causes (Table 18-3).
4. Evaluate the patient for possible psychiatric syndromes.

Table 18-3. Differential Diagnosis of Patients with Delusions and Hallucinations

Medical

Metabolic	Renal failure, hepatic failure, pancreatic disease, hyper/hyponatremia, hyper/hypocalcemia, hyper/hypoglycemia, porphyria, endocrinopathies (Addison's disease, Cushing's disease, hypo/hyperthyroidism, panhypopituitarism), dehydration, hyperosmolar states
Nutritional deficiency states	Thiamine, folate, B_{12}, niacin
Autoimmune disorders	Systemic lupus erythematosus, temporal arteritis
Drug-related	
Intoxication	"Street drugs" (alcohol, hallucinogens, heroin, inhalants, psychostimulants, MDMA and 3,4-methylene dioxymethamphetamine)
	Prescription drugs (antiarrhythmics, antibiotics, anticholinergics, antiparkinsonians, antituberculous, anti-malarial, anticonvulsants, antidepressants, anti-hypertensives, baclofen, belladonna alkaloids, chemo-therapeutic agents, cimetidine, digoxin, disulfiram, dopamine agonists, non-steroidal anti-inflamatory drugs, opiates, sedative-hypnotics, steroids, sympathomimetics)
	Over-the-counter drugs (antihistamines, anticholiner-gics, herbal remedies)
Withdrawal	Alcohol, hallucinogens, opiates, psychostimulants, sedative-hypnotics
Poisoning	Anticholinergics, carbon monoxide, heavy metals (arsenic, manganese, mercury, thallium)

Neurologic

Infection	Viral (e.g., herpes simplex virus, human immuno-deficiency virus), syphilis, parasitic, prions
Neoplasm, cerebrovascular, trauma	(especially frontal and temporal)
Degenerative	Alzheimer's disease, Pick's disease
Motor disorders	Parkinson's disease, Huntington's disease, Sydenham's chorea, Wilson's disease, idiopathic basal ganglia calcification, spinocerebellar degeneration
Seizure	Especially complex partial
Myelin disease	Adrenoleukodystrophy, metachromatic leukodystrophy, Marchiafava-Bignami disease, multiple sclerosis
Miscellaneous	Hydrocephalus, hypoxic encephalopathy, narcolepsy

Psychiatric

Psychotic disorders	Bipolar disorder, brief reactive psychosis, delusional disorder, post-partum psychosis, psychotic depression, schizoaffective disorder, schizophrenia, substance-induced psychosis
Others	Body dysmorphic disorder, borderline personality dis-order, dementia, malingering/factitious disorder, obses-sive-compulsive disorder, post-traumatic stress disorder, schizotypal personality disorder

B. Medical History

1. **Previous psychiatric disorders** should be identified and documented. Pay attention to any pre-existing psychotic or mood disorder as well as evidence of post-traumatic stress disorder or personality disorder (e.g., borderline and schizotypal) (see Chapters 13 and 56).

2. **Neurologic disorders** (e.g., seizure, degenerative disorders, neoplasms, traumatic brain injury, and stroke) often cause hallucinations and delusions. Infections and de-myelinating diseases also should be noted.

3. Multiple **medical conditions** (Table 18-3) can lead to abnormalities of perception and thought. Pay attention to endocrinopathies, autoimmune disorders, and conditions resulting in acute confusional states.

4. Document any history of illicit **drug use.** Substance-induced psychotic symptoms may persist long after the cessation of the offending drug (e.g., post-hallucinogen perceptual disorder months or years after lysergic acid diethylamide [LSD] use).

5. Document a **family history** of medical, neurologic, or psychiatric disorders that can lead to hallucinations or delusions.

C. Interview. The mental status examination often provides clues for the differential diagnosis of hallucinations and delusions.

1. Inquire about the patient's **thoughts.** Paranoid ideation occurs in many conditions, whereas **ideas of reference** (e.g., the belief that one is receiving special messages from the television or radio) and beliefs in thought manipulation or broadcasting typically are seen in schizophrenia.

2. Determine whether the patient is experiencing **hallucinations** in any sensory modality: visual, auditory, olfactory, gustatory, or tactile.

3. Ascertain the patient's level of **insight** into the delusion or hallucination. Patients with psychotic disorders typically have poor insight into their psychotic symptoms.

4. The patient's **appearance** (attention to personal hygiene, clothing, posture, and general nutritional state) may suggest an underlying psychotic thought process.

5. The patient's **eye contact** may be decreased (suggesting depression) or avoidant and hypervigilant (as in paranoia). Patients who are experiencing hallucinations may glance about the room as if responding to internal stimuli.

6. Listen for **slurred speech,** which may suggest an organic etiology (e.g., intoxication or stroke); an increased latency of response (i.e., delay before responding to questions) also can be seen in a hallucinating or delusional patient.

7. **Psychomotor activity** can be increased (as in a delusional and agitated patient) or decreased (as in a patient with depression). Tremor or bradykinesia may suggest an extrapyramidal movement disorder or be a manifestation of medication side effects.

8. The **outward display of emotion** (affect) should be differentiated from the **internally felt emotion** (mood). It is important to note whether the two are congruent with each other and are appropriate to the situation. Inquire about the neurovegetative signs of major depression: alterations in sleep, decreased interest, guilty ruminations, decreased energy, decreased concentration abilities, change in appetite, psychomotor agitation or retardation, and thoughts of suicide or death. These symptoms can be remembered by using the mnemonic SIG: E CAPS (see Chapter 15).

9. Ask the patient about **thoughts of self-harm or harming others.** Delusional or hallucinating patients may believe that they are being ordered to perform violent acts and find it difficult to resist those commands.

10. Take note of the patient's **thought processes.** Are the patient's thoughts tangential, grossly disorganized, or "loose" and difficult to follow (as seen in mania), or is there a decreased production of thoughts (as seen in depression and some forms of schizophrenia)?

11. A formal examination of the patient's **cognitive status** [e.g., the Mini-Mental State Examination (MMSE)] (see Chapter 49) is particularly useful in elderly patients to help rule out dementia.

D. Examination of the patient should include a **complete physical examination** focusing on signs of medical and neurologic conditions that are known to cause hallucinations and/or delusions (Table 18-3). For patients who are resistant to physical examination because of paranoia, it can be helpful to explain that the symptoms they are experiencing may have physical causes.

1. A thorough **neurologic exam** of cranial nerves, sensory and motor function, gait, reflexes, and cerebellar function helps rule out conditions, such as cerebrovascular accident, neoplasm, and motor disorder.

2. The commonly employed **laboratory screens** (routine chemistry panel, liver and thyroid function tests, calcium and magnesium levels, complete blood count, and levels of vitamin B_{12} and folate) usually are sufficient to detect the most common medical and neurologic conditions which may cause or exacerbate hallucinations and delusions. There is no proven utility of general laboratory screenings in patients with hallucinations or delusions. It is more helpful to test hypotheses generated by the history and physical examination, e.g., to rule out autoimmune diseases and endocrinopathies. Toxicologic screening of serum or urine is recommended, especially if the use of illicit drugs or toxic doses of prescription drugs is suspected.

3. **Neuroimaging** is indicated if there is a focal neurologic finding or if psychiatric symptoms are temporally related to physical illness (e.g., after head trauma or a cerebrovascular accident).

4. **Electroencephalography** should be performed if the history and physical examination are consistent with a seizure disorder. However, only 60–80% of all patients with a seizure disorder will have a markedly abnormal electroencephalogram (EEG).

III. Differential Diagnosis

A. **Secondary psychotic disorders** (those due to a medical illness) should be differentiated from primary psychotic disorders. An acute and late onset of psychotic symptoms, a pronounced cognitive deficit, and a lack of previous psychiatric symptoms make an organic etiology more likely.

B. **Abnormalities of the mental status** other than hallucinations or delusions can be useful diagnostically. Depressive symptoms are seen in patients with psychotic depression and bipolar disorder, pronounced cognitive deficits make a diagnosis of dementia more likely, and an impaired or fluctuating level of consciousness is a hallmark of acute confusional states.

C. **Characteristic psychotic symptoms,** such as **bizarre delusions** (e.g., a chip has been implanted in the patient's brain) and **prominent hallucinations** (e.g., hearing voices arguing about oneself) are typically seen in schizophrenia but are not pathognomonic.

D. **Auditory hallucinations,** especially voices, are the most common type of hallucination in patients with schizophrenia, and visual hallucinations are the most common type of hallucination in alcohol withdrawal states and drug intoxication. However, all sensory modalities can be altered in these conditions.

E. In the elderly, there is an increased incidence of **visual hallucinations** (e.g., Charles Bonnet syndrome) as well as persecutory and somatic delusions.

IV. Treatment Strategies

A. Conducting a search for **underlying medical conditions** is essential for the appropriate treatment of delusions and hallucinations. Correction of underlying abnormalities (e.g., abnormal glucose levels, thyroid dysfunction, and toxic levels of medication) alone often leads to normalization of mental status.

B. The clinician should **assess the severity of the psychotic symptoms.** Patients who appear to experience command hallucinations (potentially leading to dangerous or violent behavior) and patients who cannot take care of themselves should be evaluated by a psychiatrist on an emergent basis. Patients with a long history of abnormal thoughts or perceptions who are at a safe baseline may not need emergent psychiatric care, such as hospitalization.

C. Discuss with these patients their **degrees of disability** and the impact of hallucinations and delusions on their performance of daily activities. Patients who are severely distressed by hallucinations or delusions are more likely to be compliant with treatment than are patients with mild delusions or pleasant hallucinations.

D. If no treatable underlying conditions can be found, **symptomatic treatment of delusions and hallucinations** should be considered.

   1. Antipsychotic medications provide the most effective symptomatic treatment for hallucinations and delusions. Typically, an effective dose of haloperidol ranges from 2 to 10 mg/day (0.5 to 2.0 mg/day in the elderly) or the equivalent dose of other antipsychotics. Because all the traditional antipsychotics are equal in efficacy, the selection of a particular drug should be based on the patient's history of response to such medications as well as the drug's side effect profile (Table 18-4). Certain subgroups of patients may benefit from a particular antipsychotic medication.

      a. Patients with **extrapyramidal motor disorders** or a history of extrapyramidal side effects from typical antipsychotics may respond more favorably to the atypical antipsychotics risperidone, olanzapine, ziprasidone, quetiapine, or clozapine.

      b. **If agitation is prominent** or if the patient would benefit from a more sedating antipsychotic, a lower-potency neuroleptic, such as chlorpromazine, should be considered.

      c. **For patients with sensitivity to anticholinergic effects** (e.g., patients with a history of narrow-angle glaucoma, prostate enlargement, or cognitive deficits), a higher-potency antipsychotic, such as haloperidol, should be prescribed.

      d. Some reports suggest that in patients with an isolated delusional disorder, the antipsychotic pimozide has superior efficacy compared with other typical antipsychotics. Because of its calcium channel-blocking properties at higher doses, pimozide should be avoided in patients with cardiac illness.

      e. **If non-compliance is an obstacle to proper treatment** (and the patient has had minimal or no side effects from oral antipsychotic medication), a long-acting decanoate preparation of haloperidol or fluphenazine can be delivered intramuscularly on a regular schedule (monthly for haloperidol and every 2 to 3 weeks for fluphenazine).

   2. **Benzodiazepines** may be helpful in reducing the anxiety produced by delusions or hallucinations but do not provide definite symptomatic treatment. Patients

Table 18-4. Typical and Atypical Antipsychotic Drugs

Generic Name	Proprietary Name	Equivalent Dose, mg	Sedative Effect	Hypotensive Effect	Anticholinergic Effect	Extrapyramidal Effect	Weight Gain	QTc Prolongation	Prolactin Elevation
Typical Antipsychotics									
Chlorpromazine	Thorazine	100	S	S	I	W	I/S	I	S
Thioridazine	Mellaril	100	S	S	S	W	I/S	I	S
Molindone	Moban	10	W	W	W	W	W	S	NA
Perphenazine	Trilafon	8	W	W	W	I/S	W	S	NA
Trifluoperazine	Stelazine	5	W	W	W	S	I/S	W	S
Thiothixene	Navane	5	W	W	W	S	I/S	W	S
Fluphenazine	Prolixin	2	W	W	W	S	I/S	W	S
Haloperidol	Haldol	2	W	W	W	S	I/S	W	S
Atypical Antipsychotics									
Risperidone	Risperdal	NA	I	I	W	W	I	W/I	S
Olanzapine	Zyprexa	NA	I	W	S	W	S	W	W
Quetiapine	Seroquel	NA	S	S	W	W	I	W	W
Ziprasidone	Geodon	NA	I	I	W	W	W	I	W
Clozapine	Clozaril	NA	S	S	S	W	S	W	W

NOTE: S, strong; I intermediate; W, weak; NA, not available.

163

withdrawing from alcohol or sedatives and those in a confused or agitated state may benefit from the adjunctive use of benzodiazepines.

3. The **anticonvulsants**, carbamazepine and valproic acid, may be useful in controlling hallucinations and/or delusions. These medications should be considered particularly in patients with a history of head injury or suspected seizure activity. Also, patients whose symptoms of hallucinations or delusions worsen with antipsychotic treatment may benefit from a trial of an anticonvulsant. Serum drug levels should be checked to document a patient's individual range of therapeutic and/or toxic levels.

E. **Explain to the patient the expected results of treatment.** Tell the patient, "This should reduce the voices" or "This will probably help you feel less stressed about the people you feel are bothering you."

F. Whenever possible, **obtain the patient's permission to involve family members** or significant others in treatment and consult them on a regular basis (especially with paranoid patients) in the presence of the patient.

Selected References

Assad, G., & Shapiro, B. (1986). Hallucinations: Theoretical and clinical overview. *American Journal of Psychiatry, 143,* 1088–1097.

Benson, D.F., & Gorman, D.G. (1996). Hallucinations and delusional thinking. In B.S. Fogel, & R.B. Shiffer (Eds.), *Neuropsychiatry.* Baltimore: Williams & Wilkins, pp. 307–323.

Cummings, J.L. (1988). Organic psychosis. *Psychosomatics, 29,* 16–26.

Fricchione, G.L., Carbone, L., Bennett, W.I. (1995). Psychotic disorder caused by a general medical condition, with delusions. *Psychiatric Clinics of North America, 18,* 363–378.

Grunebaum, M.F., Oquendo, M.A., Harkavy-Friedman, J.M., et al. (2001). Delusions and suicidality. *American Journal of Psychiatry, 158*(5), 742–747.

Hersh, K., & Borum, R. (1998). Command hallucinations, compliance, and risk assessment. *Journal of the American Academy of Psychiatry and the Law, 26*(3), 353–359.

Zisook, S., Byrd, D., Kuck, J., & Jeste, D.V. (1995). Command hallucinations in outpatients with schizophrenia. *Journal of Clinical Psychiatry, 56,* 462–465.

CHAPTER 19

The Patient with Obsessions or Compulsions

DARIN D. DOUGHERTY AND MICHAEL A. JENIKE

I. Introduction

A. **Obsessive-compulsive disorder (OCD)** is a common but underdiagnosed disorder.
   1. The lifetime prevalence of OCD is 2–3% in the United States and 0.5–5.5% world-wide.
   2. The hallmark signs and symptoms of OCD include unwanted thoughts (obsessions) and repetitive behaviors (compulsions).
   3. Unlike patients with psychotic disorders, most patients with OCD maintain insight about the senselessness of their symptoms and are often embarrassed by them.
   4. Because OCD was once thought to be rare, many physicians and non-physician mental health professionals have not been trained to make the diagnosis of OCD, or to treat the disorder.

B. **Body dysmorphic disorder (BDD)** involves a preoccupation with an imagined or slight defect in physical appearance; it is an obsessive-compulsive spectrum disorder.
   1. In the medical setting, patients with BDD often present with dermatologic problems (from skin picking) or with requests for cosmetic surgery. Many patients with BDD undergo multiple cosmetic surgical procedures. Of course, due to the nature of their illness, they are unlikely to ever be satisfied with the results of their surgery.
   2. BDD often goes unrecognized and untreated.
   3. The symptoms of BDD dramatically reduce one's quality of life and can cause significant impairment.

II. Evaluation of the Problem

A. **General recommendations.** Since OCD commonly co-exists with other psychiatric disorders, the most efficient way to screen for it in a general medical practice is to ask specifically about obsessions and compulsions every time a patient presents with a psychiatric problem. Active screening will be necessary as these patients may not volunteer a description of their symptoms. Common conditions associated with OCD include the following:
   1. **Depression** (major depression and dysthymia)
   2. Any other **anxiety disorder** (panic disorder, generalized anxiety disorder, social phobia, or simple phobia)
   3. **Chemical dependency**
   4. **Tics** (motor or vocal)

B. **Symptomatology**
   1. **The most common obsessions include:**
      a. Themes of contamination
      b. Themes of violence, such as the fear of killing or stabbing someone and/or the fear of having hit a pedestrian while driving

      c. Sexual themes, such as homosexuality, bestiality, incest, sex with children (not pedophilia, since these are unwanted, abhorrent thoughts; these patients are not aroused by children)

      d. Blasphemous themes

      e. Somatic themes (see the section on differentiation from hypochondriasis as follows), such as fear of having cancer or HIV infection. In the medical setting, these patients may present with no risk factors for HIV infection but present for HIV testing. Often, they may request repeated testing as they do not believe negative test results.

      f. In patients with BDD, an imagined defect in physical appearance.

          i. These patients often have simultaneous concerns about more than one body part.

          ii. The most common concerns involve the hair, skin (especially the face), and nose.

          iii. The concern about an imagined defect in physical appearance is often all-consuming, occupying the patient's thoughts throughout the day.

2. **The most common compulsions include** the following:

      a. **Washing** (e.g., hand washing, long or frequent showers, washing of "contaminated" objects). In the medical setting, these patients may present with atypical dermatitis of the hands that results from frequent handwashing.

      b. **Checking** door locks, water faucets, stove burners, and light switches, along with excessive checking of work and driving back to see if they have hit someone else while driving. It may take people who check a long time to leave the house.

      c. **Counting** and other "number problems": contemplation of lucky or unlucky numbers, or doing things a certain number of times.

      d. **Repeating** other behaviors (e.g., tying shoes or walking through doors).

      e. **Hoarding** newspapers, spoiled food, wrappers, coupons, or useless clothes. By the time this comes to clinical attention, it is usually not a subtle problem.

      f. Patients with BDD often repeatedly check their appearance in mirrors and other reflecting surfaces. There may be behaviors that "conceal" a perceived defect and/or skin picking in an effort to correct the perceived imperfection. Ironically, these efforts at correcting an imperfection may cause an actual imperfection. Patients with BDD often avoid social situations and may give up working because of embarrassment about their appearance.

C. Interview. The most efficient way to screen for OCD is to ask patients with any other psychiatric disorder the following questions:

1. Do you have repeated unwanted thoughts that strike you in some way as being senseless (e.g., thoughts of contamination or violence)?

2. Do you do things over and over that strike you in some way as senseless or excessive (e.g., washing or checking)?

III. Psychiatric Differential Diagnosis

A. Delusional disorders (e.g., schizophrenia or psychotic depression). Unlike those with delusions, patients with obsessions almost always maintain a degree of insight and know that the content of their obsessions is senseless.

B. Hypochondriasis. Patients with somatic obsessions have more insight than do patients with hypochondriasis; they are more likely to understand on some level that they do not have the disease that they fear. Nevertheless, patients with OCD are unable to dismiss somatic obsession(s) without the proper treatment.

C. Major depression with ruminations. Ruminations lack the senseless quality of obsessions. "My wife left, and I miss her so much," for instance, is a repetitive, unwanted, and painful thought for the patient in this example, but it is not a senseless thought.

D. "Compulsive behaviors" (e.g., overeating, gambling, alcohol and/or drug abuse, or sexual behavior disorders). Unlike OCD, at some point in the course of these conditions, the behaviors do not strike the patient as senseless or unwanted. Instead, there is an element of pleasure involved. These patients find the consequences of their behaviors, rather than the behaviors themselves, troublesome.

E. Obsessive-compulsive personality disorder (OCPD). Only 5–15% of patients with OCD have OCPD. Unlike OCD patients, patients with OCPD do not have obsessions and compulsions as defined in this chapter. Instead, they have a life-long pattern of over-attention to detail, loss of the "big picture," rigidity, hypermorality, and an inability to express warm or loving feelings. While the symptoms bother OCD sufferers endlessly, generally it is those around a patient with OCPD who are more likely to complain about the OCPD symptoms; the patient is rarely perturbed.

IV. Diagnostic Criteria for Obsessive-Compulsive Disorder

A. Obsessions or compulsions cause significant distress; they interfere with functioning, or take up more than an hour each day.

1. Obsessions are recurrent, persistent thoughts that at some point in the illness strike the patient as senseless.
2. Compulsions are behaviors or mental rituals that are done in response to obsessions in an effort to allay the distress caused by these obsessions. At some point in the illness they strike the patient as senseless or excessive.

B. If the patient has another psychiatric diagnosis, he or she may still have OCD as long as the content of the obsessions is not restricted to the other psychiatric diagnosis. For example, a woman with a senseless thought that she is overweight who also has food-related rituals, marked weight loss, and amenorrhea may have OCD as well as anorexia nervosa (as long as she also has obsessions or compulsions that are not related to food and weight).

V. Diagnostic Criteria for BDD (an imagined defect in physical appearance)

A. The patient has a preoccupation with an imagined defect in appearance or a clear over-concern about a mild abnormality.

B. The preoccupation causes impairment in social, work, or other functioning, or causes the person distress.

C. It is not due to another psychiatric disorder, such as an eating disorder.

VI. Treatment Strategies

Optimal first-line treatment of both OCD and BDD involves serotonin reuptake inhibitors (SRIs) and behavior therapy. There are a number of alternative treatments that may be used if first-line treatments fail. In addition, patient education and involvement in a support group may be helpful.

A. First-line pharmacotherapy: SRIs

1. **These include all of the selective serotonin reuptake inhibitors (SSRIs) as well as one tricyclic antidepressant (TCA) (clomipramine).** The remaining TCAs are not effective for the treatment of OCD.

2. **Required doses are usually higher than the doses used for treatment of depression.**
   a. Fluvoxamine: up to 300 mg/day
   b. Fluoxetine: 40 to 80 mg/day
   c. Paroxetine: 40 to 60 mg/day
   d. Sertraline: up to 200 mg/day
   e. Citalopram: up to 60 mg/day
   f. Escitalopram: dose unknown
   g. Clomipramine: up to 250 mg/day
3. Each medication must be tried at a given dose for 10 to 12 weeks before it is possible to assess the efficacy of that dose. For this reason, it is usually best to advance the dose to those listed above relatively quickly so that the required 10 to 12-week trial can begin.
4. A 100% response to medication is rare. This should be addressed explicitly with the patient at the outset of treatment. However, with "only" a 50% reduction in symptom severity, the patient often feels much better and his or her ability to function may be greatly increased.
5. Length of treatment: Patients should remain on a medication for at least a year after maximum improvement has been achieved. Most will need treatment with SRIs indefinitely, as there is a high relapse rate once medication has been discontinued. It is felt that tapering medication slowly, over a few months, may reduce the risk of relapse. Patients who have had exposure therapy with response prevention have a much better chance of getting off, and staying off, medications.
6. The obsessions and compulsions often get worse under stress, even in patients who are doing better. If there is a foreseeable end to the stress, an adjustment in the dose may not be necessary.
7. Which SRI should one choose? In the few head-to-head trials that have been completed, no significant differences in efficacy have been found.
8. If the first SRI does not work, it is worth trying others.

B. **Second-line pharmacotherapy: SRI augmentation and alternative monotherapies**
   While most patients with OCD or BDD will respond to SRIs, some may require additional treatments.
   1. SRI Augmentation
      a. Controlled trials have demonstrated that SRI augmentation with neuroleptics (both conventional and atypical) can be highly effective for patients with treatment-resistant OCD or BDD.
         i. The most studied conventional neuroleptics have been haloperidol and pimozide and the most studied atypical neuroleptic has been risperidone. However, it is likely that patients will respond to other agents in each class.
         ii. Given the higher incidence of side effects with conventional neuroleptics, it may be best to initially augment an SRI with an atypical neuroleptic.
         iii. Examples and their typical dosages are:
            Pimozide: 1–3 mg/day
            Haloperidol   0.5–10 mg/day
            Risperidone   0.5–6.0 mg/day
         iv. Generally, a therapeutic trial of 4 weeks is adequate to determine if the augmentation strategy is efficacious.
      b. Although fewer controlled trials have been conducted with other agents that may be used for SRI augmentation, there is some evidence that clonazepam, buspirone, and lithium may be efficacious.

2. **Alternative monotherapies.** A small number of controlled studies suggest that three agents (clonazepam, buspirone, and MAOIs) may be effective alternative monotherapies for OCD. Data for BDD are not available. Given the small number of studies, these recommendations must be considered provisional.

   a. Clonazepam

   b. Buspirone

   c. Monoamine oxidase inhibitors (MAOIs)

      i. Some evidence suggests that use of MAOIs may be more effective in patients with co-morbid panic attacks, co-morbid social phobia, or prominent symmetry concerns.

      ii. Tranylcypromine up to 60 mg/day or phenelzine up to 90 mg/day.

      iii. As with SRIs, a trial length of 10–12 weeks is required to determine if the treatment is efficacious.

      iv. To avoid a potentially dangerous serotonergic crisis, it is essential that the MAOI not be started until an adequate washout from previously taken SRIs has been completed. This is 2–3 weeks for clomipramine or a short half-life SSRI, and 5-8 weeks for fluoxetine.

      v. Both the patient and physician must be aware of potential medication interactions and the need for a low tyramine diet.

C. First-line behavioral therapy: Exposure and response prevention. This is a form of behavior therapy that has been shown to work at least as well as medications, and it may have longer-lasting effects.

1. Patients are first carefully educated about the behavioral theory of OCD and the theory of exposure therapy with response prevention. As the assignments can be anxiety-provoking for the patients, it is important that they understand why they are doing what they are doing.

2. The patients are then asked to come into contact with the situations that they fear for a long enough time for the anxiety to diminish (exposure). Response prevention entails an agreement by these patients not to perform rituals while they are doing the exposure.

3. Individual exposure "exercises" typically last 20 minutes to 2 hours. The length may be adjusted according to the patient's response to the exposure.

4. The patient's attitude toward the anxiety is important to the success of the treatment. Ordinarily, patients try to ward off, diminish, or minimize the anxiety their obsessions arouse. During exposure therapy it is important that the patient adopt a different stance and deliberately face the anxiety—without attempting to diminish it.

5. The therapist acts as a coach or mentor. Most of the treatment is done at home or in the feared situation (as homework), not in the office sessions. The total number of hours of exposure is related to the degree and speed of treatment success.

6. **Exposure can be graded.** The patient should ideally suggest what she or he would like to try. If the exposure exercise chosen is too difficult, the patient should be encouraged to start with something easier and then build up to a more difficult assignment.

7. The texts listed at the end of this chapter are especially useful for learning how to guide patients to do this type of treatment.

D. Electroconvulsive therapy (ECT) is not an effective treatment for OCD or BDD, although it may be useful for treating co-morbid major depression.

E. Limbic system surgery (including anterior cingulotomy and capsulotomy) may be effective, if all other treatment options have failed.

F. Education about OCD
   1. Many books on OCD written for the lay public are available at bookstores.
   2. Pamphlets and other educational materials are available through the Obsessive-Compulsive Foundation, 9 Depot St., Milford CT, 06460 or http://www.ocfoundation.org.

G. Support groups
   1. The Obsessive-Compulsive Foundation can tell a patient where to find a support group near his or her home or place of work.
   2. These groups are an extremely valuable resource for education, and patients often express a sense of relief after meeting others who have the same condition.

Suggested Readings

Baer, L. (2000). *Getting control* (2nd ed.). New York: Plume.

Dougherty, D.D., Rauch, S.L., & Jenike, M.A. (2002). Treatment of obsessive-compulsive disorder. In P.E. Nathan, & J.M. Gorman (Eds.), *A guide to treatments that work* (2nd ed.). New York: Oxford University Press.

Dougherty, D.D., Baer, L., Cosgrove, G.R., et al. (2002). Prospective follow-up of 44 patients who received cingulotomy for treatment-refractory obsessive-compulsive disorder. *American Journal of Psychiatry, 159,* 269–275.

Jenike, M.A., Baer, L., & Minichiello, W.E. (Eds.). (1998). *Obsessive-compulsive disorders. Theory and management* (3rd ed.). St. Louis: Mosby.

Phillips, K. (1998). *The broken mirror*. New York: Oxford University Press.

Rapoport, J.L. (1989). *The boy who couldn't stop washing: The experience and treatment of obsessive compulsive disorder.* New York: Dutton.

Steketee, G., & White, K. *When once is not enough: Help for obsessive-compulsives.* Oakland, CA: New Harbinger.

CHAPTER 20

The Patient with Anorexia or Bulimia

JENNIFER BREMER, DAVID B. HERZOG, AND EUGENE V. BERESIN

I. Introduction

A. The Primary Care Physician's Role
Eating disorders are disabling and are associated with significant morbidity and mortality. In caring for a patient with an eating disorder, the primary care physician (PCP) has several critical tasks: recognizing the eating disorder, diagnosing and treating the medical complications, educating the patient about the medical consequences, determining when a patient requires hospitalization, and guiding the patient toward psychiatric treatment. Patients with eating disorders often do not obtain psychiatric treatment or they delay for years before starting treatment. The PCP has the opportunity to help guide these patients toward psychiatric care and thus affect an eating disorder's chronicity. The physician also may help a resistant patient realize the seriousness of her or his illness and encourage treatment.

B. Definitions
1. **Anorexia nervosa is a syndrome involving a disturbance in body image that leads to self-starvation. Patients with anorexia nervosa misperceive their bodies, which they see as being too fat. They suffer from a consuming fear of weight gain and consequently refuse to maintain their weight in a healthy range.** Anorectic patients use a variety of measures to remain underweight, including restricting food intake (restricting subtype), purging by vomiting or laxative use (binge-eating/purging subtype), and exercising excessively. The American Psychiatric Association has created criteria to help clarify these diagnoses.
2. **Bulimia nervosa is a syndrome characterized by frequent episodes of binge eating during which a bulimic patient eats large amounts of food and feels unable to control her or his food intake.** To prevent weight gain the patient then purges by vomiting, taking laxatives, taking diuretics, fasting, or exercising excessively. Weight fluctuations are typical in bulimic patients, who often are of normal weight. The American Psychiatric Association has developed criteria to clarify this diagnosis.
3. **The diagnoses of anorexia nervosa and bulimia nervosa occur along a spectrum, and it is common for patients to alternate between diagnoses during the course of illness.** Approximately half of anorexic patients have bulimic symptoms, and approximately half of bulimic patients have a history of anorexia nervosa at some point during their illness.
4. It is also common for women who do not meet the criteria for either diagnosis to have some symptoms of these eating disorders. Many women have body distortions or weight preoccupation and use restricting or binging and purging behaviors without meeting full criteria for anorexia nervosa or bulimia nervosa. Some women chew and

spit out food. Such women may be diagnosed as having an eating disorder, not otherwise specified.

C. **Clinical Picture**

1. **Anorexia nervosa commonly begins in a teenager who is overweight or sees himself or herself as being overweight. A stressor or loss,** such as the loss of a friend or family member or a departure to a new school, **may precipitate the onset of anorexia nervosa.** A comment about her weight may motivate a young woman to begin a diet which leads to starvation and escalates into an obsession with thinness. The woman may lose weight by restricting her caloric intake, purging (vomiting or the use of laxatives or diuretics), and exercising excessively. The anorectic woman may be hyperactive, with fidgeting and pacing. She usually denies her symptoms, although she appears emaciated. These patients often limit not only the amount they eat but also which food items they eat and they have obsessive-compulsive symptoms in regard to food. Women with anorexia nervosa often have personality characteristics of perfectionism, rigidity, obsessionality, compliance, dependency, cautiousness, and competitiveness.

2. **Bulimia nervosa commonly begins in a normal-weight or overweight woman who has tried various diets. The woman learns about self-induced vomiting or other purging behaviors and begins the cycle of binging and purging.** Bulimics purge through self-induced vomiting, ipecac-induced vomiting, abuse of laxatives, fasting, or excessive exercise. Bulimics usually binge and purge secretly, as they are embarrassed by their behaviors, which often contribute to their low self-esteem. Commonly, family members and friends are unaware of the illness. Bulimic patients often engage in high-risk and impulsive behaviors, including promiscuity and drug and alcohol abuse.

D. **Epidemiology**

Approximately 0.5% of adolescent and young adult women suffer from anorexia, and up to 3% of adult women have bulimia nervosa. Most of these women are between the ages of 15 and 30 years. Many others have eating disorder symptoms but do not meet the criteria for anorexia nervosa or bulimia nervosa. Only 5–10% of the eating-disordered population are males. Homosexual men may suffer from eating disorders more often than do heterosexual men.

E. **Risk Factors**

Primary risk factors associated with eating disorders include being female, dieting, and participating in activities or sports in which thinness is highly valued (e.g., modeling, ballet, gymnastics, figure skating, and competitive running). Women with a family history of anorexia nervosa or bulimia nervosa are up to three times more likely to have eating disorders than are women without a family history of eating disorders. Cultural pressure on women to be thin may contribute to the high prevalence of eating disorders in women in Western societies today. Many women with eating disorders have a history of being sexually abused.

F. **Mortality and Morbidity**

These illnesses have significant mortality, with **up to 5% of patients with anorexia nervosa dying from the disease each decade, many from suicide.** There also is significant medical morbidity from starvation and purging, as described in the section on medical complications below.

II. Evaluation of the Eating Disorders Patient

A. General Recommendations

1. So that other diagnoses are not missed, the symptoms must be treated initially as though they were caused by a medical disorder, even when an eating disorder appears likely.

B. Medical History

1. **The physician must ask specific questions, as eating disorder patients generally are good at hiding their symptoms and behaviors.** Moreover, their perceptions of normal food intake and weight usually are distorted, so details in the history are important.

2. **An eating disorder history should include the following:**
   a. Duration of illness
   b. Weight history
   c. Food intake history
   d. Calorie counts
   e. Purging history
   f. Medication use, including use of diuretics, laxatives, ipecac, and diet pills
   g. Exercise history
   h. Menstrual history

3. **Denial of symptoms is common** in patients with eating disorders. While denial often obscures the diagnosis, it also may help the physician make it. Unlike a medically ill cachectic woman, a patient with anorexia nervosa denies the severity of the weight loss or its significance and generally relishes the weight loss.

4. **A review of systems** often includes fatigue, lethargy, abdominal discomfort, bloating, constipation, cold intolerance, polyuria, hyperactivity, and insomnia.

5. **Medical records** should be obtained and other health care personnel should be contacted to clarify the diagnosis and the course of the eating disorder.

6. **Additional history** from family members and friends also is helpful in clarifying the diagnosis and the course of an eating disorder.

C. Examination of the patient. For all patients with eating disorders, weight and vital signs, including blood pressure, pulse, and temperature, should be recorded at each visit. Orthostatic blood pressure readings frequently are helpful. A baseline height also should be recorded in all, and height should be followed at each visit in children and adolescents.

1. **Anorexic patients often appear cachectic, hidden in many layers of loose-fitting clothing, with dry, pale, or yellow-tinged skin, lanugo (fine hair on the face and arms), bradycardia, hypotension, and hypothermia.**

2. **Bulimic patients are often of nearly normal weight and may have Russell's sign (abrasions on the metacarpophalangeal joints from self-induced vomiting), parotidomegaly, perimolysis (enamel loss), and signs of dehydration, including orthostatic hypotension.**

D. Routine laboratory studies should include the following:

1. Electrolytes, blood urea nitrogen (BUN), creatinine, and fasting blood glucose
2. Thyroid function tests
3. A complete blood count
4. Liver function tests
5. An electrocardiogram

Table 20-1. Selected Medical Complications of Eating Disorders

Cardiovascular

  Bradycardia
  Hypotension, orthostatic hypotension
  Arrhythmias
  Ipecac cardiomyopathy
  Congestive heart failure (during re-feeding in anorexia patients)

Dental

  Caries (in purgers)
  Perimolysis (in purgers)

Dermatologic

  Lanugo (in anorexia patients)
  Russell's sign (metacarpophalangeal area abrasion)
  Yellowish skin (carotenemic)

Endocrine/metabolic

  Electrolyte abnormalities, including hypokalemia
  Amenorrhea (in anorexia patients)
  Infertility (in anorexia patients)
  Menstrual irregularities (in bulimia patients)
  Elevated serum cortisol
  Euthyroid sick syndrome
  Hyperamylasemia (in purgers)

Gastrointestinal

  Delayed gastric emptying
  Constipation
  Elevated liver enzymes
  Gastric dilation or rupture
  Esophagitis
  Mallory-Weiss tears

Hematologic

  Anemia
  Leukopenia
  Thrombocytopenia

Hypothalamic

  Hypothermia

Renal

  Renal calculi

Skeletal

  Osteoporosis (in amenorrheic patients)

E. **Additional studies** may include **bone densitometry** in those with amenorrhea to evaluate possible osteoporosis. Brain imaging and an electroencephalogram (EEG) should be considered if the neurologic evaluation is abnormal.

F. **Medical complications.** Complications from starvation and vomiting should be considered (Table 20-1), including the following:

1. **Cardiovascular.** These patients may have bradycardia, arrhythmias, hypotension, congestive heart failure (during re-feeding in anorexia patients), cardiomyopathy (from ipecac use), decreased cardiac chamber size and thinning of the left ventricle, and mitral valve prolapse (disappears with weight gain).

2. **Cerebral.** Abnormal computed tomography scans of the brain often are seen, with lateral ventricular and cortical sulcal enlargement correlated to weight loss severity.

3. **Dental.** Caries and perimolysis occur frequently.

4. **Dermatologic**. Brittle hair and nails, lanugo-type hair on the body, yellow-tinged (carotenemic) skin, and Russell's sign (metacarpophalangeal joint area abrasions) may occur in those who vomit.

5. **Endocrine.** Because of low body fat, anorectic patients often have diminished gonadotropin secretion with consequent anovulation, amenorrhea, estrogen deficiency, and infertility. Menstrual irregularities also occur in patients with bulimia nervosa. Because of weight loss, the metabolism of the anorectic patients slows (to decrease energy use). This occurs by preferential conversion of thyroxine to inactive reverse triiodothyronine instead of active triiodothyronine. No increase in thyroid-stimulating hormone (TSH) occurs. Anorectics may have reduced vasopressin secretion from the posterior pituitary with resultant polyuria. In a patient with severe anorexia nervosa, hypoglycemia may cause coma or death.

6. **Gastrointestinal.** These patients may have delayed gastrointestinal motility (causing feelings of bloating and constipation), pancreatitis, elevated liver function tests, esophagitis, gastritis, Mallory-Weiss tears (esophageal rupture), and parotidomegaly with hyperamylasernia.

7. **Hematologic.** Anorectic patients may have reversible bone marrow depression that results in anemia without iron, folate, or vitamin B_{12} deficiency; leukopenia without immunosuppression; and thrombocytopenia.

8. **Hypothalamic.** Hypothermia is common in these patients.

9. **Metabolic.** Low serum zinc levels, and electrolyte disturbances (usually a hypokalemic, hypochloremic alkalosis) often occurs in patients who purge.

10. **Renal.** Dehydration and a lowered glomerular filtration rate may lead to renal calculi in these patients.

11. **Skeletal.** Osteoporosis occurs in anorexia patients and may not reverse with re-feeding. Pathologic fractures may occur in association with the osteoporosis.

III. Psychiatric Differential Diagnosis

A. **Physical Conditions.** A thorough history and physical examination must be performed, and a medical etiology of the disordered eating must be ruled out. The medical differential diagnosis includes the following:

1. Brain tumors involving the hypothalamic-pituitary axis
2. Addison's disease
3. Diabetes mellitus

   4. Neurologic disorders with symptoms similar to those of bulimia nervosa, including Kluver-Bucy syndrome (characterized by visual agnosia, compulsive licking and biting, placidity, hypersexuality, and hyperphagia) and Kleine-Levin syndrome (characterized by episodes of hypersomnia and hyperphagia)

B. Major Depression

C. Psychotic Disorders in which there may be delusions about food

D. Obsessive-Compulsive Disorder

E. Substance Use Disorder

F. Conversion Disorder

G. Dissociative Disorder

H. Personality Disorder

I. Anxiety Disorders: panic disorder, phobias about food

IV. Diagnostic Criteria

A. Diagnostic Criteria from *DSM-IV*

   1. *DSM-IV* **criteria for anorexia nervosa** include the following:

      a. Refusal to maintain body weight over a minimal normal weight for age and height: weight loss leading to maintenance of body weight that is less than 85% of normal weight

      b. Intense fear of gaining weight or growing fat even though one is underweight

      c. Disturbance in the way in which one's body weight or shape is experienced: undue influence of body weight or shape on self-evaluation or denial of the seriousness of the current low weight

      d. In postmenarcheal females, amenorrhea: the absence of at least three consecutive menstrual cycles

         i. **Restricting type.** In this type of anorexia nervosa, the person has not regularly engaged in binge eating or purging behavior (self-induced vomiting or the misuse of laxatives, diuretics, or enemas).

         ii. **Binge-eating/purging type.** In this type, the person has regularly engaged in binge eating or purging behavior (self-induced vomiting or misuse of laxatives, diuretics, or enemas).

   2. *DSM-IV* **criteria for bulimia nervosa** include the following:

      a. Recurrent episodes of binge eating. An episode of binge eating is characterized by both of the following:

         i. Eating within any 2-hour period an amount of food that is definitely more than what most people would eat during a similar period and under similar circumstances

         ii. A sense of lack of control over eating during the episode (i.e., a feeling that one cannot stop eating or control what or how much one is eating)

      b. Recurrent inappropriate compensatory behaviors to prevent weight gain include self-induced vomiting; misuse of laxatives, diuretics, enemas, or other medications; fasting; and excessive exercise.

      c. The binge eating and inappropriate compensatory behaviors both occur on average at least twice a week for 3 months.

      d. Self-evaluation is unduly affected by body shape and weight.

      e. The disturbance does not occur only during anorexia nervosa.

         i. Purging and non-purging subtypes

B. Co-morbid psychiatric disorders. Co-morbid psychiatric illnesses occur frequently and should be considered in the evaluation of an eating disorders patient. Up to one-half or more of patients with eating disorders meet the criteria for major depression. Patients with anorexia nervosa frequently have co-morbid anxiety disorders, including obsessive-compulsive disorder, social phobia, and simple phobias. Patients with bulimia nervosa often have co-morbid substance abuse, kleptomania, anxiety disorder, and impulsive behaviors, such as promiscuity and self-mutilation.

V. Treatment Strategies

The treatment of eating disorders requires a multi-modal, inter-disciplinary approach. As patients with eating disorders generally are resistant to treatment, it is crucial to coordinate treatment among the psychologist, psychiatrist, nutritionist, and PCP.

A. **Medical Stabilization**
   1. **Watch for other possible causes of weight fluctuations or purging.**
   2. **Assess the degree of malnutrition, dehydration, and electrolyte abnormalities to** determine whether hospitalization is necessary for medical reasons and to outline guidelines for outpatient treatment. These guidelines should include minimum acceptable weight, weight goal, recommended pace of weight gain (1 to 2 pounds per week) for underweight patients, and maintenance of safe electrolyte values.
   3. **Assess weight** while being aware that patients often use tricks to appear heavier than they are. Patients may layer clothes, water-load, carry weights in their pockets, or use other methods to make their weight look higher during physician visits. Therefore, it is generally best for the physician to take the patient's weight him or herself while the patient wears a hospital gown.
   4. **Prescribe daily multivitamins and calcium supplements (1,500 mg daily) and vitamin D** (400 IU/day) for amenorrheic patients.
   5. **Consider bone densitometry** for patients who are underweight and amenorrheic at evaluation.
   6. There is no medication that has been shown efficacious for treating osteoporosis in anorexia nervosa. Nutritional rehabilitation is the treatment of choice.

B. **Education**
   1. **Educate the patient about the medical risks of eating disorders** in an ongoing way.
   2. Specific risks should be explained. The cardiac toxicity of ipecac use should be underlined. **The risks of purging, diuretic abuse, laxative abuse, and starvation should be detailed.** The role fasting and under-eating play in inducing the binge/purge should be explained to bulimics.
   3. Parents of children and adolescents with eating disorders should be educated about eating disorders at length. Parents need to know the risks of these disorders and the benefits of early and aggressive treatment.

C. **Hospitalization**
   1. **If the patient is medically unstable** (e.g., dangerous hypokalemia, electrocardiographic changes, severe bradycardia, hypotension, or hypothermia), the patient must be hospitalized.

2. **If the patient is psychiatrically unsafe** (e.g., depression with suicidal ideation), in-patient admission is mandatory.

3. **Failure of outpatient treatment** with rapid worsening of symptoms also merits in-patient hospitalization.

4. Note that during hospitalization, the PCP should **watch for signs of re-feeding syndrome** which includes phosphate depletion and may lead to cardiac failure and cardiac arrest. The risk of this syndrome is highest in the first three weeks of re-feeding.

C. **Day treatment and/or partial hospitalization.** This is an option for a patient who can live at home but needs intensive treatment.

D. **Therapy**

1. **Cognitive-behavioral therapy** is used to diminish errors in the patient's thinking and perceptions that result in distorted attitudes and eating-disordered behaviors. The patient practices new ways of examining cognitions and self-monitors behaviors.

2. **Psychodynamic therapy** explores the underpinnings of the disorder.

3. **Group therapy offers** support to eating-disordered patients who feel isolated while offering another arena in which to explore the eating disorder.

4. **Family therapy** is especially efficacious in early-onset and short-duration anorexia. It supports parent re-feeding of children and identifies family dynamics which may be contributing to the problem.

5. **Nutritionists** can help the patient gradually learn healthier eating habits.

E. **Pharmacologic treatment** must be used carefully in patients with eating disorders. The dehydration and electrolyte fluctuations that are common in eating-disordered patients may lead to dangerous medication effects on the cardiac conduction system.

1. **Anorexia nervosa.** In controlled trials, no medication has been shown to be consistently effective in patients with acute anorexia nervosa. However the neuroleptics (e.g., olanzapine as well as haloperidol) at very low doses look promising in open trials. Also, low doses of benzodiazepines (e.g., lorazepam) before eating occasionally reduce anxiety. Fluoxetine has been found to help weight-recovered anorectics maintain weight and avoid relapse. Other selective serotonin reuptake inhibitors (e.g., sertraline, paroxetine) may also be of benefit.

2. **Bulimia nervosa.** Serotonin reuptake inhibitors (SRIs) are generally the psychotropic agents of choice in bulimia nervosa patients. These medications include fluoxetine, sertraline, and paroxetine.

3. **Co-morbidity.** Co-morbid disorders merit aggressive treatment. In eating-disordered patients with co-morbid depression, antidepressants should be considered. SRIs are generally the safest choice. Mirtazapine is another option, one which also may help insomnia. Of note, mirtazapine has a 12% incidence of weight gain as a side effect, although no studies look at this in anorexia. Nefazodone is another option but one must watch for a rare side effect of liver failure. Caution is necessary with the tricyclics (e.g., nortriptylline, desipramine), which are also effective. Also, careful prescribing of medications that can be fatal in overdose and close monitoring of suicidality are essential. Monoamine oxidase inhibitors (MAOIs) are effective in treating depression, but the dietary precautions (to avoid hypertensive crises) may add to dietary restrictions and the patient's preoccupation with food. Bupropion has been shown to increase the risk of seizures in patients with bulimia and thus is not recommended for use in bulimic patients.

VI. Conclusion

The PCP plays a central role in the treatment of eating-disordered patients. The PCP not only evaluates and treats the patient medically but also guides the patient to psychiatric treatment and guides the psychiatric treatment team in regard to the patient's weight goals and the medical need for hospitalization.

Suggested Readings

American Psychiatric Association Work Group on Eating Disorders. (2000). Practice guideline for the treatment of patients with eating disorders (revision). *American Journal of Psychiatry, 157,* 1–39.

American Psychiatric Association. (1994). Eating disorders. In *Diagnostic and statistical manual of mental disorders* (4th ed.). Washington, DC: American Psychiatric Association, pp. 539–550.

Becker, A.E., Grinspoon, S.K., Klibanski, A., & Herzog, D.B. (1999). Eating disorders. *New England Journal of Medicine, 340,* 1092–1098.

Beresin, E.V., Gordon, C.D., & Herzog, D.B. (1989). The process of recovering from anorexia nervosa. *Journal of the American Academy of Psychoanalysis, 17*(l), 103–130.

Cassano, G.B., Miniati, M., Pini, S., et al. (2003). Six-month open trial of haloperidol as an adjunctive treatment for anorexia nervosa: A preliminary report. *International Journal of Eating Disorders, 33,* 172–177.

Eisler, I., Dare, C., Russell, G.F., et al. (1997). Family and individual therapy in anorexia nervosa: A 5-year follow-up. *Archives of General Psychiatry, 54*(11), 1025–1030.

Fairburn, C.G., & Brownell, K.D. (Eds.). (2002). *Eating disorders and obesity: A comprehensive handbook* (2nd ed.). New York: Guilford Press.

Fisher, M., Golden, N.H., Katzman, D.Y., et al. (1995). Eating disorders in adolescents: A background paper. *Journal of Adolescent Health, 16*(6), 420–437.

Grinspoon, S., Thomas, E., Pitts, S., et al. (2000). Prevalence and predictive factors for regional osteopenia in women with anorexia nervosa. *Annals of Internal Medicine, 133,* 790–794.

Herzog, D.B., & Becker, A.E. (1999). Eating disorders. In A.M. Nicholi (Ed.), *The new Harvard guide to psychiatry* (3rd ed.). Cambridge, Mass.: Harvard University Press, pp. 400–411.

Herzog, D.B., Keller, M.B., Sacks, N.R., et al. (1992). Psychiatric comorbidity in treatment-seeking anorexics and bulimics. *Journal of the American Academy of Child and Adolescent Psychoanalysis, 31*(5), 810–818.

Herzog, D.B., Nussbaum, K.M., & Marmor, A.K. (1996). Comorbidity and outcome in eating disorders. *Psychiatric Clinics of North America, 19,* 843–859.

Herzog, D.B., Dorer, D.J., Keel, P.K., et al. (1999). Recovery and relapse in anorexia and bulimia nervosa: A 7.5 year follow-up study. *Journal of the American Academy of Child and Adolescent Psychiatry, 38,* 829–837.

Herzog, D.B., Greenwood, D.N., Dorer, D.J., et al. (2000). Mortality in eating disorders. *International Journal of Eating Disorders, 28,* 20–26.

Jimerson, D.C., Herzog, D.B., & Brotman, A.W. (1993). Pharmacologic approaches in the treatment of eating disorders. *Harvard Review of Psychiatry, 1,* 82–93.

Klibanski, A., Biller, B.M., Schoenfeld, D.A., et al. (1995). The effects of estrogen administration on trabecular bone loss in young women with anorexia nervosa. *Journal of Clinical Endocrinology and Metabolism, 80,* 898–904.

Lowe, B., Zipfel, S., Buchholz, C., et al. (2001). Long-term outcome of anorexia nervosa in a prospective 21-year follow-up study. *Psychological Medicine, 31*(5), 881–890.

Malina, A., Gaskill, J., McConaha, C., et al. (2003). Olanzapine treatment of anorexia nervosa: A retrospective study. *International Journal of Eating Disorders, 33,* 234–237.

Mehler, P. (2002). Diagnosis and care of patients with anorexia nervosa in primary care settings. *Annals of Internal Medicine, 134*(11), 1048–1059.

Mitchell, J.E., Seim, H.C., Colon, E., & Pomeroy, C. (1987). Medical complications and medical management of bulimia. *Annals of Internal Medicine, 107,* 71–77.

Powers, P.S., Santana, C.A., Bannon, Y.S. (2002). Olanzapine in the treatment of anorexia nervosa: An open label trial. *International Journal of Eating Disorders, 32,* 146–154.

Rigotti, N.A. (1995). Eating disorders. In K.J. Carlson, & S. Eisenstat (Eds.), *Primary care of women.* St. Louis: Mosby, pp. 443–449.

Sharp, C.W., & Freeman, C.P.L. (1993). Medical complications of anorexia nervosa. *British Journal of Psychiatry, 162,* 452–462.

Walsh, T.B. (1991). Longterm outcome of antidepressant treatment for bulimia nervosa. *American Journal of Psychiatry, 148,* 1206–1212.

CHAPTER 21

The Patient with Elevated, Expansive, or Irritable Mood

GARY S. SACHS, JEFF C. HUFFMAN, AND THEODORE A. STERN

I. Introduction

A. **Overview. Pathological mood states, including elevated, expansive, or irritable mood, are common** and may occur as part of a primary mood disorder (bipolar mood disorder). Explicit in the *DSM-IV* is the concept that a primary mood disorder is only one of the possible causes that can produce a mood episode. Other common causes of mood episodes include medical disorders (mood disorder secondary to another medical problem), substance abuse disorders (substance-induced mood disorder), and other psychiatric illnesses.

B. **Prevalence. Bipolar mood disorders are a major public health problem that tend to be underdiagnosed;** hence many patients go untreated. **The lifetime prevalence for bipolar mood disorders is about 1–4%** of the population. Among patients diagnosed in epidemiological studies only about one-third have been diagnosed by a physician. **At any point in time, only 27% of those who have been diagnosed are receiving medical treatment.** This represents the lowest percentage of any major psychiatric illness.

C. **Morbidity and mortality. The morbidity, mortality, and disability associated with bipolar mood disorder rank above nearly all other medical disorders. Moreover, the consequences of underdiagnosis and undertreatment are severe.** For example, studies of untreated bipolar patients find that **15–25% die by suicide.** Women with untreated bipolar illness have a reduction in life expectancy of 9 years. The dramatic presentation of acute episodes and complications (e.g., substance abuse, violence, and suicide) frequently heightens the impact of bipolar illness.

D. **Diagnosis. The distinguishing characteristic of bipolar mood disorder is the occurrence of a distinct period of abnormally elevated, expansive, or irritable mood.** The diagnosis of hypomania or mania is given when the abnormal mood state is persistent and is accompanied by symptoms sufficient to meet the *DSM-IV* criteria for hypomania or manic episodes (see Appendix). Bipolar illness is equally prevalent among men and women. The majority of episodes of hypomania and mania are relatively brief. Keller reported **the median duration of manic and mixed episodes was 10 and 39 weeks respectively.** A small percentage of patients experience chronic hypomania or mania.

E. **Course of illness.** The course of illness is quite variable, but some generalities are useful. **Bipolar mood disorder is always recurrent.** Bipolar disorder is characterized by episodes of disordered mood (depression and mania) interspersed with periods of inter-episode recovery. **The duration of well intervals between episodes tends to shrink progressively over the first three to five episodes.** For most patients cycle frequency will then stabilize. Many patients experience a seasonal pattern of exacerbation and remission. **A pattern of relapses mainly in the spring and fall is particularly common.** The onset of illness may occur at any time, but peak onset is between 15 and 30 years of age. New-onset is rare after the fifth decade of life, and should prompt thorough evaluation for general medical causes of mania.

F. **Classification and characteristics of elevated, expansive, or irritable mood states.** Mood disorders are distinct from the episodes that comprise them. In the *DSM-IV* episodes with prominent elevated, expansive, or irritable mood include hypomania, mania, and mixed episodes. Patients with unipolar disorder may also present with irritability and agitation, but in the absence of other symptoms of mania, the episodes would not be considered to be hypomanic or manic.

(For full *DSM-IV* criteria, see appendix to this chapter.)

II. Evaluation of the Problem

A. **General Recommendations**
   1. **Ensure safety: Assess the risk for violence, provocative behavior, risk-taking, and suicide. In general, most acutely manic patients require hospitalization.** Some patients with mild episodes can be managed on an outpatient basis with close medical follow-up and with support from family or friends.

B. **Examination of the Patient**
   1. **Medical History**
      a. **A general medical history should be taken that focuses on ruling out causes of mania that require additional treatment or affect selection of medication** (See section IV.B). *DSM-IV* skirts the issue by defining secondary mania as due to a medical condition or substance use without saying how it can be determined when mania is due to another condition. Treatment to control symptoms of mood elevation may be the same for primary and secondary mania, but secondary mania may require other specific treatments.
      b. *Neuropsychiatric assessment*
         i. Physical examination. Emphasis is placed on evaluation of neurological and endocrine systems. **In the absence of psychotic features (e.g., hallucinations), primary mood disorders do not involve alteration in cranial nerves, reflexes, or sensation.**
         ii. **Routine laboratory evaluation focuses on ruling out other medical causes of mood disturbance. There are no laboratory tests diagnostic of bipolar mood disorder.** Complete blood count, serum chemistries, thyroid function tests (e.g., TSH), and screening for toxic substances are usually indicated at the time of evaluation.
         iii. Additional labs may also be indicated based on the clinical presentation. **Any patient who has psychotic symptoms should have at least one electroencephalogram (EEG) and a brain imaging study, such as CT or MRI.** Other studies, such as erythrocyte sedimentation rate (ESR) or antinuclear antibodies (ANA), may be useful in patients with a history of rashes or other inflammatory symptoms. Treatment need not be delayed to obtain these tests. Instead, treatment may be initiated using agents least likely to cause untoward effects given the suspected pathology.
      c. **Interview**
         i. **The first objective is to obtain a history of the present illness sufficient to establish the current mood state** (e.g., depression, mania, hypomania, or mixed state). This is often difficult when the patient is acutely ill. During episodes, pa-

tients rarely complain of the symptoms that comprise hypomania or mania, but are more likely to endorse symptoms when asked a direct question (e.g., "This week, how many hours have you actually been sleeping?" rather than "This week, have you had problems with sleep?"). Even with direct questions, denial of symptoms should be expected, not because patients are necessarily attempting to deceive the physician, but because a patient with mood elevation is, in general, insensitive to problems. Many patients with mania do, however, report their mood as depressed, and are very aware when they are feeling irritable or annoyed.

ii. **Do not rule out mania solely on the patient's self-report.** Additional sources of history are essential.

iii. **Brief periods of abnormal mood elevation should be regarded as significant.** Diagnosis of a bipolar illness should be entertained for a patient when he or she (or another historian) reports periods of elevated, expansive, or irritable mood clearly recognized as abnormal, not simply better than periods of low mood.

iv. **Accuracy of diagnosis is improved by a brief systematic inquiry into mood and the symptoms associated with acute episodes.** Useful screening questions include the following:

  (a) How many days in the past 10 days has your mood been depressed? (How many of those days has your mood been depressed most of the day?)

  (b) How many days in the last 10 days have you had any period when your mood has been abnormally elevated even briefly?

  (c) How many days in the last 10 days have you had any period when you were abnormally or excessively irritable even briefly?

  (d) How many days in the last 10 days have you had any period when you were abnormally or excessively anxious?

  (e) Have you ever been so "hyper" that you weren't your normal self or it got you into trouble?

  (f) Did you do anything this month that you or people who know you would regard as unusual behavior?

v. **If the history is indicative of a current episode then determine the following:**

  (a) Onset of illness

  (b) Presence of chronic medical problems

  (c) Medication use

  (d) Recent change in diet and hydration

  (e) History of infection

  (f) History of head trauma/loss of consciousness

  (g) Sleep pattern

  (h) Menstrual regularity

  (i) Plans for conception, delivery, and lactation

  (j) Family history of psychiatric illness.

vi. **Diagnose which mood disorder is present by reviewing for the most severe (current or prior) episode.**

  (a) If positive for mania, the diagnosis is bipolar I (note that the diagnosis of bipolar I does not require a depressive episode).

  (b) If positive for hypomania and ≥ one depressive episode the diagnosis is bipolar II.

  (c) If negative for subsyndromal episodes of mood elevation, the diagnosis is unipolar depression.

  (d) If none of the preceding, consider bipolar disorder, not otherwise specified (BP NOS), cyclothymia, or another non-mood disorder diagnosis.

    d. **Rule out potentially contributory or life-threatening medical conditions:** A neuropsychiatric evaluation with physical examination, vital signs, and routine laboratories is sufficient to screen for the following conditions or agents listed.

        i. Intoxication/withdrawal states (substance-induced mania)

            Alcohol/benzodiazepines/barbiturates
            Stimulants: amphetamine, methylphenidate, caffeine, cocaine
            Phencyclidine (PCP)
            Steroids
            Anticholinergics
            Other iatrogenic agents: antidepressants, sympathomimetics, oral contraceptives, thyroxine, L-dopa, and many others

        ii. Endocrine/metabolic

            Thyrotoxicosis
            Cushing's disease
            Hypoglycemia
            Hyperparathyroidism
            Hyperprolactinemia
            Electrolyte imbalance (especially of sodium and calcium)

        iii. Nutritional deficiency

            "Megaloblastic madness"
            Wernicke's syndrome
            Hypoxia

        iv. Damage to brain tissue

            Encephalitis (syphilis, human immunodeficiency virus [HIV] infection)
            Post-viral (influenza)
            Stroke (usually right-sided, especially of the right thalamus)
            Temporal lobe epilepsy
            Trauma
            Subcortical dementias (e.g., Huntington's disease, Parkinson's disease, and Wilson's disease)
            Multiple sclerosis
            Systemic lupus erythematosus

III. Psychiatric Differential Diagnosis

It may be exceedingly difficult or impossible to differentiate between mania and the conditions listed below. Errors commonly result from taking the approach that one and only one condition is present and then coming to a premature diagnostic conclusion. Cross-sectional evaluation is far less reliable than is longitudinal assessment. The diagnosis of mania cannot be ruled out on initial evaluation even when a patient presents with classic symptoms of schizophrenia. Furthermore, with the exception of schizophrenia and schizoaffective disorders, the following disorders are also commonly co-morbid; the majority of bipolar patients will meet criteria for one or more of these disorders.

A. Schizophrenia: Chronic psychotic symptoms without prominent mood symptoms; often there is no intra-episode recovery.

B. Schizoaffective disorder: Combined psychotic and mood symptoms, but psychotic symptoms persist in the absence of mood symptoms for at least two weeks.

C. Substance abuse and withdrawal syndromes: Sedative (alcohol/benzodiazepine/barbiturate) withdrawal, cocaine/amphetamine/PCP intoxication.

D. Anxiety disorders: Panic disorder, generalized anxiety disorder. Severe, persistent anxiety can simulate chronic hypomania.

E. Personality disorders: Mood lability from borderline personality disorder can simulate symptoms of rapid-cycling bipolar disorder.

F. Attention-deficit/hyperactivity disorder: The inattention, impulsivity, and hyperactivity characteristic of this disorder can resemble hypomania or mania.

IV. Treatment Strategies (see Figure 21-1)

A. General Approach

Accurate assessment of the current episodes and the patient's illness form the basis for selecting and staging treatment. For example, a bipolar patient may present with major depression. Simply initiating antidepressant therapy without regard to a history of bipolar illness may result in iatrogenic mania.

Avoid discounting symptoms attributed to situational or geographic stressors. Among *DSM-IV* disorders, mania is the most reliable psychiatric disorder. Course of illness and response to treatment are likely to be the same whether or not a psychosocial stressor can be identified as a precipitant for the episode.

1. **Perform a baseline medical evaluation** (see the preceding section)
2. **Eliminate mood-elevating agents** (where possible)

   During manic, hypomanic, or mixed episodes, antidepressants are likely to exacerbate mania and should be tapered. Therapies directed against Parkinsonism (e.g., L-dopa), asthma (e.g., theophylline), or arthritis (e.g., cortisone) that have mood-elevating properties should also be minimized.

3. **Encourage good mood hygiene. Among the most important elements of good mood hygiene is assuring adequate sleep.** Patients and their families should also be made aware that common-sense practices can impact the course of illness. Situations with high levels of stress, conflict, or excessive stimulation often escalate behavioral symptoms because manic patients are typically overreactive. Therefore, in interactions with a manic patient, confrontations, ultimatums, and threats are generally counterproductive.

4. **Optimize mood-stabilizing therapies. Treatments with mood-stabilizing properties (see Table 21-1) are effective during the acute phase of treatment.** Therapies that may be effective during acute episodes of elevated mood include the following:

   a. **Lithium:** The oldest and best-studied mood stabilizer, lithium is effective for both acute and maintenance treatment of bipolar disorder. However, in severe mania, adjunctive treatment is often required because treatment with lithium may require several days or weeks before its full effect is seen.

      Dosing: initial: 300 mg b.i.d. (300 mg t.i.d. for severe mania)
      Initial target dose: 900–1,200 mg/day. (target serum level: between 0.6 and 1.0 mEq/liter)

Ensure safety and evaluate the etiology of symptoms:
• inquire about thoughts of harm to self and others
• obtain collateral information from family, friends, other caregivers
• evaluate for substance intoxication/withdrawal
• evaluate for general medical conditions that could cause symptoms

Utilize mood-stabilizing medications to treat symptoms
(and use adjunctive treatments as needed)

Initial Treatment:
• Lithium or divalproex
    (Lithium possibility preferred for euphoric mania)
    (Divalproex possibly preferred for mixed, rapid-cycling, or secondary mania)
• For severe mania or mania with psychotic symptoms:
    Add atypical antipsychotic: olanzapine or risperidone

symptoms persist*

Options:
1. Add/increase atypical antipsychotic (olanzapine/risperidone)
2. Add mood-stabilizing benzodiazepine (usually clonazepam)
3. Increase lithium/divalproex
    (if sufficient time has passed for these agents to reach steady state)

symptoms persist*

Options:
1. Consider above options
2. Add second first-line mood-stabilizing agent (lithium/divalproex)
3. Add adjunctive mood-stabilizing agent:
    carbamazepine, oxcarbazepine, topiramate, or lamotrigine
4. Evaluate for ECT
    (especially in severe, refractory mania and in pregnancy)

symptoms persist*

Options:
1. Consider above options
2. Add second atypical antipsychotic:
    olanzapine, risperidone, quetiapine, clozapine
3. Add typical antipsychotic
4. Add other potentially mood-stabilizing agent:
    thyroid hormone, clondine, calcium channel blocker, beta-blocker

* in persistent or refractory mania, continue ongoing evaluation for general medical conditions, substance use disorders, and co-morbid psychiatric disorders that may be contributing to symptoms or reducing effectiveness of treatment.

Figure 21-1. Mania treatment algorithm.

b. **Divalproex:** Another first-line mood stabilizing agent. Divalproex is possibly better than lithium for dysphoric mania, mixed episodes, and rapid-cycling bipolar disorder. It can be rapidly loaded in acute mania.

>   Dosing: initial: 250 mg b.i.d. (however, it can be loaded 20mg/kg/day in acute mania)
>   Initial target dose: 1,000–1,250 mg/day (target level: greater than 50 µg/ml; usually 50–100 µg/ml)

c. **Carbamazepine and oxcarbazepine:** Carbamazepine is a well-established, second-line mood-stabilizing agent. Its use has been somewhat limited by its adverse effects and metabolic properties. Carbamazepine induces liver metabolism, and it decreases levels of oral contraceptives, divalproex, phenytoin, and other medications. Furthermore, carbamazepine has been associated with aplastic anemia, leukopenia, SIADH, and Stevens-Johnson syndrome.

   Oxcarbazepine is a metabolite of carbamazepine. It appears to have lower rates of hematologic and dermatologic adverse events, and somewhat less of an effect on induction of enzymes. However, its mood-stabilizing properties are less well established.

>   Dosing for carbamazepine: initial: 200 mg b.i.d. (200 mg t.i.d. in acute mania)
>   Initial target dose: 800–1,000 mg/day (target level: 8–12 µg/ml)
>   Oxcarbazepine dosing: roughly 1.5 times that of carbamazepine (e.g., initial dose 300 mg b.i.d.).

d. **Atypical antipsychotics:** Can be used adjunctively with mood-stabilizing agents in severe mania. There is also growing evidence (especially with olanzapine) for their use as monotherapy during acute manic episodes. However, there is limited evidence for their efficacy as monotherapy maintenance treatment for bipolar disorder. Olanzapine and risperidone are the best-studied atypical antipsychotics for the treatment of elevated mood.

>   Dosing (olanzapine): initial: 5–10 mg per day (10–15 mg per day for acute mania)
>   Initial target dose: 10–15 mg per day
>   Dosing (risperidone): initial: 0.5–1 mg b.i.d. (1–2 mg b.i.d. for acute mania)
>   Initial target dose: 2–4 mg per day

e. **Topiramate:** A newer anticonvulsant with possible mood-stabilizing properties. Open-label trials have found it to be superior to placebo in acute mania, usually as an add-on to existing treatments. Topiramate appears to have the additional benefit of causing weight loss in many patients.

>   Dosing: initial: 50 mg/day (50–100 mg b.i.d. in acute mania)
>   Initial target dose: 100–200 mg/day

f. **Lamotrigine:** Another new anticonvulsant with apparent mood-stabilizing properties. Double-blind studies have found lamotrigine to have significant efficacy in the treatment of bipolar depression; however, slow upward titration (required because of the elevated risk of Stevens-Johnson syndrome with rapid dose escalation) makes lamotrigine less attractive as an antimanic agent. However, recent trials have found lamotrigine to be especially effective in patients with rapid-cycling bipolar disorder, and it may be effective as monotherapy in patients with this subtype.

Dosing: initial: 25 mg/day

Initial target dose: 100 mg/day (divided b.i.d.)

Note: In patients taking divalproex, lamotrigine doses should be reduced by 50% (e.g., initial dose: 12.5 mg/day)

Many patients present with acute episodes despite their being prescribed maintenance treatment with one or more mood-stabilizing therapy. In such cases, the therapy may be simply ineffective, partially effective, or the patient may have been non-compliant with therapy. Drawing a serum drug level and charting the patient's mood will clarify this issue. It is important to assure that the patient is receiving an adequate dose of medication as quickly as possible.

5. **Implement a specific treatment plan.**

   a. **Determine the need for antipsychotic treatment. Lithium, valproate, and carbamazepine all appear to be less effective for treatment of psychotic mania than nonpsychotic mania.** Although these agents may be sufficient for milder cases, **the presence of acute psychotic symptoms (e.g., hallucinations, delusions, or extreme agitation) often warrants additional treatment with an antipsychotic agent.** Atypical antipsychotic agents (e.g., risperidone, olanzapine, or quetiapine) have become the antipsychotic treatments of choice for psychotic mania. They can be initiated before, or concurrently with, antimanic agents.

6. **Follow an algorithm for treatment of mania and be cognizant of recommended sequencing of therapies.** Figure 21-1 displays an algorithm for the treatment of an acute mood episode with elevated, expansive, or irritable mood. The algorithm proceeds from the initial treatment with lithium or divalproex and proceeds stepwise, adding treatments based on the severity of a patient's symptoms and the need for safety.

   Treatment of bipolar disorder can be separated into four phases (acute, continuation, maintenance, discontinuation).

   a. **The acute phase** begins when the patient is diagnosed and treatment is initiated to control manic symptoms. Treatments are added, as required, by the acuity of the patient's symptoms and their response to treatment. Each therapeutic trial is carried out to one of three endpoints:

      i. Discontinuation because the patient is unable to tolerate adverse effects.

      ii. Discontinuation because the patient fails to respond to a trial at maximal dose (with augmentation strategies, if indicated).

      iii. The patient enjoys a sustained remission.

   b. **The continuation phase** begins with remission of the acute symptoms. During this phase the tasks are as follows:

      i. Continue successful acute therapies at full therapeutic dosage.

      ii. Adjust dosage as needed to sustain remission and to manage adverse effects. Manic patients are known to tolerate large doses of medication with little complaint, but when mania remits, this changes and dosages of lithium, valproate, carbamazepine, and antipsychotic medications must be changed accordingly. These changes may reflect state-dependent changes in drug metabolism. Lithium levels and complaints of side effects tend to increase after remission of acute mania. Carbamazepine levels, however, drop after 8 to 12 weeks of treatment owing to enzyme induction. Return of symptoms after a period of remission warrants at least closer follow-up and may justify an increase in one of the acute-phase treatments.

      iii. **Choose an appropriate duration for the acute phase. Generally a desirable duration for the continuation phase is double the duration of the last known manic**

episode. When no information is available, the continuation-phase treatment can be sustained for a period of 6 to 12 weeks after the patient has achieved remission.

   c. **The maintenance/discontinuation phase** begins with declaration of recovery from the acute episode. Now the focus of therapeutic effort shifts from control of acute symptoms to prevention of illness recurrence.

      i. **Gradually taper acute-phase treatments** (discontinuation).

      ii. **Maintain therapies at therapeutic doses targeting the prevention of the next episode of mania or depression (maintenance).**

      iii. **Monitor clinical status and laboratories.**

      iv. **Manage treatment-emergent adverse effects.**

      v. **Assure that serum levels remain in the therapeutic range.**

      vi. **Monitor for early signs of recurrence.** A patient who has enjoyed a prolonged remission of symptoms may present with several symptoms that fall short of meeting the diagnostic criteria for mania or depression, but that represent a clear change from a previously smooth course. Such "roughening" may herald relapse. Roughening with hypomanic symptoms is particularly worrisome and is an indication for closer follow-up and in most cases increased dosage of antimanic prophylaxis.

      vii. **Maintenance treatment should be recommended for at least one year after the first and any subsequent manic episodes. Expert consensus supports long-term maintenance treatment for any patient who has experienced three or more episodes.** When a decision to discontinue maintenance treatment is made, patients should be informed that their risk of relapse is high and that abrupt discontinuation is associated with early relapse of mania. **Based on data from studies of lithium discontinuation, a slow taper of mood-stabilizing medications is preferable.** Therefore, in the absence of a medical imperative a reasonable taper schedule would reduce the maintenance daily dosage of mood-stabilizing medication by 25–33% each month.

B. Selecting a Mood-Stabilizing Treatment

   1. **Assessment of the patient provides the basis for choosing an antimanic agent.** It is extremely helpful to include the patient and patient's family in the process of drug selection and education. At present, according to evidence-based guidelines, lithium and divalproex are the most appropriate initial first-line treatments for mania. In addition, carbamazepine, olanzapine, and electroconvulsive therapy (ECT) are widely accepted among psychiatrists as appropriate therapies for acute mania.

   2. **Although mood-stabilizers are effective for many patients, response is commonly incomplete.** Therefore, it is frequently necessary to augment treatment. Although seldom effective alone, benzodiazepines, thyroxine, and psychotherapy are commonly used to enhance response to a primary mood-stabilizing regimen.

   3. **Patient education is important in improving compliance and treatment outcome.** The tables included here summarize the information necessary to initiate treatment and they can be discussed with patients (see Table 21-1).

V. Appendix

A. Criteria for *DSM-IV* Episodes with Elevated, Expansive, or Irritable Mood

   1. ***DSM-IV* criteria for manic episode**

     a. A distinct period of abnormally and persistently elevated, expansive, or irritable mood, lasting at least 1 week (or any duration if hospitalization is necessary).

Table 21-1. Pharmacologic Treatments for Elevated, Expansive, or Irritable Mood

	Significant Contraindications	Major Drug Interactions	Most Common Adverse Effects	Most Worrisome Adverse Effects	Initiating Maintenance Therapy	Follow-up Laboratories	Patient Education
L **I** **T** **H** **I** **U** **M**	• Renal impairment • Complicated fluid or salt balance • Acute MI • Myasthenia gravis • Pregnancy	• Diuretics • NSAIDs • Carbamazepine • Ca⁺⁺ channel blockers • ACE inhibitors • Metronidazole • Neuroleptics	• GI irritation • Sedation • Tremor Other important effects • Weight gain • Edema • Acne • Psoriasis • Polyuria • Polydipsia	• Acute intoxication • Seizure • Coma • Death • Intoxication sequelae: Renal Cardiac CNS Other: • Thyroid inhibition • Arrhythmias • Renal dysfunction • Teratogenicity	Pre-treatment laboratories: • CBC • Electrolytes • TSH • Creatinine • BUN • Urinalysis • EKG if > 35 or clinically indicated Initial dosage: 300 mg b.i.d. (300 mg t.i.d. for acute mania)	Laboratories Titration: Q week: • Li level • BUN • Creatinine Routine: • Lithium 1–4 months for 1 year then every 4–6 months Q 6–12 months or when clinically indicated: • TFTs • Creatinine • BUN • Urinalysis • CBC	**Expect (one or more)** • GI irritation • Sedation • Mild tremor • Thirst • Increased WBC **Report** • Moderate tremor • Slurred speech • Muscle twitching • Change in fluid balance • Memory impairment • Rash • Edema **Discuss** • Lab rationale • Weight control • Importance of sodium • Potential teratogenicity

VALPROATE				+ Pretreatment	Titration	Expect
• Impairment of liver function • Blood dyscrasia	• Pregnancy • Inhibits hepatic metabolism • Increases levels of: • Aspirin • Anti-coagulants • Fatty acids • Lamotrigine	• Tremor • Dizziness • Sedation • Nausea/-vomiting • GI pain • Headache • Elevated LFTs	• Marrow suppression • Thrombocy-topenia • Prolongation of coagulation time • Pancreatitis Other important: • Hair loss • Weight gain • Teratogenicity	• CBC with differential • Platelets • LFTs: Initial Dosage: 250 mg b.i.d. More gradual titration can min-imize side effects (500 mg b.i.d. or 20 mg/kg/day for acute mania)	• Establish level of at least 50 Determine weekly until stable: • Drug levels, CBC, and LFTs **Routine** • Monthly until 6 months • Thereafter q 6–12 months	(transiently) • Sedation • Tremor • GI symptoms **Report** • Easy bruisability • Abdominal swelling • Rash • Jaundice • Edema (facial) **Discuss** • Weight control program • Common drug interactions • Potential teratogenicity • Use of vitamins/minerals (folate, Se, Zn)

(continued)

Table 21-1. Pharmacologic Treatments for Elevated, Expansive, or Irritable Mood (Continued)

	Significant Contraindications	Major Drug Interactions	Most Common Adverse Effects	Most Worrisome Adverse Effects	Initiating Maintenance Therapy	Follow-up Laboratories	Patient Education
O L A N Z A P I N E	• Diabetes mellitus • Obesity • Pregnancy	• Levels increased with: • Ritonavir • Ciprofloxacin • Fluvoxamine	• Sedation • Dizziness • Increased appetite • Headache Other important: • Weight gain • Constipation • Dry mouth	• Diabetes mellitus (including new-onset DKA) • Extrapyramidal symptoms (rare): • Dystonia • Parkinsonism • Akathisia/restlessness	Pretreatment laboratories: • None required Initial dosage: • 5–10 mg qhs • (10–15 mg qhs for acute mania)	None required • Monitor weight at follow-up visits • Consider fasting glucose q 3–6 months	Expect • Sedation • Dizziness • Dry mouth • Increased appetite Report • Stiffness of arms, legs, or neck • Difficulty speaking or swallowing • New-onset tremor, slowed movements, or ataxia • Persistent restlessness or need to move • Polydipsia/polyuria • Memory impairment/confusion Discuss • Weight control • Risk of diabetes • Potential teratogenicity *(continued)*

CARBAMAZEPINE

	Drug Interactions	CNS / GI / Other important	Hematologic / Dermatologic	Pretreatment	Titration	Expect / Report / Discuss
• Impairment of cardiac, renal, or liver function • Pregnancy • Prior hematological dyscrasia	• Induces P450 isoenzymes • Reduces levels of: • Neuroleptics • Divalproex • Oral contraceptives • Many others • Increased levels of CBZ with: • H2 blockers • Erythromycin • Isoniazid • Propoxephene • Valproate • Ca+ channel blockers • Lithium	**CNS** • Dizziness • Sedation • Unsteady gait • Incoordination • Cognitive impairment • Blurred vision/diplopia **GI** • Nausea • Anorexia • Pain • Elevated LFTs	**Hematologic** • Aplastic anemia • Agranulocytosis • Thrombocytopenia • Hepatitis **Dermatologic** • Rash (pruritic, erythematous) • Erythema multiforme or nodosum • Toxic epidermal necrolysis • Stevens-Johnson **Other important** • Hyponatremia • Altered thyroid function • Edema • Arrhythmia, AV block • Alopecia • SLE • Potential teratogenicity	**Pretreatment** • CBC with differential • Platelets • LFTs • Urinalysis Useful • EKG • Electrolytes • Reticulocyte count **Initial Dosage (mg):** • 200 mg b.i.d. (More gradual titration can minimize side effects) • 200 mg t.i.d. (for acute mania)	**Titration** (to clinical response not level) • q 7–14 days • CBC • Drug level • LFTs for 2–3 months and stable dose • Routine monthly × 6 months • Drug level • CBC • LFTs • Electrolytes • Thereafter 6–12 months CBC • Drug level • LFTs • Electrolytes • TFTs	**Expect** • Sedation • GI symptoms • Lightheadedness **Report** • Rash • Jaundice • Incoordination • Irregular heartbeat • Facial edema **Discuss** • Importance of weight control program • Common drug interactions • Potential teratogenicity • Use of vitamins/minerals (folate, Se, Zn)

   b. During the period of mood disturbance, three (or more) of the following symptoms have persisted (four if the mood is only irritable) and have been present to a significant degree:
       i. Inflated self-esteem or grandiosity
      ii. Decreased need for sleep (e.g., feels rested after only 3 hours of sleep)
     iii. More talkative than usual, or pressure to keep talking
      iv. Flight of ideas or subjective experience that thoughts are racing
       v. Distractibility (e.g., attention too easily drawn to unimportant or irrelevant external stimuli)
      vi. Increase in goal-directed activity (either socially, at work or school, or sexually) or psychomotor agitation
     vii. Excessive involvement in pleasurable activities that have a high potential for painful consequences (e.g., engaging in unrestrained buying sprees, sexual indiscretions, or foolish business investments)
   c. The symptoms do not meet criteria for a mixed episode (which requires simultaneous depression).
   d. The mood disturbance is sufficiently severe to cause marked impairment in occupational functioning, in usual social activities, or in relationships with others, or to necessitate hospitalization to prevent harm to oneself or others, or there are psychotic features.
   e. The symptoms are not due to the direct physiological effects of a substance (e.g., a drug of abuse, a medication, or another treatment) or a general medical condition (e.g., hyperthyroidism).
       i. NOTE: Manic-like episodes that are clearly caused by somatic antidepressant treatment (e.g., medication, electroconvulsive therapy, or light therapy) should not count toward a diagnosis of bipolar I disorder.
      ii. This is a significant change from *DSM-III-R,* which stated, "It cannot be established that an organic factor initiated and maintained the disturbance." NOTE: Somatic antidepressant treatment (e.g., drugs, ECT) that apparently precipitates a mood disturbance should not be considered an etiologic organic factor.
 2. *DSM-IV* **criteria for hypomanic episode**
   a. A distinct period of persistently elevated, expansive, or irritable mood, lasting throughout at least 4 days, that is clearly different from the usual non-depressed mood.
   b. (same as for mania)
   c. The episode is associated with an unequivocal change in functioning that is uncharacteristic of the person when not symptomatic.
   d. The disturbance in mood and the change in functioning are observable by others.
   e. The episode is not severe enough to cause marked impairment in social or occupational functioning, or to necessitate hospitalization, and there are no psychotic features.
   f. The symptoms are not due to the direct physiological effects of a substance (e.g., a drug of abuse, a medication, or other treatment) or a general medical condition (e.g., hyperthyroidism).
      NOTE: Hypomanic-like episodes that are clearly caused by somatic antidepressant treatment (e.g., medication, ECT, or light therapy) should not count toward a diagnosis of bipolar II disorder.
 3. *DSM-IV* **criteria for mixed episode**
   a. The criteria are met both for a manic episode and for a major depressive episode (except for duration) nearly every day during at least a 1-week period.

    b. The mood disturbance is sufficiently severe to cause marked impairment in occupational functioning, in usual social activities, or in relationships with others, or to necessitate hospitalization to prevent harm to oneself or others, or there are psychotic features.

    c. The symptoms are not due to the direct physiological effects of a substance (e.g., a drug of abuse, a medication, or another treatment) or a general medical condition (e.g., hyperthyroidism).

        NOTE: Mixed episodes that are clearly caused by somatic antidepressant treatment (e.g., medication, ECT, or light therapy) should not count toward a diagnosis of bipolar I disorder.

B. The *DSM-IV* definition of mood disorders

  1. **Substance-induced mood disorders**

    a. Characterized by a prominent and persistent disturbance in mood that is judged to be a direct physiological consequence of a drug of abuse, a medication, another somatic treatment for depression, or exposure to a toxin.

        NOTE: This now includes antidepressant-induced episodes.

  2. **Mood disorders due to a general medical condition**

    a. Characterized by a prominent and persistent disturbance in mood that is judged to be a direct physiological consequence of a general medical condition (e.g., hypothyroidism, Cushing's disease, frontal lobe tumor).

  3. **Mood disorder not otherwise specified**

    a. Included for coding disorders with mood symptoms that do not meet the criteria for any specific mood disorder and in which it is difficult to choose between depressive disorder not otherwise specified and bipolar disorder not otherwise specified (e.g., acute agitation).

Suggested Readings

American Psychiatric Association. (1994). *Diagnostic and statistical manual of mental disorders* (4th ed.). Washington, DC: American Psychiatric Association.

Bowden, C., Brugger, A., Swann, A., et al. (1994). Efficacy of divalproex vs lithium and placebo in the treatment of mania. *Journal of the American Medical Association, 271,* 918–924.

Bhana, N., & Perry, C.N. (2001). Olanzapine: A review of its use in the treatment of bipolar I disorder. *CNS Drugs, 15,* 871–904.

Calabrese, J.R., Suppes, T., Bowden, C.L., et al. (2000). A double-blind, placebo-controlled, prophylaxis study of lamotrigine in rapid-cycling bipolar disorder. *Journal of Clinical Psychiatry, 61,* 841–850.

Chengappa, K.N., Gershon, S., & Levine, J. (2001). The evolving role of topiramate among other mood stabilizers in the management of bipolar disorder. *Bipolar Disorders, 3,* 215–232.

Fava, G., & Kellner, R. (1991). Prodromal symptoms in affective disorders. *American Journal of Psychiatry, 148,* 823–830.

Hirschfeld, R.M.A., Bowden, C.L., Gitlin, M.J., et al. (2002). Practice guideline for the treatment of patients with bipolar disorder (revision). *American Journal of Psychiatry, 159*(suppl 4), 1–50.

Kukopulos, A., Reginaldi, P., Laddomada, G., et al. (1980). Course of the manic-depressive cycle and changes caused by treatments. *Pharmakopsychiatrie Neuro-Psychopharmakologie, 13,* 156–167.

Sachs, G.S. (1989). Adjuncts and alternatives to lithium therapy for bipolar affective disorder. *Journal of Clinical Psychiatry, 50*(suppl 12), 31–39.

Sachs, G.S., Grossman, F., Ghaemi, S.N., et al. (2002). Combination of a mood stabilizer with risperidone or haloperidol for treatment of acute mania: A double-blind, placebo-controlled comparison of efficacy and safety. *American Journal of Psychiatry, 159,* 1146–1155.

Sachs, G.S., Printz, D.J., Kahn, D.A., et al. (2000). The Expert Consensus Guideline Series: Medication Treatment of Bipolar Disorder 2000. *Postgraduate Medicine,* Special issue #1, 1–104.

Sachs, G.S. (1996). Bipolar mood disorder: Practical strategies for acute and maintenance phase treatment. *Journal of Clinical Psychopharmacology,* suppl 16, 32s–47s.

Viguera, A.C., Cohen, L.S., Baldessarini, R.J., et al. (2002). Managing bipolar disorder during pregnancy: Weighing the risks and benefits. *Canadian Journal of Psychiatry, 47,* 426–436.

Wehr, T.A., & Goodwin, F.K. (1987). Can antidepressants cause mania and worsen the course of affective illness? *American Journal of Psychiatry, 144*(11), 1403–1411.

Yatham, L.N. (2002). The role of novel antipsychotics in bipolar disorders. *Journal of Clinical Psychiatry, 63*(suppl 3), 10–14.

CHAPTER 22

The Patient with Memory Problems or Dementia

WILLIAM E. FALK

I. Introduction

Dementia is a syndrome characterized by a clinically significant decline in memory and at least one other area of cognitive function. Dementia usually develops over months or years, as opposed to delirium, which evolves over days to weeks and typically impairs arousal and attention more than it impairs memory.

A. The clinician must **determine the specific cause of a dementia to assess the prognosis** and course and to initiate the appropriate treatment. Important questions to consider include the following:

1. Is it the result of a primary dementing disorder, such as **dementia of the Alzheimer's type (DAT)?**
2. Is it secondary to a general **medical or neurologic** condition?
3. Is it due to **medications or alcohol?**
4. Is there more than one contributing factor to the cognitive difficulties?

B. More than 80 specific disorders can cause dementia. Some, like DAT, are fairly common, while most are exceedingly rare (Table 22-1).

1. **Not all dementias are progressive.** Some are static, and **a few are reversible.**
2. The clinician should establish a specific diagnosis and should never attribute a significant decline in cognition to "old age." A specific diagnosis is essential in planning treatment and helping the patient and family understand what to expect in the future.

C. The border between memory deficits associated with aging and those associated with early dementia can be indistinct. With **age-associated memory impairment,** there is a slowing of the ability to learn new information compared to younger individuals, but not an overt memory impairment once information is retained, and there is no impairment to occupational or social functioning. A new descriptor, mild cognitive impairment, is used when an individual experiences a decline in cognition compared to age-matched controls. The clinician should follow minor memory complaints over time and observe whether they worsen and affect the patient's ability to function in work and social settings, which would suggest a progression to DAT.

II. Terminology

A. Dementia means a decline in cognitive function, that is, mentation. *DSM-IV* criteria **require** the presence of **an acquired deficit in memory as well as at least one other area of impaired higher cortical function.**

1. **Aphasia** is difficulty with language (e.g., speaking, reading, writing, or repeating).
2. **Apraxia** is inability to carry out motor tasks despite intact motor function.
3. **Agnosia** is failure to recognize a familiar object despite intact sensory function.
4. **Executive dysfunction** includes impairments of abstraction as well as planning, sequencing, monitoring, and stopping complex behaviors.

Table 22-1. Dementia: Diagnosis by Categories with Representative Examples

Degenerative
- Dementia of the Alzheimer's type
- Frontal lobe dementia with or without neuron disease
- Pick's disease
- Dementia with Lewy Bodies
- Corticobasal degeneration
- Huntington's disease
- Wilson's disease
- Parkinson's disease
- Multiple system atrophy
- Progressive supranuclear palsy

Psychiatric
- Pseudodementia of depression

Vascular
- Vascular dementia
- Binswanger's encephalopathy
- Amyloid dementia
- Diffuse hypoxic/ischemic injury

Obstructive
- Normal-pressure hydrocephalus
- Obstructive hydrocephalus

Traumatic
- Chronic subdural hematoma
- Dementia pugilistica
- Post-concussion syndrome

Neoplastic
- Tumor, malignant: primary or secondary
- Tumor, benign, e.g., frontal meningioma
- Paraneoplastic limbic encephalitis

Infectious
- Chronic meningitis (e.g., tuberculous)
- Post-herpes encephalitis
- Focal cerebritis/abscesses
- HIV dementia

Infectious (*continued*)
- HIV-associated infection
- Syphilis
- Lyme encephalopathy
- Subacute sclerosing panencephalitis
- Creutzfeldt-Jakob disease
- Progressive multifocal leukoencephalopathy
- Parenchymal sarcoidosis
- Chronic systemic infection

Demyelinating
- Multiple sclerosis
- Metachromatic leukodystrophy

Autoimmune
- Systemic lupus erythematosus
- Polyarteritis nodosa

Drugs/Medications
- Anticholinergics
- Antihistamines
- Anticonvulsants
- Beta-blockers
- Sedative-hypnotics

Substance abuse
- Alcohol
- Inhalants
- Phencyclidine (PCP)

Toxins
- Arsenic
- Bromide
- Carbon monoxide
- Lead
- Mercury
- Organophosphates

SOURCE: Adapted with permission from Schmahmann, J.D. (1995). Neurobehavioral manifestations of focal cerebral lesions. Presented at the Massachusetts General Hospital course in Geriatric Psychiatry, Boston.

B. Additional essential features include the following:
   1. There is a significant **impairment of social or occupational function.**
   2. There is a notable **decline** from a previous level **of function.** This criterion separates patients with mental retardation from those with dementia.
   3. The impairment should be present in the **absence of delirium.** However, delirium can be superimposed on dementia. In fact, demented patients are at greater risk for experiencing delirium from any given insult than are those with normal cognition.
   4. The condition cannot be accounted for by another Axis I disorder, such as major depression.

III. Epidemiology

A. Advanced age is a risk factor for most types of dementia, particularly DAT.
   1. **The overall prevalence of dementia in people over 60 years of age currently is estimated to be 15%,** or more than 3 million people, in the United States.
   2. The prevalence is approximately 1% at age 60 and it doubles every 5 years thereafter.
   3. **By age 85, the prevalence may be as high as 50%.**
   4. Although there are somewhat higher rates of vascular dementia and lower rates of DAT in men, the overall incidence of dementia is equivalent in men and women.
   5. As the average life expectancy of men and women continues to expand, the number of people affected by dementia will grow. Thus, we can anticipate an epidemic of dementia in the twenty-first century.

B. A familial pattern of transmission occurs with certain dementing disorders.
   1. Some disorders have well-known patterns of transmission, for example, the autosomal dominant **Huntington's disease.**
   2. **Early-onset DAT** occurs frequently in families and can be associated with several different chromosome mutations.
   3. The presence of **homozygote apoliproprotein E4 alleles** occurs more frequently in patients with DAT than in those without it. The utility of this observation requires further study before it can become clinically relevant.

IV. Evaluation

A. Brain failure deserves at least as much attention as does the failure of any other organ (Fig. 22-1).
   1. The clinician should never diagnose a patient with "senility" or "cerebral arteriosclerosis." These terms tend to be nihilistic and do not transmit meaning.
   2. **All dementias are treatable** even if they are not reversible or curable. Although the majority (50–70%) of dementias are diagnosed as DAT, a disorder that is not curable, there is much the clinician can do to help afflicted patients and their families.
   3. **The evaluation requires a reliable history** (cognitive, psychiatric, medical, and family), **complete medical and neurologic examinations, appropriate laboratory testing, and assessment of mental status and cognitive function.**

B. History: general issues
   1. Although the patient's observations are important, **the history is best obtained by interviewing family members or close friends.** Relying solely on the patient's report is unwise; it may be inaccurate and certainly will be incomplete.
   2. Generally, the clinician should conduct at least a portion of the interview with family members away from the patient to minimize distress and enhance accuracy.

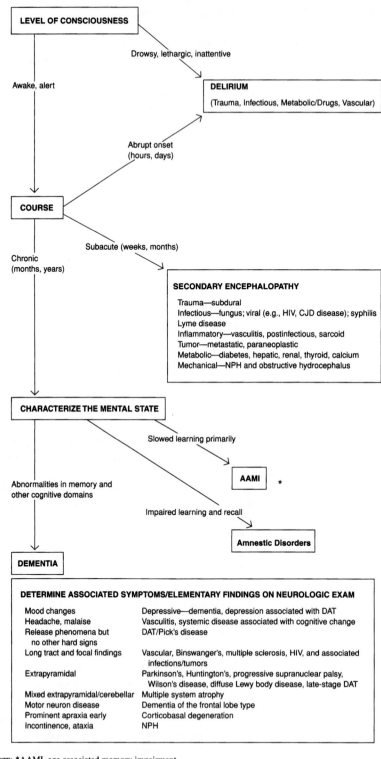

NOTE: *AAMI, age associated memory impairment

Figure 22-1.   An algorithm for dementia diagnosis.

C. Cognitive history

1. It is important to **determine whether the initial symptoms came on gradually,** as typically occurs with DAT, **or abruptly,** as usually occurs with vascular dementias. Delirium generally has an acute onset as well; however, if it results from certain conditions, such as a gradually developing drug toxicity, the onset may be subacute or even insidious.

2. The manner in which symptoms have progressed over time also provides important diagnostic information. For example, **stepwise deterioration is more characteristic of vascular dementia, while gradual decline is typical of DAT.**

3. The clinician should elicit carefully the **time of onset and the nature of behavioral changes.** This information can be important in differentiating various types of dementia. For example, disinhibited and inappropriate behavior is characteristic of the early stages of Pick's disease, whereas **the early symptoms of DAT often involve increased apathy and a decline in the ability to learn new information.**

4. The clinician must always **ask about the patient's functional status.** This information can be obtained easily by asking about a patient's typical day, including work and leisure activities. Alternatively, scales have been developed to cover functional status in a structured way.

   a. **The Activities of Daily Living Scale** surveys six basic areas of function: **bathing, dressing, toileting, transferring, continence, and feeding.** The interviewer simply determines whether the patient can perform these tasks independently or requires assistance.

   b. **The Instrumental Activities of Daily Living Scale** provides a sense of the patient's ability to perform more complex tasks, such as **ambulating, using the telephone, shopping, preparing meals, performing housework, making simple home repairs, doing laundry, self-administering medication, and managing money.** Whether these tasks can be performed independently, with assistance, or not at all gives the clinician a sense of how autonomously the patient can function.

   c. To assess more subtle deficits in function, the clinician must know what hobbies or other areas of interest the patient has had and how well those activities can now be performed. In addition, a social and occupational history is useful in assessing pre-morbid intelligence and education.

D. Psychiatric history

1. The clinician should inquire about past mood or psychotic symptoms.

2. Although cognitive changes can be seen in depression, the history and mental status examinations usually allow the clinician to separate depression from dementia or determine that both are present (Table 22-2).

3. Nonetheless, lack of energy, diminished motivation, sleep disturbance, and appetite changes all can be seen in both depression and dementia.

4. Some patients may have a long history of a psychotic disorder, such as schizophrenia. These patients may appear superficially to have a primary dementing disorder when in fact they do not. Obtaining the history of past psychotic episodes is critical.

E. Medical history

1. The practitioner should **assess whether surgical procedures** (e.g., gastrectomy predisposing to vitamin B_{12} deficiency) **or medical illnesses** (e.g., hypertension or lupus) **have contributed** to the symptoms of cognitive dysfunction. In addition, **deficits in hearing and vision should be noted.**

Table 22-2. Clinical Features of Delirium, Depression, and Dementia of the Alzheimer's Type

	Delirium	*Depression*	*Dementia of the Alzheimer's Type*
Onset	Abrupt	Relatively discrete	Insidious
Initial symptoms	Difficulty with attention and disturbed consciousness	Dysphoric mood or lack of pleasure	Memory deficits: verbal and/or spatial
Course	Fluctuating over days to weeks	Persistent, usually lasting months if untreated	Gradually progressive, over years
Family history	Not contributory	May be positive for depression	May be positive for DAT*
Memory	Poor registration	Patchy/inconsistent	Recent memory worse than remote
Memory complaints	Absent	Present	Variable: usually absent
Language deficits	Dysgraphia	Increased speech latency	Confrontation naming difficulties
Affect	Labile	Depressed/irritable	Variable: may be neutral

NOTE: *DAT, dementia of the Alzheimer's type.

2. **Questions about head injury (e.g., concussions), cigarette usage, toxin exposure, and blood transfusions and other human immunodeficiency virus risks are important.**

3. The clinician should question the patient carefully about **nutritional status, alcohol and cigarette usage, and drug history,** including prescribed, over-the-counter, and illicit drugs. Ideally, the clinician should request that all medications be brought to the evaluation. Medications are implicated in a significant number of cases of dementia. Common offenders include anticholinergics, antihypertensives, antihistamines, sedative-hypnotics, psychotropics, and narcotic analgesics.

4. The clinician should **assess associated medical symptoms** (e.g., difficulty walking, sensory loss) for clues about underlying medical problems. Associated symptoms may lead to a particular diagnosis. For example, incontinence and gait apraxia are seen in normal pressure hydrocephalus.

F. **Family history.** The family history can be helpful in making the diagnosis. Certain dementing disorders have definite genetic modes of transmission, while in other cases (e.g., the majority of patients with DAT) there is likely to be a complex interaction between genetics and other factors.

G. Physical and neurologic examination

1. The clinician should **carry out a careful general medical assessment** focused on, but not limited to, the cardiovascular and respiratory systems.
2. The **neurologic examination** must be complete to uncover any focal abnormalities, primitive reflexes, or signs of particular neurologic disorders, including assessment of gait and vibration and position sense.
3. **Vision and hearing evaluations** also should be performed carefully.

H. Psychiatric mental status examination

1. The patient's current mood state should be assessed to **determine whether a treatable depression is causing or contributing to cognitive difficulties.**
   a. The clinician should inquire about depressed mood directly and, if it is acknowledged by the patient or a family member as being present, ask further questions about neurovegetative signs and other depressive symptoms (see Chapter 14).
   b. A depressed patient may have **suicidal thoughts.** Inquiry about them does not increase the risk of a patient acting on those thoughts; if anything, it may diminish the patient's urge to carry them out.
   c. An elevated, expansive, or inappropriately **inflated mood** may suggest **manic symptoms** or disinhibition associated with frontal lobe disorders.
   d. **Irritability** can be seen in many dementing disorders as well as in depression and mania.
2. **Psychotic symptoms also should be noted.**
   a. Although late-onset schizophrenia and delusional disorders occur, patients with these disorders typically have had psychotic symptoms since early life.
   b. With frontal lobe disorders, changes in behavior or personality may precede notable memory deficits.

I. Cognitive testing

1. Important data about cognitive function can be obtained during the interview. Difficulties with memory, word-finding, and abstraction may be apparent. The clinician must be sensitive to the patient's limitations in attending to task and concentrating (signs of delirium) to evaluate the validity of the patient's assessments of memory and other functions.
2. To assure that important areas of cognition are evaluated, a short structured instrument, such as the **Mini-Mental State Examination,** is very useful. It is also helpful in following the course of illness or the response to treatment (see Table 23-3).
3. Additional tests of cognitive function (such as generating words in a category [e.g., animals] in one minute and learning an extended word list then recalling it after a delay) can be administered when indicated. Having the patient over time, draw a clock face and set the hands at a particular time (e.g., at 10 past 11 or 10 to 2), can be informative as can asking the patient to copy a clock face if he or she has difficulty spontaneously drawing it. In addition, patients can be asked to perform simple acts of praxis: brushing their teeth, combing their hair, writing or sending a letter. Interpreting proverbs, naming recent presidents, and discussing current events also provide information about a patient's ability to abstract, recall and use information.
4. Referral for neuropsychological testing may be useful and is essential when deficits are mild or difficult to characterize.

Table 22-3. Recommended Laboratory Studies for a Dementia Work-up

Blood studies
  Complete blood count (CBC)
  Vitamin B_{12}
  Folate
  Sedimentation rate (ESR)
  Glucose
  Calcium
  Phosphorus
  Magnesium
  Electrolytes
  Liver function tests (LFTs) (e.g., SGPT, bilirubin, alkaline phosphase)
  Thyroid function tests (TFTs) (thyroid-stimulating hormone [TSH] as screen)
  Creatinine, blood urea nitrogen (BUN)
  Cholesterol (high-density lipoprotein/low-density lipoprotein)
  Triglycerides
  Syphilis serology (e.g., RPR)
Urinalysis
Other studies
  Electrocardiogram (ECG)
  Computed axial tomography (CT) or magnetic resonance imaging (MRI)
Representative additional studies based on history and physical findings
  Chest x-ray (CXR)
  Electroencephalography (EEG)
  Non-invasive carotid studies
  Human immunodeficiency virus (HIV) testing
  Rheumatoid factor (RF), antinuclear antibody (ANA), and other autoimmune disorder screens
  Lumbar puncture (LP)
  Drug levels
  Heavy metal screening

J. Laboratory studies

1. For DAT, the most common dementing disorder, there are no definitive laboratory studies available; some may become available in the near future as research in this area progresses.

2. Routine hematologic and urine studies are listed in Table 22-3. Additional tests are indicated if the initial work-up is uninformative, if a particular diagnosis is suspected, or if the presentation is atypical. The yield from these studies will be low, but they still should be carried out. The clinician routinely should obtain recently performed laboratory test results so that those tests will not be repeated needlessly.

V. Diagnosis

The diagnosis of the dementia syndrome is described in terminology, above. *DSM-1V* provides additional diagnostic criteria for various specific dementing disorders.

A. The diagnostic criteria for DAT include gradual onset and progressive decline as well as the absence of other central nervous system and systemic conditions known to cause dementia.

1. **Progressive memory impairment, disorientation, and language difficulties**—particularly in word-finding and confrontation naming—are very common. **Visuospatial difficulties** are also common and can lead to early problems with driving, dressing, and self-care.

2. **Psychiatric symptoms** occur frequently but often are overlooked.
   a. **Depressive and anxiety symptoms** usually are seen early in the course of DAT.
   b. **Paranoid delusions and visual hallucinations** also occur, particularly when cognitive symptoms are moderate to severe.
   c. **Changes in personality** (e.g., from docility to agitation) and accentuation of personality characteristics commonly occur.

3. **Focal neurologic signs** typically are present only late in the course of the disorder. If they occur early, the diagnosis of DAT should be questioned. For example, if extrapyramidal symptoms and hallucinations occur early, the diagnosis may be a disorder related to DAT called Dementia with Lewy Bodies (DLB) and the patient's function may go downhill more rapidly.

B. Vascular dementia, previously known as multi-infarct dementia, is a condition in which infarcts are not the only cause of dementia and it accounts for about 20% of cases of dementia; emboli, hemorrhages, infections and inflammatory vascular diseases, and diffuse white matter disease (e.g., Binswanger's encephalopathy) all can cause cognitive decline.

1. The diagnosis requires the **presence of focal neurologic signs or symptoms** or **laboratory evidence of cerebrovascular disease.**

2. Vascular dementia usually has a **fluctuating course,** with the prognosis depending on the type of underlying disorder and the response to treatment interventions, particularly focusing on addressing underlying risk factors, such as atrial fibrillation or hypertension.

C. Dementia resulting from other medical conditions includes a broad range of disorders, such as **structural lesions; trauma; infections; endocrine, metabolic, and/or nutritional disorders; and autoimmune disorders.** In addition, certain conditions that principally affect brain tissue are included in this *DSM-1V* diagnostic area. Examples include **Pick's disease,** dementia associated with **Parkinson's disease, Creutzfeldt-Jakob disease, and DLB.**

1. **Pick's disease** is a rare disorder that initially affects functions (e.g., executive function and behavior) associated with the frontal lobes. The onset typically occurs under the age of 60, and there may be no memory deficits early in the course. The absence of classic Pick bodies on post-mortem studies of some patients has led authorities to characterize the disorder as **frontotemporal dementia,** with Pick's disease being only one subtype of this family of dementias.

2. Dementia principally characterized by cognitive slowing and decreased executive function eventually occurs in approximately one-third of patients with **Parkinson's disease.** Mood and psychotic symptoms also occur frequently and can be worsened by the medications used to treat the parkinsonian symptoms.

3. **Creutzfeldt-Jakob disease** is a rare, rapidly progressive infectious disorder caused by a virus-like entity called a prion. Personality and cognitive changes may precede a variety of neurologic symptoms, including myoclonus. Electroencephalography may show a characteristic wave pattern, and early in the disease a brain biopsy may be necessary to establish a definitive diagnosis.

4. DLB may be more prevalent than previously recognized. Post-mortem studies reveal the presence of cortical and subcortical Lewy Bodies in up to 28% of dementia cases, although they can also be detected in cases of DAT and Parkinson's disease. In addition to cognitive decline (which can be fluctuating), visual hallucinations, delusions, depression, parkinsonian symptoms and falls can be seen. Patients may also be unusually sensitive to adverse effects of typical neuroleptics.

D. **Substance-induced persisting dementia** is diagnosed when history, examination, or laboratory data show that cognitive deficits consistent with dementia probably are caused by substance use. This diagnosis cannot be made if the symptoms are present only in periods of acute intoxication or withdrawal.

1. The most common cause of this type of disorder is **chronic alcohol use.**

2. **Sedatives, hypnotics, inhalants, toxins, poisons,** and other agents also can cause chronic cognitive deficits.

3. Elimination of the offending agent may result in only partial improvement or no improvement at all.

E. **Patients can have more than one cause of cognitive decline.** A fairly common example of dementia resulting from multiple etiologies is the co-existence of DAT and vascular dementia. However, the clinician should inquire carefully about the presence of inappropriate medication usage in patients with other dementing disorders, which would exacerbate these symptoms.

VI. Differential Diagnosis

A. In the medical setting, the two most important disorders requiring differentiation from dementia are delirium (see Chapter 23) and depression (see Chapter 14). Table 22-2 lists the differences among these three entities. However, the clinician must remember that dementia predisposes to delirium and that depression occurs frequently with DAT.

1. In some studies, less than half the patients with **delirium** were identified in a general hospital setting. Furthermore, medically ill patients who have an untreated delirium have a very high 6-month mortality rate. Aside from a history of attentional difficulties and labile affect, simple pencil and paper procedures can be helpful in the diagnosis of delirium. The clinician can ask the patient to write sentences, both dictated and spontaneous. Degradation in the quality of handwriting and difficulty in the completion of the task are highly suggestive of delirium. Patients with mild to moderate dementia usually have well-maintained handwriting and can follow simple dictation easily.

2. **Depression** in the elderly often is **accompanied by complaints of severe memory impairment and dysfunction in self-care activities.** These complaints usually are out of proportion to the test results obtained, which may be quite good if the patient is given sufficient time and encouragement. For depressed patients, there can be variability of test results at different points in time, and such patients may perform better on more difficult tasks than they do on easier ones.

B. Drugs and alcohol intoxication also must be considered in the differential diagnosis. If the symptoms (ataxia, slurred speech, or incoordination) are blatant, the diagnosis is easy to make. However, particularly with habituation or chronic low-dose usage, the symptoms may be subtle, with impaired short-term memory being the only prominent sign.

VII. Care for the Patient with Dementia

A. The importance of determining etiology cannot be overemphasized. The clinician should "think of zebras when hoofbeats are heard." This does not mean that every patient requires arcane laboratory studies, but it does mean that the clinician needs to consider carefully all aspects of the history and physical findings before arriving at a diagnosis. The approach to the treatment of a dementing disorder depends on the specific diagnosis that is established as well as the troublesome symptoms and signs that must be managed. Treatment can be divided into four broad categories: surgical and medical interventions, behavioral treatments, pharmacotherapy, and management of the family and milieu.

1. An example of a **surgical intervention** is the benefit achieved by the shunting of cerebrospinal fluid in patients **with normal-pressure hydrocephalus.** Similarly, when patients with frontal subdural hematomas have them drained, they may experience an improvement in cognition and behavior.

2. **Reversible medical disorders** that cause dementia should be corrected. For example, thyroid repletion in a myxedematous patient usually will improve cognitive function. However, in some conditions, damage has already been done and repletion may provide marginal improvement at best. However, further deterioration of cognition and other nervous system functions may be prevented by the treatment.

3. Sometimes the **reduction or elimination of drugs,** particularly those which affect the central nervous system (e.g., beta-blockers and certain antihypertensives) can be helpful. For example, patients with Parkinson's disease and psychotic symptoms secondary to the use of dopamine agonists may require dosage adjustments to reduce the psychotic symptoms. Another example is barbiturate-induced cognitive decline. Elimination of the sedative is essential, since the cognitive symptoms caused by the drug most likely will remit after its cessation. However, care must be taken to avoid a withdrawal syndrome or another medical complication caused by too abrupt a discontinuation of a drug.

4. **Identification of co-existing medical conditions** that have a deleterious effect on the patient's cognition is critical, particularly in patients with well-diagnosed primary DAT and other dementias. For example, the aggressive treatment of a urinary tract infection improves not only physical comfort but also intellectual functioning (since infection in a patient with DAT often causes delirium). Pain also may have a negative effect on cognition. A patient whose DAT was manageable at home can become severely aggressive and more confused because of the discomfort of an impacted bowel. A patient with presumed vascular dementia may show some improvement in cognition after congestive heart failure is treated.

5. The clinician should review carefully all the **medications** (including over-the-counter agents) a patient currently takes and eliminate any that are unnecessary. In addition, the clinician should be careful not to miss a history of alcohol abuse.

B. Four pharmacologic agents, all acetyl cholinesterase (Ach E) inhibitors, have been approved by the U.S. Food and Drug Administration for cognitive enhancement in DAT. While none of them stop the progression of the dementia, each may slow the rate of decline by six months to a year. All can have cholinergic side effects, such as nausea, headaches, and bradycardia.

1. **Tacrine (Cognex)** is the prototype of this class, but its four-times-a-day dosing, gradual titration upward, frequent blood monitoring (for reversible elevation of liver enzymes), and high rate of side effects limits its current use, as better choices are available.

2. **Donepezil (Aricept)**, a reversible and specific inhibitor of Ach E, tends to have a low incidence of gastrointestinal side effects and no hepatotoxicity. Dosing usually occurs in two steps: 5 mg once per day for four to six weeks, then 10 mg, once per day thereafter.

3. **Rivastigmine (Exelon)** is an inhibitor of AcheE that is metabolized at its site of action (not in the liver), thereby minimizing any drug–drug interactions. It is also an inhibitor of butyryl cholinesterase, providing a theoretical but unproven advantage in late-stage disease, but it also may cause more gastrointestinal side effects than other drugs in this class, particularly at higher doses. The regimen starts at 2 mg twice a day gradually increasing to a maximum of 6 mg twice a day; reaching maximum therapeutic dose may take several months.

4. **Galantamine (Reminyl)**, a reversible AchE inhibitor also is a selective enhancer of nicotinic activity which may have theoretical but unproven boosting effects on acetylcholine as well as other neurotransmitters. It is initiated at a dose of 4 mg twice a day to a maximum dose of 12 mg twice a day, or over a period of 2–3 months.

C. Other agents

1. While **Vitamin E** (an antioxidant) at 2000 IU per day has been shown to slow the course of the disease somewhat, not all patients can tolerate this much and a dose of 400 IU b.i.d. is probably adequate. Although relatively benign, patients on coumadin should be monitored for alteration of bleeding parameters.

2. There is little evidence that **gingko biloba** provides significant benefit. In addition, **anti-inflammatory drugs** and **estrogen** are unlikely to be helpful once a diagnosis is established (however, both may be prophylactic in individuals at high risk for developing DAT).

3. Other treatments (such as agents that modulate neurotransmitters other than acetylcholine and vaccines) remain under study.

D. Treatment of behavioral symptoms is at least as important as treatment of cognitive decline.

1. **Behavioral management** often is highly effective in reducing certain symptoms. The basic approaches are well known but bear repeating.

    a. **Patients with dementia require frequent re-orientation to their environments.** The provision of a clock and a calendar will assist in this regard. Having familiar pictures can be reassuring. A soothing environment with comfortable lighting can have a calming effect.

    b. **Effective communication with the patient is also important.** Speaking "just loudly enough" is a critical first step. Decreased hearing acuity affects all elders, but this does not mean that one has to shout at them.

    c. **The content of what is said to the patient should be simple** and to the point. If the patient has considerable expressive language difficulties, questions should be framed so that a yes or no response will be adequate.

    d. **Reassurance and distraction are the preferred responses** to patients who are easily distressed or become paranoid.

2. **Pharmacotherapy: general rules**

    a. **Make sure that the benefits of treatment outweigh the risks.** The Food and Drug Administration "has not approved any medication" for the treatment of agitation and psychosis associated with dementia. Pharmacotherapy should be reserved for symptoms that are not responsive to the medical corrections and behavioral interventions noted above. Furthermore, certain symptoms (e.g., the motor restlessness and wandering seen in DAT) are poorly responsive to drug therapies.

    b. **The patient should be monitored closely for any improvement or decline in functioning.**

    c. When medication is prescribed, the physician should **start low, escalate doses slowly, and stay the course of treatment.** One should avoid changing medications too quickly on the basis of complaints of minor side effects or lack of efficacy over too short a period of time.

    d. Clinicians should attempt to keep the regimen simple. However, **polypharmacy** is appropriate if a synergistic and/or additive beneficial effect can be achieved. Complex regimens require **consultation** with specialists.

    e. **Take very good care of the caregivers.** There is a high incidence of stress and depression in the care providers of demented patients.

3. **Target symptoms**

    a. **Hallucinations** (particularly visual) and **delusions** (paranoid and other types) frequently occur in patients with DAT and other dementias. The clinician should treat these symptoms only if they cause the patient distress or are potentially dangerous to the patient or others.

       i. Clinicians should recognize that all AchE inhibitors can have a beneficial effect on psychotic symptoms and agitation in DAT, and may also mitigate these symptoms for DLB patients.

      ii. Risperidone (Risperdal) may be better tolerated than are older, traditional antipsychotic agents because of its relatively benign side effect profile. Dosing with risperidone at 0.25 mg per day to start and with gradual titration upward to 1–1.5 mg can be quite helpful. Higher doses are rarely necessary and may cause extrapyramidal signs.

     iii. Alternative novel agents include **olazapine (Zyprexa)** at doses of 2.5–10 mg per day and **quetiapine (Seroquel)** 25–200 mg per day. Both are somewhat more sedating than risperidone, and upward dose titration should be cautious.

     iv. When these drugs fail, **high potency typical neuroleptics,** such as haloperidol, are generally effective. Starting with 0.25 to 0.5 mg of haloperidol (or equivalent dose of similar agents like trifluoperazine or perphenazine), the dose can be gradually increased to 2–3 mg per day. However, these agents must be used with extreme caution if DLB is suspected because cases of severe side effects and death have been reported.

      v. **Low-potency agents,** such as thioridazine and chlorpromazine, have marginal utility as a result of their sedative and postural hypotensive side effects, which often are seen at all but extremely low doses.

      vi. Refractory cases should prompt a referral for consultation.

  b. **The depressive component of any dementia** should be assessed and treated aggressively. If it is unclear how much affective symptoms are contributing to cognitive dysfunction, a therapeutic trial of an antidepressant should be employed.

    i. The choice of an agent is based principally on the side effects it produces; thus, tertiary amine **tricyclics** (e.g., amitriptyline and imipramine) should be avoided. Nortriptyline has been used effectively in patients with depression after a stroke and generally is well tolerated. **The selective serotonin reuptake inhibitors** (SSRIs) (e.g., fluoxetine, paroxetine, sertraline, and citalopram) and **bupropion** have favorable side-effect profiles and should be considered despite the paucity of literature on their use in patients with depression associated with dementia.

    ii. When anergy and lack of motivation are prominent symptoms of the dementia, **psychostimulants** can be tried. For example, methylphenidate, starting at a dose of 2.5 mg t.i.d. and gradually increasing the dose, can be prescribed safely for most patients.

    iii. Finally, in severely depressed patients who have not responded to other treatments, **monoamine oxidase inhibitors** (MAOIs) and electroconvulsive therapy could be considered.

  c. **Agitation** can take the form of motor restlessness, verbal outbursts, and physical aggression.

    i. Before one institutes any medication, reversible causes of agitation, such as infection and drug effects, should be investigated. Several atypical and psychotics are now approved by the Food and Drug Administration for the treatment of these symptoms in the context of dementia, but many classes of medications (including **neuroleptics, benzodiazepines, antidepressants, beta-blockers, and mood stabilizers**) have been tried, and some studies suggest that cholinesterase inhibitors may diminish agitation.

    ii. **Neuroleptics** are the most widely used agents for agitation, but their efficacy is generally considered only fair. Recommendations for their use with hallucinations and delusions also apply for treating agitation.

    iii. **Benzodiazepines** have also been used to treat agitation associated with dementia; however, the risk of worsening cognition and inducing behavioral disinhibition should be weighed against possible benefit, particularly before one prescribes long-acting agents (e.g., diazepam and clonazepam) or prescribes them for protracted periods. The short-acting lorazepam (in an oral dose of 0.25 to 1 mg) is often quite helpful when it is administered before an uncomfortable, potentially frightening procedure, such as a lumbar puncture or magnetic resonance imaging (MRI).

    iv. Reports of **buspirone** used for the treatment of agitation exist, but buspirone usually requires at least a few weeks to achieve a modest benefit.

    v. Among the antidepressants, **trazodone** has been the subject of most case reports documenting behavioral improvement in agitated demented patients. In our experience, trazodone has been modestly effective for agitation but quite useful for nocturnal insomnia. Beginning at doses of 25 to 50 mg per day, trazodone can be increased to as much as 400 mg a day as tolerated. Although generally well tolerated, it can induce postural hypotension and priapism.

    vi. **Beta-blockers** (e.g., propranolol and pindolol) have been beneficial in the treatment of agitation associated with dementias of various etiologies. However, the risk of side effects may outweigh the potential benefits; a very gradual dosage escalation is necessary, particularly in geriatric patients.

vii. **Lithium carbonate, carbamazepine, and valproic acid** have all been reported to improve agitation associated with dementia. Of the three, valproic acid may hold the most promise, since the doses found to be effective are low and side effects are minimal and well tolerated. A starting dose is 125 mg once or twice a day, with therapeutic doses ranging from 250 to 500 mg twice a day. Blood levels should be obtained periodically to guide dosing.

VIII. Summary and Recommendations

A. As the population ages, the number of people with dementing disorders is increasing dramatically; most will have DAT or vascular dementia. Although neither syndrome is curable, both have treatable components, as have all other dementias, whether they are reversible, static, or progressive. The role of the primary care physician (PCP) in the diagnosis and management of these disorders will become more important in the future.

B. Family members are the hidden victims of progressive dementia. They typically appreciate the physician's communication about the diagnosis and the expected course of the disorder. They can benefit from advice about how best to relate to the patient, how to restructure the home environment, and how to seek out legal and financial guidance if appropriate. They may require very assertive assistance from the physician in regard to the issue of driving. Family members also should be made aware of the assistance available to them through organizations, such as the Alzheimer's Association.

C. Referral to a neuropsychiatric consultant is recommended in a number of circumstances:

1. **When the cause of impairment is unclear** despite an initial screening work-up
2. **When the presentation is atypical** or is associated with unusual neurologic or psychiatric symptoms
3. **When the patient has a history of a major psychiatric disorder** and it is unclear how this history affects the presentation
4. **When psychiatric and/or behavioral symptoms do not respond** to usually effective treatments
5. **When family members or the PCP needs additional expert advice** about diagnosis and management
6. **When research protocols that are potentially helpful** to the patient are available

Suggested Readings

Cummings, J.L., Vintners, H.V., Cole, G.M., & Khachaturian, Z.S. (1998). Alzheimer's disease: Etiologies, pathophysiology, cognitive reserve, and treatment opportunities. *Neurology, 51,* S-2–S-17.

Daly, E.J., Falk, W.E., & Brown, P.A. (2001). Cholinesterase inhibitors for behavioral disturbance in dementia. *Current Psychiatry Reports, 3,* 251–258.

Diagnostic and statistical manual of mental disorders (4th ed., Primary Care Version). (1994). Washington, D.C.: American Psychiatric Association.

Felicion, O., & Sandson. T.A. (1999). The neurobiology and pharmacotherapy of Alzheimer's Disease. *Journal of Neuropsychiatry and Clinical Neuroscience, 11,* 19–31.

Geldmacher, D.S., & Whitehouse, P.J. (1996). Evaluation of dementia. *New England Journal of Medicine, 335,* 330–336.

Helmuth, L. (2002). New Alzheimer's treatments that may ease the mind. *Science, 297,* 1260–1263.

Hardy, J., & Selkoe, D.J. (2002). The amyloid hypothesis of Alzheimer's disease: Progress and problems on the road to therapeutics. *Science, 297,* 353–356.

Peterson, R.C., Stevens, J.C., Ganguli, M., et al. (2001). Practice parameter: Early detection of dementia: Mild cognitive impairment (an evidence-based review). *Neurology,* 133–142.

in t'Veld, B.A., Ruitenberg, A., Hofman, A., et al. (2001). Nonsteroidal anti-inflammatory drugs and the risk of Alzheimer's disease. *New England Journal of Medicine, 345,* 1515–1521.

CHAPTER 23

The Patient with Neuropsychiatric Dysfunction

STEPHAN HECKERS AND ROGER C. PASINSKI

I. Introduction

Primary care physicians (PCPs) often are called on to bridge the disciplines of medicine, neurology, and psychiatry in dealing with a patient who has behavioral abnormalities. Behavioral abnormalities that reflect alterations of normal brain function are obvious in patients with neurologic disorders, such as hyperkinetic and hypokinetic movement disorders and generalized seizures. The behavioral manifestations of simple and complex partial seizures and medical conditions, such as thyroid disease and liver failure, are less obvious. Even more complex are the neural substrates of functional psychoses, mood disorders, anxiety disorders, and dementia.

II. General Evaluation

The neuropsychiatric evaluation combines medical, neurologic, and psychiatric skills and includes documentation of the history, examination of the patient, and often the ordering of additional tests.

A. **Specific features of the neuropsychiatric evaluation**
 1. **History.** The history is often difficult to obtain, since the patient's attention, memory, thinking, cooperation, or motivation may not allow the collection of even the most basic details. However, it is very helpful to learn about the onset and course of symptoms and the duration of neuropsychiatric dysfunction. Family members and professional caretakers may be able to provide valuable historic data.
    a. **An acute onset of behavioral change** should always lead to a thorough search for traumatic events, including physical (e.g., traumatic brain injury), chemical (e.g., hypoxia during a stroke), and psychological (e.g., stress during a disaster) insults. Even if a clear injury to the brain cannot be documented, it is still possible that impaired function developed as a reaction to an acute event. Several psychiatric symptoms, such as depression, anxiety, and even amnesia, can present shortly after a traumatic event. Often overlooked are the neuropsychiatric sequelae (such as depression and anxiety after a stroke) of a medical condition that present some time after the initial symptoms have disappeared.
    b. **The age of onset of several neuropsychiatric disorders,** including autism, schizophrenia, mania, and dementia, is relatively well defined. In considering a diagnosis that is rare (e.g., late-onset schizophrenia or early-onset dementia) other, more prevalent conditions should be ruled out.
    c. **The course and temporal pattern** (e.g., stable, progressively deteriorating, episodic, ictal) of the expression of symptoms can provide clues for the diagnosis of specific disorders, such as seizures and dementia. However, a disorder such as bipolar disorder may have a protean time course and often requires detailed charting of individual episodes on a time axis.
    d. **The differential diagnosis** of many neuropsychiatric symptoms is extensive and requires a thorough work-up.

2. **Baseline mental functioning of the patient.** It is crucial to assess the degree of deficits, such as memory loss, language difficulties, and impaired judgment, and determine how it differs from the pre-morbid level of functioning.

3. **Findings of the physical and mental status examination.** It is helpful to organize the pattern of behavioral abnormalities along the lines of cortical and subcortical structures (Table 23-1). However, the behavioral affiliations of brain regions, such as the frontal lobe, are numerous, and lesions can produce markedly different perturbations of behavior.

4. **Think in a circular and comprehensive rather than a linear fashion.** If the patient demonstrates deficits in one behavioral domain, related functions should be examined (see Table 23-1).

B. Medical History

The history of present illness should document recent surgical procedures or medical problems. For example, delirium is often seen post-operatively, after a myocardial infarction, or with infections (especially when fever is present). Depression frequently is seen after stroke or can accompany a malignancy. Particularly challenging are paraneoplastic syndromes, such as limbic encephalitis, if the neuropsychiatric deficits pre-date the onset of other signs of the underlying malignancy. Any previous neurologic event or recurrent psychiatric illness, such as psychotic disorder, anxiety, mood disorder, and drug abuse, should be documented. Current drug use, including prescription, over-the-counter, herbal/alternative, and illicit drugs, should be documented.

C. Examination

1. **Physical examination. Abnormal vital signs,** especially fever and tachycardia, should prompt a thorough search for systemic or central nervous system (CNS) abnormalities that could explain the neuropsychiatric dysfunction. If **signs of meningeal irritation** (neck stiffness, Kernig's sign, or Brudzinski's sign) are present, computed tomography (CT) of the head and lumbar puncture should be performed. During the general physical examination, particular attention should be paid to the stigmata of medical conditions that are known to cause impairment of mental functions (Table 23-2).

2. **Neurologic examination.** The examination of the **cranial nerves** should include a funduscopic examination and the testing of extraocular movements, the sensory and motor function of the face, and the gag reflex. Tests of smell are important in patients with a history of traumatic brain injury if an orbitofrontal process (stroke or tumor) is suspected and in patients who report olfactory or gustatory hallucinations. **Abnormal muscle tone and abnormal movements** of the face and limbs may be seen in patients with extrapyramidal movement disorders and patients treated with psychotropic medications. Muscle strength should be tested for symmetry and weakness. **Examination of reflexes** typically includes deep tendon reflexes, Babinski's reflex, and primitive reflexes (snout, grasp, glabellar, and palmomental reflexes as frontal release signs). Coordination can be tested easily with the finger-nose-finger test or the heel-shin-heel test. Gait and stance also should be assessed.

3. **Laboratory tests.** Tests that can rule out many medical conditions that may lead to neuropsychiatric dysfunction include electrolytes, calcium, glucose, kidney, liver and thyroid function, complete blood count, levels of vitamins B_{12} and folate, arterial blood gases or oxygen saturation, syphilis serology (such as the rapid plasma reagin

Table 23-1. Mapping of Behavioral Abnormalities

Region	Language	Affect	Behavior Memory	Other	Motor
Frontal	Motor aphasia [L] Confabulation	Apathy Inappropriate, disinhibited Motor aprosodia [R]	Impaired working memory	Impaired attention Poor planning, insight Reduplicative paramnesia	Paresis Abulia Echopraxia Perseveration Frontal release signs
Parietal	Dyslexia [L] Dysgraphia [L]	Sensory aprosodia [R]		Impaired attention [R] Dyscalculia [L]	Dyspraxia [R]
Temporal	Sensory aphasia [L]		Impaired encoding/ recall of information	Prosopagnosia [L,R] Finger agnosia [L]	
Striatum	Dysarthria Left caudate nucleus: fluent aphasia				Extrapyramidal movement disorder
Thalamus	Confabulation Anterolateral thalamus: logorrheic aphasia		Impaired encoding/ recall of information	Impaired attention	

NOTE: [L] and [R] indicate the left (dominant) and right (non-dominant) hemispheres, respectively; in some right hemisphere-dominant left-handed subjects, the hemispheric asymmetry is reversed.

DEFINITIONS: abulia, lack of will or motivation; agnosia, lack of sensory ability to recognize objects; aphasia, impairment of language function from brain damage; aprosodia, lack of pitch, rhythm, and modulation in speech; dysarthria, disturbance of articulation; dyscalculia, difficulty computing; dysgraphia, difficulty writing; dyslexia, difficulty reading; dyspraxia, difficulty executing purposeful movements; echopraxia, involuntary imitation of movements made by another person; prosopagnosia, difficulty recognizing faces; reduplicative paramnesia, (Capgras syndrome), delusion that a person has been replaced by an imposter.

Table 23-2. Clues from the General Physical Examination to the Etiology of Neuropsychiatric Dysfunction

Area	Sign	Etiology/Diagnosis
General appearance	Cyanosis	Cardiorespiratory failure
	Pallor	Anemia
Vital signs	Fever	Meningitis, encephalitis
	High blood pressure with bradycardia	Increased intracranial pressure
	Tachycardia	Hyperthyroidism
Skin	Café au lait spots	Neurofibromatosis
	Butterfly rash	Systemic lupus erythematosus
HEENT	Trauma, bruises	Epi- or subdural hematoma, closed head injury, increased intracranial pressure
	Papilledema	
	Oral thrush	HIV/AIDS
Neck	Stiffness	Meningitis, subarachnoid hemorrhage
Lymph nodes	Enlargement, tenderness	Lymphoma, malignancy, HIV/AIDS
Thyroid	Enlargement	Hyper- or hypothyroidism
Chest	Rales	Pneumonia, COPD
		Congestive heart failure
	Wheezing	Reactive airway disease, COPD
Cardiac	S3, enlargement	Congestive heart failure
	Murmur	Endocarditis
Abdomen	Hepatomegaly	Liver disease
Genitalia	Testicular mass	Malignancy
	Pelvic mass	
Extremities	Edema	Congestive heart failure, liver failure, renal failure

[RPR]), and antibodies against the human immunodeficiency virus (HIV). Screening for drugs (illicit, therapeutic, and over-the-counter) in serum and urine is often essential but requires the permission of the patient except in an emergency.

III. Evaluation of Behavioral Domains

A. **Level of consciousness.** An alert patient responds promptly and appropriately to sensory stimulation. Fluctuation of the level of consciousness between alertness, drowsiness, and stupor is a hallmark of acute confusional states (delirium) and may be detected only on repeated examinations. Hyperalertness can be seen in drug-induced states and severe anxiety. Any acute alteration in the level of consciousness requires a prompt examination of vital signs and core neurologic functions to rule out life-threatening situations.

B. Appearance and psychomotor activity. The patient's posture, hygiene, and clothing may provide valuable information about the patient's affect, thinking, and reality testing. The patient's attitude toward the way in which the physician and the patient engage in the interview may provide information about the patient's personality structure. Abnormal motor behavior can be due to cortical, basal ganglia, cerebellar, or lower motor neuron disease. Repetitive movements may represent tremor, dyskinesia, or tics. Psychomotor retardation often is seen in depression, but also can be due to hypokinetic movement disorders (e.g., Parkinson's disease), degenerative diseases (e.g., Alzheimer's disease), stroke, or catatonia. Waxy flexibility (where the patient remains in a position modeled by the examiner) sometimes is seen in a patient in a catatonic state. Increased psychomotor activity to the degree of agitation is seen in anxious or psychotic patients as a side effect of psychotropic medication (akathisia), mainly neuroleptics and selective serotonin reuptake inhibitors (SSRIs), and in patients with the hyperactive form of delirium.

C. Speech. The flow, volume, and rate of speech should be noted. Pressured speech often accompanies a manic state, whereas a decreased rate of speech may be due to depressed mood and unexpected pauses may represent the psychotic symptom of thought blocking. If speech is not coherent or goal-directed, more formal language testing (see Language as follows) and detailed examination of the thought process are warranted. **Prosody,** or the affective modulation of speech, often is impaired in patients with right hemisphere lesions, with parietal lesions more likely to affect the perception (sensory aprosodia) and frontal lesions more likely to affect the production (motor aprosodia) of affectively modulated speech. However, aprosodia also is seen in patients with depression and hypokinetic movement disorders. Abnormalities of the larynx, tongue, or mouth can lead to **dysarthria,** a pure motor dysfunction which should be differentiated from **aphasia.**

D. Affect. The outward display of emotion (affect) should be differentiated from the **internally felt emotion (mood).** Affect is normally appropriate to the situation and congruent with mood and thinking. Inappropriate and incongruent affect is seen in patients with schizophrenia, with mania, or after frontal lobe damage. Pseudobulbar palsy can result in markedly inappropriate and incongruent affect, so-called pathologic laughter or pathologic crying. The range of affect and appropriate modulation can be restricted to a consistently dysthymic or anhedonic level, as in depression, or to a consistently elevated level, as in mania and frontal lobe damage. The mnemonic SIG: E CAPS summarizes the major behavioral representations of affect (sleep, interest, feelings of guilt, energy, concentration, appetite, psychomotor activity, suicidal ideation) that typically are altered in depression and it is helpful in differentiating mild (up to four symptoms) from more severe forms of depression. Irritability, distractibility, and decreased need for sleep typically are seen in manic states.

E. Thought. Thinking is assessed appropriately by listening to the patient talk freely. The **thought process** should be coherent, logically organized, and goal-directed. Loosely organized and incoherent speech (flight of ideas and loose associations), an excessive use of words in response to a question that fails to end with the appropriate answer (circumstantiality) or not answering at all (tangentiality) are typically seen in mania. Also consider aphasia in a patient with incoherent speech (see Language). Poverty of thought with lack of associations is seen in depression, in some forms of schizophrenia, after frontal lobe damage, and in basal ganglia disorders, such as Parkinson's disease. The **thought content** is the material of the patient's conversation. Excessively recurring themes may indicate a preoccupation or delusion. Delusions are often of a persecutory nature (see Chapter 26). It is important to question the patient about the character of his or her thoughts and rule out clearly psychotic symptoms, such as thought insertion or withdrawal and ideas of reference (e.g., the television is sending messages specifically to the patient).

F. **Perception.** The correct reception and interpretation of sensory input can be altered by abnormalities of the peripheral sensory organs, their projections to unimodal cortical areas, and higher-order cortical areas and subcortical structures. Sensory deficits can occur at any of these levels. Illusions typically occur with abnormalities of the sensory organs, in drug-induced states, and in acute confusional states. Hallucinations often are seen in psychotic disorders but also can be found in patients with seizure, stroke, or tumor and secondary to drug intoxication or withdrawal (see Chapter 18).

G. **Cognition.** The Mini-Mental State Examination (MMSE) (Table 23-3) can be used for a quick assessment of cognitive skills. Scores should be adjusted according to the patient's age and education level (Crum et al., 1993).

1. **Orientation.** The patient should be oriented to person, place, and time. Orientation to person is almost always preserved, even in acute confusional states. Non-aphasic patients who are disoriented to person should be evaluated for a dissociative disorder or malingering. Orientation to place (ask for the name of the city, building, floor, and type of room) or time (ask for the year, month, day, and time of day) is often impaired in dementia, delirium, and amnestic disorders. Orientation changes rapidly in acute confusional states, and answers should be recorded to determine the degree of impairment.

Table 23-3. Mini-Mental State Examination and Instructions

Patient _____

Examiner _____

Date _____

MINI-MENTAL STATE EXAMINATION

Maximum score	Score	Orientation
5	( )	What is the (year) (season) (date) (day) (month)?
5	( )	Where are we: (state) (county) (town) (hospital) (floor).
		Registration
3	( )	Name 3 objects: 1 second to say each. Then ask the patient all 3 after you have said them. Give 1 point for each correct answer. Then repeat them until the patient learns all 3. Count trials and record.
		Trials _____
		Attention and Calculation
5	( )	Serial 7's. 1 point for each correct. Stop after 5 answers. Alternatively spell "world" backwards.

Table 23-3. *(Continued)*

		Recall
3	( )	Ask for the 3 objects repeated above. Give 1 point for each correct.
		Language
9	( )	Name a pencil and watch (2 points)
		Repeat the following: "No ifs ands or buts." (1 point)
		Follow a 3-stage command:
		"Take a paper in your right hand, fold it in half, and put it on the floor" (3 points)
		Read and obey the following:
		Close your eyes (1 point)
		Write a sentence (1 point)
		Copy design (1 point)
		Total score
		ASSESS level of consciousness along a continuum

Alert	Drowsy	Stuporous	Comatose

INSTRUCTIONS FOR ADMINISTRATION OF MINI-MENTAL STATE EXAMINATION

Orientation

1. Ask for the date. Then ask specifically for parts omitted, e.g., "Can you also tell me what season it is?" One point for each correct.

2. Ask in turn "Can you tell me the name of this hospital?" (town, county, etc.). One point for each correct.

Registration

Ask the patient if you may test his or her memory. Then say the names of 3 unrelated objects, clearly and slowly, about one second for each. After you have said all 3, ask the patient to repeat them. This first repetition determines the patient's score (0-3) but keep saying them until the patient can repeat all 3, up to 6 trials. If the patient does not eventually learn all 3, recall cannot be meaningfully tested.

Attention and Calculation

Ask the patient to begin with 100 and count backwards by 7. Stop after 5 subtractions (93, 86, 79, 72, 65). Score the total number of correct answers.

If the patient cannot or will not perform this task, ask the patient to spell the word "world" backwards. The score is the number of letters in correct order. e.g., dlrow = 5, dlorw = 3.

Recall

Ask the patient if he or she can recall the 3 words you previously asked him or her to remember. Score 0–3.

Language

Naming: Show the patient a wristwatch and ask him or her what it is. Repeat for pencil. Score 0–2.

(continued)

Table 23-3. *(Continued)*

Repetition: Ask the patient to repeat the sentence after you. Allow only one trial. Score 0 or 1.

3-Stage command: Give the patient a piece of plain blank paper and repeat the command. Score 1 point for each part correctly executed.

Reading: On a blank piece of paper print the sentence "Close your eyes" in letters large enough for the patient to see clearly. Ask the patient to read it and do what it says. Score 1 point only if the patient actually closes his or her eyes.

Writing: Give the patient a blank piece of paper and ask him or her to write a sentence for you. Do not dictate a sentence, it is to be written spontaneously. It must contain a subject and verb and be sensible. Correct grammar and punctuation are not necessary.

Copying: On a clean piece of paper, draw intersecting pentagons, each side about 1 inch, and ask the patient to copy it exactly as it is. All 10 angles must be present, and 2 must intersect to score 1 point. Tremor and rotation are ignored.

Estimate the patient's level of sensorium along a continuum, from being alert on the left to being comatose on the right.

SOURCE: Adapted from Folstein, M.F., Folstein, S.E., & McHugh, P.R. (1975). Mini-mental state: A practical method for grading the cognitive state of patients for the clinician. *Journal of Psychiatric Research, 12,* 189–198.

---

2. **Attention.** The attentional matrix provides the background for all other cognitive faculties and includes vigilance, perseverance, concentration, and resistance to interference. The reticular activating system, the thalamus, and the association cortical areas, primarily those of the frontal lobes, all contribute to the attentional matrix. Serial recitation tasks (such as the serial sevens) and the digit span test (repeating a string of numbers forward or backwards; 6 ± 1 correct numbers in one string is normal) are very helpful and easy to use tests to assess attention. Patients with frontal lobe damage, delirium, or metabolic encephalopathy often score very poorly on these tests. However, anxious and depressed patients also may do poorly. Poor attention is seen in patients with dementia and in children, adolescents, and adults with attention deficit disorder. One form of impaired attention—**unilateral neglect**—is seen after lesions of the parietal cortex, cingulate cortex, frontal eye field, thalamus, or striatum. Simple bedside tests (e.g., asking the patient to bisect lines of varying lengths drawn on a piece of paper or cancel all the letters of one type on a piece of paper covered with many different letters) often are preferable to sensory extinction on one side after bilateral sensory stimulation.

3. **Language.** The disruption of language function interferes significantly with the everyday functioning of the patient. The assessment should include testing of repetition, comprehension, naming, reading, and writing. Spontaneous speech should be classified as fluent or nonfluent. If language deficits are found, it is always helpful

to look for additional neurologic deficits (paresis, apraxia, visual deficits) to localize the lesion.

   a. **Repetition** can be tested with sentences such as "No ifs, ands, or buts." Repetition is impaired in all four major aphasic disorders involving perisylvian structures (Broca's area in motor aphasia, Wernicke's area in sensory aphasia, both areas in global aphasia, and the arcuate fasciculus connecting the two areas in conduction aphasia) (Table 23-4). Paraphasic errors made while repeating should be recorded. Correct repetition does not indicate comprehension of the language.

   b. **Comprehension** can be tested by asking the patient to perform one-, two-, or three-step tasks. Alternatively, especially when the patient is apraxic, simple yes-no questions or commands to point to body parts may be used. If a temporoparietal lesion involves Wernicke's area or its vicinity (as in lesions resulting in sensory transcortical aphasia), comprehension will be impaired.

   c. **Naming** usually is assessed by confrontation naming of objects or body parts. Alternatively, words from a given category, such as animals, can be requested; normal subjects should be able to name about 12 in 1 minute. Word-finding difficulties (dysnomia) also are seen in metabolic encephalopathy, as a side effect of psychotropic medications, and in exhaustion, anxiety, and depression. It is important to rule out other language deficits.

   d. **Reading** should be tested by asking the patient to read individual words, sentences, or paragraphs. Alexia is the inability to comprehend written material; it is associated with **agraphia** if there is a lesion is in the left inferior parietal lobule.

   e. **Writing** tests should include dictation of sentences rather than just phrases such as "I'm fine." Purely mechanical agraphia caused by motor dysfunction should be excluded. Aphasia typically is associated with agraphia, but agraphia is not always associated with aphasia.

4. **Memory.** Short-term memory can be tested by asking the patient to encode a list of three or four words and then testing immediate and delayed recall after 5 minutes. Remote memory can be tested by asking for past events or famous people. Impaired memory is seen in psychiatric disorders and as a result of a neurologic insult. In

---

Table 23-4. Differential Diagnosis of the Main Types of Aphasia

Type of Aphasia	Repetition	Comprehension	Speech
Global	Impaired	Impaired	Non-fluent
Wernicke's	Impaired	Impaired	Fluent
Broca's	Impaired	Intact	Non-fluent
Conduction	Impaired	Intact	Fluent
Transcortical			
Motor	Intact	Intact	Non-fluent
Sensory	Intact	Impaired	Fluent

patients with psychogenic amnesia, personal events cannot be recalled, but non-personal information from the same time period often is spared. Psychotic disorders and depression often lead to impaired encoding of memory. It is always important to distinguish between amnesia, an isolated memory deficit, and more global neuropsychiatric dysfunctions, such as dementia and delirium, that also affect cognitive domains other than memory. Hippocampal damage from hypoxia and hypoglycemia and damage to the thalamus, mamillary bodies, and periventricular structures caused by thiamine deficiency (i.e., Wernicke-Korsakoff syndrome) are well-known causes of amnestic syndromes.

5. **Visuospatial skill.** Drawing intersecting geometric figures or drawing a clock (with the hands indicating, for example, "10 to 2") are simple tests of visuospatial skills. Demented or confused patients and those with lesions of the association cortex in the parietal, temporal, and frontal lobes typically show significant impairment. However, damage of the visual pathways from the retina to the primary visual cortex also can result in impairment. Damage to the parietal lobe of the non-dominant hemisphere is especially likely to produce visuospatial deficits. Such patients also may show dyspraxia, or difficulty executing purposeful movements, such as brushing the teeth, combing the hair, and dressing.

H. **Abstracting abilities.** Testing for abstract similarities (What do a plane and a car have in common?), interpretation of proverbs, or practical judgment (How many slices are in a loaf of bread?) is a helpful probe to determine abstracting abilities affiliated with the dorsolateral frontal cortex. Patients with frontal lobe damage also tend to perseverate, often adhere concretely to the material presented, and have difficulty shifting attention. However, frontal lobe deficits may not be apparent during formal testing in the office but instead be determined by assessing the patient's level of functioning at home. Bilateral frontal lobe damage may lead to **abulia,** or the lack of motivation to speak, move, or act. Other syndromes associated with frontal lobe damage are **reduplicative paramnesia** (Capgras' syndrome), the delusion that a person has been replaced by an imposter, and **echopraxia,** the involuntary imitation of movements made by another person.

I. **Insight and judgment.** Neurologic insults that lead to **unilateral neglect** or **anosognosia** typically cause impaired awareness and insight. Psychiatric conditions, such as mood disorders, schizophrenia, dementia, and amnestic disorders, also produce poor insight. To assess the quality of the patient's insight, ask the patient how much the observed deficits affect him or her or the people around him or her.

IV. Summary

Patients with neuropsychiatric dysfunction present a complex diagnostic and management challenge to the PCP. At times, the diagnosis can be made easily and quickly from an abnormal blood test or a very specific clinical finding. More often, consultation with a psychiatrist or neurologist will be required, as well as brain imaging and neuropsychological testing. With a good foundation in the general principles of neuropsychiatry, the physician can streamline and optimize the evaluation and consultation process.

Suggested Readings

Crum, R.M., Anthony, J.C., Basset, S.S., & Folstein, M. (1993). Population-based norms for the Mini-Mental State Examination by age and education level. *Journal of the American Medical Association, 269,* 2386–2391.

Damasio, A.R. (1992). Aphasia. *New England Journal of Medicine, 326,* 531–539.

Fogel, B.S., & Schiffer, R.B. (1996). *Neuropsychiatry.* Baltimore: Williams & Wilkins.

Folstein, M.F., Folstein, S.E., & McHugh, P.R. (1975). "Mini-Mental State": A practical method of grading the cognitive state of patients for the clinician. *Journal of Psychiatric Research, 12,* 189–198.

Hier, D.B., Gorelick, P.B., & Shindler, A.G. (1987). *Topics in behavioral neurology and neuropsychology.* Boston: Butterworth.

Mesulam, M.M. (Ed.). (2000). *Principles of behavioral neurology.* New York: Oxford University Press.

Mesulam, M.M. (1986). Frontal cortex and behavior. *Annals of Neurology, 19,* 3211–3325.

CHAPTER 24

The Patient with Seizures

STEPHAN HECKERS AND ANDREW J. COLE

I. Introduction

Approximately 5–10% of the population will experience at least one seizure during their lifetimes. The incidence of seizures is highest during childhood and after age 60. Complex partial seizures are the most common seizure type, accounting for about one-third of newly diagnosed cases.

II. Evaluation

A. General Recommendations

1. **Seizure or epilepsy?**

It is important to distinguish patients with a single seizure from those with recurrent unprovoked seizures, that is, those who have epilepsy. Only 30% of patients who have an unprovoked seizure will experience a second seizure. The 2-year recurrence rate is about 40%; it is highest in those with symptomatic seizures (i.e., secondary to a prior brain injury or neurologic syndrome) and those with an abnormal electroencephalogram (EEG). Seizures may recur in people who do not have epilepsy, for example, because of alcohol withdrawal.

2. **Classification of seizures**

Depending on the origin of a seizure (the seizure focus), the clinical symptoms vary considerably. A **simple partial seizure** is due to seizure activity limited to a single brain area (Table 24-1). The symptoms may include motor, sensory, autonomic, and psychic phenomena, but not an alteration in consciousness (Table 24-2). If this type of seizure spreads to closely connected areas and results in impaired consciousness, it is called a **complex partial seizure** (Table 24-1). Many but not all complex partial seizures originate in the temporal lobes. Widespread seizure activity involving the entire cortical mantle either originates from a partial seizure (secondarily generalized) or lacks a focal onset (represents a primary generalized seizure), arising from abnormal thalamocortical interactions (Tables 24-1 and 24-3).

Table 24-1. Seizure Types

| | Consciousness | |
Seizure Onset	Normal	Impaired
Focal	Simple partial	Complex partial
Generalized	—	Generalized

Table 24-2. Clinical Features of Partial Seizures

Feature	Examples
Motor	
Oral	Lip smacking, chewing, swallowing
Upper extremity	Hand clasping, grabbing, picking, tapping, dystonia
Lower extremity	Walking, running, kicking
Vocalization	Grunts, repetition of words or phrases
Sexual	Pelvic thrusting, masturbatory movements
Sensory (hallucination/illusion)	
Olfactory	Unpleasant smell (ammonia, burning rubber, garbage, feces)
Visual	Pattern, geometric shapes, flashing light, formed images, metamorphosia (sudden distortion of a common object), micropsia/macropsia (objects become smaller/larger)
Auditory	Ringing, buzzing, voice
Gustatory	Metallic or foul taste
Vertiginous	Dizziness, nausea
Somatosensory	Headache, focal pain, discomfort, tingling, numbness
Autonomic	
Epigastric	Nausea, "like an elevator ride," abdominal pain
Flushing	Hot sensation
Pupillary changes	Spontaneous unilateral pupillary dilation
Cardiac	Chest pain, tachycardia
Psychic	
Experiential	Illusion of familiarity or unfamiliarity: déjà vu/vécu (already seen/experienced), jamais vu/vécu (never seen/experienced)
Affective	Fear, panic attacks, sadness, depression, sudden crying, explosive laughter
Dysmnesic	Memory flashbacks, memory loss
Compulsive	Forced thinking, rituals

3. **Goals of the evaluation process**
   a. Classification of the seizure type (Table 24-1 and 24-3) and identification of the cause are imperative. However, a definitive structural or functional brain abnormality can be found in only one-third of patients with seizures.
   b. Careful evaluation of the treatment options for idiopathic seizures is required. If deemed necessary, treatment should be efficacious and have as few side effects as possible.

Table 24-3. Classification of Seizure Types

I. Generalized seizures

   A. Tonic-clonic (grand mal) seizures

      1. Primary (idiopathic or familial)

      2. Secondary (due to structural lesion, infection, drug intoxication, metabolic imbalance)

      3. Grand mal status epilepticus

   B. Absence (petit mal) seizures

      1. With impaired consciousness only

      2. With one or more of the following: atonic or tonic components, automatisms, autonomic components

   C. Myoclonic seizures (sudden, brief, involuntary movements)

   D. Clonic seizures (rhythmic contractions of all muscles)

   E. Tonic seizures (sustained muscular contraction, opisthotonus)

   F. Atonic seizures (drop attacks, without warning signs)

II. Partial (focal) seizures (see Table 24-2)

   A. Simple partial seizures: consciousness not impaired

      1. Motor

      2. Sensory

      3. Autonomic

      4. Psychic

   B. Complex partial seizures: consciousness impaired

      1. Simple partial onset followed by impaired consciousness

      2. With impairment of consciousness at onset

      3. With automatisms (impaired attention, perception, and memory with apparently normal or automaton/robot-like motor behavior)

   C. Partial seizures evolving into secondarily generalized seizures

---

   c. Education of the patient and the patient's family about seizures should include information about risk factors and precipitants of seizures such as alcohol, fever, and sleep deprivation as well as the manifestations and treatment of particular seizure types. The clinician may facilitate a discussion of lifestyle planning (e.g., job selection) and should discuss with the patient whether the seizure disorder limits the patient's ability to drive a car. Legislation about driving restrictions for patients with epilepsy varies considerably among the states, and the physician may want to follow published recommendations (Spudis et al, 1986; Krumholz et al, 1991).

   d. Referral to a neurologist should be considered for seizure patients with an acute insult to the central nervous system (CNS) (symptomatic seizures), patients with recurrent unprovoked seizures (epilepsy), and patients who have a poor response to treatment with antiepileptic drugs. Referral to a psychiatrist should be considered for seizure patients with prominent behavioral abnormalities, such as depression, anxiety, hallucinations, and personality changes, and for patients with psychogenic non-epileptic seizures.

B. Medical History

The pregnancy and delivery history is helpful in the assessment of congenital or acquired abnormalities. The physician should ask about possible risk factors, including abnormal gestation, febrile seizures, head injury, encephalitis, meningitis, stroke, and a family history of epilepsy. If there is evidence of epilepsy, the physician should document the onset and course of the epileptic disorder. Particular attention should be paid to a history of drug abuse or dependence. Seizures can occur in a patient in the intoxicated state (e.g., with cocaine) or the withdrawal state (e.g., from alcohol, benzodiazepines, or barbiturates). The use of prescription drugs that are known to lower the seizure threshold (Table 24-4) should be documented.

Table 24-4. Drugs Associated with Seizures

Anesthetics	Psychotropics	Illicit drugs
Enflurane*	Antidepressants	Amphetamine
Etomidate*	Amitriptyline	Cocaine**
Lidocaine	Amoxapine*	Phencyclidine**
Procaine	Bupropion*	Miscellaneous drugs
Antimicrobials	Clomipramine	Baclofen
Imipenem-cilastatin	Desipramine	Beta-blockers
Isoniazid*	Doxepin	Contrast agents**
Metronidazole	Nortriptyline	Cyclosporine
Quinolones	Imipramine	Insulin
Penicillins*	Maprotiline**	Meperidine**
Antineoplastics	Lithium	Narcotics (except
Chlorambucil*	Neuroleptics	meperidine)
Busulfan*	Chlorpromazine*	Propranolol
	Clozapine**	Theophylline*
	Haloperidol	
	Perphenazine	
	Thiothixene	

Drugs Associated with Seizures After Withdrawal

Ethanol

Benzodiazepines

Barbituates

Flumazenil-induced benzodiazepine withdrawal

NOTE: Seizures are typically observed in patients taking high doses or overdoses of these drugs. The estimated frequency of seizures is as follows:
No asterisk: Rare (< 1% and typically < 0.1%)
*Occasional (1–3%)
**Common (> 3%)

C. Interview

Most patients have impaired awareness or frank loss of consciousness during seizures and have difficulty remembering the event. It is very helpful to find a witness who can describe the patient's seizure.

1. Establish the frequency, severity, and duration of the seizures.
2. Try to get a clear picture of the clinical features of the seizure. Pay special attention to the onset of the attack and the sequence of the seizure events. Such information may provide evidence of focality.
3. Without putting words into the patient's mouth, ask about the presence of warning signs or auras (Table 24-2). An **aura** is a simple partial seizure with sensory or autonomic phenomena that may develop into a complex partial seizure with or without secondary generalization.
4. Determine whether there are provocative factors, such as alcohol use, sleep deprivation, or photic stimulation.
5. Document the response to previous treatment with antiepileptic drugs.
6. Ask about specific signs that can help classify the seizure type, such as automatisms, myoclonus, and focal neurologic abnormalities, that point to a seizure focus in one hemisphere.

D. Examination

1. **Physical examination.** In the majority of patients, the neurologic examination is essentially normal. The clinician should look for obvious developmental asymmetries compatible with structural brain lesions and focal neurologic or cognitive abnormalities suggestive of acquired disease. Attention should be paid to evidence of an unrecognized co-existing disease (e.g., stroke, infection, endocrine or metabolic disturbance, and tumor) that could be related to the onset of seizures.

2. **Use of the electroencephalogram.** The first EEG obtained in patients with seizures shows epileptiform discharges (spikes or sharp waves) in 50%. Only 1–2% of normal adults show such abnormalities. However, even with repeated EEG recordings, abnormalities are found in only 60–90% of adults with epilepsy. Sleep deprivation, recordings made during sleep, hyperventilation, and photic stimulation may increase the yield. Referral to an epileptologist for more invasive or extensive uses of EEG should be considered for several groups of patients.

   a. If there is a high suspicion of complex partial seizures and the standard EEG is not diagnostic, specially placed electrodes (e.g., sphenoidal leads and nasopharyngeal leads) help document abnormalities in structures, such as the amygdala and hippocampus.

   b. Simultaneous video and EEG recording is extremely helpful in studying and documenting psychogenic seizures or non-epileptic paroxysmal events and localizing a seizure focus before surgery.

   c. High-quality ambulatory EEG recordings are particularly helpful in the diagnosis of seizures in children.

   d. When the EEG reveals a seizure focus or a characteristic pattern, it may support specific diagnoses (e.g., temporal lobe epilepsy, three-per-second spike and wave pattern in absence seizure) and have therapeutic implications (e.g., choice of the appropriate antiepileptic drugs and referral to surgery).

3. **Imaging.** Magnetic resonance imaging (MRI) is the procedure of choice for anatomic imaging in patients with seizure disorders and is particularly useful in evaluating foreign tissue lesions, cortical dysplasia, developmental abnormalities, gliosis, and

neuronal loss as manifested by atrophy within specific structures. The use of computed tomography (CT) should be confined to the acute management of seizures in the emergency room, if there is a question of intracranial hemorrhage, and to the evaluation of calcified lesions or bony abnormalities that may not be well appreciated on MRI. Positron emission tomography (PET) imaging and single photon emission computed tomography (SPECT) are also useful in examining patients with focal seizures.

4. **Other laboratory tests.** Abnormalities in electrolytes, glucose, calcium, and magnesium and in liver and renal function often contribute to the occurrence of seizures. A lumbar puncture should be performed if a CNS infection is suspected. History or an examination suggesting recent use of drugs should lead to screening for illicit drugs in serum or urine (especially if cocaine is suspected) (Table 24-4).

III. Differential Diagnosis

A. Seizures with a known underlying brain abnormality should be differentiated from idiopathic seizures. Only 30% of patients with seizures have an identifiable neurologic or systemic disorder.

B. Several seizure types can be distinguished on the basis of the phenomenology, site of focus, etiology, or age at onset of seizure.

1. **Tonic-clonic (grand mal) seizures** (i.e., the "classic fit") typically start with a tonic phase during which the patient stiffens, becomes rigid, and loses consciousness; this is followed by a clonic phase of rhythmic jerking limb movements. Bowel and bladder incontinence are common. Post-ictally, patients are briefly unarousable and then lethargic and confused and often prefer to sleep.

2. **Complex partial seizures that originate in the temporal lobe** are the most common seizure type in adults and typically originate in mesial temporal lobe structures (amygdala, hippocampus, and parahippocampal gyrus). Auras and automatisms (such as picking at clothes, a glazed stare, head turning, and lip smacking) are seen frequently. Ictal symptoms range from motor, sensory, and autonomic phenomena to perceptual abnormalities, experiential (e.g., déjà vu, jamais vu) phenomena, and even prolonged confusion and fugue states (Table 24-2). Post-ictal confusion, sedation, and amnesia for the event are typical. Complex partial seizures with prominent motor symptoms or automatisms are not difficult to diagnose. More subtle affective or perceptual abnormalities that are reported by the patient, but are not obvious to the examiner, are more difficult to ascertain and often are misdiagnosed as pseudoseizures or psychiatric disorders.

3. **Frontal lobe seizures** often are short-lived, are followed by a very brief or no post-ictal period, often occur at night, and tend to produce prominent motor symptoms (thrashing limbs, loud and obscene vocalizations). EEG changes are often minimal. These seizures have a proclivity to develop into status epilepticus.

4. **Post-traumatic seizures** typically occur within the first year after the injury; however, 10% occur more than 5 years after the injury. The risk for this type of seizure correlates with the level of consciousness, the extent of injury, the occurrence of hemorrhage, and the loss of brain substance.

5. **Epilepsia partialis continua** (simple partial status) is a syndrome of unremitting motor seizures, often clonic-myoclonic jerks, without a loss of consciousness. They are seen in patients with chronic inflammatory CNS processes, stroke, metastases, metabolic encephalopathy, or hyperosmolar hyperglycemia.

6. **Childhood epilepsy** often has a particular age of onset, for example, **infantile spasms** before 6 months of age and **childhood absence** between the ages of 4 and 12.

C. The recognition of **non-epileptic seizures** is a major challenge for clinicians. These non-epileptic attacks include the following categories:

1. **Pseudoseizuures** (psychogenic non-epileptic seizures) result from a somatization or conversion disorder and should be recognized as a genuine psychiatric illness. Diagnosis involves recording the patient's typical attacks and doing a detailed assessment of psychosocial stresses and underlying psychopathology. Some clues that make pseudoseizure more likely than true seizure include variation of the clinical features from one episode to the next, lack of self-injury, resistance to the attempt to open the patient's eyes, recollection of events after the seizure, and unchanged reflexes during the seizure (Table 24-5).

2. Pseudoseizures should be differentiated from **malingering,** or the conscious creation of non-epileptic seizures as a means to achieve a secondary gain.

3. **Syncope** of vasovagal or cardiogenic origin also may mimic epileptic attacks. This is particularly true during the period of maximal ischemia, when several clonic jerks may be observed by bystanders, leading to the erroneous diagnosis of a seizure disorder. Prodromal events, such as a feeling of warmth, nausea, diaphoresis, and a gradual fading of consciousness, are important historic elements that usually can be remembered by patients who suffer syncopal events.

D. **Psychiatric presentations of seizures.** Simple partial seizures can produce affective and perceptual perturbations (Table 24-2) without alteration of consciousness that mimic the symptoms of psychiatric disorders, such as schizophrenia, depression, mania, and panic disorder. Features more consistent with seizures include a sudden onset of

---

Table 24-5. Differential Diagnosis: Pseudoseizure versus Seizure

Pseudoseizure	*Seizure*
Gradual ictal onset over minutes	Sudden onset, often preceeded by aura
Prolonged duration (> 5 min)	Brief duration (< 5 min)
Clinical features vary from one seizure to another	Stereotypic seizures
Thrashing, crying, pelvic thrusting, side-to-side movements; lack of self-injury; intermittent, out-of-phase jerking	Partial seizure: bizarre, complex motor automatisms
	Rhythmic, in-phase jerking leading to tonic-clonic seizure
Bilateral motor activity with preserved consciousness	Bilateral motor activity typically with impaired consciousness
Unchanged reflexes	Abnormal reflexes during seizure
Frequent seizures despite therapeutic plasma levels of antiepileptic drugs	Typically a decrease in the frequency of seizures with therapeutic plasma levels of antiepileptic drugs
No post-ictal confusion or lethargy	Post-ictal confusion or lethargy often seen

attacks and a time-limited-course of symptoms. Personality changes, including irritability, altered sexual interest, hyperreligiosity, and viscosity of character ("interpersonal stickiness"), can be seen in the inter-ictal period. It is debated whether such inter-ictal behavioral changes are related to the focal abnormality seen during the seizure.

IV. Diagnostic Strategies

As in other branches of medicine, an appropriate diagnosis relies first on the history and examination; however, uniquely in the field of epilepsy, it often requires recording of the attacks of interest for analysis. Every experienced epileptologist has been fooled into thinking that genuine epileptic attacks were pseudoseizures and that pseudoseizures were genuine epileptic attacks. This distinction can be made with certainty only with video/ EEG recording and appropriate analysis. Application of these technological diagnostic strategies may be cost-effective and of benefit to the patient (Chabolla et al, 1996).

V. Treatment Strategies

A. General information

1. **When to treat.** Treatment of first seizures reduces the relapse rate, but the decision to institute treatment should be made individually, weighing the risks of toxic side effects against the potential benefits. Since 60–70% of patients with an unprovoked seizure will not have another seizure, ongoing treatment is not always required. If EEG and imaging studies have not demonstrated any abnormality, it is reasonable to observe the patient without administering antiepileptic drugs until seizure activity recurs (typically during the first 3 months). Patients with an increased risk for a second seizure (structural lesions, pre-existing neurologic deficit, or post-ictal Todd's paresis) may benefit from early treatment with an antiepileptic drug.

2. **How to treat.** The selection of the anticonvulsant drug depends on the seizure type, the presence of liver and renal dysfunction, the use of other similarly acting medications, and the presence of co-morbid mood disorders (Table 24-6). Seizures refractory to medication may be amenable to surgical treatment.

B. Pharmacologic treatment

1. **Antiepileptic drugs**
   a. Valproate, phenytoin, carbamazepine, lamotrigine, and topiramate are all effective for **tonic-clonic seizures.** Valproate should be started at 250 mg twice a day to avoid gastrointestinal side effects, then slowly increasing to 500 mg twice a day. Lamotrigine should be started at 25 mg each day, and gradually increased to 300-500 mg per day to reduce the risk of serious rash. Topiramate should be started at 25 mg b.i.d. and gradually increased to 200 mg twice a day to reduce acute adverse cognitive events.
   b. Carbamazepine, phenytoin, valproate, lamotrigine, topiramate, levtiracetam, phenobarbital, and primidone **are all effective in reducing** the frequency of partial seizures. Phenytoin (starting at 5 mg/kg of body weight) and carbamazepine (starting at 100 mg b.i.d. and advancing to 200 t.i.d. to avoid side effects, such as ataxia and diplopia) are first-line drugs, although newer agents are gradually coming into wider early use. After 3 to 4 weeks, carbamazepine induces its own metabolism and the dose has to be adjusted to achieve a therapeutic level.
   c. Ethosuximide (starting at 500 mg per day), valproate, and lamotrigine are first-line drugs for **absence seizures.** Ethosuximide is ineffective against generalized convulsive seizures.

Table 24-6. Antiepileptic Drugs

Drug	Seizure Type Primary GTCS	Secondary GTCS	Partial Seizure	Absence Seizure	Maintenance Dose mg per day	Therapeutic Levels µg/ml
Phenytoin		1	1	X	300–500	10–20
Carbamazepine	X	1	1	X	400–1,600[a]	4–12
Valproic acid	1	2	2	1	750–3,000	50–100
Ethosuximide	X	X	X	1	750–1,500	40–100
Lamotrigine	1	2	2	1	300–500	3–12
Gabapentin	X	2	2	X	1,200–3,600	5–20
Phenobarbital		3	3		30–180	10–40
Primidone		3	3		500–1,000	4–12.5
Felbamate	[b]	[b]	[b]		2,400–3,600	NA
Topiramate	2	2	2	NA	200–400	4–10
Levtiracetam	NA	2	2	NA	2,000–4,000	NA
Oxcarbazepine	X	2	2	X	600–1,200	NA
Tiagabine	X	3	3	X	16–56	NA
Zohisamide	2	2	2	NA	400	NA

[a]After 4-6 weeks of treatment, autoinduction may necessitate a dosage adjustment.
[b]Use restricted to the most severe cases because of risk of aplastic anemia and hepatic failure.
X: Indicates use may be contraindicated.
NA: Insufficient information available.
GTCS: generalized tonic-clonic seizure.
NOTE: 1,2,3, indicate first-, second-, and third-line drugs.

    d. Newer antiepileptic drugs (lamotrigine, levtiracetam, topiramate, gabapentin, and, rarely, felbamate) should be considered for adults with focal seizures when first-line anticonvulsants are no longer effective or cause intolerable side effects.

    e. About 70% of seizure patients are well controlled on monotherapy. The remaining nonresponders may respond to dual (80% response) or triple therapy (85% response). No consensus exists for the use of multiple anticonvulsants; their use depends on the patient's aversion to drugs and their tolerance for risk.

2. **Long-term laboratory monitoring.** The efficacy of anticonvulsants correlates with the serum level of the drug, not the drug dose. The "therapeutic range" (Table 24-6) is only a guide that indicates the probabilities of efficacy and toxicity but does not predict the occurrence of idiosyncratic side effects. Serum levels may also help assess compliance, since only 70% of patients take antiepileptics as prescribed.

3. **Special conditions**

    a. **Status epilepticus** describes a convulsive or non-convulsive seizure lasting longer than 10 minutes or recurrent seizures without recovery of consciousness between attacks. About 65,000 cases occur each year in the United States. **Convulsive status** is a medical emergency that results in death in 7–10% of affected adults. The outcome depends on the duration of the status. Immediate intervention is essential, including the following steps:

    i. Protect the airways and support breathing and circulation.

    ii. Establish intravenous (IV) access and send off laboratory tests (including chemistry panel, toxicologic screen, arterial blood gases, and complete blood cell count) immediately.

    iii. If there is an uncertain history, an IV glucose solution should be administered.

    iv. Several drugs are effective: IV lorazepam 0.1 mg/kg (i.e., up to 7 mg for a 70-kg person but no faster than 2 mg/minute) is preferred over IV diazepam 0.2 mg/kg (i.e., up to 14 mg for a 70-kg person but no faster than 5 mg/minute) because of its longer half-life. Either of these should be followed immediately with IV fosphenytoin, a water-soluble phenytoin preparation, 20 mg/kg (1,400 mg for a 70-kg person at up to 150 mg/minute), or with phenytoin 20 mg/kg (1,400 mg for a 70-kg person at a rate of 50 mg/minute). IV phenytoin is highly basic (pH 12) and can cause local necrosis if it extravasates, thus fosphenytoin is preferred. If there is no response, additional phenytoin, phenobarbital, or pentobarbital should be given and urgent neurological consultation should be obtained.

    v. Imaging of the brain with CT should be performed to rule out intracranial bleeding or stroke. Lumbar puncture is indicated if an infection is suspected.

Non-convulsive status presents as a confusional state with bizarre behavior, hallucinations, delusions, or even catatonia. The underlying abnormality (generalized absence seizures or complex partial seizures) can be diagnosed by generalized or focal EEG changes. Typically, a good response can be observed to diazepam (5 to 10 mg IV) or lorazepam (1 to 2 mg IV) followed by IV phenytoin (20 mg/kg at a rate of 50 mg/minute).

  b. **Intractable seizures** are defined as epilepsy that remains uncontrolled after an adequate trial (3 months) of available antiepileptic drugs used singly and in combination. Risk factors include being younger than 2 years of age at onset and having frequent generalized seizures, brain damage, a severe EEG abnormality, or a low IQ. Anatomic and functional imaging may document specific causes, such as mesial temporal sclerosis.

  c. Although **seizure prophylaxis** often is initiated in patients with tumors or after a stroke, intracranial hemorrhage, or craniotomy, there is no good data to support this practice. Because anticonvulsants carry the risk of severe adverse events, prophylaxis in patients who have not had seizures is not indicated.

  d. More than 90% of women who receive antiepileptic drugs have a successful **pregnancy** outcome. Valproate and more recently carbamazepine have been associated with neural tube defects in offspring of about 1–2% of mothers who take these drugs. It is now recommended that all women of childbearing age under treatment for epilepsy receive supplemental folate. Monotherapy should be chosen if possible. If valproate or carbamazepine is used, amniocentesis and ultrasound examinations during pregnancy should be considered during week 18 to week 22.

  e. **Withdrawal of antiepileptic drugs** can be considered when a patient is seizure-free for at least 2 years. However, the advice of an experienced neurologist should be obtained, as certain epileptic syndromes have a high rate of recurrence. Most seizures recur within the first year after the cessation of treatment. Factors that predict an unsuccessful withdrawal include an abnormal neurologic exam and difficulty establishing effective seizure control with the initial antiepileptic drug regimen.

C. Epilepsy surgery. Surgical ablation of an epileptogenic focus is a last resort for medically refractory patients with seizures arising from accessible brain regions. Surgical procedures include anterior temporal lobectomy and extratemporal removal, most commonly in the frontal lobe and less often in the parietal or occipital region. Palliative procedures, such as corpus callosotomy, may be performed in patients with intractable drop attacks or atonic seizures. Overall, 65% of patients become seizure-free and 80% experience a significant decrease in seizures after temporal lobectomy. The outcome is not as satisfactory after an extratemporal operation, with 20% of the patients becoming seizure-free and more than 50% having fewer seizures. Patients who may qualify for epilepsy surgery should be referred to a medical facility that can perform the extensive pre-operative diagnostic studies as well as the surgery.

Acknowledgments

The authors thank Dr. Roger Snow for helpful suggestions during the preparation of the manuscript.

Selected References

Brodie, M.I., & Dichter, M.A. (1996). Antiepileptic drugs. *New England Journal of Medicine, 334,* 168–175.

Britton, J.W., & So, E.L. (1996). Selection of antiepileptic drugs: A practical approach. *Mayo Clinic Proceedings, 71,* 778–786.

Cascino, G.D. (1994). Epilepsy: Contemporary perspectives on evaluation and treatment. *Mayo Clinic Proceedings, 69,* 1199–1211.

Chabolla, D.R., Krahn, L.E., So, E.L., & Rummans, T.A. (1996). Psychogenic nonepileptic seizures. *Mayo Clinic Proceedings, 71,* 493–500.

Delgado-Escueta, A.V., & Janz, D. (1992). Consensus guidelines: Preconception counseling, management, and care of the pregnant woman with epilepsy. *Neurology, 42,* 149–160.

Dichter, M.A., & Brodie, M.J. (1996). New antiepileptic drugs. *New England Journal of Medicine, 334,* 1583–1590.

Dodson, W.E., DeLorenzo, R.J., Pedley, T.A., et al. (1993). Treatment of convulsive status epilepticus: Recommendations of the Epilepsy Foundation of America's working group on status epilepticus. *Journal of the American Medical Association, 270,* 854–859.

Engle, J. (1996). Surgery for seizures. *New England Journal of Medicine, 334,* 647–652.

First Seizure Trial Group. (1993). Randomized clinical trial on the efficacy of antiepileptic drugs in reducing the risk of relapse after a first unprovoked tonic-clonic seizure. *Neurology, 43,* 478–483.

Garcia, P.A., & Alldredge, B.K. (1994). Drug-included seizures. *Neurologic Clinics of North America, 1,* 85–99.

Krumholz, A., Fisher, R.S., Lesser, R.P., & Hauser, W.A. (1991). Driving and epilepsy: A review and reappraisal. *Journal of the American Medical Association, 265,* 622–626.

Mattson, R.H., Cramer, J.A., & Collins, J.F. (1992). Comparison of valproate with carbamazepine for the treatment of complex partial seizures and secondarily generalized tonic-clonic seizures in adults. *New England Journal of Medicine, 327,* 765–771.

Mattson, R.H., Cramer, J.A, Collins, J.F., et al. (1985). A comparison of carbamazepine, phenobarbital, phenytoin, and primidone in partial and secondarily generalized tonic-clonic seizures. *New England Journal of Medicine, 313,* 145–151.

Rosentein, D.L., Nelson, J.C., & Jacobs, S.C. (1993). Seizures associated with antidepressants: A review. *Journal of Clinical Psychiatry, 54,* 289–299.

Spudis, E.V., Penry, J.K., & Gibson, P. (1986). Driving impairment caused by episodic brain dysfunction: Restrictions for epilepsy and syncope. *Archives of Neurology, 43,* 558–564.

Stevens, J. (1988). Psychiatric aspects of epilepsy. *Journal of Clinical Psychiatry, 49*(Suppl 4), 49–57.

Tisher, P.W., Holm, J.C., Greenberg, M., et al. (1993). Psychiatric presentations of epilepsy. *Harvard Review of Psychiatry, 1,* 219–228.

CHAPTER 25
The Patient Following Closed Head Injury

FELICIA A. SMITH AND KATHY M. SANDERS

I. Introduction

A. **Nearly 10 million head injuries occur in the United States yearly.** Ninety percent of these injuries are considered mild to moderate. **Closed head trauma results from non-penetrating blows to the head, either with or without loss of consciousness.** The yearly incidence of brain injury and post-concussion syndrome is 350 per 100,000. This is greater than the incidence of dementia, epilepsy, multiple sclerosis, Parkinson's disease, schizophrenia, and stroke combined! Because of the apparent minimal injury sustained in closed head trauma, patients are expected to recover rapidly and completely. However, **although the majority of symptoms experienced by patients in the initial post-concussive phase resolve by 3 to 6 months, some patients show significant neuropsychological impairments several years after their injury.**

1. **Acceleration/deceleration forces** may cause significant neuronal damage from shear forces. Microscopic disruption of cerebral vasculature and nerve fibers results in a wide variety of neuropsychological deficits.

2. The primary brain injury in **closed head injury typically occurs in the anterior temporal lobes and on the inferior surface of the frontal lobes.**

3. Complex and heterogenous neurobehavioral impairments, involving cognitive, somatic, and emotional symptoms, may follow closed head injury.

4. Higher rates of mood and anxiety disorders have been seen after closed head injury.

5. **The personal cost of closed head injury and its recovery involves changed personality, disrupted relationships, extensive medical care (for the management of the acute injury and rehabilitation), and economic losses due to unemployment.**

6. Neurocognitive deficits cause more morbidity than do physical deficits with regard to returning to work and social activities.

II. Evaluation of the Problem

A. **General Recommendations**

1. Maintain a high degree of clinical suspicion that cognitive-behavioral symptoms are due to a previous head injury. Expect head injury sequelae until proven otherwise.

2. A thorough assessment of mood, anxiety, and personality changes should be a routine part of post-head injury screening, as should a comprehensive cognitive-behavioral evaluation.

3. In general, most of the neurocognitive and behavioral symptoms associated with closed head injury resolve within 6 months. However, cognitive deficits and personality changes may persist for several years.

4. Psychosis following head injury is rare; it may be significantly delayed in its onset when it does occur.

Table 25-1. Neurobehavioral Symptoms of Post-concussive Syndrome

Somatic	Cognitive	Emotional
Headache	Diminished concentration	Irritability
Dizziness	Memory problems	Anxiety
Fatigue	Perseveration	Mood lability
Sleep disturbance	Poor planning	Hypochondriasis
Photophobia	Dyspraxia	Depression
Hypersensitive to noise	Vacuous appearance	Personality changes
Tinnitus	Poor motivation	Apathy
Blurred vision	Poor attention	Aggression
Diminished libido		Avoidance
Decreased tolerance to alcohol		Disinhibition

B. Medical History

1. Concomitant substance abuse disorders, which may or may not be remembered by the patient, often co-exist in patients who have suffered head trauma.
2. Additionally, substance abuse may affect the degree of damage sustained in a closed head injury owing to underlying effects on cerebral blood flow and neurotransmitter response to injury and recovery.
3. Suspect a head injury when there has been a significant history of physical injuries, motor vehicle accidents, falls, or fights.
4. In general, mild head injuries result from traffic injuries, falls, fights, sports injuries, and work-related accidents.
5. Older patients, or those with evidence of arteriosclerosis, may suffer more significant cognitive and neurobehavioral impairments following mild head trauma.
6. Rapid return to work or involvement in stressful activities after a mild head injury may bring out subtle cognitive deficits not previously noted.

C. Interview

1. Components of the interview should elicit a significant history of head trauma. Searching for head injuries sustained in childhood is important because post-concussion disorder may have long-term ramifications.
2. Search for athletic injuries, episodes of loss of consciousness and their etiology (e.g., substance abuse blackouts), and risk-taking behaviors (e.g., bungee jumping, motor-cycle riding, or rollerblading in traffic).
3. Elicit a history of subtle personality changes.
   a. Determine if the patient's significant others complain of a change in behavioral style (e.g., vacuous, non-engaging, or apathetic)
   b. Ask about irritability and impulsivity.
4. Look for changes in pre-morbid job function.
   a. Determine if there has been a decline in work capabilities.
   b. Inquire about the patient's inability to handle the pace of work or to carry out several tasks simultaneously.

5. Be aware of attempts to obtain secondary (e.g., litigious) gain.
   a. Determine if the symptoms vary from visit to visit.
   b. Evaluate whether symptoms appear exaggerated.
   c. Consider whether there are true impairments but the patient seems more incapacitated than objective findings warrant.
   d. Assess whether there is little or no follow-up on the patient's part for treatment and rehabilitation recommendations.
   e. Determine if there is pressure from the patient or family to document and apply for disability.

D. Examination of the Patient
   1. Objective evidence of impairment in memory, concentration, and tolerance of visual and auditory stimulation should be evaluated.
      a. Neuropsychological testing that focuses on attention, concentration, and memory impairment will further specify and quantify deficits. (See Chapter 23, Neuropsychiatric Dysfunction.)
      b. Neurocognitive testing, coupled with personality and stress testing, will be useful in designing an individualized rehabilitation program.
   2. Use of the electroencephalogram (EEG) and magnetic resonance imaging (MRI) of the brain will help establish the impact of significant head injury.
      a. Although the EEG may be normal, focal abnormalities in the EEG, when present, support an organic basis of symptomatology.
      b. Frontal intermittent rhythmic delta activity (FIRDA) is a non-specific indicator of metabolic disruption in the brain.
   3. MRI may show subtle lesions in the frontal and temporal lobe regions, and in the periventricular white matter. Findings may not be deficit-specific.
   4. In general, clinical improvement is reflected in normalization of the EEG and MRI.

III. Psychiatric Differential Diagnosis

A. The differential diagnosis of a post-concussive disorder includes dementia, mild neurocognitive disorder following head trauma, somatization disorder, factitious disorder, and malingering. In all cases, the differential is based on the presence of a complex constellation of cognitive, somatic, and behavioral symptoms found in a patient following a concussion. Other diagnoses are limited to symptoms found in only one or two of these symptom categories. The most difficult diagnosis to make is that of malingering. Confirmation of this diagnosis (and proving that secondary gain is creating or exaggerating impairments) takes time and consistent re-evaluation of symptoms.
   1. Despite the fact that memory impairment and other measurable cognitive and behavioral impairments may result from head injury, dementia due to head trauma is not classified as a post-concussive disorder. When only cognitive impairment follows a head injury, the diagnosis is dementia.
   2. A mild neurocognitive disorder may follow head injury or result from some other medical condition. It lacks the complexity of a post-concussion disorder with cognitive, somatic, and behavioral symptoms.
   3. Somatization disorder may result in similar behavioral and somatic symptoms, but lacks measurable cognitive impairments.
   4. Factitious disorder (with an underlying dynamic to assume the sick role) may result in a symptom complex that may look like a post-concussive disorder.

5. Malingering should be suspected in cases where compensation and legal issues predominate. Secondary gain may influence the course and progression of symptoms following a closed head injury.

B. Rule out major depression, bipolar disorder, post-traumatic stress disorder, adjustment disorder with mixed emotional and behavioral features, and organic personality disorder. It is important to note, however, that there is evidence for causal association between head injury and mood and anxiety disorders.

IV. Diagnostic Criteria

Research criteria have been developed (see following, from Appendix B of *DSM-IV-TR* for post-concussional disorder. These criteria will help develop and refine our understanding of post-concussive syndromes.

A. A history of head trauma that caused significant cerebral concussion. Note: the manifestations of concussion include loss of consciousness, post-traumatic amnesia, and, less commonly, post-traumatic onset of seizures. The specific method of defining this criterion needs to be established by further research.

B. Evidence from neuropsychological testing or quantified cognitive assessment of difficulty in attention (concentrating, shifting focus of attention, performing simultaneous cognitive tasks) or memory (learning or recalling information).

C. Three (or more) of the following occur shortly after the trauma and last at least three months:
1. Fatigue
2. Disordered sleep
3. Headache
4. Vertigo or dizziness
5. Irritability or aggression on little or no provocation
6. Anxiety, depression, or affective lability
7. Changes in personality (e.g., social or sexual inappropriateness)
8. Apathy or lack of spontaneity

D. The symptoms in Criteria B and C have their onset following head trauma or else represent a substantial worsening of pre-existing symptoms.

E. The disturbance causes significant impairment in social or occupational functioning and represents a significant decline from a previous level of functioning. In school-aged children, the impairment may be manifested by a significant worsening in school or academic performance dating from the trauma.

F. The symptoms do not meet criteria for dementia due to head trauma and are not better accounted for by another mental disorder (e.g., amnestic disorder due to head trauma, personality change due to head trauma).

V. Treatment Strategies

A. Rehabilitation in a multifactorial, multidisciplinary, and collaborative approach to patient evaluation and treatment planning is the basis of treatment of brain-injured patients, and is best accomplished by a case management team.
1. **Neuropsychiatric assessment** over time and in response to treatment should include psychiatric, psychological, behavioral, occupational, and vocational evaluations. (See Chapter 23, Neuropsychiatric Dysfunction.)

2. **Brain-injury treatment centers** are best equipped for this comprehensive evaluation and for observation over time. (See Chapter 9, Principles of Behavioral Therapy.)

3. **Behavioral techniques** are valuable in managing aggressive outbursts or other inappropriate social behavior.

4. **Vocational counseling and skills retraining** to assist patients who have memory and concentration impairments provide specific strategies to work with and around such deficits.

5. **Stress management and coping skills** are particularly useful psychological interventions that take into account pre-morbid functioning, reaction to the injury, and response to deficits sustained from the injury. Pre-morbid personality or psychopathology will worsen in response to brain injury. Psychological and cognitive approaches work synergistically with psychopharmacology for optimal recovery.

6. **Family therapy and couples counseling** will be useful for the patient with significant personality changes after head injury. (See Chapter 59, The Family in Crisis.)

B. **Psychopharmacology of the head-injured patient is symptom-based and is generally used when depression, aggression, or psychosis complicates recovery.**

1. **General caveats** include the following:

a. Brain-injured patients are more sensitive to side effects of medications and to the effects of lowering the seizure threshold caused by use of psychotropic medications.

b. As with geriatric patients, start with low doses and gradually increase doses over time.

c. Co-administration of effective doses of anticonvulsants and psychotropics (that lower the seizure threshold) is protective.

2. **Treatment of affective illness**

a. The use of antidepressants for head-injured patients should follow the same principles as are followed for the treatment of depression in the non-injured brain. (See Chapter 14, Approach to the Patient with Depression.) Side effects may limit drug choice. Tricyclics lower the seizure threshold and usually require upward dose titration for therapeutic effects. The selective serotonin reuptake inhibitors may cause more side effects in patients with brain injury than seen in the un-injured population.

b. Use of psychostimulants or electroconvulsive therapy are other treatment options.

c. Treatment of mania will likely require use, in therapeutic doses, of lithium carbonate, carbamazepine, or valproic acid.

d. Mood lability may be managed with doses of antidepressants and/or anticonvulsants that are in general lower than are typically used for major depression.

3. **Treatment of psychosis** responds to the use of neuroleptics.

a. Brain-injured patients are more susceptible to the sedating, hypotensive, and extrapyramidal side effects of neuroleptics.

b. Some neuroleptics (particularly low-potency agents with anticholinergic side effects) are likely to lower the seizure threshold.

c. Use low starting doses.

4. **Treatment of aggression** is a challenging and multifactorial problem faced during both acute and chronic rehabilitation phases after brain injury.

a. Acute aggression is best managed with antipsychotic or neuroleptic medication.

b. When sedation is a desired result of medication, benzodiazepines and other sedative hypnotics may be employed.

c. **The chronic management of aggression requires a comprehensive treatment plan** for observation of the target behaviors and response to interventions.

d. Pharmacologic management includes use of antidepressants, buspirone, anticonvulsants, lithium carbonate, neuroleptics, and β-blockers.

Suggested Readings

Bohnen, N., & Jolles, J. (1992). Neurobehavioral aspects of postconcussive symptoms after mild head injury. *Journal of Nervous and Mental Disease, 180,* 683–692.

Bohnen, N., Twijnstra, A., & Jolles, J. (1993). Persistence of postconcussional symptoms in uncomplicated, mildly head-injured patients: A prospective cohort study. *Neuropsychiatry Neuropsychology and Behavioral Neurology, 6,* 193–200.

Corrigan, P.W., & Yudofsky, S.C. (Eds.). (1996). *Cognitive rehabilitation for neuropsychiatric disorders.* Washington, DC: American Psychiatric Press.

Cummings, J.L., & Trimble, M.R. (2002). *Concise guide to neuropsychiatry and behavioral neurology* (2nd ed.). Washington, DC: American Psychiatric Press.

Deb, S., Lyons, I., Koutzoukis, C., et al. (1999). Rate of psychiatric illness 1 year after traumatic brain injury. *American Journal of Psychiatry, 156*(3), 374–378.

Diagnostic and statistical manual of mental disorders (4th ed., Text Revision). (2000). Washington, DC: American Psychiatric Association.

Frieboes, R.M., Muller, U., Marck, H., et al. (1999). Nocturnal hormone secretion and the sleep EEG in patients several months after traumatic brain injury. *Journal of Neuropsychiatry and Clinical Neuroscience, 11*(3), 354–360.

Fujii, D.E., & Ahmed, I. (2001). Risk factors in psychosis secondary to traumatic brain injury. *Journal of Neuropsychiatry and Clinical Neuroscience, 13*(1), 61–69.

Goldstein, F.C., Levin, H.S., Goldman, W.P., et al. (2001). Cognitive and behavioral sequelae of closed head injury in older adults according to their significant others. *Journal of Neuropsychiatry and Clinical Neuroscience, 7*(3), 373–383.

Leininger, B., Gramling, S., Farrell, A., et al. (1990). Neuropsychological deficits in symptomatic minor head injury patients after concussion and mild concussion. *Journal of Neurology Neurosurgery and Psychiatry, 53,* 293–296.

Max, J.E., Robertson, B.A., & Lansing, A.E. (2001). The phenomenology of personality change due to traumatic brain injury in children and adolescents. *Journal of Neuropsychiatry and Clinical Neuroscience, 13*(2), 161–170.

Ponsford, J. (1990). Psychological sequelae of closed head injury: Time to redress the imbalance. *Brain Injury, 4,* 111–114.

Significant Achievement Awards: Creating a continuum of care for a previously unserved population—McHenry County (Ill.) traumatic brain injury case management program. (1998). *Psychiatric Services, 49,* 1344–1345.

Silver, J.M., Hales, R.E., & Yudofsky, S.C. (1992). Neuropsychiatric aspects of traumatic brain injury. In S.C. Yudofsky, & R.E. Hales (Eds.), *Textbook of neuropsychiatry* (2nd ed.). Washington, DC: American Psychiatric Press.

Silver, J.M., Hales, R.E., & Yudofsky, S.C. (Eds.). (1994). *Neuropsychiatry of traumatic brain injury.* Washington, DC: American Psychiatric Press.

Slagle, D.A. (1990). Psychiatric disorders following closed head injury: An overview of biopsychosocial factors in their etiology and management. *International Journal of Psychiatry and Medicine, 20,* 1–35.

Van Reekum, R., Cohen, T., & Wong, J. (2002). Can traumatic brain injury cause psychiatric disorders? *Journal of Neuropsychiatry and Clinical Neuroscience, 12*(3), 316–327.

CHAPTER 26

The Patient with Headache

CLAUDIA BALDASSANO AND THEODORE A. STERN

I. Introduction

Headache is one of the most frequent complaints in a medical practice, and nearly everyone has experienced a headache. Typically, those with headaches treat themselves, but those that consult a physician are often worried about some dire underlying cause. Proper diagnosis is essential so that timely and effective therapy can be provided.

II. Evaluation of the Problem

A. **General recommendations.** Many factors are involved in categorizing and making a diagnosis of headache. It is rare for any test to demonstrate an abnormality that is not suspected from the history or the physical examination. The physical examination and the neurologic examination, the response to medications, and follow-up observations are crucial factors for making the proper diagnosis and for directing effective treatment.

B. **Medical history.** Head injury or trauma preceding a headache may be significant historical features. Diseases of the eyes, ears, nose, and sinuses also may cause headaches. Infections in the head and neck should alert one to the possibility of an intracranial abscess. A recent onset of headache and confusion should alert one to central nervous system (CNS) infection or disease. Hypertension may exacerbate migraines or tension headaches, particularly if the hypertension is labile. Constant headaches in obese females should lead one to consider the diagnosis of pseudotumor cerebri. Smoking and alcohol consumption predispose individuals to cluster headaches.

C. **Interview.** Obtaining a good headache history from a patient is the most important step in making an accurate diagnosis. Identification of the severity and character of the headache pain, the precipitating and alleviating factors, the duration of the headache syndrome, the temporal associations, the typical onset and offset, the ameliorating or exacerbating factors, the impact of medications, and the prodromal symptoms (if any) is essential to making the proper diagnosis and to guiding further evaluation.

   1. **Epidemiology**
      a. **Migraine headaches**
         i. The prevalence in females is approximately 20%, and that in males is about 6%.
         ii. After puberty, migraines are more common in females than in males, but in children there is a slight preponderance among males.
         iii. Ninety percent of afflicted persons have their first attack by age 40.
         iv. A family history is present in up to 90% of migraine sufferers.
         v. A higher incidence of duodenal ulceration and elevated gastric acid levels is found in those with migraines.

     b. **Cluster headaches**

        i. The ratio of males to females is 5:1.

        ii. The estimated prevalence of cluster headaches ranges from 0.4–0.8% and most individuals start to develop attacks before the age of 25.

        iii. Rarely is there a family history of cluster headaches.

        iv. A higher incidence of duodenal ulceration and elevated gastric acid levels is present among those with cluster headaches.

        v. Cluster headaches are strongly related to tobacco smoking and cluster headaches are often triggered by alcohol consumption.

2. **Characteristics of Headaches**

    a. **Migraine Headaches**

        i. Migraines are usually unilateral in the frontotemporal area.

        ii. Migraines often are experienced behind the eyes.

        iii. Episodes are usually severe and throbbing.

        iv. **Photophobia and sonophobia** (sensitivity to sound) are common features.

        v. **Nausea and vomiting** are common features.

        vi. Chills, polyuria, diarrhea, urticaria, and a feverish sensation also occur.

        vii. The headache typically last from 4 to 24 hours.

        viii. Foods, such as aged cheese, red wine, chocolate, and peanuts can precipitate migraines.

    b. **Tension Headaches**

        i. Tension headaches are usually generalized.

        ii. They may be concentrated in the frontal, nuchal, or occipital area.

        iii. They are often described as "bandlike" or feeling like a "tight hat."

    c. **Cluster Headaches**

        i. Cluster headaches are by far **the most painful type of recurrent headache.**

        ii. They typically are manifested by stereotyped attacks.

        iii. Despite readily recognizable features, cluster headaches often are misdiagnosed as trigeminal neuralgia or as sinus or dental disease.

        iv. Often retroorbital and in the temporal region, they are usually unilateral; they may switch sides from one cluster to the next.

        v. Pain may uncommonly be localized to the cheek or jaw.

        vi. The onset of cluster headaches occurs quickly, with pain intensifying very rapidly and peaking in 5 to 10 minutes.

        vii. Injected conjunctiva, nasal blockage, profuse sweating, facial flushing on the side of the headache, ptosis, and miosis on the side of the pain are common.

        viii. Photophobia may occur, though it develops less commonly than it does with migraines.

        ix. Facial swelling may occur.

        x. Smoking tobacco and drinking alcohol can precipitate headache.

    d. **Headaches from Organic Disease** (e.g., mass lesion or infection)

        i. Headaches from mass lesions are constant in nature, but may be intermittent.

        ii. These headaches usually are not as severe as the pain of migraines.

        iii. Such headaches are often associated with nausea and vomiting.

    e. **Psychogenic Headaches**

        i. Heaviness, fullness, or tightness about the scalp often is present.

        ii. These headaches usually occur daily without periods of relief.

        iii. Often an underlying depression is present.

f. **Headaches from Aneurysms and Arteriovenous Malformations**

    i. **Intracranial aneurysms** are rarely responsible for headaches unless they rupture, and aneurysms are never the cause of migraine headaches (the incidence of migraines in patients who have ruptured an aneurysm is 5%, which is similar to the incidence in the general population).

    ii. **Arteriovenous malformations (AVMs)** rarely cause pain before they rupture. Very large lesions can be associated with ipsilateral or bilateral throbbing headaches, but only rarely do they cause a migraine-like syndrome. AVMs should be suspected when the triad of seizures, headaches, and focal neurologic deficits is present.

g. **Headaches from a Subarachnoid Hemorrhage**

    i. Rupturing of an intracranial aneurysm or AVM results in a subarachnoid hemorrhage.

    ii. The headache typically is described as explosive in onset and of an overwhelming intensity. The headache rapidly generalizes and may be associated with neck and back pain.

    iii. Vomiting may be an associated feature.

    iv. Loss of consciousness usually intervenes.

h. **Sinus Headaches**

    i. Maxillary sinusitis gives rise to pain and tenderness over the cheek. Frontal sinus disease gives rise to frontal pain. Sphenoidal and ethmoidal sinusitis causes pain behind and between the eyes and it may be referred to the vertex.

    ii. Pain is worsened by bending forward or by coughing.

3. **Onset and Duration of the Headache Syndrome**

a. **Migraine Headaches**

    i. Usually migraines start during the teenage years.

    ii. Often migraines improve in a person's thirties and forties.

    iii. Migraines are exacerbated or relieved during menstruation, pregnancy, and menopause.

b. **Tension Headaches**

    i. These headaches usually begin after the age of ten.

    ii. They are usually exacerbated during times of stress or at the end of the day.

c. **Cluster Headaches**

    i. Usually are seen in males (in their twenties through sixties).

    ii. Cluster headaches come in clusters and last for weeks to months.

    iii. Cluster headaches may be seasonal.

    iv. A positive family history of cluster headaches is usually absent.

d. **Organic Headaches**

    i. These headaches do not fit the classic patterns suffering of migraine, tension, or cluster headaches.

    ii. There may be a sudden appearance of headache in a person without a previous history of headaches.

e. **Psychogenic Headaches**

    i. There is no specific age of onset for these headaches.

4. **Precipitating and Ameliorating Factors**

a. **Migraine Headaches**

    i. Alcoholic beverages, chocolate, aged cheese, and monosodiurn glutamate may precipitate migraine.

    ii. Hypoglycemia may trigger migraines ("hunger headaches").

    iii. Menstrual periods may exacerbate headaches.

        iv. Oral contraceptives and estrogens aggravate or induce headaches.

        v. Reserpine and vasodilating antihypertensive agents, such as hydralazine and nitrates, often induce headaches.

        vi. Indomethacin may cause migraines.

        vii. Weekends and vacations and the time after a stressful menstrual period may induce migraine.

        viii. Bright lights (particularly sunlight), weather changes, pollution, and carbon monoxide exposure may induce a migraine attack.

        ix. The headache often is relieved by sleep and by vomiting.

    b. **Tension Headaches**

        i. These headaches occur during stressful periods.

        ii. They are often relieved by relaxation techniques and by neck massage.

    c. **Cluster Headaches**

        i. These headaches may be precipitated by alcohol ingestion.

        ii. Headache-onset often occurs during the night or 1 to 2 hours after going to sleep.

        iii. Cluster headaches are not relieved by sleep.

        iv. Almost invariably, those with cluster headaches are unwilling to lie down because doing so increases the intensity of the headache.

        v. Unlike patients with migraines, these patients are restless and prefer to pace during an attack.

        vi. Cold weather and being outdoors may help those who suffer from cluster headaches.

    d. **Organic (e.g., Brain Tumor) Headaches**

        i. These headaches may be worse when the patient first arises in the morning.

        ii. Coughing or straining may exacerbate these headaches.

  5. **Prodrome**

    a. **Migraine Headaches**

        i. Migraine headaches are classified as classic (preceded by a visual or olfactory aura) or common (no prodrome).

        ii. The most common prodromes are visual, such as flashing lights, field cuts, and scintillations.

        iii. Any neurologic symptoms can be part of a prodrome.

    b. Other headache syndromes usually do not have prodromes.

D. Examination of the patient must include a neurological examination, a funduscopic examination (that searches for papilledema) and a physical examination of the head (that searches for tenderness, masses, or bruits) may offer clues to the presence of organic factors, particularly if the patient is symptomatic during the examination.

  1. Evaluate for **focal signs** which may be indicative of a structural lesion, such as a brain tumor or an AVM. Any asymmetry in the examination should prompt further evaluation. A careful funduscopic examination is essential to look for papilledema.

  2. Evaluate for **autonomic dysfunction** during the headache, such as nasal congestion, tearing, and injection of the eye, which may lead to the diagnosis of cluster headaches.

  3. Evaluate for **scalp tenderness,** which may indicate migraine headaches.

  4. Evaluate for **temporal artery tenderness,** as temporal arteritis in the elderly may present with headaches. One sometimes can see an inflamed temporal artery that is exquisitely tender to palpation.

  5. Evaluate for **increased intraocular pressure** by palpating the globe. This is important in the elderly who present with eye pain, red eye, and vomiting, as glaucoma can have headache as the presenting complaint.

6. Evaluate for **hypertension,** as it can lead to exacerbation of the headache syndrome, although it rarely is the etiologic cause.

7. Evaluate for **cervical arthritis,** which can present as headache in the elderly. Neck stiffness or neck mobility that exacerbates the headache may be a clue.

8. Evaluate for **papilledema** in a young obese female who present with headaches, as pseudotumor cerebri is not an uncommon cause of constant headaches in young people.

9. Evaluate for a **cranial bruit** which can be seen with an AVM.

E. **Performance of ancillary tests.** Although it is unusual for any test to identify an abnormality not suspected by the history and physical examination, special tests may confirm the presence of specific diagnosis.

1. CT and MRI may detect masses.

2. A lumbar puncture may allow for identification of infection.

3. An elevated erythrocyte sedimentation rate may suggest a giant cell arteritis.

III. Psychiatric Differential Diagnosis

In the evaluation of a headache patient, the physician must deal not only with the symptom of the headache but also with the patient. **Emotional factors play a role in the perception of, and reaction to, pain,** and the doctor must not lose sight of the fact that the patient is feeling pain. Depression commonly presents with headaches and other somatic complaints. Complaints of daily, constant, and unremitting headache should alert the physician to the possibility of major depression. Treatment strategies should be directed toward optimizing treatment for major depression, and this usually results in resolution of the headache syndrome.

IV. Treatment Strategies

A. **Acute Treatment for Migraines.** The most commonly used medications for abortive treatment of migraines are a new class of medication called triptans. Triptans are 5-HT agonists. Although they cannot prevent migraines, they are used to stop the headache and its associated symptoms. Drugs in this class need to be taken early in the headache cycle to be most effective. They should only be prescribed after a thorough examination that in part serves to rule out contraindications (see below).

1. Triptans: sumatriptan, zolmitriptan, naratriptan, rizatriptan, almotriptan, frovatriptan, eletriptan

a. Sumatriptan (Imitrex) (100 mg tab, 6 mg subcutaneous, or 5 mg or 20 mg nasal spray); Dose: 100 mg PO given immediately; may repeat in 2 hours not to exceed 200 mg/day or 6 mg subcutaneously, may repeat in 1 hour not to exceed 12 mg/day or 20 mg nasal spray or 5 mg nasal spray—one spray, may repeat in 2 hours, not to exceed 40 mg/day.

b. Zolmitriptan (Zomig) (oral disintegrating tablet (Zomig-ZMT) 2.5 mg tab or 5 mg tab). After 2 hours, may repeat not to exceed 10 mg/24-hour period.

c. Naratriptan (Amerge) (tab: 1, 2.5 mg); dose: 2.5 mg, may repeat in 4 hours, maximum 5 mg/24 hours.

d. Rizatriptan (Maxalt) (tab: 5, 10 mg); dose: 5 to 10 mg, may repeat in 2 hours, maximum 30 mg/24 hours.

e. Almotriptan (Axert) (tab 6.25, 12.5 mg); dose: 12.5 or 25 mg/24 hours.

f. Frovatriptan (Frova) (tab 2.5 mg); dose 2.5 mg/24 hours.

g. Eletriptan (Relpax), pending FDA approval.

h. **Contraindications and warnings for triptans (5-HT $_{1B/1D}$ agonists):** Because of the potential of this class of compounds (5-HT $_{1B/1D}$ agonists) to cause coronary vasospasm, these agents should not be given to patients with documented ischemic or vasospastic coronary artery disease (CAD). It is strongly recommended that tripans not be given to patients in whom unrecognized CAD is predicted by the presence of risk factors (e.g., hypertension, hypercholesterolemia, smoking, obesity, diabetes, strong family history of CAD, being female with surgical or physiological menopause, or being male over the age of 40 years) unless a cardiovascular evaluation provides satisfactory clinical evidence that the patient is reasonably free of CAD and ischemic myocardial disease or other significant underlying cardiovascular disease. These agents are also contraindicated in pregnancy and when breastfeeding.

i. **Potential Interactions with triptans:**

MAOIs and triptans (rizatriptan, sumatriptan, and zumitriptan) are contraindicated with MAOIs because they increase the levels of these triptans which could lead to a hypertensive crisis. There are no known interactions between MAOIs and the other triptans.

Propranolol raises the level of rizatriptan; therefore, dosage of rizatriptan should be halved when co-administered with propranolol.

Caution is recommended when co-prescribing triptans with SSRIs because of a theoretical concern of causing a serotonin syndrome. The risk of this complication is low and is based on a few anecdotal case reports.

2. Cafergot (two tabs PO stat, then one tab PO every 5 hours if needed up to a maximum of six tabs per attack).
3. Aspirin (325 to 650 mg) or acetaminophen (350 to 1,000 mg).
4. lbuprofen (600 to 800 mg).
5. Fiorinal (used with caution, as it may be habit-forming) (1 to 2 tabs PO every 4 hours).
6. Droperidol 2.5 mg IV x 1.

B. Prevention of migraines

Some migraines have identifiable triggers. Keeping a daily log often helps the patient to identify these often undetected triggers. Lipophilic beta-blockers (e.g., propranolol), cyproheptadine (Periactin), and anticholinergic tricyclics (e.g., amitriptyline) are used effectively to prevent headaches. Possible triggers include sleep deprivation or too much sleep, oral contraceptives, stress, excitement, emotional upset, fluorescent lights, and flashing lights.

C. Prophylactic Treatment for Migraines

Substances with proven efficacy include the beta-blockers metoprolol and propranolol, the calcium channel-blocker flunarizine, several 5-HT antagonists, and amitriptyline. Recently antiepileptic drugs (valproic acid, gabapentin, topiramate) were evaluated for the prophylaxis of migraine. The use of botulinum toxin is under investigation.

1. Propanolol (40 to 320 mg).
2. Tricyclic antidepressants (standard antidepressant dosages).
3. Calcium channel-blockers (e.g., verapamil, 180 to 320 mg).
4. Phenytoin (100 mg PO t.i.d., target therapeutic range of 10 to 20 mEq/L).
5. Methylsergide (1 to 2 mg PO t.i.d.); should not be used for prolonged periods because it is associated with retroperitoneal fibrosis. It should be reserved for refractory cases.
6. Pizotifen (start with 0.5 mg PO qhs; may increase to 3 to 6 tablets qhs if necessary).

7. Sodium valproate (250 mg PO qd; target therapeutic range of 50 to 100 mEq/L). Patients should be directed to avoid triggers of migraines, such as caffeine, chocolate, alcohol, skipped meals, and sleep deprivation. Each patient should be directed to keep a careful diary to establish triggers, which may be individualized.
8. Gabapentin (Neurontin) has been shown in recent clinical trials to offer migraine prevention at doses of 1,800 mg–2,400 mg/day.
9. Topiramate (Topimax) has been shown in recent clinical trials to offer migraine prevention with the target dose of 100 mg b.i.d.

D. Treatment of Cluster Headaches
1. 100% nasal oxygen may abort the headache.
2. Sublingual or parenteral ergots (ergotamine tartrate 2 mg sublingually immediately; repeat every 30 minutes up to 6 mg per 24 hours).
3. Steroids (medrol dose pack).
4. Indomethacin (25 to 50 mg PO t.i.d.).
5. Lithium carbonate may be helpful prophylactically (300 mg PO qd; target therapeutic range of 0.7 to 1.2 mEq/L).
6. Topirimate has been shown to be effective in small case series; dose 100 mg b.i.d.

E. Treatment of Tension Headaches
1. Acetaminophen or aspirin.
2. Ibuprofen (600 to 800 mg PO t.i.d.).
3. Narcotics should not be used in tension headaches.
4. Neck massage and heat.

F. Treatment of Psychogenic Headaches
1. Antidepressants (therapeutic dosages for major depression).
2. Relaxation techniques.

Suggested Readings

Dalessio, D.J. (1987). *Woff's headache and other head pain* (4th ed.). New York: Oxford University Press.

Diamond, S. (Ed.). (1991). Headache. *Medical Clinics of North America, 75*(3), 50–75.

Ferrari, M.D. (1993). Sumatriptan in the treatment of migraine. *Neurology, 43*(suppl 3), S43–S47.

Kaufman, D.M. (1995). *Clinical neurology for psychiatrists* (4th ed.). Philadelphia: WB Saunders, pp. 197–220.

Kunkel, R.S. (1979). Evaluating the headache patient: History and workup. *Headache, 19*(3), 122–126.

Lipton, R.B., Hamelsky, S.W., & Dayno, J.M. (2002). What do patients with migraine want from acute migraine treatment? *Headache, 42*(suppl 1), 3–9.

Matthew, N.T. (2001). Antiepileptic drugs in migraine prevention. *Headache, 41*(suppl 1), 18–25.

Norris, E.R., & Samuels, M.A. (2000). Headache. In T.A. Stern, & J.B. Herman (Eds.), *Psychiatry update and board preparation.* New York: McGraw-Hill, pp. 301–304.

Pascual, J. (2002). Clinical benefits of early triptan therapy for migraine. *Headache, 42*(suppl 1), 10–17.

Samuels, M.A. (1997). *Video textbook of neurology for the practicing physician.* Boston: Butterworth-Heinemann.

Singer, E.J. (1996). Neuropsychiatric aspects of headaches. In H.I. Kaplan, & B.J. Sadock (Eds.), *Comprehensive textbook of psychiatry VI* (6th ed., pp. 251–257). Baltimore: Williams and Wilkins.

CHAPTER 27
The Patient with Disordered Sleep

Jeffrey B. Weilburg and James M. Richter

I. Introduction

Complaints about sleep, most often insomnia, are reported by 36% of adults in the United States. Insomnia is reported by 20% of general medical outpatients during routine visits, and is regarded as a chronic or significant problem by 10% of medical outpatients.

 Sleep disorders are associated with significant morbidity, poor daytime function, and injuries or death from motor vehicle accidents. Insomnia is associated with approximately the same reduction in health-related quality of life as occurs with depression and congestive heart failure. Sleep disorders are associated with an estimated cost of $15 billion per year in the United States.

II. Terminology and Classification

A. Terminology

The most common and clinically useful classification schema for sleep disorders are those provided in the *Diagnostic and Statistical Manual,* 4th ed. *(DSM-IV)* (and its primary care companion, the *DSM-IV PC*) and by the International Classification of Sleep Disorders (ICSD).

1. The ICSD classification system offers a comprehensive nosology of sleep disorders. An abstract of the ICSD schema is found in Table 27-1.

Table 27-1. International Classification of Sleep Disorders

I. Dyssomnias

  A. Intrinsic sleep disorders

    1. Psychophysiological insomnia

    2. Sleep state misperception

    3. Idiopathic insomnia

    4. Narcolepsy

    5. Recurrent hypersomnia

    6. Idiopathic hypersomnia

    7. Post-traumatic hypersomnia

    8. Obstructive sleep apnea syndrome

    9. Central sleep apnea syndrome

    10. Central alveolar hypoventilation syndrome

    11. Periodic limb movement disorder

(continued)

Table 27-1. *(Continued)*

  12. Restless legs syndrome
  13. Intrinsic sleep disorder (not otherwise specified)
 B. Extrinsic sleep disorders
  1. Inadequate sleep hygiene
  2. Environmental sleep disorder
  3. Altitude insomnia
  4. Adjustment sleep disorder
  5. Insufficient sleep syndrome
  6. Limit-setting sleep disorder
  7. Sleep-onset association disorder
  8. Food allergy insomnia
  9. Nocturnal eating (drinking) syndrome
  10. Hypnotic-dependent sleep disorder
  11. Stimulant-dependent sleep disorder
  12. Alcohol-dependent sleep disorder
  13. Toxin-induced sleep disorder
  14. Extrinsic sleep disorder (not otherwise specified)
 C. Circadian rhythm sleep disorders
  1. Time zone change (jet lag) syndrome
  2. Shift-work sleep disorder
  3. Irregular sleep–wake pattern
  4. Delayed sleep phase syndrome
  5. Advanced sleep phase syndrome
  6. Non–24-hour sleep–wake disorder
  7. Circadian rhythm sleep disorder (not otherwise specified)
II. Parasomnias
 A. Arousal disorders
  1. Confusing arousals
  2. Sleepwalking
  3. Sleep terrors
 B. Sleep–wake transition disorders
  1. Rhythmic movement disorder
  2. Sleep starts
  3. Sleep talking
  4. Nocturnal leg cramps
 C. Parasomnias usually associated with REM sleep
  1. Nightmares
  2. Sleep paralysis
  3. Impaired sleep-related penile erections

Table 27-1. *(Continued)*

---

    4. Sleep-related painful erections
    5. REM sleep-related sinus arrest
    6. REM sleep behavior disorder
  D. Other parasomnias
    1. Sleep bruxism
    2. Sleep enuresis
    3. Sleep-related abnormal swallowing syndrome
    4. Nocturnal paroxysmal dystonia
    5. Sudden unexplained nocturnal death syndrome
    6. Primary snoring
    7. Infant sleep apnea
    8. Congenital central hypoventilation syndrome
    9. Sudden infant death syndrome
   10. Benign neonatal sleep myoclonus
   11. Other parasomnia (not otherwise specified)

III. Sleep disorders associated with medical/psychiatric disorders
  A. Associated with mental disorders
    1. Psychoses
    2. Mood disorders
    3. Anxiety disorders
    4. Panic disorder
    5. Alcoholism
  B. Associated with neurological disorders
    1. Cerebral degenerative disorders
    2. Dementia
    3. Parkinsonism
    4. Fatal familial insomnia
    5. Sleep-related epilepsy
    6. Electrical status epilepticus of sleep
    7. Sleep-related headaches
  C. Associated with other medical disorders
    1. Sleeping sickness
    2. Nocturnal cardiac ischemia
    3. Chronic obstructive pulmonary disease
    4. Sleep-related asthma
    5. Sleep-related gastroesophageal reflux
    6. Peptic ulcer disease
    7. Fibrositis syndrome

SOURCE: Abstracted from ICSD, 1990.

2. The *DSM-IV* and *DSM-IV PC* systems are complaint-based. Clinicians will find these systems most useful if the nature of the patient's complaint is clarified at the outset. Complaints may be lumped into several basic categories:
   a. **Insomnia** (trouble falling or staying asleep, or non-restorative sleep)
   b. **Hypersomnia** (excessive sleepiness)
   c. **Parasomnias** (problems related to behaviors or physiologic events that occur during sleep)
   d. **Sleep–wake schedule-related problems** (mismatch between endogenous circadian rhythm generators and exogenous demands on sleep timing)
   e. **Other** (abnormal muscle activity related to sleep)

This chapter utilizes elements of the systems employed by both the *DSM-IV* and the ICSD.

III. Insomnia

A. **Diagnosis. Insomnia is a difficulty in the initiation or maintenance of sleep,** or of **non-restorative sleep,** that is associated with clinically significant distress or functional impairment in daytime function.

1. **Typical complaints.** Patients with insomnia typically complain of malaise, "not enough sleep," and they report feeling tired and fatigued. They often manifest mild to moderate impairment in concentration and psychomotor function on objective testing during the day.

2. **Etiology. No single physiologic basis of insomnia exists.** Perceptual and psychological factors often play an important role. Patients who are anxious, angry, or frustrated, or who are under situational stress, or depressed, often experience insomnia. People who are likely to overestimate the time it takes to fall asleep or the time they spent awake after sleep onset may also, especially during times of emotional distress, be prone to complaints of insomnia.

   Establishing the diagnosis requires careful attention to history. Interviewing family members and significant others about psychiatric and substance abuse problems that patients neglect to report can be helpful. Pursuit of underlying medical problems suggested by history is important (see Table 27-2), but no routine laboratory screening is indicated. Keeping a log of sleep (time in bed, estimated time asleep, arousals, time awake, level of alertness upon arousal, mood, events, and drug or alcohol use during the day) for 2 weeks is also often useful to clarify the history.

   Polysomnography (all-night monitoring of the electroencephalogram [EEG], respiration, muscle activity, and other physiologic parameters), performed in the sleep laboratory, is the definitive diagnostic test for insomnia. Patients with primary or severe insomnia often demonstrate **prolonged sleep latency** (an inability to fall asleep in less than 30 minutes) and sleep that is shallow or fragmented by multiple arousals during polysomnographic study. Patients with insomnia secondary to depression tend to manifest specific changes (a shortened rapid eye movement [REM] latency) in sleep physiology. Some patients who complain of insomnia appear to have objectively normal sleep. **Polysomnography** for the work-up of insomnia is **only** indicated when a primary disorder of sleep, like sleep apnea, is suspected, or when refractory cases are encountered, and **should probably be ordered only after consultation with a sleep specialist has been obtained.**

Table 27-2. Medical Causes of Insomnia

Medications which can produce insomnia

Sedatives: barbiturates, benzodiazepines, narcotics (withdrawal, long-term abuse)

Stimulants: amphetamines, methylphenidate, pemoline, caffeine (in OTC agents, e.g., Anacin, Excedrin)

Antidepressants: phenelzine, tranylcypromine, protriptyline, desipramine, imipramine, amoxapine, fluoxetine (by direct stimulant properties, and in some by induction of periodic leg movements of sleep [PLMS]; tricyclic withdrawal)

Antipsychotics: phenothiazines, butyrophenones (induction of PLMS)

Anti-asthmatics: decongestants (pseudoephedrine, phenylephrine, phenyl propanolamine) theophylline, terbutaline, albuterol, metaproteranol

Anti-hypertensives: beta-blockers (propranolol, atenolol, pindolol), alpha-methyl dopa, diuretics, reserpine, clonidine (by induction of nightmares, or PLMS)

Cimetidine (by induction of nightmares or PLMS)

Thyroxine, steroids, birth control pills (induction of nightmares, PLMS), progesterone

Anti-neoplastics: medroxyprogestrone, leupride, goserelin, pentostatin, daunorubicin, alpha interferon.

Medical problems which can produce insomnia

Non-specific symptoms: pain of any source, cough, pruritus, dyspnea, fever

Cardiovascular disease: angina, congestive heart failure

Pulmonary disease: chronic obstructive pulmonary disease, asthma, hypoventilation secondary to polio, scoliosis, or other conditions (alveolar hypoventilation)

Gastrointestinal disease: duodenal ulcer, hiatal hernia and reflux syndromes, hepatic failure

Neurologic disease: migraine and cluster headache, Parkinson's disease, Alzheimer's and related dementias, stroke, tumor (of the thalamus, hypothalamus, brain stem, third ventricle), head injury, meningoencephalitidies (viral, bacterial, or fungal)

Musculoskeletal disease: fibromyalgia, arthritis (including degenerative, rheumatoid, and autoimmune types)

Renal disease: uremia, nephrolithiasis, polyuria

Endocrine disease and changes: hyper- and hypothyroidism, use of exogenous steroids, endogenous hyper- or hypoadrenalism, diabetic peripheral neuropathy

Pregnancy

B. **Types of Insomnia.** Insomnia is often divided into two basic types: transient and persistent.

1. **Transient insomnia** is a common response to situational stressors; patient education, emotional support, and attention to proper sleep hygiene (see Table 27-3) are indicated. In selected cases short-term (two to four nights) treatment with benzodiazepines is often useful. Table 27-4 lists medications commonly used to treat insomnia.

Table 27-3. Rules of Proper Sleep Hygiene

1. Use the bed for sleeping and lovemaking only; avoid eating, reading, or watching television in bed
2. Leave the bed and the bedroom if unable to fall asleep (after 15 to 30 minutes); read or perform a quiet, non-stimulating activity (no television); return to bed only when sleepy
3. "Wind down" with a quiet activity 1 hour before bedtime; **no exercise in the evening**
4. Keep a regular bedtime and wake-up time, including on weekends
5. Avoid naps (one nap of 30 minutes is acceptable)

---

2. **Persistent insomnia** requires a diligent attempt to determine and treat the underlying problem. **Psychiatric consultation to address and manage possible confounding axis II or substance abuse disorders may be indicated.**

C. **Treatment.** Combination of non-pharmacologic techniques with monitored use of medication is often helpful for patients with chronic insomnia.

1. **Non-pharmacologic treatments**

   a. **Behavioral techniques,** including various methods of relaxation and meditation, can be learned by self-help tapes or manuals, or by consultation with mental health clinicians. Sleep restriction therapy (a specific method of graded matching of time spent in bed to actual sleep) is useful for more persistent or severe cases, and usually requires consultation with a sleep disorders center.

Table 27-4. Medications Commonly Used for Insomnia

Name	Onset of action	Duration of action	Half-life in hours (includes metabolites)	Usual dose (mg)
Clonazepam (Klonopin)	Intermediate	Long	15–50	0.5–1.0
Estazolam (ProSom)	Intermediate	Intermediate	10–24	1–2
Flurazepam (Dalmane)	Rapid-intermediate	Long	24–150	15–30
Lorazepam (Ativan)	Intermediate	Intermediate	10–20	1
Quazepam (Doral)	Rapid-intermediate	Long	35–150	15
Temazepam (Restoril)	Slow-intermediate	Intermediate	8–20	15
Triazolam (Halcion)	Rapid	Short	1.5–6	0.125–0.5
Zolpidem (Ambien)	Rapid	Short	2.4–3	10
Diphenhydramine (Benadryl)	Intermediate	Intermediate	3.5–9.5	50
Zalepon (Sonata)	Rapid	Short	1	5–10

---

      b. **Psychotherapy** to reduce anxiety, anger, or depression, and to help patients better handle situational stress, is often helpful.

      c. **Lifestyle alterations,** such as obtaining regular aerobic exercise (best performed before 4 PM), omitting caffeine (including chocolate in some individuals), alcohol, and cigarettes, eating the evening meal at least 3 hours before bed, and attending to the rules of sleep hygiene, are also indicated.

   2. **Medications**

      a. **Sedating antidepressants,** such as trazodone, nortriptyline, paroxetine, or low doses of mirtazapine, may be used for patients with concomitant affective or anxiety disorders.

      b. **The long-term use of benzodiazepines,** although controversial, is common in practice, and may be appropriate for those patients with insomnia secondary to an anxiety disorder. Benzodiazepines should be used with caution or avoided in patients with past or current histories of alcohol or substance abuse, personality disorders, or sleep-related breathing disorders. Careful monitoring of prescriptions, to avoid dose escalation, is indicated when these agents are used for more than four weeks.

      c. Melatonin remains incompletedly studied; some authors suggest that 2 mg at bedtime may be effective.

      d. **Sedating antihistamines** can be used as alternatives to benzodiazepines; however, they may cause delirium in the elderly or in those with a compromised central nervous system (CNS).

      e. **Chloral hydrate, short-acting barbiturates, and ethchlorvynol** are less effective and more toxic than other agents and should be used rarely, if ever, and then under closely monitored conditions.

D. Insomnia Secondary to Psychiatric Problems. This category is generally considered to be the most common type of insomnia, followed by insomnia secondary to substance use or abuse.

   1. Patients with **affective or anxiety disorders** frequently feel and function poorly during the day and suffer from insomnia at night. Insomnia may be the first symptom of depression, and may predict the development of depression. Treatment of the underlying psychiatric disorder typically relieves the problem; when insomnia becomes prominent treatment of it as a target symptom can be useful.

   2. Patients with **character disorders** may become angry when deprived of the rest to which they feel entitled; they may have increased trouble falling asleep once angered which result in a self-reinforcing negative cycle. A search for external solutions and the perfect sleeping pill, rather than attempts to resolve their inter- and intrapersonal sources of distress is common. Such patients may demand increasingly large doses of hypnotics and place themselves at risk for drug dependence and addiction.

E. Insomnia Secondary to Substance Abuse. This condition may result from use of even small amounts of substances, such as caffeine and nicotine. The use of an alcoholic beverage as a "nightcap" or home remedy for insomnia is common. However, since alcohol used in this way tends to produce increased sleep-related respiratory disturbances, disrupted shallow sleep in the early morning, and next day rebound insomnia, its use should be discouraged. Significant disruption of sleep architecture and complaints of insomnia are common in alcoholic and stimulant-abusing patients. Proper discontinuation of the offending agents is the first step in treatment.

F. Insomnia Secondary to Medical Conditions. Insomnia secondary to pain (of any source), or conditions such as prostatism, and esophageal reflux are commonplace. See Table 27-2 for a list of medical conditions causing insomnia.

G. **Insomnia Secondary to Sleep Apnea or Central Alveolar Hypoventilation.** These conditions are less common than is excessive sleepiness and may be worsened by injudicious use of sedatives (including benzodiazepines).

H. **Primary Insomnia.** Primary insomnia may begin during childhood; some patients have a positive family history of sleep problems.

IV. Hypersomnia

Hypersomnia, or excessive daytime sleepiness, is characterized by falling asleep inappropriately during the day or by prolonged episodes of sleep. Patients may fall asleep during conversation or while carrying out potentially hazardous activities, such as driving. Patients with true hypersomnia often deny the extent of their somnolence, especially when inattention, cognitive decline, or memory disturbance are present. Once suspected, excessive sleepiness can be documented by testing in the sleep laboratory (as with the Multiple Sleep Latency Test or the Maintenance of Wakefulness Test).

Hypersomnia often results from a primary sleep problem, such as sleep apnea or narcolepsy, or from inadequate amounts of nocturnal sleep. In both sleep apnea and narcolepsy there is an inability to obtain restorative sleep; thus, simply achieving more sleep is not curative. If snoring, breath-holding, obesity, or other signs and symptoms of chronic obstructive pulmonary disorder or sleep apnea are evident the work-up for breathing-related sleep disorders should be undertaken. For patients who consistently sleep less than 7 hours per night, and try to catch up on weekends, a 2-week trial of sleep extension is warranted.

A. **Sleep Apnea**
   1. **Diagnosis.**
      a. Sleep apnea is noted in approximately 2–4% of adults; this is probably an underestimate of its true prevalence, as it is often unrecognized. An episode of sleep apnea is defined as the complete cessation of respiration lasting a minimum of 10 seconds, which causes a reduction in oxyhemoglobin saturation. An hypopnea is a minimum of one-third reduction in airflow.
      b. **Sleep apnea is diagnosed when more than five episodes of apnea or hypopnea per hour of sleep** are found on the polysomnogram. Home sleep monitors for the diagnosis are in development, but have not yet been widely accepted. Three subtypes of sleep apnea have been recognized: central, obstructive, and mixed.
         i. In **central sleep apnea** no respiratory effort is made until arousal supervenes.
         ii. In **obstructive sleep apnea,** which occurs in 1–4% of adults, the negative pressure in the airway during inspiration causes airway collapse. Cessation of respiration despite respiratory effort leads to loud snorts and snores; total body movements typically follow. An abnormal decrease in the tone of the oropharyngeal musculature, excessive tissue mass in the pharynx and tongue (found in some obese patients), malposition of the jaw or tongue, or a narrow airway all contribute to the problem. Patients often experience dry mouth, morning headache, mental dullness, irritability, and impotence, and are at elevated risk of developing cardiac arrhythmias, pulmonary and systemic hypertension, right heart failure, and stroke. One-fourth to one-third of patients with moderate to severe apnea die within 8 to 10 years of their diagnosis.
         iii. The most common type is the **mixed type.** Mixed episodes begin with a relatively brief period of central apnea and progress as respiratory effort is made to an obstructive phase.

The severity of sleep apnea is determined by the **respiratory index** (the number of apneic episodes per hour), the extent of the oxygen desaturation (oxygen nadir and number of desaturations below 85%), the sleep fragmentation caused by respiratory events, and the presence of associated cardiac arrhythmias.

Obstructive and mixed types of sleep apnea tend to occur in males and post-menopausal females.

2. **Treatment.** Obese patients with obstructive sleep apnea need to **lose weight** and **avoid alcohol and sedatives** (which reduce the activity of the upper airway muscula-ture and extend the duration of apneic episodes). There is a high prevalence of hyper-tension in patients with sleep apnea, so blood pressure should be monitored and reduced appropriately. Most patients benefit from use of **continuous positive air-way pressure (CPAP)** which "splints" the upper airway and prevents the frequent arousals and persistent episodic oxyhemoglobin desaturation. Use of CPAP appears to prevent the long-term morbidity and mortality associated with sleep apnea and produces near normal levels of wakefulness by providing restorative sleep. Uvulopat-latopharyngeoplasty and related procedures are effective in the relief of snoring, but their use for apnea treatment is uncertain. **Tracheostomy** is effective, but is typically reserved for CPAP treatment-failures. No medications are clearly beneficial for apnea. In some cases medications, such as protriptyline, appear useful.

B. Narcolepsy

1. **Diagnosis. The classic tetrad of narcolepsy** is characterized by the following:
   a. **Sleep attacks:** irresistible, usually brief (10 to 60 minutes), refreshing episodes of sleep that often occur several times each day.
   b. **Cataplexy:** the sudden bilateral loss of motor tone, often in the knees, sometimes in the arms, face, jaw, or any voluntary muscles, without impaired consciousness, usually triggered by emotion. Episodes tend to last from seconds to minutes and can evolve into a sleep attack.
   c. **Sleep paralysis:** the appearance of episodes of total muscular paralysis at sleep onset or awakening.
   d. **Hypnogogic or hypnopompic hallucinations:** vivid visual and auditory phenomena occurring while falling asleep or on waking up.
   e. While not part of the classic tetrad, **disordered nocturnal sleep,** associated with a high incidence of parasomnias, abnormal movements, and other primary sleep disorders, is frequently present in narcoleptics.

2. **Etiology.** The recurrent intrusion of elements of rapid eye movement (REM) sleep into the transition between sleep and wakefulness, at various times during the day, produces narcoleptic symptoms. **A mutation in the gene coding for the production of a neurotransmitter, hypocretin, is probably a causative factor.**

3. **Prevalence.** Narcolepsy occurs in approximately 0.05% of the population. Onset tends to develop in the second decade of life. Roughly one-third of patients have a family member with excessive daytime sleepiness.

4. **Treatment.** Treatment is directed toward relief of daytime sleepiness and REM-related phenomena. **Stimulants** tend to improve alertness. **Prophylactic naps,** when feasible, can reduce the total daily dose of stimulants required. **Antidepressants** are the treatment of choice for cataplexy, sleep paralysis, and hypnogogic hallucinations due to their ability to suppress REM sleep. Adjunctive use of a short- to intermediate-acting benzodiazepine may consolidate nocturnal sleep and permit lower doses of both stimulants and antidepressants to be used.

V. Parasomnias

Parasomnias are abnormal behavioral or physiologic events which occur during sleep related to activation (autonomic, motoric, or cognitive). Complaints of sleep disrupted by abnormal behavior, rather than by insomnia or hypersomnia, result. Sleep terrors, nightmares (dream anxiety attacks), bedwetting (enuresis), teeth grinding (bruxism), sleep paralysis, and sleepwalking (somnambulism) are examples. See Table 27-1 for a complete list of parasomnias. Consultation with a sleep disorders specialist is often advisable for diagnosis and treatment of clinically significant parasomnias.

VI. Sleep-Wake Schedule Disorders

Sleep–wake schedule or circadian rhythm disorders occur when there is a mismatch between the endogenous sleep–wake cycle and a person's schedule. The problem may be exogenous, as in shift workers who must stay awake during the night, or in travelers who cross time zones (jet lag), or may be endogenous, as in delayed sleep phase syndrome (falling asleep too late) or advanced sleep phase syndrome (falling asleep too early). As for parasomnias, consultation with a sleep disorders specialist for assistance with diagnosis and treatment is advisable.

VII. Other Sleep Disorders

Restless legs syndrome, an "achey" or "crawling" paresthesia in the legs that appears at night, often around bedtime, has been found in 25–30% of patients in family practice settings. It is partially relieved by movement, so patients feel a need to pace about which interferes with going to sleep. **Periodic leg movements of sleep,** sometimes called **nocturnal myoclonus,** are brief involuntary movements of the limbs during sleep that appear every 20 to 40 seconds. The movements disrupt sleep continuity and produce nocturnal arousals (sometimes unknown to the patient) or actual awakenings and are associated with hypersomnia. Both restless legs syndrome and periodic leg movements of sleep are associated with a variety of conditions (renal failure, diabetes, chronic anemia, peripheral nerve injuries, uncomplicated pregnancy); with the use of various medications (antidepressants, neuroleptics, lithium, and diuretics); during narcotic withdrawal; or without co-morbid conditions. Treatment may include use of benzodiazepines, dopamine agonists, and narcotics.

VIII. Conclusion

Insomnia is the most common sleep problem seen in primary care settings. Work-up and treatment can, in general, be accomplished by primary care providers. Management of patients with hypersomnias, parasomnias, and sleep–wake schedule problems often require specialty consultation.

Suggested Readings

Diagnostic and statistical manual of mental disorders (4th ed., primary care version). (1995). Washington, DC: American Psychiatric Association.

Kupfer, D.J., & Reynolds, C.F. III (1997). Current concepts: Management of insomnia. *New England Journal of Medicine, 336,* 341–346.

Strollo, P.J., & Rogers, R.M. (1996). Current concepts: Obstructive sleep apnea. *New England Journal of Medicine, 334,* 99–104.

Diagnostic Classification Steering Committee (Thorpy, M.J., chairman). (1990). *ICSD—International classsification of sleep disorders: Diagnostic and coding manual.* Rochester, Minn.: American Sleep Disorders Association.

Weilburg, J.B., & Hopkins, H.S. (1997). Insomnia. In A. Gelenberg, E. Bassuk, & S. Schoonover (Eds.), *Practitioners guide to psychoactive drugs* (4th ed.). New York: Plenum.

CHAPTER 28
The Patient with Dizziness

CLAUDIA BALDASSANO AND THEODORE A. STERN

I. Introduction

Dizziness and other sensations of imbalance are among the most common complaints among medical outpatients. Terms used to describe these complaints frequently mean different things to different people. **Vertigo** implies the illusory sensation of turning and spinning. **Dizziness** is more vague and implies light-headedness or a feeling of uneasiness in the head. Because the physical examination and all diagnostic testing may be normal in these patients, the diagnosis hinges primarily on the history.

II. Evaluation of the Problem

A. **General Recommendations.** It is incumbent on the physician to distinguish true vertigo from dizziness or other types of pseudovertigo in an anxious patient. The goal of the clinician is to **decide if it is peripheral** (labyrinthine, cochlear, or vestibular), **central** (brainstem or cerebellum), or **systemic** (e.g., cardiovascular or metabolic). A careful history and examination usually provide the basis for separating these different etiologies.
1. **Complaint of "dizziness"**
   a. **Encompasses a gamut of symptoms. Try to elicit exactly what the patient is feeling and experiencing; attempt to let the patient tell the story without your offering possible terms.** For example, the patient's complaint may actually be of clumsiness that represents cerebellar dysfunction. Symptoms that a patient often refers to as "dizziness" include:
      i. Vertigo
      ii. Unsteadiness
      iii. Imbalance
      iv. Spinning
      v. Fainting
      vi. Clumsiness
      vii. Blurred vision
      viii. Staggering
      ix. Passing out
      x. Swaying

B. **Medical History**
1. A history of **episodic disequilibration** accompanied by diplopia, slurred speech, perioral numbness, dimming of vision, and occasional drop attacks **suggests transient vertebrobasilar episodes.**
2. Dizziness after head trauma suggests **cuprolithiasis.**
3. Symptoms that occur after ear surgery or a blow to the ear suggest a **perilymph fistula.**

4. The presence of deafness and hearing loss may suggest a **cerebellopontine angle mass.**

5. Exacerbation of vertigo by head turning or by head positioning suggests a peripheral etiology, such as **labyrinthitis.**

6. Hyperacusis and aura suggest **migraine headache.**

7. New-onset vertigo in the setting of an upper respiratory tract infection or a flu-like syndrome suggests a **peripheral labyrinthitis** which should be confirmed by examination.

8. Dizziness on exertion may suggest **cardiopulmonary illness.** If this is ruled out, consider primary **autonomic dysregulation.**

C. **Examination of the patient.** Every patient with a disorder of equilibrium or true vertigo should receive a screening general physical examination and a careful neurologic examination.

1. **General Medical Examination**

a. Patients with symptoms that suggest **pre-syncope or actual syncope** must have particular attention paid to the cardiovascular system.

b. Whenever the symptomatology is associated with **loss of consciousness or lightheadedness,** one should consider **cardiac dysrhythmia.**

c. Attention should be paid to systemic conditions that can give rise to a general feeling of **malaise or weakness** that may be interpreted by the patient as a disorder of balance.

2. **Neurologic Examination**

a. **Visual field defects,** such as unsuspected bitemporal or homonymous field defects, from tumors or infarcts may cause a patient to run into objects or to feel disoriented in space.

b. **An altered corneal sensation** may be a sign of an unsuspected cerebellopontine angle mass.

c. **Hearing** should be tested with a tuning fork, as cerebellopontine angle tumors can present with hearing loss and vascular or peripheral causes of vertigo can lead to hearing loss.

d. **Abnormalities of cranial nerves IX through XII** suggest the differential diagnosis of multiple cranial neuropathies, such as collagen vascular disease, tumors of the base of the skull, and nasopharyngeal carcinoma.

e. The presence of **spontaneous or induced nystagmus** is of the utmost importance in the examination of a dizzy patient.

f. **Sensory examination** may reveal a significant **peripheral neuropathy,** leading to a diagnosis of diabetes or toxic neuropathy. **Loss of posterior column function,** such as proprioception and vibration, may indicate that the patient has a **vitamin B deficiency.**

g. Any **limb or truncal ataxia** should be interpreted as a clear sign of a neurologic etiology. Unsteadiness during a Romberg test with the eyes open and only a slight exaggeration of instability with the eyes closed suggest a **cerebellar etiology.**

III. Psychiatric Differential Diagnosis

Anxiety and depression may present as complaints of dizziness or imbalance. Of course, these are important considerations in the evaluation of any patient with these complaints, but to make the diagnosis, one must gather more information to confirm the diagnosis. During a panic attack, patients often complain of feeling light-headed, but to make the diagnosis, other symptoms of panic, such as tachycardia, diaphoresis, and a feeling of impending doom, must also be elicited. **Hyperventilation** as part of an anxiety syndrome can produce vertigo or light-headedness.

IV. Diagnostic Criteria

Causes of dizziness can be divided into three broad categories: peripheral vestibulopathy, central neurologic disorders, and systemic conditions.

A. **Peripheral causes of vertigo** result from dysfunction of vestibular end organs (i.e., the semicircular canals, the utricle, and the saccule).

1. **Vestibuloneuronitis, labyrinthitis, and viral neurolabyrinthitis**
   a. These conditions imply an inflammatory process.
   b. The terms are used interchangeably.
   c. Sudden episodes of true vertigo last from hours to days and often are associated with vomiting.
   d. These episodes may be provoked by head turning.
   e. They may recur in weeks to months, and when the symptoms recur, patients often complain of a sensation of light-headedness or floating.
   f. Seasonal outbreaks suggest that there may be an infectious etiology, but this remains unproved.
   g. Latency and fatigability may occur on the Bárány maneuver.

2. **Benign Positional Vertigo**
   a. Symptoms are associated with certain head positions.
   b. Rotational vertigo is of brief duration and is episodic in nature.
   c. The symptomatology is most severe in the morning and lessens as the day goes on.
   d. It presumably is due to cuprolithiasis of the posterior semicircular canal; the stone moves freely with head turning.
   e. Latency and fatigability occur on the Bárány maneuver.

3. **Post-traumatic Vertigo**
   a. This condition usually occurs immediately after head trauma; it implies end-organ damage in the absence of other CNS signs, and it may be related to fracture of the temporal bone.
   b. The interval between the trauma and the symptoms may be days or even weeks.
   c. Symptoms are similar to those of benign positional vertigo and labyrinthitis.
   d. The prognosis is usually good.

4. **Drug Toxicity**
   a. Patients with dizziness from vestibulotoxic drugs are presumed to have persistent injury to the end organ.
   b. Aminoglycosides are the agents most often associated with this condition.

5. **Meniere's Syndrome**
   a. This syndrome is characterized by attacks of severe vertigo and vomiting, tinnitus, fluctuating hearing loss, and a feeling of aural fullness and pressure. Spontaneous recovery occurs in hours to days.
   b. Episodes may be so severe that some patients will fall to the ground.
   c. Consciousness is not lost, although some patients may have an altered awareness of their surroundings.

B. **Central Causes of Vertigo** (dysfunction of the eighth cranial nerve, the vestibular nuclei within the brainstem, and their central connections)

1. **Brainstem ischemia or infarction**
   a. Brainstem transient ischemic attacks (TIAs) should be accompanied by neurologic signs or symptoms, in addition to vertigo or dizziness, for a clear diagnosis to be entertained.

      b. Associated symptoms often include clumsiness, weakness, loss of vision, diplopia, peri-oral numbness, ataxia, drop attacks, and dysarthria.

      c. Crossed signs provide good evidence of brainstem dysfunction.

  2. **Multiple sclerosis**

      a. Those afflicted with this condition may have signs and symptoms, such as dysequilibration, that are suggestive of brainstem ischemia or tumors.

      b. The diagnosis can be made only after documentation of disseminated CNS lesions.

  3. **Cerebellopontine angle tumors**

      a. Tumors of the cerebellopontine angle rarely present with vertigo alone.

      b. The most common symptoms include progressive hearing loss, tinnitus, and a feeling of dysequilibration (which is reported more often than is vertigo).

      c. The most common tumors found in this location include schwannomas, meningiomas, epidermoids, and metastases.

C. Systemic Causes of Vertigo

  1. **Drugs** (including anticonvulsants, antihypertensives, analgesics, and tranquilizers) commonly cause dizziness or a feeling of imbalance.

  2. **Hypotension/autonomic dysregulation**

      a. Postural hypotension is a common cause of dizziness.

      b. It is also a common side effect of antihypertensives.

      c. Exertional dizziness may be secondary to autonomic dysregulation. Patients may complain of feeling foggy or spacey with mild to moderate exercise.

  3. **Multiple afferent sensory loss**

      a. The combination of **multiple sensory deficits** can produce disorientation or disequilibration that is interpreted as dizziness or vertigo.

      b. The vestibular system functions to provide spatial orientation, visual fixation, and postural tone. A combination of multiple sensory deficits can produce disequilibration.

      c. This often occurs in the elderly, in whom vision, hearing, and proprioception may all be impaired.

V. Treatment Strategies

Treatments depend on the etiology and diagnosis. Meclizine, diazepam, and lorazepam may be helpful in patients with labyrinthitis. In patients with benign positional vertigo, vestibular rehabilitation may be helpful. Referral to a physical therapist for vestibular rehabilitation or training your patients to perform simple exercises may improve symptoms and function. The patient should be instructed to position his or her head in the direction that causes vertigo and keep it there for 5 seconds. This should be repeated every hour for a few hours each day. If the etiology of dizziness is psychiatric in nature, treatment with selective serotonin reuptake inhibitors (SSRIs) may be helpful; if dizziness occurs when major depressive disorder is not readily apparent, then treatment with an SSRI is still a reasonable option.

Suggested Readings

Baloh, R.W. (1984). *Dizziness, hearing loss and tinnitus: The essentials of neuro-otology.* Philadelphia: Davis.

Brown, J.J. (1990). A systematic approach to the dizzy patient. *Neurology Clinics of North America, 8,* 209–224.

Staab, J.P., Ruckenstein, M.J., Solomon, D., & Shepard, N.T. (2002). Exertional dizziness and autonomic dysregulation. *Laryngoscope, 112*(8), 1346–1350.

Staab, J.P., Ruckenstein, M.J., Solomon, D., & Shepard, N.T. (2002). Serotonin reuptake inhibitors for dizziness with psychiatric symptoms. *Archives of Otolaryngology and Head and Neck Surgery, 128*(5), 554–560.

Troost, B.T. (1989). Nystagmus: A clinical review. *Review of Neurology (Paris), 145,* 417–428.

CHAPTER 29

The Patient with Multiple Physical Complaints

LORI CALABRESE AND THEODORE A. STERN

I. Introduction

A. Patients who present with multiple, unexplained physical complaints (i.e., patients who somatize) make up a significant proportion of primary care practice today.

1. Thirty-eight percent of primary care patients complain of symptoms that have no serious medical basis.
2. Almost half (46%) of new complaints, or new symptoms, contain some element of somatization. Fully 10% of these represent pure somatization.

B. Somatization is the tendency to experience and to report bodily symptoms that have no physiologic explanation, to misattribute symptoms to disease, and to seek medical attention for them.

1. In many patients with this tendency, somatization becomes a form of chronic illness behavior.
2. In the most severe cases, somatization becomes the focus of the patient's life, and the sick role becomes the patient's predominant mode of relating to the world.

C. Somatization differs from malingering or factitious disorders. A patient who somatizes complains frequently of bodily symptoms he or she experiences; the patient does not lie about the symptom or feign physical signs (e.g., fever or vomiting) to simulate disease.

D. Recurrent somatization (i.e., recurrent multiple unexplained physical complaints) warrants evaluation for the presence of somatoform disorders. **Somatoform disorders are psychiatric disorders characterized by the presence of physical symptoms in the absence of demonstrable pathology or known pathophysiology.**

1. The list of *DSM-IV* somatoform disorders is shown in Table 29-1.
2. The four most common somatoform disorders seen in primary care practice, in descending order of frequency: are pain disorder, hypochondriasis, somatization

---

Table 29-1. Somatoform Disorders

Somatization disorder

Hypochondriasis

Conversion disorder

Pain disorder

Body dysmorphic disorder

Undifferentiated somatoform disorder

Somatoform disorder not otherwise specified

---

disorder, and conversion disorder. The approach to the patient with pain will be discussed in Chapter 33. This chapter will focus on identifying and differentiating three major types of somatization, each associated with its own somatoform disorder.

II. Evaluation of the Somatizing Patient

A. General Recommendations

1. The evaluation of the patient who presents with multiple, unexplained physical complaints will differ, depending on whether the patient is new or established.

2. **For a new patient presenting with current or previous multiple somatic complaints, history is paramount; it should always focus on determining whether the current complaint has a physiologic basis.** The history should also elucidate whether a pattern of somatization exists. It should include the following:

   a. The current complaint

   b. The occupational or social nature and extent to which the current complaint limits the patient's functioning. ("I haven't worked in months. How could I possibly work feeling like this?")

   c. A detailed medical history of previous physical complaints, medical diagnoses, and operations. Medical history should be verified by obtaining comprehensive medical records from previous physicians and inpatient/outpatient settings.

   d. The names of all other physicians whom the patient considers current treaters, and those with whom the patient has terminated treatment within the past year.

   e. The extent to which the patient's current complaint, and history of previous complaints, is accompanied by a fear or conviction that the complaint portends disease. For example, a patient with recurrent, unexplained abdominal pain may fear that the pain represents occult pancreatic cancer.

   f. A history of significant childhood illnesses and the degree of impairment associated with them.

   g. A history of impairment or dysfunction caused by physical ailments among family members whom the patient witnessed during childhood (e.g., a father chronically out of work because of back pain).

   h. The patient's history of psychiatric symptoms (e.g., depression, anxiety, obsessions or compulsions) and their response to treatment. Psychiatric hospitalizations (including precipitants and treatments) should be included.

   i. The family history of psychiatric disorders or symptoms

   j. Medications used to address the current complaint, including over-the-counter medications, homeopathic remedies, chiropractic medicine, and alternative medicine practices (e.g., acupuncture); also, a history of previous medications and treatments for previous complaints (e.g., physical therapy or frequent antibiotics)

   k. The history of prescription narcotic and NSAID use, as well as the history of illicit drug use

   l. Finally, a determination of whether cash or other awards might be forthcoming or dependent on the outcome of the office visit (e.g., disability or release from financial obligations). Such a history may suggest that the presenting complaint is being feigned or exaggerated for the purposes of obtaining something else (i.e., that the patient is malingering).

3. **The emotional tenor of the patient is often a clue to his or her individual pattern of somatization.** Some patients present with a blasé or indifferent manner that makes eliciting specific information about the symptom (e.g., exactly what, where, when,

how often, how long) almost impossible. Others appear hostile, impatient, and argumentative from the moment they walk through the door, exasperated by each question, rebutting each finding. Both types of patients may be coaxed into providing an extensive history when history-taking is approached matter-of-factly using "best possible care" as a goal, (e.g., "In order to give you the best possible care, I need to ask a lot of questions about your symptoms and health, and about your family's as well").

4. **A physical exam should be performed to determine whether physical signs are present that support the physical complaint.**

5. **The approach to a known patient in your practice with multiple somatic complaints will depend on the type of unexplained complaints the patient usually manifests** (e.g., neurological complaints only, multi-system complaints, or one or more physical complaints overshadowed by a marked fear or conviction of occult disease).

B. **Medical History**

1. **The purpose of the medical history** in a patient with multiple, unexplained physical complaints is three-fold:

   a. **First, to determine whether the patient is reporting a symptom he or she is experiencing, whether the complaint has been elaborated, or whether accompanying signs have been produced.** Multiple, unexplained symptoms suggest somatoform disorders; egregious fakery (even when it is done in a sophisticated way) suggests malingering. In the borderland between these two scenarios are situations in which a patient who presents with multiple feigned complaints is *presumed* to be not consciously aware of faking; this situation suggests factitious disorder.

   b. **Second, the medical history is necessary to determine whether there is a physiological basis for the current complaint.** A common error is to assume that a somatizer will present always and only with somatization. These individuals are not immune to serious medical disease. The most difficult task is the determination of which symptoms warrant further diagnostic work-up, and which ones represent underlying somatization.

   c. **Finally, the medical history helps determine whether the patient's longitudinal history suggests a common somatization syndrome and warrants a diagnosis or provisional diagnosis of one of the somatoform disorders.**

2. **The most important consideration in elevating the patient's somatization to the level of a disorder is whether the patient experiences significant functional impairment because of it** (e.g., lost days at work, marital difficulties, or strained relationships with children).

C. **Interview**

1. A new patient interview should be structured like any diagnostic intake, with the modifications suggested in II.A.2.

2. The interview of an established patient for whom one is considering a diagnosis of somatoform disorder should **consider the following:**

   a. **Conversion disorder** and **somatization disorder** are much more prevalent among women than men, and somatization disorder occurs four times as often in women of low social class with marked emotional distress compared to men. **Hypochondriasis** is equally prevalent among men and women.

   b. Conversion and somatization symptoms begin at an early age, often during teenage years. The onset of hypochondriasis peaks in early adulthood, usually in the mid-30s.

3. **The interview should not occur during the physical examination** (a risk in inpatient settings). A completed interview will allow the physician to focus the physical examination.

D. Examination of the Patient

1. **The physical examination of the patient with medically unexplained complaints should be limited to the body system(s) involved in the complaint prompting the office visit, and focused on the identification of objective physical signs**.

2. **A neurologic exam is required for patients who present with a loss or change in voluntary motor or sensory functioning** that suggests a neurologic condition but defies medical explanation. The absence of confirmatory neurological findings indicates conversion disorder.

   a. Sociodemographic factors influence the nature of the presentation; more sophisticated patients present with more sophisticated symptoms.

   b. Psychological factors, usually involving extreme stress, are associated with the onset and exacerbation of these pseudoneurological symptoms. Often these factors can be discovered by asking questions about concurrent stressful events, recent or upcoming life changes, and recent losses.

   c. Personality traits displayed during the examination can include passive or dependent traits, shallow seductiveness, or abrupt mood swings. Patients may appear anxious about the outcome of the examination, but often appear indifferent during the interview and physical examination. Emotional indifference is especially important to note in patients whose symptoms suggest right parietal lesions, where true lesions may be accompanied by *la belle indifference.*

   d. A careful neurologic exam will reveal non-physiological or non-anatomical signs (e.g., sensory loss precisely over one side of the body).

3. **Hypochondriacal patients** are unique in the spectrum of somatizing patients: whether they **present with one recurrent symptom or many during the course of their somatizing, the physical complaint is accompanied by profound bodily preoccupation, persistent fear of disease, and a strong but non-delusional conviction of having a disease.** These three cognitive features are the crux of hypochondriasis.

   a. The patient often describes the symptom(s) in an obsessive, all-inclusive fashion, presenting a difficult-to-interrupt monologue. Gastrointestinal and cardiovascular symptoms are most commonly reported.

   b. Bodily preoccupation is evident in the patient's excessive focus on the meaning and authenticity of each symptom and with his or her health in general. Social history frequently reveals that the patient has made friends based on common medical problems.

   c. The patient's fear of occult disease may not be forthcoming, and should always be asked about directly, (e.g., "What do you think the abdominal bloating means?" "What are your fears or concerns?").

   d. It is often difficult to tease out the difference between a conviction of disease and a delusion in patients who appear to be hypochondriacal. Although hypochondriacal patients don't respond to diffident reassurance, they can be persuaded to consider that their symptom might "mean" something other than what they imagine, even if only momentarily. A patient whose belief is delusional (i.e., false, fixed, and idiosyncratic), will hold it unshakably.

   e. Hypochondriacal patients tend to have experienced physician rebuttals, dismissals, and exasperation more frequently than other types of somatizing patients. This is because they come to each medical encounter prepared to insist that "something" is definitely wrong but just hasn't been identified yet. They are often hostile, demanding, and dissatisfied with their medical care.

4. **Patients with multiple somatic complaints suggestive of somatization disorder present a host of physical symptoms and complicated medical histories in vague but dramatic ways.** Their histories encompass several volumes of medical charts and usually stretch out over multiple physicians and hospitals. **However, their attention is often focused on the subjective suffering caused by their symptoms and the negative consequences the symptoms pose.** The vagueness they display in their inability to describe their symptoms or history is often the result of alexithymia (i.e., difficulty distinguishing between feelings and bodily sensations of emotional arousal, difficulty identifying and describing feelings, and a cognitive style that is characterized by preoccupation with external events and their details).

III. Psychiatric Differential Diagnosis

A. **The differential diagnosis of any patient presenting with medically unexplained complaints should always include a search for true medical illness** that might "explain" the complaint.

1. **Systemic medical disorders should be considered,** including multiple sclerosis, systemic lupus erythematosus, acute intermittent porphyria, endocrine disorders (e.g., hyperparathyroidism), and chronic systemic infections (e.g., brucellosis).

2. **Sleep disorders should be considered** in patients who present with complaints of fatigue and daytime hypersomnolence among their somatic complaints.

3. In patients presenting with isolated or recurrent non-anatomic neurological complaints, other neurologic disorders should also be considered, including myasthenia gravis, uncommon seizure disorders (e.g., atonic seizures in children and temporal lobe epilepsy), and dystonias.

B. **Differential diagnosis involves identification of co-morbid Axis I and Axis II disorders.**

1. **Co-morbid psychiatric disorders are frequent in patients with medically unexplained complaints.** Major depression, anxiety disorders, and alcohol and drug abuse are prevalent. Among patients with somatization disorder, two-thirds have symptoms of other psychiatric disorders, and one-third meet criteria for at least one other psychiatric diagnosis.

2. **Major depression occurs in over half of somatizers, and is frequently missed in patients presenting with hypochondriacal symptoms.** In differentiating the two, one should ask if the hypochondriacal symptoms have an episodic course. Are they appearing for the first time in an elderly person? Does the patient acknowledge some of the cognitive symptoms of depression (e.g., believing that he or she is worthless, deserves to be sick, or isn't worth treating)?

3. **Anxiety disorders occur in 86% of patients with hypochondriasis,** among whom panic disorder is the most prevalent and especially important to identify in patients presenting with recurrent cardiovascular complaints.

4. **Psychotic and obsessive-compulsive disorders (OCD) should be included in the differential diagnosis of patients presenting with hypochondriasis;** the strength of the patient's conviction of illness can sometimes appear to border on the delusional, and the obsessive attention to bodily details and preoccupation raises the question of OCD. If you cannot cleanly rule out either of these two disorders, refer the patient for specialty consultation; the treatment of psychosis and OCD differ, and both differ vastly from the treatment of hypochondriasis.

5. **Conversion disorder** (i.e., a loss or change in voluntary motor or sensory functioning that suggests a neurological condition but defies explanation) **must be differentiated from dissociative episodes** in patients with dissociative disorders. Some of the clinical confusion may arise because patients with both disorders share a high incidence of borderline intellectual functioning, borderline personality disorder, and childhood physical and sexual abuse. However, dissociative episodes do not involve altered motor or sensory functioning, whereas that is the defining characteristic for conversion disorder.

6. **The incidence of personality disorders among patients with somatoform disorders is quite high.**
   a. The incidence of personality disorders among patients with conversion disorder has not been well studied. However, passive-dependent traits and histrionic traits have been reported in 9–40% and 4–21% of these patients, respectively.
   b. Sixty-five percent of patients with hypochondriasis have concurrent personality disorders.
   c. Seventy-two percent of patients with somatization disorder have personality disorders, predominantly obsessive-compulsive personality disorder. Their excessive attention to bodily functions and their need to control both their bodily functions and their relationships with their physicians contribute to their somatization. Notably, histrionic personality disorder, often mistakenly assumed to be quite prevalent, is much less common.

C. **Unexplained physical complaints must be differentiated as either true or feigned.** Feigned complaints suggest malingering and factitious disorders, and are addressed in other chapters.

D. **Medically unexplained complaints in chronic somatizers fall into four basic categories,** which nicely approach the four most common *DSM-IV* somatoform disorders. Perhaps the most difficult feat in the differential diagnosis of one of these disorders is ruling out the others.
   1. **Pain disorder:** This disorder is distinguished from the other somatoform disorders because it involves recurrent complaints of medically unexplained pain only.
   2. **Conversion disorder:** This disorder is distinguished from the other somatoform disorders because it involves presentations of only pseudoneurological symptoms. However, these episodes can recur and differ in their presentations. They occur in patients with hypochondriasis (though rarely) and patients who go on to meet the criteria of somatization disorder. Once a patient has met the criteria for somatization disorder, any other conversion episodes are considered to be part of the somatization disorder.
   3. **Hypochondriasis:** Cognitive doubts, apprehensions, misattributions, and fear of disease distinguish this from other somatoform disorders. The triad of bodily preoccupation, disease fear, and disease conviction is central to the diagnosis of hypochondriasis, and must be present for the diagnosis to be made. These are the true symptoms of the disorder; the physical symptoms that give rise to them may be consistent for any given patient, or vary across body systems and time.
   4. **Somatization disorder:** This is the most comprehensive disorder in its symptoms, yet the least frequently assigned. Although the diagnostic criteria listed in Table 29-2 include pain symptoms and pseudoneurological symptoms, somatization disorder is by definition more inclusive than either of these disorders. A patient with conversion disorder may go on to develop somatization disorder over time if all of the diagnostic criteria for the latter are met. However, once a diagnosis of somatization disorder is

---

Table 29-2. Somatization Disorder Symptoms

Patients experience *each* of the following four criteria at some time during the course of the disorder:

1. *Two* gastrointestinal symptoms

Bloating	Diarrhea
Nausea (other than motion sickness)	Multiple food sensitivities
Vomiting (except during pregnancy)	

2. *One* pseudoneurological symptom

Amnesia	Fainting or loss of consciousness
Difficulty swallowing	Seizure(s) or other fit(s)
Blindness	Difficulty walking
Blurred or double vision	Paralysis or muscle weakness
Deafness or mutism/aphonia	Urinary retention

3. *Four* pain symptoms

Headache	Rectal/perineal pain
Back pain	Dysmenorrhea
Joint pain	Dyspareunia
Extremity pain	Dysuria
Abdominal pain	

4. *One* sexual symptom

Sexual indifference	Menorrhagia
Erectile or ejaculatory dysfunction	Metrorrhagia
	Hyperemesis gravidarum

---

made, any further episodes of conversion or pseudoneurological symptoms are simply referred to as an exacerbation of the somatization disorder. The diagnosis of somatization and hypochondriasis may be made concurrently; 21–38% of patients with hypochondriasis also have somatization disorder.

IV. Diagnostic Criteria

A. **Conversion disorder is an unexplained loss or change in voluntary motor or sensory functioning that suggests a neurological condition.** The *DSM-IV* diagnostic criteria are as follows:

1. A loss of physical functioning or a change in voluntary motor or sensory functioning that suggests a neurological (or other medical) condition but defies medical explanation.
2. The symptoms are experienced by the patient, not intentionally produced.
3. The symptoms are presumed to be associated with psychological factors.
4. The disorder is not a culturally sanctioned response to stress.
5. The symptoms may present as a single episode, or as recurrent episodes.
6. The symptoms cause significant distress or impaired functioning.

B. Hypochondriasis is an excessive, pervasive concern about one's health that involves bodily preoccupation, disease fear, and disease conviction. It can be a limited and transient response to stress, a primary disorder in its own right, or a symptom manifested as a result of another underlying psychiatric disorder (e.g., major depression). The *DSM-IV* **diagnostic criteria for primary hypochondriasis are as follows:**
1. The patient displays a non-delusional fear or conviction of disease.
2. Disease fear or conviction arises from the patient's misinterpretation of physical symptoms as evidence of disease and persists despite negative work-up(s) and reassurance.
3. The symptoms must persist for at least 6 months.
4. Disease fear or conviction causes significant distress or impaired functioning.

C. Somatization disorder involves a history of multiple unexplained physical complaints over many years that results in frequent treatment-seeking or significant functional impairment. The behavior may be understood as an idiom for personal and social distress. **The *DSM-IV* diagnostic criteria are as follows:**
1. The symptoms must begin by age 29 and result in disproportionate social or occupational dysfunction.
2. The symptoms are not intentionally feigned.
3. They cannot be caused by alcohol, drugs, or medication, or be fully explained by a known physical disorder.
4. The symptoms themselves appear in Table 29-2.

V. Treatment Strategies

A. The gold standard in the treatment of patients with multiple, unexplained physical complaints is a long-term empathic relationship with a primary care physician (PCP).

B. The goals of treatment for somatizing patients, including those with somatoform disorders **are:**
1. Care for the patient, not necessarily "cure" the somatization.
2. Rule out concurrent physical disorders.
3. Remove any conversion, or pseudoneurological symptoms.
4. Maintain or improve the patient's overall functioning.

C. The clinical approach to the patient depends on whether the pattern of medically unexplained complaints suggests conversion disorder, hypochondriasis, or somatization disorder.
1. **The treatment for patients with conversion disorder involves providing support and reassurance combined with indirect or direct suggestions** (e.g., physical therapy retraining or behavioral techniques). For example, it is not helpful to tell a patient with conversion paralysis, "There's nothing wrong with your legs." Confrontation does them no favor. Instead, it is more effective to say, "I know exactly what's wrong here. Fortunately, this is something that came upon you very quickly, so we can expect it to resolve quickly, too. I will prescribe a series of physical therapy exercises. By tonight, you will be able to bear weight again; by tomorrow you will be able to walk with assistance, and by tomorrow night, you'll be able to walk again on your own."
   a. **Working with the patient to identify precipitant stressors once the episode has resolved may prevent future episodes or mitigate disability associated with symptom recurrence.** The number of patients who develop recurrent pseudoneurological symptoms within 1 year is 20–24% and 20% go on to develop full-blown somatization disorder within 4 years of their index episode.

    b. Psychiatric referral may be necessary to confirm the diagnosis of conversion disorder, identify and treat concurrent psychiatric disorders, particularly psychotic disorders and Axis II personality disorders, and provide psychotherapy. Patients with protracted symptoms or enormous secondary gain may benefit from cognitive-behavioral techniques; others with the capacity for introspection and confrontation may benefit from insight-oriented psychotherapy.

2. **Patients with hypochondriasis benefit from a comprehensive treatment approach described in Table 29-3.** Unlike other forms of somatization, hypochondriasis involves significant cognitive distortions, disease fear, and disease conviction; it's more about the meaning attached to physical symptoms than the bodily symptoms themselves. A trial of an SSRI (e.g., citalopram, fluoxetine, sertraline, or paroxetine) may relieve some of the ruminative thinking that accompanies this disorder. Cognitive-behavioral therapy (CBT) provided by a skilled therapist can lead to dramatic improvements in functioning.

    a. Psychiatric consultation may be required to differentiate this disorder from obsessive-compulsive disorder (OCD), anxiety disorders (e.g., panic disorder), and delusional disorders. Unfortunately, because these patients are convinced that their symptoms portend serious physical disease, they are very resistant to psychiatric consultation.

    b. Patients are more amenable to psychiatric consultation when they are prepared for it; if consultation is indicated, the patient should be told that the psychiatrist will provide the PCP with specific recommendations about how to reduce the distress the patient experiences.

3. **Somatization disorder has proven itself responsive to psychiatric case consultation,** as shown by repeated studies in medical settings. Psychiatric consultations that provide specific management suggestions to the PCP have proved effective in reducing costs associated with both hospitalization and outpatient specialty care, and in improving the patient's overall functioning. The consultation recommendations to PCP have been summarized in Table 29-4. This 10-point plan should serve as a guideline for primary care treatment.

Table 29-3. Treatment of Hypochondriasis

Schedule regular, brief appointments.

Inquire about symptoms and inquire about the patient's fear and beliefs about his or her illness.

Perform focused physical examinations.

Provide explanations and information.

- Provide accurate information about objective signs on the physical exam.
- Explain cognitive misattributions or perceptual distortions (i.e., teach the patient the model for his or her dysfunction).
- Correct misunderstandings about previous diagnoses.

Investigate objective findings further, not subjective complaints.

Make benign recommendations when appropriate (e.g., physical exercise, dietary changes, physical therapy).

Prepare the patient for any psychiatric consultation you recommend.

Table 29-4. Treatment of Somatization Disorder

The Ten-Point Plan:

1. Diagnose somatization disorder early and deliver the diagnosis to the patient.
2. Try to become the patient's only physician and minimize the patient's contact with other healthcare professionals.
3. Identify psychosocial cues or precipitants to new symptom complaints, but avoid premature confrontation.
4. Plan regularly scheduled appointments of set length at 2 to 6 week intervals.
5. Set the agenda (i.e., develop a prioritized problem list and stick to it).
6. Do conservative diagnostic work-ups: investigate objective findings, not subjective complaints.
7. Avoid spurious diagnoses and rebut the patient's rebuttals.
8. Do not treat what the patient does not have.
9. Provide an explanatory model of the symptom process: use the "stress" idiom.
10. Prepare the patient for psychiatric consultation or for psychiatric treatment by setting the agenda or identifying contingencies to continued treatment.

---

a. Further psychiatric consultation may help to diagnose and treat concurrent psychiatric illness, and provide psychotherapy for selected patients.

b. Although psychotherapy alone is not a treatment for somatization, individual psychotherapy may benefit some patients who need help with the emotional consequences of having recurrent and distressing physical symptoms. CBT may be useful for others in focusing on identification of automatic thoughts, or cognitive errors, and in correcting repeated cognitive distortions that give rise to the escalating conviction that the symptom represents disease.

c. Psychotropic medications should be avoided unless they are used to target clear, co-morbid psychiatric disorders.

Suggested Readings

Bass, C., Peveler, R., & House, A. (2001). Somatoform disorders: Severe psychiatric illnesses neglected by psychiatrists. *British Journal of Psychiatry, 179,* 11–14.

Creed, F., & Guthrie, E. (1993). Techniques for interviewing the somatising patient. *British Journal of Psychiatry, 162,* 467–471.

Noyes, R., Langbehn, D.R., Happel, R.L., et al. (2001). Personality dysfunction among somatizing patients. *Psychosomatics, 42,* 320–328.

Per, F., Rosendal, M., & Toft, T. (2002). Assessment and treatment of functional disorders in general practice: The extended reattribution and management model—An advanced educational program for nonpsychiatric doctors. *Psychosomatics, 43*(2), 93–131.

Reid, S., Wessely, S., Crayford, T., et al. (2002). Frequent attenders with medically unexplained symptoms: Service use and costs in secondary care. *British Journal of Psychiatry, 180,* 248–253.

Smith, G.C., Clarke, D.M., Handrinos, D., et al. (2000). Consultation—Liaison psychiatrists' management of somatoform disorders. *Psychosomatics, 41,* 481–489.

Warwick, H.M. (1995). Assessment of hypochondriasis. *Behavioral Research Therapy, 33,* 845–853.

CHAPTER 30

Behavior Problems of Children and Adolescents

MICHAEL S. JELLINEK

I. Introduction

A. Children and adolescents develop through a complex interaction of their biology and environment. Built-in structures evolve and change in the context of experience, family, health, risks, opportunities, and culture. **The challenge in primary care is to understand these many continuously interacting factors, assess the child's development as they integrate the experience and biology, try to optimize a child's long-term development, and relieve a child's emotional suffering.**

II. Prevalence

Studies of prevalence suggest that 12% or more of all children have psychosocial difficulties.

A. What should be defined as a "difficulty," and thus worthy of being considered, counted, or acted upon? If defined by *DSM-IV-TR* for disorders, then the prevalence would be higher, and more than 12% of children would have one or more diagnoses (called "comorbidity," e.g., depression and anxiety, attention-deficit disorder [ADD], and oppositional disorder).

B. **Primary care clinicians are better served by defining disorders based on developmental expectations and impairment or dysfunction** in conjunction with formal *DSM-IV* criteria.

C. **Accidents, a leading cause of death in children and adolescents, are often secondary consequences of psychosocial stressors.** Fires, falls from windows, drowning, and motor vehicle accidents are all more likely in the context of psychosocial dysfunction.

D. **Children with chronic disease are about twice as likely to have a psychosocial disorder** (those suffering from epilepsy are at highest risk). Psychosocial functioning also has an impact on compliance and is associated with heavier use of primary care services.

E. Recent events in the United States (e.g., the World Trade Center terrorist attack), and unfortunate events around the world, have increased the awareness and the prevalence of acute and chronic stress reactions in children. The combination of increased vulnerability, the presence of heightened security, and ever-present media coverage have as yet an unknown impact on children.

III. Recognition

A. **The goal of recognition is to provide help, preferably, at an early and effective point,** to the primary care clinician in investing clinical time. For example, rather than review symptoms of diabetes in every child, a urine screening test helps the primary care clinician determine which children need further evaluation. Screening tests are not designed to yield diagnoses among children, and it would be reductionistic to use them instead of comprehensive clinical judgment. Like most efforts at recognition, such as growth charts or urine dipsticks, **psychosocial screening is a starting point for further questions and assessment.**

B. Primary care physicians (PCPs) in busy office practices have had difficulty identifying children and adolescents with psychosocial dysfunction. Studies indicate that **less than 30% of children with substantial dysfunction are recognized, and of these less than half are referred.** Referral rates of children seen by pediatricians to mental health services range nationally from 1–4%. Often recognition depends on parental complaint or school report of overt behavioral problems; early recognition, prevention, and less overt dysfunction (such as adolescent depression, or family factors such as divorce) are much less likely to be addressed. **Several approaches to recognition are helpful:**

1. **Interviewing focused on key, high-risk issues** offers the advantage of face-to-face interaction, building a relationship with the child and family, and communicating an interest in psychosocial issues. The pressures of time, however, make this approach difficult and more costly. A format and sequence for psychosocial questions throughout development is available through the Public Health Service manual *Bright Futures: Mental Health.* Examples of this focused questioning include the following guidelines:

   a. **At intake, ask all parents for a family history of psychiatric disorder and at annual visits ask about any parental discord or divorce.**
   b. **For newborns, assess parental coping, family supports, and maternal depression.**
   c. **For infants, review temperamental characteristics of the baby and the mother's ability to cope with these traits.**
   d. **For toddlers, ask about the child's autonomy and ability to separate.**
   e. **For early school-aged children, ask about social functioning in first grade.**
   f. **For those of elementary school age, ask about academic ability and extracurricular activities.**
   g. **For adolescents, ask about autonomy (parents), mood, and substance use (adolescent patient).**

C. The Child Behavior Checklist (CBCL) developed by Achenbach is the best validated and studied **behavioral questionnaire completed by parents for children age 4 to 16 years.** The CBCL consists of two distinct item groups: behavior problems and social competency. Scoring by cutoff score or by subscales is available. The main drawback of the CBCL is length (over 100 items) with administration, scoring, and interpretation often requiring approximately 20 minutes (quite long for a busy office setting).

D. The Pediatric Symptom Checklist (PSC, Table 30-1) is **a 35-item questionnaire given to the parent at time of check-in and usually completed in several minutes in the waiting room.** The PSC is scored by assigning two points to every "often," one point to each "sometimes," and no points to "never" answers; adding the points yields the total score. If the PSC score is 28 or above, then there is an approximately 70% likelihood that the children has substantial psychosocial dysfunction. If the screening is below cutoff, then there is a 95% likelihood the child does not have serious difficulties.

1. **For children under school age, a cutoff score of 24 or above indicates a high likelihood for dysfunction,** the lower cutoff score resulting from the "never" answers to the school-based questions not relevant to this age group. There is pilot work currently under way to define a specific pre-school version of the PSC, the PPSC.

Table 30-1. Pediatric Symptom Checklist (PSC)

Please mark under the heading that best describes your child:

	Never	Sometimes	Often
1. Complains of aches and pains	___	___	___
2. Spends more time alone	___	___	___
3. Tires easily, has little energy	___	___	___
4. Fidgety, unable to sit still	___	___	___
5. Has trouble with a teacher	___	___	___
6. Less interested in school	___	___	___
7. Acts as if driven by a motor	___	___	___
8. Daydreams too much	___	___	___
9. Distracted easily	___	___	___
10. Is afraid of new situations	___	___	___
11. Feels sad, unhappy	___	___	___
12. Is irritable, angry	___	___	___
13. Feels hopeless	___	___	___
14. Has trouble concentrating	___	___	___
15. Less interested in friends	___	___	___
16. Fights with other children	___	___	___
17. Absent from school	___	___	___
18. School grades dropping	___	___	___
19. Is down on him- or herself	___	___	___
20. Visits doctor with doctor finding nothing wrong	___	___	___
21. Has trouble sleeping	___	___	___
22. Worries a lot	___	___	___
23. Wants to be with you more than before	___	___	___
24. Feels he or she is bad	___	___	___
25. Takes unnecessary risks	___	___	___
26. Gets hurt frequently	___	___	___
27. Seems to be having less fun	___	___	___
28. Acts younger than children his or her age	___	___	___
29. Does not listen to rules	___	___	___
30. Does not show feelings	___	___	___
31. Does not understand other people's feelings	___	___	___
32. Teases others	___	___	___
33. Blames others for his or her troubles	___	___	___
34. Takes things that do not belong to him or her	___	___	___
35. Refuses to share	___	___	___

2. **The PSC works virtually as well in adolescent populations** with the limitation that a parent-completed questionnaire cannot report an adolescent's intrapsychic symptoms, such as depression, that a parent may not know; however, because the test focuses on dysfunction, the test is still generally valid and useful.

IV. Clinical Perspectives

A. **Children who have major difficulties in one area of functioning often demonstrate symptoms and difficulties in other areas of their daily functioning.** For example, if they are having school difficulties secondary to attention-deficit/hyperactivity disorder (ADHD), symptoms such as motoric activity or impulsivity will be evident at home and may interfere with other activities. Even less overt disorders, such as learning disabilities or difficulties in peer relationships, will often manifest as depressed mood at home, tension with siblings, or low self-esteem.

B. **Focused preventative interventions often can have a meaningful impact.** One should encourage participation in an activity (e.g., sports or art), build a positive relationship with an adult, and develop a series of competencies and peer relationships to support resiliency in the face of stress. Tracking and reassessing are key in primary care.

C. A new manual, *DSM-PC (The Classification of Child and Adolescent Mental Diagnoses in Primary Care: Diagnostic and Statistical Manual for Primary Care, Child and Adolescent Version)* has been released that takes a developmental approach and creates three categories: normal variation, problem, and disorder (the latter category uses *DSM-IV* criteria).

1. **Normal variation acknowledges that children have different temperaments, personalities, and developmental paths, and come from a range of families and cultures.**

2. **Problems are defined as a broad range of issues, some that fit into psychiatric diagnostic categories and many others that do not,** but are nevertheless clinically relevant to PCPs (e.g., reacting "normally" to a stressor, needing support during a divorce, adapting to a chronic disease, or not compling with a necessary medical regimen).

3. **Disorders are conditions meeting *DSM-IV* criteria.**

D. **A key component of *DSM-IV* and *DSM-IV-TR* is the extent of impairment or severity.** Severity will influence prevalence (the assessment of severity may determine what is to be counted) and is critical in clinical management. Some presentations, such as psychosis or a serious suicide attempt, are clearly severe. Other conditions, however, such as depression, can vary widely in severity and in mild cases will be managed in primary care settings, some with support and reassurance; severe cases will be referred for possible hospitalization. **Severity assessment usually includes the following:**

1. **Symptoms—number, frequency, duration, and number of sites (home, school)**

2. **Functioning**—impact on functioning in major developmental areas including family, friends, school, activities, and self-esteem

3. **Burden of suffering**—intensity of suffering, duration, limitations on family, activities, or expectations, danger to self and others, and intrusiveness into developmental tasks or daily activities

E. Risk and Protective Factors

There are a number of biological and environmental factors that may put children at greater risk or may serve to protect children from adversity (see Table 30-2). Although each risk factor on its own has a profound or overwhelming impact, these factors also work in concert. **Research suggests that children facing three or more risk factors have a very high likelihood of psychosocial dysfunction.** In primary care settings, clinicians should also focus on enhancing protective factors to enhance growth and balancing risks, as a prevention strategy.

Table 30-2. Children's Well-Being: Risk and Protective Factors

	Protective—Decreased Impact of Stress	Risk—Increased Impact of Stress
Health	Good health	Chronic disease/ill health
Temperament	e.g., Pleasant mood	e.g., Negative mood; irritable
Cognitive status	Normal IQ (particularly verbal)	Learning disability/low IQ
Emotional health	Good mental health function	Pre-existing emotional disorder
Self-esteem	High; confident	Low self-esteem; self-doubting
Sociability	Good peer relations; pro-social	Poor peer relations
Child reaction to stress	Perceives stress as limited; does not blame self	Perceives continued threat; blames self
Connectedness	Committed to family, religion, school, friends, or activity	Isolated; not invested
Quality of attachment	High quality, high continuity; securely attached	Low quality, discontinuous; ambivalent, insecurely attached
Parent competence	Competent	Incompetent
Family resources	Adequate economic resources	Poverty/discrimination
Quality, stability, safety of environment	Adequate, stable, safe	Inadequate, unstable, unsafe; frequent moves
Family relationships	Good communication; little conflict	Poor communication; much conflict
Emotional and physical health of caregivers	Caregivers in good emotional and physical health	Mental illness; physical illness in caregivers
Availability/access to community resources	High access	Low access

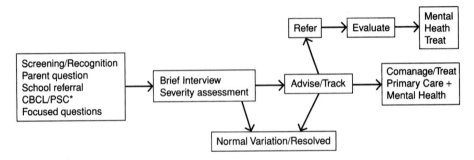

Figure 30-1. Practice flow chart. CBCL, Child Behavior Checklist; PSC, Pediatric Symptom Checklist.

V. Brief Evaluation

After recognition (following the flow chart, Figure 30-1), the primary care clinician must assess the nature of the distress and its severity.

A. **Confirm screening findings or further define the nature of the parent or school complaint, and elaborate symptoms.**

B. **Add the context of the family history of psychiatric disorders and current family functioning** (e.g., discord/divorce, relationship with child, key losses).

C. **Assess the child's daily functioning:**
1. **Family relationships**—warmth, activities, expectations, discipline, and recent losses
2. **Activities/play**—age-appropriate interests, special weakness or strength
3. **Separation experience,** daycare or school-ability to tolerate and function
4. **Friendships**—quality, number, and social acceptance
5. **Mood, self-esteem, developmentally appropriate autonomy**

D. **For young children, observe and focus questioning with parents.**

E. **For children, use confirmatory questions, if possible without parents present.**

F. **For adolescents, perform a separate interview to confirm symptoms, to assess substance use, and to explore issues of depression and sexual relations.**

G. **Conduct a focused review of potentially relevant risk/protective factors.**

H. **Confirm the safety of the child in the current settings.**

I. **Complete a severity assessment based on previously mentioned data;** rate as mild, moderate, or severe.

VI. Clinical Decision-Making

Following the flow chart (Fig. 30-1), the primary care clinician can decide that the parental, school, or screening concern is one of the following:

A. A normal variation or mild and resolving problem requires no further action.

B. A problem that should be further evaluated at the primary care level, tracked at follow-up intervals (determined by the nature and severity of the problem), referred at this time, or involved with co-management with mental health and school personnel.

C. A disorder requiring tracking of primary care treatment or referral for comprehensive evaluation, or emergency referral.

VII. Treatment Strategies

Of the psychosocial issues clinicians will face, many resolve or benefit from guidance. However, moderate to severe dysfunction requires a serious effort at treatment. After more specific primary care or subspecialist evaluation, any required treatment plan should be "comprehensive":

A. Consider all areas of daily functioning as areas to integrate into a treatment plan. Parent counseling, support from the child's teacher, use of community resources (YMCA, camp, teams), and approaches that build self-esteem should be considered.

B. Use medication appropriately.

C. Consider a variety of therapies (individual, family, behavioral).

D. Involve out-of-home services, including hospitalization, partial or day hospitals, and foster care, as indicated.

E. Provide focused treatment for substance abuse and learning disabilities.

VIII. What to Expect When You Refer

The current state of the mental health referral system is chaotic. Many managed care plans limit and control mental health services, especially for children and adolescents. Under capitation, the primary care clinician has more control, but may face financial disincentives. **The best option is to select a few responsive and communicative providers. Although somewhat more costly initially, using a highly trained individual for the evaluation may be the best service to the child and be the most cost effective over time.**

IX. Innovative Office Models

Managed care and capitation, especially for groups of PCPs in stable communities, may offer opportunities for innovative practice. For example, in-house mental health services, such as a social worker, psychologist, or part-time traveling psychiatrist, may allow many opportunities as quick referral, co-management, teamwork, and alignment of financial incentives. Larger practices may have a sufficient number of patients for preventive (cost-effective) group programs concerning divorce, attention-deficit/hyperactivity disorder, or adolescent development.

X. Primary Care Providers

PCPs face the difficult task of addressing prevention and early recognition of psychosocial dysfunction in the context of productivity demands. **Time is money, and the cost-offset of accident prevention, optimization of development, help with parenting, and referral for necessary mental health services are all hard to measure and may take years to emerge fully.** Monthly financials noting "number of patients" seen and "referrals" sent are more readily measurable and influential, but must be balanced against the child or family's immediate and long-term needs.

PCPs can also advocate with managed care companies and insurers to make mental health services more accessible.

Suggested Readings

Achenbach, T.M. (1991). *Manual for the child behavior checklist 4–18 and 1991 profile.* Burlington, VT: University of Vermont Department of Psychiatry.

American Academy of Pediatrics. (1996). *The classification of child and adolescent mental diagnoses in primary care: Diagnostic and statistical manual for primary care (DSM-PC), child and adolescent version.* M.L. Wolreich, M.E. Felice, & D. Drotar (Eds.). Elk Grove Village, IL: American Academy of Pediatrics.

American Psychiatric Association. (2000). *Diagnostic and statistical manual of mental disorders* (4th ed., Text Revision). Washington, DC: American Psychiatric Press.

Bernal, P., Estroff, D.B., Aboudarham, J.F., et al. (2000). Psychosocial morbidity: The economic burden in a pediatric health maintenance organization sample. *Archives of Pediatric and Adolescent Medicine, 154,* 261–266.

Biederman, J., & Steingard, R. (1990). *Psychopharmacology of children and adolescents: A primer for the clinician.* Washington, DC: Pan American Health Organization, World Health Organization.

Costello, E.J. (1986). Primary care pediatrics and child psychopathology: A review of diagnostic, treatment, and referral practices. *Pediatrics, 78,* 1044–1051.

Earls, F. (2001). Community factors supporting child mental health. *Child and Adolescent Psychiatric Clinics of North America, 10*(4), 693–709.

Earls, F., & Carlson, M. (2001). The social ecology of child health and well-being. *Annual Review of Public Health, 22,* 143–166.

Eisenberg, L. (1995). The social construction of the human brain. *American Journal of Psychiatry, 152*(11), 1563–1575.

Hack, S., & Jellinek, M.S. (1998). Historical clues to the diagnosis of the dysfunctional child and other psychiatric disorders in children. *Pediatric Clinics of North America, 45*(1), 25–48.

Hobbs, N., Perrin, J.M., & Ireys, H.T. (1985). *Chronically ill children and their families.* San Francisco: Josey-Bass, Inc.

Jellinek, M., Patel, B.P., & Froehle, M.C. (Eds.). (2001). *Bright futures in practice: Mental health-Volume 1, Practice Guide.* Arlington, VA: National Center for Education in Maternal and Child Health.

Jellinek, M.S., Murphy, J.M., Pagano, M.E., et al. (1999). Use of the pediatric symptom checklist (PSC) to screen for psychosocial problems in pediatric primary care: A national feasibility study. *Archives of Pediatric and Adolescent Medicine, 153,* 254–260.

Jellinek, M.S. (1994). The outpatient milieu. *Journal of Child and Adolescent Psychiatry, 33*(2), 277–279.

CHAPTER 31

The Patient with Attention-Deficit Hyperactivity Disorder

TIMOTHY E. WILENS, JOSEPH BIEDERMAN,
AND THOMAS J. SPENCER

I. Introduction

A. Diagnostic Features

The essential feature of Attention-Deficit Hyperactivity Disorder (ADHD) is a persistent pattern of inattention and or hyperactivity-impulsivity that is more frequent and severe than is typically observed in individuals at a comparable level of development. Inattentiveness may be manifest as difficulties sustaining attention on school or work-related tasks, difficulties following through on instructions, and distractbility. Hyperactivity may be manifest by fidgeting, or squirming in one's seat, and impulsivity may be manifest by impatience, difficulty in delaying responses, blurting out answers before a question has been completed, and frequent interruptions. Redundancy has been built into the diagnostic criteria to account for the frequency of these symptoms in the population. **The symptoms have to be associated with impairment in functioning and must be present in at least two settings** (e.g., home and school). Although many individuals are diagnosed after the symptoms have been present for a number of years, **the symptoms must have started before the age of seven years to qualify for this diagnosis.** This latter issue is critical for the diagnosis of adults; adults must clearly show childhood-onset of symptoms to qualify for this diagnosis.

B. Subtypes

Depending on the symptoms that predominate, *DSM-IV* recognizes a predominantly inattentive subtype, a predominantly hyperactive-impulsive subtype, and a combined subtype. *DSM-IV* also recognizes the category termed ADHD Not Otherwise Specified (NOS) for patients who do not meet full diagnostic criteria.

C. Prevalence

ADHD is a heterogeneous disorder of unknown etiology estimated to affect 5% of children and 2% of adults. It is one of the major clinical and public health problems in the United States because of its associated morbidity and disability in children, adolescents, and adults. Its impact on society is enormous in terms of the financial cost, the stress to families, the impact on academic and vocational activities, as well as the negative effects on self-esteem.

D. Course

Data from cross-sectional, retrospective, and follow-up studies indicate that **approximately half of youth will continue to manifest either full criteria for ADHD or prominent symptoms of ADHD into adulthood. Over time, hyperactive and impulsive symptoms diminish while inattentive symptoms persist.**

Predictors of persistence include family history of ADHD, psychiatric co-morbidity, and psychosocial adversity (e.g., family conflict, poverty).

E. Etiology and Pathophysiology

Although its etiology remains unknown, data from family-genetic, twin, and adoption studies, as well as segregation analysis suggest a **genetic origin** for some forms of this disorder. The etiologic role of heavy metals remains uncertain. Recent work suggests that **alcohol intake and maternal smoking during pregnancy, perinatal injuries, and psychosocial adversity could be additional risk factors for ADHD.** While the underlying neural and pathophysiological substrate of ADHD remains unknown, an emerging **neuropsychological and neuroimaging literature points to abnormalities in frontal networks** as its underlying neural substrate (fronto-striatal dysfunction) **and to catecholamine dysregulation** as its underlying pathophysiological substrate. Data suggesting candidate genes for the dopamine transporter and post-synaptic D_4 receptor have been reported.

F. Co-morbidity

In recent years, evidence has been accumulating regarding **high levels of psychiatric and cognitive (i.e., learning disability) co-morbidity between ADHD and a number of disorders** (including mood, anxiety, oppositional and conduct disorder) in prepubescent youth with the addition of substance abuse in adolescents and young adults. It indicates that ADHD is most likely a group of conditions, rather than a single homogeneous clinical entity, with potentially different etiologic and modifying risk factors and different outcomes.

G. Gender Distribution

Although **the disorder is more common in males than in females,** little doubt remains that ADHD affects both genders; however, it tends to be under-identified in females. Females with ADHD share with their male counterparts prototypical features of the disorder (e.g., high rates of school failure and cognitive impairments, and high levels of familiality) but, they tend to be less aggressive than males. This last characteristic may account for the **under-identification and under-treatment of females with ADHD.** This under-identification of ADHD in females may have substantial clinical and educational implications, i.e., it deprives them of highly effective treatment programs.

H. Medical History and Laboratory Findings

There are no physical features, laboratory, or psychological tests that have been established as diagnostic in the clinical assessment of ADHD. Although minor physical anomalies, e.g., hypertelorism, arched palate, low set ears, and physical injury, may occur at higher rate than in the general population, none of these characteristics is diagnostic. Although some tests, such as the continuous performance test (CPT), that require effortful mental processing have been noted to be abnormal in groups of individuals with this disorder compared with controls, they have little diagnostic utility in individual patients.

I. Differential Diagnosis

In early childhood it is important to distinguish symptoms of ADHD from age-appropriate behaviors in very active children. Also important to distinguish are symptoms of inattention in children with low IQ and in children with autism or pervasive developmental disorders. **Symptoms of inattentiveness, hyperactivity, and**

impulsivity can be present in other mental disorders, such as mood disorders, as well as in individuals with other metabolic or neurologic conditions. School failure needs to be differentiated from learning disabilities, psychosocial stressors, or acute onset of a mood disorder. Behavioral problems in school age children need to be differentiated from conduct and oppositional defiant disorder. Although these conditions need to be considered in the differential diagnosis of ADHD, it is important to remember that they are not mutually exclusive with ADHD, in other words, they commonly co-exist.

J. Prognostic Factors

Positive prognostic factors include ADHD without additional learning or psychiatric disorders, good intellectual abilities, history of prior accomplishments, and a supportive environment. **Poor prognostic factors include severe mood lability, severe impulsivity or aggression, psychiatric co-morbidity, and limited cognitive abilities.**

H. Evaluation of the Problem

The diagnosis of ADHD at any age is based on a careful psychiatric history (anamnesis) and psychiatric examination. It is common for the symptoms *not* to be evident during the interview since they tend to express themselves in unstructured situations, such as school or work. Since children with ADHD tend not to be good historians, information should be gathered from a parent or a caretaker and whenever possible supplemented by reports of teachers.

II. Treatment Strategies

A. General Principles

A comprehensive treatment approach to the ADHD patient should attempt to address the three main areas of potential dysfunction: biological, psychosocial, and educational. Potentially useful psychotherapeutic efforts in the management of ADHD patients include behavioral and cognitive-behavioral interventions, e.g., training in self-instruction, parent instruction, self-evaluation, attribution, social skills, and anger management. Since at least 30% of ADHD children may suffer from learning disabilities, and since learning disorders are not drug-sensitive, learning-disabled ADHD patients require additional educational support including tutoring, placement in special classes, and consideration of specialized schools in refractory cases. **The pharmacotherapy of ADHD, although not curative, can help improve abnormal behaviors in school or work and, equally important, the individual's social and family life.** The medications employed for the treatment of ADHD include the stimulants, antidepressants, and antihypertensive medications.

B. Stimulants

Stimulants are sympathomimetic drugs structurally similar to endogenous catecholamines. **The most commonly used compounds in this class include methylphenidate (Ritalin, Concerta, Metadate), amphetamine compounds (Adderall), D-amphetamine (Dexedrine), and magnesium pemoline (Cylert).** These drugs are thought to act both in the central nervous system (CNS) and peripherally by preventing re-uptake of catecholamines (dopamine > norepinephrine) into pre-synaptic nerve endings, and thus preventing their degradation by monoamine oxidase.

Table 31-1. Medications Used in Attention-Deficit Hyperactivity Disorder

Medication (Generic)	Medication (Brand)	Daily Dose (mg/kg)	Daily Dosage Schedule	Common Adverse Effects
Stimulants				
Methylphenidate	Ritalin	0.3–2.0		• Insomnia,
	Focalin		Twice to four times	• Decreased appetite/weight loss
	Metadate CD	(0.6–1.0)	Once	• Possible reduction in growth velocity with chronic use
	Concerta			• Stomach aches
	Ritalin LA			• Headaches
				• Dysphoria
Amphetamine	Dexedrine	0.3–1.5	Twice or three times	• Rebound phenomena (short-acting preparations)
Dextroamphetamine	Adderall			
Mixed amphetamine salts	Adderall XR		Once	
Magnesium pemoline	Cylert	1.0–3.0	Once or twice	• Same as other stimulants
				• Abnormal liver function tests
Antidepressants				
Tricyclics (TCA)				
Imipramine	Tofranil	2.0–5.0	Once or twice	• Dry mouth, constipation
Desipramine	Norpramine			• Weight loss
Nortriptyline	Pamelor	1.0–3.0		• Vital sign and ECG changes

Bupropion	Wellbutrin	3–6	Three times	• Irritability, insomnia
	Wellbutrin SR		Once or twice	• Risk of seizures (in doses > 6 mg/kg)
	Wellbutrin XL		Once	• Contraindicated in bulimics
Venlafaxine	Effexor	0.5–3	Two	• Nausea
				• Sedation
				• GI distress
Antihypertensives				
Clonidine	Catapress	3–10 mcg/kg	Twice or three times	• Sedation, dry mouth, depression
				• Confusion (with high dose)
				• Rebound hypertension
				• Localized irritation with patch
Guanfacine	Tenex	30–100 mcg/kg	Twice	• Similar to clonidine but less sedation
				• Insomnia, irritability reported
Noradrenergic agents				
Atomoxetine	Not available	< 1.2 mg/kg	Once or twice	• Nausea
				• Headaches
				• Stomach aches

Dosing recommendations are not FDA-approved.

Immediate-release methylphenidate and D-amphetamine are both short-acting compounds with an onset of action within 30 to 60 minutes and a peak clinical effect usually seen between 1 and 3 hours after administration. Therefore, multiple daily administrations are required for a consistent daytime response. **Slow-release preparations, with a peak clinical effect between 1 and 5 hours, are available for methylphenidate and D-amphetamine and can often allow for a single dose to be administered in the morning that will last for the entire school day.**

Extended-release stimulants are now available for both methylphenidate (Metadate CD, Ritalin LA, Concerta) and amphetamine (Adderall XR). Magnesium pemoline is an older, long-acting compound. Typically these compounds have a rapid onset of action so that clinical response will be evident soon after a therapeutic dose has been obtained and will last from 8 to 12 hours. The extended release preparations of stimulants are preferred to shorter-acting formulations to enhance compliance, reduce the peaks and troughs of the medication, reduce the need for in-school dosing, reduce stigma, and potentially reduce diversion.

Although the safety and efficacy of stimulant drugs has been amply documented in more than 250 controlled studies with more than 6,000 children, adolescents, and adults, as many as 30% do not respond to these drugs. Although methylphenidate is by far the most studied stimulant medication, **the literature provides little evidence of differential response to the various available stimulants, although some patients may respond preferentially to one or another stimulant.**

1. **Spectrum of effects**

   Stimulant treatment diminishes behavior prototypical of ADHD, including motoric overactivity, impulsivity, and inattentiveness. Stimulants can also be effective in patients with ADHD in whom hyperactivity is not a significant clinical problem. In addition to improving core symptoms of ADHD, stimulants also improve associated behaviors, including on-task behavior, academic performance, and social function. These effects appear to be dose-dependent and cross-situational, including home, clinic and school. In adults, occupational, driving, and marital dysfunction often improve with stimulant treatment.

   Observational studies also demonstrate stimulant-enhanced social skills in school, within families and with peers, including improved maternal-child and sibling interactions. Studies also find that families of stimulant-responsive children are more amenable to psychosocial interventions. Investigations of peer relationships in ADHD children show that those treated with stimulants have increased abilities to perceive peer communications, self-perceptions, and situational cues. In addition, these children show improved modulation of the intensity of behavior, with improved communication and greater responsiveness with fewer negative interactions. These findings support the importance of treating ADHD children beyond school hours (to include evenings, weekends, and vacations), should problems exist at these times.

2. **Dosing**

   Due to their short half-life, the short-acting stimulants should be given in divided doses throughout the day, typically 4 hours apart. The extended release stimulants are given once a day in the morning. The total daily dose ranges from 0.3 mg/kg/day to 2 mg/kg/day (1.5 mg/kg/day for amphetamine) in the various age groups. The starting dose is generally 2.5 to 5 mg/day of immediate release, given in the morning, with the dose being increased if necessary every few days by 2.5 to 5 mg in a divided dose schedule. Extended-release preparations can be sequenced initially and should be started at the lowest dose level available (e.g., 18 mg of Concerta). Because of the well-documented dose-response relationship, the stimulants should be titrated upward for optimal outcome (improved ADHD symptoms with minimal adverse effects). Due to the anorexogenic effects of the stimulants, it may be beneficial to administer the medicine during or after meals.

3. **Drug-drug interactions**

The interactions of the stimulants with other prescription and non-prescription medications are generally mild and not a source of concern. Whereas co-administration of sympathomimetics (e.g., pseudoephedrine) may potentiate the effects of both medications, the antihistamines may diminish the stimulant's effectiveness. Caution should be exercised when using stimulants and antidepressants of the monoamine oxidase inhibitor (MAOI) type because of the potential for hypertensive reactions with this combination. The concomitant use of stimulants and tricyclic antidepressants (TCAs) or serotonergic reuptake inhibitors (SRIs) appears to be well tolerated without known drug interactions.

4. **Adverse effects**

The most commonly reported side effects associated with the administration of stimulant medication are appetite suppression and sleep disturbance. The sleep disturbance that is most commonly reported is delay of sleep onset. This usually occurs when stimulants are administered in the late afternoon or early evening. Although less commonly reported, mood disturbances, ranging from increased tearfulness to a full-blown major depression-like syndrome, can be associated with stimulant treatment. Other infrequent side effects include headaches, abdominal discomfort, increased lethargy, and fatigue. Mild increases in pulse and blood pressure of unclear clinical significance have been observed with stimulants in youth and adults. A rare stimulant-associated toxic psychosis has been observed, usually in the context of either a rapid rise in the dosage or very high doses. The reported psychosis in children in response to stimulant medications resembles a toxic phenomenon (e.g., visual hallucinosis) and is dissimilar from the exacerbation of the psychotic symptoms present in schizophrenia. Administration of magnesium pemoline has been associated with hypersensitivity reactions involving the liver accompanied by elevations in liver function studies (SGOT and SGPT) after several months of treatment. Thus, baseline liver function studies and repeat studies are recommended with the administration of this compound.

Although stimulants routinely produce anorexia and weight loss, their effect on growth in height is less certain. Although early reports indicated that children with a personal or family history of tic disorders were at greater risk for developing a tic disorder when exposed to stimulants, recent work has increasingly challenged this view. Recent data indicate that youth with ADHD and tics can be treated with stimulants with close observation for the approximate 30% who manifest exacerbation in their tics. Similar uncertainties remain about the abuse potential of stimulants in ADHD children. **Despite the concern that ADHD may increase the risk of abuse in adolescents and young adults (or his or her associates), the aggregate literature suggests that stimulant-treated ADHD children have lower substance abuse in later life.**

C. Antidepressants

1. Bupropion hydrochloride

Bupropion is a novel-structured antidepressant of the aminoketone class related to the phenylisopropylamines but pharmacologically distinct from known antidepressants. Although bupropion seems to have both indirect dopamine agonist and noradrenergic effects, its specific site or mechanism of action remains unknown. **Bupropion has been reported to be better than placebo in reducing ADHD symptoms.** The response of ADHD to bupropion appears to be delayed for up to 6 weeks and sustained. **Bupropion may be particularly helpful for youth with ADHD and co-morbid mood disorders** as it may have antidepressant activity and may not activate mania.

Dosing for ADHD appears to be similar to that recommended for depression (daily dosing of 300 mg/day for children and 400 mg/day for adolescents of the sustained release preparation in divided doses). Bupropion is rapidly absorbed, with peak plasma levels usually achieved after 2 hours, with an average elimination half life of 14 hours (range = 8–24 hours).

Side effects include rashes, nocturia, irritability, anorexia, and insomnia. **It appears to have a somewhat higher rate of drug-induced seizures relative to other antidepressants, particularly in daily doses higher than 6 mg/kg and in patients with a previous history of seizures and eating disorders.**

2. Tricyclic antidepressants

Tricyclic antidepressants (TCAs) include the tertiary amines (amitriptyline, imipramine, doxepin, and trimipramine), and the secondary amines (desipramine, nortriptyline, and protriptyline). The mechanism of action appears to be due to the blocking effects of these drugs on the re-uptake of brain neurotransmitters, especially norepinephrine and serotonin. However, these agents have variable effects on pre- and post-synaptic neurotransmitter systems, resulting in differing positive and adverse effect profiles.

Imipramine and desipramine are the most studied TCAs in ADHD, followed by a handful of studies on other TCAs. Outcomes in both short and long-term TCA studies have been equally positive. Improvement of ADHD symptoms can be maintained when daily doses of TCAs are titrated upward over time. Statistically and clinically significant results with desipramine have been demonstrated in ADHD youth (dosing to 5 mg/kg/day) and adults (dosing to 200 mg/day). Recently, nortriptyline has been found to be useful in ADHD at doses of 2 mg/kg/day.

The available literature seems to indicate that TCAs are slightly less efficacious than stimulants in controlling ADHD. Despite higher weight-corrected dosing, children often have lower plasma TCA levels than adults. Although high doses (up to 5 mg/kg) of imipramine and desipramine have been used to treat school phobia, major depressive disorder, and ADHD in children, TCA-treatment should always be individualized in an attempt to use the lowest effective dose.

A baseline ECG should be completed. Treatment of children with a TCA should be initiated with a 10 mg or 25 mg dose, depending on the weight of the child and increased slowly every 4 to 5 days by 20–30%. When a daily dose of 2 mg/kg/day (nortriptyline) or 3 mg/kg of other TCAs (or a lower effective dose) and the youth is found to be responding to the medication at six weeks follow-up, an electrocardiogram (ECG) should be obtained. **TCA serum level monitoring is**

useful to signal compliance and to avoid toxicity. However, subjective adverse effects, e.g., dry mouth or dizziness, are unrelated to drug serum levels.

Common short-term adverse effects of the TCAs include anticholinergic effects, e.g., dry mouth, blurred vision, and constipation. However, there are no known deleterious effects associated with chronic administration of these drugs. Gastrointestinal symptoms and vomiting may occur when these drugs are discontinued abruptly. **TCA treatment has been associated with asymptomatic, minor, but statistically significant increases in heart rate and ECG measures of cardiac conduction times.**

The potential benefits of TCAs in the treatment of ADHD have been clouded by rising concerns about their safety stemming from reports of sudden unexplained death in four ADHD children treated with desipramine. However, the causal link between desipramine and these deaths remain uncertain. Because of this uncertainty, prudence mandates that TCAs should be used as second-line treatment for ADHD in juveniles and only after carefully weighing the risks and benefits of treating or not treating an affected child.

3. **Monoamine oxidase inhibitors (MAOIs)**

The monoamine oxidase inhibitor (MAOI) antidepressants have also been studied for the treatment of ADHD. The MAOIs are comprised of two types: MAOI-As preferentially metabolize norepinephrine, epinephrine, and serotonin. MAOI-Bs preferentially metabolize phenylethylamine (PEA), an endogenous amphetamine-like substance, and N-methylhistamine. Both MAOI-A and Bs metabolize tyramine and dopamine. In addition, irreversible MAOIs are susceptible to the "cheese effect" whereas the reversible MAOIs are less susceptible. MAOIs (MAOI-A [clorygline] and a mixed MAOI-A/B [tranylcypromine sulfate]) have reduced ADHD symptoms with minimal adverse effects. In a recent open study, selegiline was evaluated in 29 children with both ADHD and tics. Results showed that 90% of the children improved in their ADHD symptoms with no serious adverse effects; only 2 patients showed an exacerbation of tics. However, **major general limitations to the use of MAOIs are the dietary restrictions of tyramine-containing foods (e.g., most cheeses), pressor amines (i.e., sympathomimetic substances), or drug interactions (e.g., most cold medicines, amphetamines), which can induce a hypertensive crisis or the serotonergic syndrome when MAOIs are combined with predominantly serotonergic drugs.** Daily doses should be carefully titrated based on response and adverse effects and range from 0.5 to 1.0 mg/kg. While dietary restrictions and potential drug–drug interactions complicate the use of MAOIs in ADHD, nonetheless, they may be important to consider in treatment refractory patients.

4. **Selective serotonin reuptake inhibitors (SSRIs) and atypical antidepressants**

Selective serotonin reuptake inhibitors (SSRIs) (fluoxetine, paroxetine, sertraline, citalopram, and fluvoxamine) while not systematically evaluated in the treatment of ADHD, **do not appear to be useful for the core symptoms of the disorder.** Although the role of the novel atypical antidepressant venlafaxine in the treatment of ADHD remains uncertain, two recent open studies reported on the beneficial effects of this compound in the treatment of ADHD adults with prominent mood symptoms. Venlafaxine has a medium half-life of approximately 5 hours. The usual dose range is 2.0 to 5.0 mg/kg daily given in three divided doses. Venlafaxine lacks significant activity at muscarinic/cholinergic, alpha-adrenergic, and histaminergic sites thus has fewer effects (sedation, anticholinergic) than other antidepressants.

5. **Antihypertensive agents**

Clonidine is an imidazoline derivative with alpha-adrenergic agonist properties which has been primarily used in the treatment of hypertension. At low doses, it appears to stimulate inhibitory, pre-synaptic autoreceptors in the CNS. **Beneficial effects of clonidine in the treatment of ADHD have been reported in four pediatric studies** with daily doses of up to 4 to 5 mcg/kg (average 0.2 mg/day). Clonidine is a relatively short-acting compound with a plasma half-life ranging from approximately 5.5 hours (in children) to 8.5 hours (in adults). Daily doses should be titrated and individualized. Usual daily doses range from 3 to 10 mcg/kg, given generally in divided doses, twice or three times daily. Initial dosage can more easily be given in the evening hours or before bedtime due to sedation.

The most common short-term adverse effect of clonidine is sedation. It can also produce, in some cases, hypotension, dry mouth, depression, and confusion. Clonidine is not known to be associated with long-term adverse effects. In hypertensive adults, abrupt withdrawal of clonidine has been associated with rebound hypertension. Thus, it requires slow tapering when discontinued. **Clonidine should not be administered concomitantly with beta-blockers since adverse interactions have been reported with this combination.** While concerns linger about the co-administration of clonidine with stimulants, a recent multisite study of clonidine plus methylphenidate demonstrated clinical efficacy (combined or is better than individual agents) without evidence of cardiotoxicity.

Recent controlled **studies of the longer-acting, more selective alpha$_{2a}$ agonist, *guanfacine*, in children and adolescents with ADHD report beneficial effects on hyperactive behaviors and attentional abilities.** In these studies, youth with tics plus ADHD were found to manifest improvement in both domains. Side effects are similar to clonidine, although less sedation has been reported.

A small open study of propranolol in ADHD adults with temper outbursts found some improvement in ADHD symptoms at daily doses of up to 640 mg/day. Another report indicated that beta-blockers may be helpful in combination with the stimulants. The dose range of propranolol is approximately 2–8 mg/kg/day. Short-term adverse effects of propranolol are usually not serious and generally abate upon cessation of drug administration. Propranolol can cause bradycardia and hypotension as well as increase airway resistance and is contraindicated in asthmatic and certain cardiac patients. There are no known long-term effects associated with chronic administration of propranolol. Since abrupt cessation of this drug may be associated with rebound hypertension, gradual tapering is recommended.

6. **Other agents**

A recently approved agent, atomoxetine, has been shown in more than eight controlled studies including children, adolescents, and adults to be very useful in the treatment of ADHD (Michelson et al., 2001, 2002). Atomoxetine is a highly specific presynaptic noradrenergic re-uptake inhibitor that has little effect on other neurotransmitter systems and is unscheduled.

Atomoxetine has been positioned to be among first-line agents for ADHD. Moreover, studies completed also indicate that it is useful in stimulant non-responders or in those who are intolerant to the adverse effects of stimulants. ATMX has been demonstrated efficacious in all subtypes of ADHD. Currently under study, ATMX may be particularly useful in ADHD co-morbid with mood, anxiety, or tic disorders.

ATMX is readily absorbed and peaks 1–2 hours after administration. The pharmacokinetics of ATMX are similar in children, adolescents, and adults. Results from dose-ranging studies indicate an optimal dose of 1.2 mg/kg/day. In children and adolescents (< 70 kg), ATMX should be initiated at a total daily dose of 0.5 mg/kg and increased after two weeks to 1.2 mg/kg/day. In older children and adults, ATMX should be started at 40 mg and increased after two weeks to 80 mg and then ultimately to a maximum of 100 mg in those who have not had a maximal effect. Studies suggest that ATMX can be given either once or twice daily with similar efficacy and tolerability.

Atomoxetine is metabolized hepatically—though the current dosing guidelines take into account slow and rapid metabolizers. Drug interactions of agents that inhibit the P450 2D6 system (e.g. paroxetine, fluoxetine) should be expected—dosing of ATMX concomitantly may not need to exceed 0.5 mg/kg/day for efficacy under these conditions.

Atomoxetine is generally well tolerated. Side effects of somnolence, insomnia, stomach aches, headaches, nausea, vomiting, and weight loss/appetite suppression have been reported. ATMX also has mild effects on elevating blood pressure and pulse but does not require routine monitoring in youth. However, adults receiving ATMX should have their blood pressure/pulse monitored at baseline and on drug. Longer-term data suggests continued effectiveness and tolerability of ATMX. Similar to stimulants, participants on ATMX experienced transient lack of weight gain over the first six months; although these participants had expected gain in height. Atomoxetine can be discontinued abruptly without tapering.

D. Treatment Strategies

Although monotherapy is always preferred, in clinical practice many ADHD patients require multiple treatments. Combined pharmacological approaches can be used for the treatment of co-morbid ADHD, as augmentation strategies for patients with insufficient response to a single agent and for the management of treatment emergent adverse effects. Examples of combined treatment include the use of an antidepressant plus a stimulant for ADHD and co-morbid depression, the use of clonidine to ameliorate stimulant-induced insomnia, and the use of lithium plus an anti-ADHD agent to treat ADHD co-morbid with bipolar disorder.

1. Treatment of refractory patients

Despite the availability of various agents for the management of the ADHD patient, **a sizable number of individuals either do not respond to, or are intolerant of the adverse effects of medications used to treat their ADHD.** In managing medication non-responders, several therapeutic strategies are available. If psychiatric adverse effects develop concurrently with a poor medication response, alternate treatments should be pursued. Severe psychiatric symptoms, such as psychosis or mania, that emerge during the acute phase of treatment can be problematic, irrespective of the efficacy of the medication for ADHD. These symptoms may require reconsideration of the diagnosis of ADHD and careful reassessment of the presence of co-morbid disorders. If reduction of dose or change in preparation (i.e., regular vs. slow-release stimulants) do not resolve the problem, consideration should be given to alternative treatments. Emerging data indicate the importance of treating co-morbidity with ADHD (e.g., mood lability, anxiety) to enhance ADHD responsivity. Concurrent non-pharmacological interventions, e.g., behavioral or cognitive therapy, may assist with symptom reduction.

2. **Practical guidelines**

   At any age, the pharmacotherapy of ADHD should be part of a treatment plan in which consideration is given to all aspects of the patient's life. However, a recent multisite, multimodal study highlights the fundamental importance of treating ADHD pharmacologically for the longer-term benefit of the patient. The administration of medication to patients with ADHD should be undertaken as a collaborative effort with the patient, with the physician guiding the use and management of efficacious anti-ADHD agents. **The use of medication should follow a careful evaluation of the patient including psychiatric, social, and cognitive assessments. Careful attention should be paid to the onset of symptoms, longitudinal history of the disorder, and differential diagnosis including medical/neurological, as well as psychosocial and educational factors contributing to the clinical presentation.** Issues of co-morbidity with learning disabilities and other psychiatric disorders, as well as specific academic needs should be addressed. Patients with ongoing abuse of or dependence on psychoactive substances should generally not be treated until appropriate addiction treatments have been undertaken and the patient has maintained a drug- and alcohol-free period. Other concurrent psychiatric disorders also need to be assessed and, if possible, the relationship of the ADHD symptoms to these other disorders delineated.

   The ADHD patient and his or her family need to be familiarized with the risks and benefits of pharmacotherapy, the availability of alternative treatments, and the likely adverse effects. Certain adverse effects can be anticipated based on known pharmacological properties of the drug (i.e., appetite change, insomnia), while other more infrequent effects are unexpected (idiosyncratic) and are difficult to anticipate based on the properties of the drug. Short-term adverse effects can be minimized by introducing the medication at low initial doses and titrating slowly. Idiosyncratic adverse effects generally require drug discontinuation and selection of alternate treatment modalities.

   Treatment should be started at the lowest possible dose; this usually is the lowest manufactured dose. Once pharmacotherapy is initiated, frequent (e.g., weekly) contact with the patient and family is necessary during the initial phase of treatment in order to carefully monitor response to the intervention and adverse effects. Evaluation of adverse effects should include both subjective reports from the patient and family (e.g., stomach aches, appetite changes) as well as appropriate evaluation of objective measurements (e.g., heart rate, blood pressure changes). Following a sufficient period of clinical stabilization (e.g., 6–12 months), it is prudent to re-evaluate the need for continued psychopharmacological intervention. Withdrawal symptoms should be distinguished from the exacerbation of the disorder for which the psychotropic was prescribed. To minimize withdrawal reactions, it is important to discontinue medications gradually.

Selected References

Barkley, R. (1998). *Attention-deficit/hyperactivity disorder: A handbook for diagnosis and treatment* (2nd ed.). New York: Guilford Press.

Biederman, J., Faraone, S., & Mick, E. (2000). Age-dependent decline of ADHD symptoms revisited: Impact of remission definition and symptom subtype. *American Journal of Psychiatry, 157,* 816–817.

Biederman, J., Newcorn, J., & Sprich, S. (1991). Comorbidity of attention deficit hyperactivity disorder with conduct, depressive, anxiety, and other disorders. *American Journal of Psychiatry, 148,* 564–577.

Faraone, S.V., Biederman, J., Weiffenbach, B., et al. (1999). Dopamine D4 gene 7-repeat allele and attention deficit hyperactivity disorder. *American Journal of Psychiatry, 156,* 768–770.

Faraone, S.V., Biederman, J., Mick, E., et al. (2000). Family study of girls with attention deficit hyperactivity disorder. *American Journal of Psychiatry, 157,* 1077–1083.

Gadow, K., Sverd, J., Sprafkin, J., et al. (1999). Long-term methylphenidate therapy in children with comorbid Attention-Deficit Hyperactivity Disorder and Chronic Multiple Tic Disorder. *Archives of General Psychiatry, 56,* 330–336.

Michelson, D., Faries, D., Wernicke, J., et al. (2001). Atomoxetine in the treatment of children and adolescents with attention-deficit/hyperactivity disorder: A randomized, placebo-controlled, dose-response study. *Pediatrics, 108,* E83.

Michelson, D., Allen, A., Busner, J., et al. (2002). Once-daily atomoxetine treatment for children and adolescents with ADHD: A randomized, placebo-controlled study. *American Journal of Psychiatry, 159,* 1896–1901.

Multimodal Treatment Group: A 14-month randomized clinical trial of treatment strategies for attention-deficit/hyperactivity disorder, The MTA Cooperative Group. Multimodal Treatment Study of Children with ADHD. *Archives of General Psychiatry, 56,* 1073–1086.

Spencer, T., Biederman, J., Wilens, T., et al. (1996). Pharmacotherapy of attention deficit disorder across the life cycle. *Journal of the American Academy of Child and Adolescent Psychiatry, 35,* 409–432.

Spencer, T.J., Biederman, J., Harding, M., et al. (1996). Growth deficits in ADHD children revisited: Evidence for disorder-associated growth delays? *Journal of the American Adademy of Child and Adolescent Psychiatry, 35,* 1460–1469.

Wilens, T., Spencer, T. (2000). The stimulants revisited. In C. Stubbe (Ed.), *Child and adolescent psychiatric clinics of North America.* Philadelphia: Saunders, pp. 573–603.

Wilens, T., Faraone, S., Biederman, J., & Gunawardene, S. (2002). Does the stimulant pharmacotherapy of ADHD beget later substance abuse: A metaanalysis of the literature. *Pediatrics, 11,* 179–185.

Zametkin, A., Liotta, W. (1998). The neurobiology of attention-deficit/hyperactivity disorder. *Journal of Clinical Psychiatry, 59,* 17–23.

CHAPTER 32

The Patient with Chronic Medical Illness

GREGORY L. FRICCHIONE AND EDWARD MARCANTONIO

I. Introduction

A. Illness often leads to an acute crisis, which increases patient vulnerability and diminishes patient confidence.

B. The outcome of an acute crisis strongly influences a patient's adaptation to chronic medical illness.

C. Chronic conditions can result in frustration and isolation.

D. Physicians are often perceived as not giving enough information or support.

II. The Crisis of Medical Illness

A. Adaptive Tasks Related to a Medical Illness
1. Adjusting to pain
2. Adjusting to the hospital environment
3. Adjusting to a decreased level of functioning (loss of independence)
4. Adjusting to procedures used for evaluation and treatment
5. Adjusting to many medical team members (a crisis of trust)

B. Personal Adaptive Tasks
1. Maintaining psychological equilibrium
2. Maintaining a healthy measure of self-esteem
3. Maintaining supportive attachments to family members and friends
4. Maintaining an orientation to the future

C. Crisis Model (Figure 32-1) and Attributional Style
1. Appraisal or perception of an illness is the beginning point in the coping process.
2. After this, specific situation-based beliefs can predict the particular coping strategy adopted.
3. Appraisal involves making casual attributions regarding the illness.
4. Attributions can be optimistic or pessimistic and have an impact on the perceived meaningfulness of life.
5. Pessimism can lead to negative emotions, which appear to worsen outcomes (e.g., cardiac disease).
6. Pessimistic attributional styles correlate with helplessness, resignation, and avoidance as determined by a meta-analysis of 27 coping studies (Roesch & Weiner, 2001).
7. Attributions may guide cognitions and illness behaviors and help predict coping strategies.
8. Coping has a direct effect on psychosocial adjustment to illness.

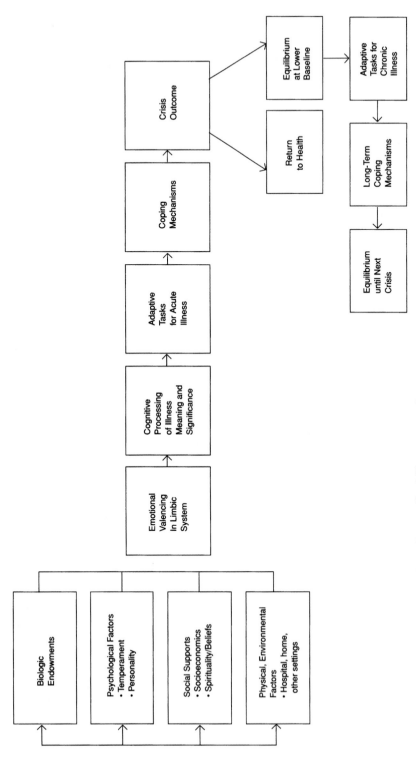

Figure 32-1. A crisis approach to the medical illness experience. [SOURCE: Adapted from Moos, R.H., & Tau, V.D. (1977). The crisis of physical illness: An overview. In R. Moos (Ed.), *Coping with physical illness.* New York: Plenum Press, pp. 3–21.]

D. Adaptation to an illness requires coping mechanisms

1. **Using denial** to avoid the seriousness of an illness. This can be adaptive as long as adherence is not jeopardized.
2. **Using suppression or displacement** to deal with distressing emotions, such as anger
3. **Seeking medical information** and using one's intellect resourcefully
4. **Asking for, and accepting, reassurance** from loved ones, as well as from medical caretakers
5. **Mastering the technical procedures** associated with a particular illness
6. **Constructing realistic and incremental goals**
7. **Preparing mentally** for a variety of outcomes
8. **Re-framing of the illness** and its meaning in the context of one's life

E. Management

1. Recognition of normal grief responses to illness and the losses that pertain to this situation
2. Familiarity with adaptive tasks and coping mechanisms
3. Provision of information
   a. Be available to respond to questions.
   b. Dispel myths.
   c. Help with the anticipation of physical and mental challenges.
   d. Serve as a referral source for support in the community, e.g., agencies, self-help groups, and associations.
4. Establishing a therapeutic alliance
   a. Acknowledge emotional issues.
   b. Provide reassurance, understanding, and solace.
   c. When appropriate, recommend strategies that foster independence and self-esteem, instead of battling for control and compliance.
5. Understanding the social context of the patient
   a. Increase family and community involvement and support for the patient.
   b. The stress-illness equation:

$$\text{Propensity to illness} = \frac{\text{Life stress (allostatic loading)}}{\text{Social support}}$$

   c. Social Course Model (Ware, 1999):
      i. Chronic illness leads to social marginalization and role constriction, as well as impoverishment and isolation.
      ii. This is opposed by acts of resistance directed towards social reintegration.
      iii. An oscillation by marginalizing and integrating is experienced by those with chronic illness.
6. Understanding one's personal reactions to an illness
   a. Guards against countertransference (the response of a physician to a patient based on past responses to important persons in the physician's life).
   b. Enables the caregiver to understand the origin of caring in the attachment behavior all people share, making it easier to provide the solace that patients require from their physicians.

III. The Chronic Illness Experience

A. The Meaning of Chronic Illness

1. While anxiety regarding survival may be reduced, there is still a lingering sense of vulnerability as well as mourning for lost health and for potentially lost interpersonal roles and functions.
2. The personal significance of these losses plays a large role in determining the overall adaptation of a patient to chronic illness.

B. Chronic Illness and Defense Mechanisms

1. **Denial**-like processes
   a. Denial involves the following:
      i. Perceiving symptomatology or a problem
      ii. Repudiating a portion of the meaning of the perception
      iii. Substituting a less threatening version for the repudiated portion
      iv. Re-orienting oneself to accommodate the reviewed reality

   Denial can be maladaptive when it hinders the search for the attention to medical problems or compliance with treatment, for example, a woman with breast cancer who fails to see her doctor for a breast lump.

2. **Intellectualization**
   a. Intellectualization is defined as the attempt by a patient to overcome his or her fear of the unknown—namely, the illness—by trying to learn everything known about it.
   b. Implied is the hope that knowledge will somehow relieve the patient of vulnerability.
   c. Intellectualization can often be adaptive by binding anxiety.
   d. It can often be maladaptive by leading to obsessive indecisiveness.

3. **Regression**
   a. When threatened with illness, a patient may revert to earlier behavior patterns that are immature in nature.
   b. This often involves **overdependency** as a way to gain attention even if it is not associated with true caring.
   c. Regressing to a dependent position also offers **relief from responsibilities**. This may be adaptive when a patient is acutely ill; however, it is often maladaptive in the chronically ill, as it will reduce a patient's functional level.

4. **Displacement**
   a. In an effort to diminish anxiety, patients claim that others besides themselves are worried or that a less threatening symptom is on their minds.

5. **Projection**
   a. In this primitive defense, the illness has distressed the patient so much that his or her anger about being vulnerable is intolerable.
   b. This anger is projected onto someone else, frequently the physician, as the alleged source of the distress.

6. **Projective Identification**
   a. The frustration of chronic illness can lead a patient to incite his or her distressful emotions in the person closest to him or her.
   b. This can relieve some of the patient's distress.

7. **Introjection**
   a. Instead of blaming the illness on others, as in the projective defense, patients who use introjection interpret an illness as self-punishment for past wrongs.

b. This sense of self-punishment flows from a patient's understanding himself or herself as the cause of the illness.

c. Depression becomes the predominant mood in maladapting patients.

C. Chronic Illness and Adjustment Reactions

1. Anxiety

a. Anxiety often stems from the fear of dying and it is related to the stress-response systems, in particular the sympathetic nervous system's fight-or-flight response.

b. Chronic illness can lead to a state of chronic vulnerability that is reflected in anxiety states, particularly if a patient's defense mechanisms are incapable of binding anxiety.

2. Depression

a. Depression stems from the experience of loss (of role, functional level, and confidence).

b. Chronic illness is particularly hard to battle as a source of depression because it can inexorably chip away at a person's self-image, self-esteem, and self-worth.

c. Depression can lead to what is called a "giving up-given up state." Major depression may crystallize in the chronic mentally ill population. Its prevalence in the medically ill is from 6–14%. Katon (2001) described four adverse effects of major depression in those with chronic medical illness: increased mortality, higher symptom burden, decreased quality of life and functionality, and increased medical utilization and costs.

3. Anger

a. Anger stems from the rage a person feels when the vulnerability imparted by the experience of illness impinges on a person's sense of autonomy and self-sufficiency.

b. Chronic illness at any point in the life cycle, such as adolescence, can lead to anger, since it stunts normal yearnings for independence.

c. Anger is a reaction against unwanted feelings of helplessness.

4. Regressive Dependency

a. Some patients receive so much secondary gain (attention from loved ones and caregivers, freedom from "making a living," or compensation) that they become overdependent in the context of chronic illness.

b. Dependency needs can reach a point where they are insatiable, and lead to interpersonal conflicts over dependency-independency.

5. Treatment Non-compliance

a. Sometimes chronically ill patients are destabilized by dysregulation of mood and behavior to the point where they will express their attempts at independence (despite vulnerability) in a maladaptive fashion: e.g., not complying with the recommended medical regimen (see Chapter 74).

b. This non-compliance may be designed to be a temporary respite, an angry rebellion against the vulnerability of illness (reaction formation), a depressive withdrawal from the struggle, or a signal that more support is desired.

IV. Personality Types and Illness Behavior and Effects on the Chronic Illness Experience

A. Personality and Illness

1. In the context of the crises and vulnerabilities of chronic illness, certain individuals react by regressing to an earlier, less mature personality style, or become accentuated caricatures of their present personality styles. Both situations can be problematic for the patient and the physician, and lead to chronic illness behaviors.

B. Hints for the Use of Personality Typing

1. **Resist the impulse to label the patient,** especially early on; patients are usually mixtures of various personality types.
2. Getting to know a patient over time is the best way to know that patient's personality.
3. Management recommendations must be part of an individualized treatment approach that takes into account the biopsychosocial features of the patient.
4. Personality characteristics of the medically ill are not carved in stone. As medical crises abate and anxiety lessens, a patient's personality often matures or stabilizes.

C. Personality Types (see Kahana and Bibring, 1964)

1. **Dependent, Overdemanding Reaction**
   a. Oral personality
   b. Management issues
      i. Each patient expresses demands for special attention
      ii. The patient makes extraordinary dependency demands
      iii. The patient reacts impulsively with a reduced tolerance for frustration
   c. Meaning of illness
      i. The patient has an infantile wish for total care
      ii. Separation and/or abandonment anxiety exists
   d. Medical management
      i. Attempt to meet reasonable demands
      ii. Set limits in a three-step process:

         • Point out the unacceptable behavior.
         • Explain why it is unacceptable.
         • Offer healthier alternatives.

      iii. Avoid the tendency to be punitive in response to demands outside mutually set limits.
      iv. Offer positive feedback when a limit is maintained.

2. **Orderly, Controlled Personality**
   a. Compulsive personality
   b. Management issues
      i. The patient will demand explanations with excruciating precision and detail.
      ii. Challenging and oppositional attitudes will be displayed.
      iii. The patient may become non-compliant.
   c. Illness meaning. The patient will fear vulnerable feelings.
   d. Medical management
      i. Provide early information, if available, regarding the diagnosis and treatment.
      ii. Provide structured, organized care.

3. **Dramatizing, Emotionally-Involved Personality**
   a. Hysterical personality
   b. Management issues
      i. The patient will make demands for attention.
      ii. The patient will be rejection-sensitive when demands are not met, leading to jealousy of other patients and dysphoria.
      iii. The patient will worry excessively about pending medical procedures, especially those which may affect the patient's body image.
      iv. The patient may, by contrast, exhibit "la belle indifference" to illness, which can delay important treatment.

    c. Illness meaning

       i. The patient fears a change in body image or aging secondary to illness.

       ii. The patient exhibits neediness and attention-seeking behavior.

    d. Medical management

       i. Provide care with a calm, warm, but firm approach.

       ii. Provide medical information in a non-detailed reassuring way.

       iii. Use suggestibility to aid therapeutics.

       iv. Provide an atmosphere in which the patient can express fears and vulnerabilities.

4. **Long-Suffering, Self-Sacrificing Personality**

    a. Masochistic personality

    b. Management issues

       i. The patient presents with obvious suffering.

       ii. The patient rejects efforts to have suffering relieved, always opting for the sick role.

    c. Illness meaning

       i. The patient believes that only through suffering is love or caring for him or her deserved.

       ii. The patient will exhibit neediness and attention-seeking behavior.

    d. Medical management

       i. Validate, rather than minimize, the suffering patient.

       ii. Re-frame improvement, in the medical condition with the theme that suffering will continue in that relative health will bring the added responsibility of caring for others.

5. **Guarded, Complaining Personality**

    a. Paranoid personality

    b. Management issues

       i. The patient presents in a suspicious, accusatory manner.

       ii. The patient is vigilant in perceiving any disapproval.

       iii. The patient tends to blame others in a hypercritical way.

    c. Illness meaning

       i. The patient is in a site of vulnerability, making him or her even more suspicious about being hurt.

    d. Medical management

       i. Provide a cordial, respectful approach, acknowledging the patient's desire for security and control.

       ii. Avoid over-involvement.

       iii. Avoid argumentative struggles while also avoiding the tendency to give short shrift to the patient.

       iv. Provide recognition of the patient's emotional state while not validating or contradicting the patient's experience.

6. **Superior-Feeling Personality**

    a. Narcissistic personality

    b. Management issues

       i. The patient presents in an egotistical manner.

       ii. The patient displays entitlement, expecting special treatment.

       iii. The patient detracts from others to try to elevate himself or herself.

    c. Illness meaning

       i. The patient, when ill, has a breach in the veneer of invulnerability to contend with.

       ii. The patient responds with increasing demands.

    d. Medical management

       i. Take a respectful, self-assured approach to patient care.

       ii. Provide reassurance of the patient's inherent value as a human being.

7. Uninvolved, Aloof Personality

    a. Schizoid personality

    b. Management issues

       i. The patient may have eccentric beliefs regarding the illness and its management.

       ii. The patient may lack attachment skills, making caretakers uncomfortable.

       iii. The patient may shy away from interactive therapies and strategies.

    c. Illness meaning

       i. The patient may become fearful of losing autonomy and becoming engulfed.

       ii. The patient may react to others as parts of a threatening environment.

    d. Medical management

       i. Respect the patient's desire for privacy.

       ii. Provide non-intrusive support without an expectation of social feedback.

D. Illness Behavior

  1. Evidence suggests that there is traumatogenic potential in chronic diseases related to exacerbations. When coupled with stressful life events, maladaptive illness behavior over the life course may arise as a result of cumulative adversity. (Alonzo, 2000)

  2. Patients with chronic illness may develop certain chronic behaviors associated with the experience of illness. These behaviors reflect the psychological, sociocultural, and spiritual influences that bear on the emergence of illness as well as the psychosocial and spiritual effects of an illness. Abnormal illness behaviors usually emerge from over-dependency on the physician and over-elaboration of physical symptoms in relation to the pathophysiology present (Mayou, 1989). This often stems from a patient's need for caring.

  3. Somatoform disorder represents a type of abnormal illness behavior which often is seen and treated by primary care doctors. Management includes the following:

    a. Give the primary care doctor the primary responsibility.

    b. Perform a thorough medical evaluation but try to keep it simple and try to avoid surgery.

    c. Legitimize the reality of the patient's symptoms, but do not assign diagnostic labels.

    d. Re-formulate your goals in terms of improving the patient's functions and illness behavior.

    e. Have regular primary care follow-up visits, for example, 20 minutes every 2 to 4 weeks, to diminish the patient's fear of abandonment.

    f. Don't stress that the patient is perfectly healthy. The patient still needs care.

    g. Encourage the expression of feelings.

    h. Simplify the drug regimen; try to wean the patient from addictive substances.

    i. Use antidepressants if they are warranted.

    j. Obtain a psychiatric consultation.

V. Medical Supportive Psychotherapy

A. Supportive Psychotherapy

  1. Establish and maintain a positive treatment alliance.

  2. Strengthen the patient's mature defenses and discourage the maladaptive ones.

  3. Contribute to more positive yet realistic frames of thought.

4. A supportive and active therapeutic alliance will reduce a patient's anxiety; the physician will serve as a real object and enhance reality in the therapeutic relationship.

5. A priority is to improve or at least to maintain the patient's self-worth and function.

B. Family Interventions

1. Provide information about the chronic illness.

2. Offer advice about potential family responses.

3. Serve as a resource for community supports.

4. Help the patient make decisions that are based on risks and benefits.

5. Acknowledge the emotional responses of the family.

6. While acceptance may not be possible, stress that a level of adaptation to chronic illness is part of the required long-term coping process.

7. Warn the patient against making abrupt family changes.

8. Make a home visit if possible to assess the patient's environment firsthand.

9. Suggest periodic "re-fueling" for caretakers, rest and relaxation.

VI. Chronic Illness and the Origin of Caring

A. By definition, those with a chronic illness are incurable, and they seek care from physicians.

B. The origin of caring involves "transitional relatedness" (Horton, 1981): the willingness and ability of the physician to be a resolute source of caring for those who, by virtue of illness, are thrust into a transitional zone where the threat of separation and the longing for attachment co-exist.

Suggested Readings

Abram, H.S. (1970). Survival by machine: Psychological aspects of chronic hemodialysis. *Psychiatric Medicine, 1,* 37–50.

Alonzo, A.A. (2000). The experience of chronic illness and post-traumatic stress disorder: The consequences of cumulative adversity. *Social Science and Medicine, 50,* 1475–1484.

Bertram, S., Kurland, M., Lydick, E., et al. (2001). The patient's perspective of irritable bowel syndrome. *Journal of Family Practice, 50,* 521–525.

Buckley, P. (1986). Supportive psychotherapy: A neglected treatment. *Psychiatric Annals, 16,* 515–521.

Fricchione, G.L. (1993). Illness and the origin of caring. *Journal of Medical Humanities, 14,* 15–21.

Gordon, G. (1987). Treating somatizing patients. *Western Journal of Medicine, 147,* 88–91.

Horton, P.C. (1981). *Solace: The missing dimension in psychiatry.* Chicago, Ill.: University of Chicago Press.

Kahana, R.J., & Bibring, G.L. (1964). Personality types in medical management. In N.E. Zinberg (Ed.), *Psychiatry and medical practice in a general hospital.* New York: New York International University Press, pp. 108–123.

Katon, W.J. (2001). The depressed patient with comorbid illness. Program and abstracts of the 154th Annual Meeting of the American Psychiatric Association, May 5–10; New Orleans, La. Industry Symposium, Part 2, 438.

Leahey, M., & Wright, L.M. (1995). Intervening with families with chronic illness. *Family Systems in Medicine, 3,* 60–69.

Mayou, R. (1989). Illness behavior and psychiatry. *General Hospital Psychiatry, 11,* 307–312.

Moos, R.H., & Tau, V.D. (1977). The crisis of physical illness: An overview. In R. Moos (Ed.), *Coping with physical illness.* New York: Plenum Press, pp. 3–21.

Roesch, S.C., & Weiner, B. (2001). A meta-analytic review of coping with illness. Do casual attributions matter? *Journal of Psychosomatic Research, 50,* 205–219.

Ware, N.C. (1999). Toward a model of social course in chronic illness: The example of chronic fatigue syndrome. *Culture, Medicine, and Psychiatry, 23,* 303–331.

Wells, K.B., Stewart, A., Hays, R.D., et al. (1989). The functioning and well-being of depressed patients: Results from the Medical Outcomes Study. *Journal of the American Medical Association, 262,* 914–919.

CHAPTER 33

The Patient with Acute or Chronic Pain

MENEKSE ALPAY

I. Introduction

A. Overview

1. **Origin of the term pain:** *Poena* (from Latin), meaning punishment.
2. **Definition:** "An unpleasant sensory and emotional experience arising from the actual or potential tissue damage or described in terms of such damage" (International Association for the Study of Pain).
3. **Scope of the problem**
   a. Pain is the most common symptom reported to physicians.
   b. Billions of dollars are spent each year on pain-relieving remedies and devices.
   c. Pain is challenging to treat due to its complex nature. A multi-disciplinary approach is required to control pain and restore function.

B. Components of pain

1. Localizing discriminative component, nociception
2. Endogenous system of analgesia
3. Psychiatric component (e.g., affective state, personality, prior conditioning)

C. Nociception

1. Nociception results from the activation of nociceptors with intact peripheral afferent pain receptors.
2. It may occur concurrently with pain from damaged nerves.
3. Broken down into somatic pain, involving activation of nociceptors in peripheral tissues, and visceral pain, involving activation of nociceptors in organ tissues.
   a. **Somatic pain is usually well localized, attributable to certain anatomical structures or areas, and characteristically described as stabbing, aching, or throbbing.**
   b. **Visceral pain is usually poorly localized, not necessarily attributable to the involved organ (i.e., referred pain), and is characteristically described as dull, crampy, and poorly localized.**
4. Conduction of nociception
   a. **Peripheral conduction of nociception**
      i. Skin-originated pain is usually used as the model for nociception. Nociceptors in the skin transduce mechanical, thermal, and chemical stimuli into action potentials. Nociceptors are stimulated by the liberation of prostaglandins (PGs), arachidonic acid, histamine, and bradykinin during the injury. Aspirin, acetaminophen, steroids, and non-steroidal anti-inflammatory agents (NSAIDs) act at this very first step.
      ii. Subsequently, axons transmit the pain to the spinal cord, where their cell bodies are located in the dorsal root ganglia. **Nerve blocks interrupt the entire peripheral nerve conduction and are helpful in thoracic, lumbar, and abdominal pain.**

b. **Central conduction of nociception**
 i. Fibers carrying nociceptive information enter the dorsal root and either ascend or descend one to three segments before synapsing with the neurons of spinothalamic tract of the substantia gelatinosa in the gray matter. Substance P (11-aminoacid polypeptide) is released from the fibers at many of these synapses. **Capsaine, which is extracted from red hot pepper, inhibits nociception by inhibiting substance P, the major pain neurotransmitter.**
 ii. Stimulation of peripheral nerve fibers not only excites some neurons but also inhibits others at the dorsal horn level. This inhibition of nociceptive nerve fibers may explain the effects of acupuncture and transcutanous electrical nerve stimulation (TENS). In addition, pain within the dorsal horn may be affected by mechanisms through effects of the brain stem, limbic system, and cortex.
 iii. The spinothalamic tract crosses to the other side and ascends towards the thalamus. At the level of the brain stem more than half of this tract synapses in the reticular activating system (this part is also called the spinoreticular tract), the limbic system, and in other brain stem regions. **The close relationship of pain, affect, and sleep is explained by these synapses. Other projections go to the periaqueductal gray (PAG), which plays an important role in the brain's endogenous system of analgesia.**
 iv. Subsequently, the thalamic nuclei project to the somatic sensory cortex of the parietal lobe as well as to the entire cortex. These projections serve to alert rather than to localize the pain, and they are also involved in the affective component of pain. **Producing lesions in thalamus may relieve intractable pain.** With the examination of the segmental innervation, the affected nerve root(s) can be determined.

c. **Descending analgesic pain pathway**
 i. This pathway starts in the PAG (replete with high levels of endogenous analgesics) and then descends via the brainstem to the spinal cord's dorsal horn.
 ii. The neurons in the brainstem use serotonin to activate endogenous analgesics in the dorsal horn.
 iii. This causes inhibition of nociception at the level of dorsal horn, since neurons containing enkephalins (endogenous opiates) synapse with spinothalamic neurons.
 iv. Additionally there are noradrenergic neurons projecting from the locus ceruleus (the main noradrenergic center in the CNS) to the dorsal horn that inhibit the dorsal horn neurons' response to nociceptive stimuli.
 v. **The effect of tricyclic antidepressants (TCAs) is indicated by increasing serotonin and noradrenaline, thereby inhibiting nociception at the level of dorsal horn.**

D. **The endogenous analgesic system**
1. There at least 18 endogenous peptides with opiate-like activity in the CNS, that are products of three precursor proteins: proopiomelanocortin (precursor of beta endorphin and adrenocorticotropic hormone), proenkephaline (precursor of metenkephaline and leuenkephaline), prodynorphine (the precursor of dynorphin and related peptides).
2. These endogenous opiates have different affinities for the three major central opiate receptors.
 a. μ-receptors: affecting analgesia, respiratory depression, constipation, miosis, and dependence. (Exogenous opiates generally act at these receptors).
 b. κ-receptors: affecting spinal analgesia, sedation, and miosis.

    c. δ-receptors: affecting spinal analgesia, hypotension, and miosis.

    d. In addition to these well-known effects, there are also psychotomimetic effects (e.g., psychosis) of opiates in the CNS. These are thought to be due to binding to glutamate receptors (glutamate being the major excitatory amino acid in the CNS), NMDA receptors, and sigma receptors. These effects are not reversed by naloxone, an opiate antagonist.

E. Psychiatric component of pain:

1. Practitioners of psychiatry and neurology treat suffering; they often treat the same conditions and deal with disorders that have few objective markers. In addition, they prescribe antidepressants, anticonvulsants, benzodiazepines, neuroleptics, stimulants, and α-2 agonists (Table 33–1).

Table 33-1. DEA Guidelines for the Prescription of Controlled Substances

1. A prescription for a controlled substance is lawful only if issued for a legitimate medical purpose by an individual practitioner acting in the usual course of professional practice. Prescriptions under the law may not be issued for narcotic drugs for the purpose of detoxification or maintenance of narcotic addicts.

2. All prescriptions for controlled substances must bear the following information:

    a. Name of patient

    b. Home address of patient

    c. Name of practitioner

    d. Address of practitioner

    e. Registration number of practitioner

    f. Name of the drug, strength, and quantity of the medicine to be dispensed

    g. Directions for use

3. All prescriptions must be dated with the day when issued to the patient and must be signed manually on that day by the practitioner.

4. It is illegal under both Federal and State law to issue a prescription for other than a legitimate *bona fide* medical need or to date a prescription other than the date when it is issued to the patient and signed by the practitioner.

5. Schedule II controlled substances require written prescriptions prior to dispensing. They may not be refilled. A Schedule II drug may be dispensed in an emergency by a pharmacist upon oral prescription of a practitioner if the quantity is limited to the emergency period, if the prescription is reduced immediately to writing by the pharmacist and contains all the information required of written prescriptions except the signature of the prescriber, if the pharmacist knows the prescriber, or makes a reasonable effort to verify the order's validity, and if the prescriber issues to the pharmacist a written prescription within 48 hours of the oral order. If the pharmacist does not receive a written prescription from the prescriber within 72 hours, he or she must by law notify the DEA regional office.

6. A controlled substance prescription must be for no more than 30 days of medicine.

SOURCE: From Borsook, D., Lebel, A.A., & McPeek, B. (1995). *MGH handbook of pain management.* Boston: Little, Brown & Co.

2. Mood and anxiety disorders are commonly co-morbid with pain.
   a. Depressive disorders are found in 30–87% of pain patients. Major depression is found in 8–50% of pain patients, while dysthymia may be seen in > 75% of patients with chronic pain.
   b. Anxiety disorders (panic disorder, generalized anxiety disorder, post-traumatic stress disorder) are found in > 50% of patients with chronic pain.
3. Somatoform disorders (body dysmorphic disorder, conversion disorder, hypochondriasis, somatization disorder, pain disorder) do not involve the conscious production of symptoms.
   a. DSM-IV changed its terminology from somatoform pain disorder to pain disorder and it avoids using the terms "psychogenic" or "idiopathic" pain. Pain is a major part of the clinical presentation and it causes significant impairment in function. These include:
      i. Pain disorder with psychological factors (acute and chronic)
      ii. Pain disorder with both psychological factors and a general medical condition
4. Other psychiatric states that may be co-morbid with pain
   a. Factitious disorders which involves the intentional production or feigning of physical or psychological symptoms (unconscious motivation, conscious production)
   b. Malingering that involves the intentional production or feigning of physical or psychological symptoms that is motivated by clear external incentives (conscious motivation, conscious production)
5. Psychoactive Substance Use Disorders. In these conditions dependence and abuse may develop as a result of chronic pain.
6. Personality disorders
7. Adjustment disorder

II. Major Classes of Pain

A. Acute pain
1. Acute pain is usually related to an identifiable injury or disease and is self-limited, resolving over hours to days or in a period that is associated with a reasonable period for healing.
2. Acute pain is usually associated with objective autonomic features, such as tachycardia, hypertension, diaphoresis, mydriasis, or pallor.

B. Continuous pain in the terminally ill (e.g., cancer pain).
1. This type of pain originates from well defined tissue damage; it is a variant of nociceptive pain.
2. Stress, sleep deprivation, depression, and pre-morbid personality may exacerbate this type of pain.

C. Chronic (behavioral) pain
1. This type of pain does not have a well-defined neurological mechanism.
2. Chronic pain, by definition, persists beyond the normal time of healing or more than 6 months.
3. Characteristic features include vague descriptions of pain (despite forceful assertions of its existence) and an inability to describe the pain's timing and localization.
4. Unlike acute pain, chronic pain typically lacks signs of heightened sympathetic activity, which may be owing to chronic adaptation of the autonomic nervous system.

5. Depression, anxiety, and pre-morbid personality problems are common in afflicted patients.

6. Usually a major problem is the lack of motivation to improve.

7. It is usually helpful to establish the presence of a dermatomal pattern, and the presence of neuropathic pain; in addition, assessment of pain behavior is crucial.

D. Neuropathic pain

1. Neuropathic pain is caused by an injured or dysfunctioning central or peripheral nervous system, which results in the characteristic description of spontaneous, sharp, shooting, and burning pain.

2. Burning pain usually occurs in a dermatomal distribution (Figures 33-1 and 33-2).

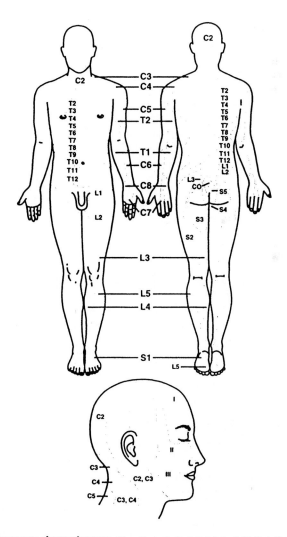

Figure 33-1. Sensory dermatomes. [From Borsook, D., Lebel, A.A., & McPeek, B. (1995). *MGH handbook of pain management.* Boston: Little, Brown & Co.]

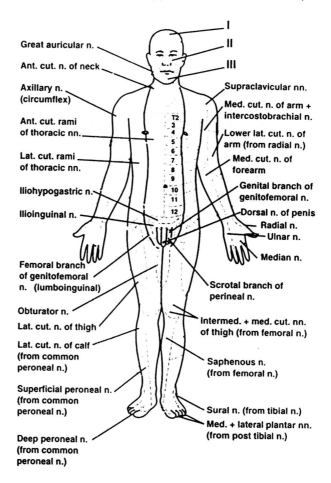

Figure 33-2. Sensory innervation of the skin. [From Borsook, D., Lebel, A.A., & McPeek, B. (1995). *MGH handbook of pain management.* Boston: Little, Brown & Co.]

3. Many other names are given to neuropathic pain or its specific syndromes, including neurogenic pain, deafferentation syndrome, diabetic neuropathy, central pain syndrome, trigeminal neuralgia, and post-herpetic neuralgia.
   a. Hyperalgesia is an increased response to noxious stimuli (pressor or heat).
   b. Allodynia is pain from a stimulus that is not normally painful, such as light touch or a breeze of cool air.
   c. Hyperpathia is pain from a painful stimulus with a delay, persistence beyond stimulation, and distribution beyond the area of stimulation.

E. **Reflex sympathetic dystrophy (RSD)**
   1. RSD produces sympathetically maintained pain, or a complex regional pain syndrome; it is a syndrome of pain in an extremity that is mediated by sympathetic overactivity that does not involve a major nerve. It leads to sensory, autonomic, motor, and trophic changes.
   2. The syndrome is usually caused by an injury, although the cause is unknown in approximately 10% of cases. It may be caused either by microtrauma or

macrotrauma, such as from a sprain, fracture, or contusion. Iatrogenic causes, such as amputation, lesion resection, myelography, and IM injection, are also evident. It may be related to a variety of conditions, such as myocardial infarction, shoulder-hand syndrome, herpes zoster, cerebrovascular accidents, diabetic neuropathy, a herniated disc, degenerative disk disease, neuroaxial tumors or metastases, multiple sclerosis, or poliomyelitis.

    a. The sensory component often includes reports of spontaneous pain and evoked pain in the affected extremity.

    b. Autonomic manifestations include changes in skin blood flow (marbled, hyperemic to cyanotic skin color, edema, and asymmetrical skin temperature between affected and unaffected limbs).

    c. Motor changes involve weakness, decreased range of motion, tremor, hypotonia, atrophy, and dystonias (rare)

    d. Trophic changes are seen in approximately 30% of cases; rarely do they occur within first 10 days of initial symptoms. These changes include disturbed nail growth, increased hair growth, palmar/planter fibrosis, thin glossy skin, hyperkeratosis, and distal osteoporosis.

  3. The clinical course starts with an acute phase that involves pain, edema, and warm skin (which may last up to 6 months). Subsequently, dystrophic changes dominate the picture, with cold skin and trophic changes (3 to 6 months after the untreated acute phase). Over time, irreversible atrophic changes (atrophy and contractures) develop.

  4. There may be symptomatic improvement with inhibition of sympathetic output; thus, sympathetic blockade may be both diagnostic and therapeutic.

F. Idiopathic pain, previously referred to as "psychogenic pain," refers to a spectrum of poorly understood pain states that do not imply or exclude a psychological component.

  1. Typically there is no evidence of an associated organic etiology or anatomical pattern of symptoms; associated symptoms are often grossly out of proportion to any identifiable organic pathology.

  2. Examples include myofascial pain syndrome, fibromyalgia, fibrositis, muscular rheumatism, psychogenic rheumatism, rheumatoid modulating disorder, and chronic idiopathic pain syndrome.

III. Analgesic Therapies

A. Overview

  1. Analgesic therapy often involves treatment of nociceptive and non-nociceptive features.

  2. Significant psychopathology may preclude analgesia; therapies from several disciplines may each offer partial analgesia.

  3. Assessment and encouragement of function is often the best strategy for effective treatment.

  4. The Pain Verbal analog scale and McGill Pain Questionnaire are useful instruments for the quantification of pain.

B. Pharmacological approaches vary depending on whether pain is acute or chronic (Table 33-2)

  1. Opioid pharmacotherapy

  2. Non-opioid pharmacotherapy

Table 33-2. Non-steroidal Anti-inflammatory Drugs

Drug	Dosage (mg)	Dose Interval (hours)	Maximum Daily Dose (mg/d)	Peak Effect (hours)	Half-Life (hours)
Diclofenac	25–75	6–8	200	2	1–2
Etodolac acid	200–400	6–8	1,200	1–2	7
Fenoprofen	200	4–6	3,200	1–2	2–3
Flurbiprofen	50–100	6–8	300	1.5–3.0	3–4
Ibuprofen	200–400	6–8	3,200	1–2	2
Indomethacin	25–75	6–8	200	0.5–1.0	2–3
Ketoprofen	25–75	6–8	300	1–2	1.5–2.0
Ketorolac[a]					
Oral	10	6–8	40	0.5–1.0	6
Parenteral	60 load, then 30	6–8	120 (use no longer than 5 d)		
Meclofenamic acid	500 load, then 275	6–8	400		
Mefanamic acid	500 load, then 250	6	1,250	2–4	3–4
Nabumetone	1,000–2,000	12–24	2,000	3–5	22–30
Naproxen	500 load, then 250	6–8	1,250	2–4	12–15
Naproxen sodium	550 load, then 275	6–8	1,375	1–2	13
Oxaprozin	60–1,200	Every day	1,800	2	3–3.5
Phenylbutazone	100	6–8	400	2	50–100
Piroxicam	40 load, then 20	24	20	2–4	36–45
Sulindac	150–200	12	400	1–2	7–18
Tolmetin	200–400	8	1,800	4–6	2

[a] Use no longer than 5 days.

SOURCE: From Borsook, D., Lebel, A.A., & McPeek, B. (1995). *MGH handbook of pain management.* Boston: Little, Brown & Co.

C. Non-pharmacological approach
1. Invasive techniques: nerve blocks, implantable devices, and neurosurgery
2. Non-invasive techniques: physical therapy, acupuncture, massage, biofeedback, cognitive-behavioral therapy, relaxation techniques, and hypnosis

D. Treatment of Acute Pain
1. Acute pain is usually treated medically; initially one should treat the underlying disorder.

2. It is useful to follow the WHO Analgesic Ladder as a guideline (Fig. 33-3)
3. Severe acute pain, typically requires use of strong oral opioids, such as hydromorphone, levorphenol, or morphine. These may be delivered by patient-controlled analgesia (PCA) (Table 33-3) or by an epidural route, either with or without local anesthetics (see Table 33-4 for information regarding use of opioids).

E. Treatment of Chronic Pain. This usually requires a multi-disciplinary approach since long-standing pain has diffuse effects on many physical and psychological systems (see multi-disciplinary approach following).

1. **Neuropathic pain:** This type of pain is typically treated with agents that decrease nerve firing (Table 33-5) such as anticonvulsants (carbamazepine, phenytoin, gabapentin, clonazepam) or antiarrythmics (lidocaine, mexilitine, or tricyclics). Response may also be seen with other analgesics, such as opioids or NSAIDs. Nerve blockade and nerve transection rarely offer persistent relief.

2. **Chronic regional pain syndrome (RSD)** (Table 33-6): Initial treatment is with conservative therapy, mild analgesics, and physical therapy. Sympathetic interruption may be both diagnostic and therapeutic. Direct sympatholysis usually involves lumbar sympathetic or stellate ganglion block or systemic drug challenge with sympatholytic agents (phentolamine or phenoxybenzamine).

3. **Idiopathic Pain or Pain that Fails Conventional Therapy**
   a. This type of pain requires a multi-disciplinary approach, which may include the following: anesthesia, psychiatry, behavioral medicine, surgery/neurosurgery, physiatry, physical therapy, occupational therapy, nursing, pharmacy, social work, and case management.

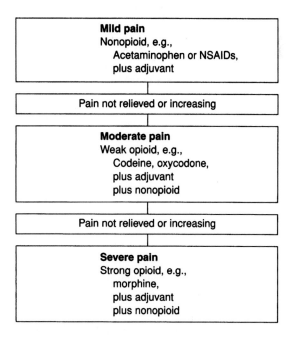

Figure 33-3.   The analgesic ladder. [From Borsook, D., Lebel, A.A., & McPeek, B. (1995). *MGH handbook of pain management.* Boston: Little, Brown & Co.]

Table 33-3. Adult Patient Controlled Analgesia (PCA)

| | *Drug* | | |
Requirements	*Morphine*	*Dilaudid*	*Meperidine*
mg/ml	1	0.5	10
Demand dose (ml)	1	0.5	1
Range (ml)	0.5–2.0	0.5–2.0	0.5–2.0
Lockout interval	6 minutes	10 minutes	6 minutes
Basal rate (ml/hour)			
Day	0	0	0
Night	0.5	0.5	0.5
Hourly limit (ml)	< 12	< 6	< 10
Loading dose (mg)			
(every 5 minutes until comfortable)	2 mg	0.5 mg	2.0 mg
Maximum loading dose (mg)	10–15 mg	2–4 mg	75–150 mg

NOTE: These suggested dosages are based on those required by a healthy, 55 to 70 kg, opioid-naive adult; adjustments must be made according to the condition of the patient, his or her prior opioid use, and the recent (preoperative) use of opioids.

SOURCE: From Borsook, D., Lebel, A.A., & McPeek, B. (1995). *MGH handbook of pain management.* Boston: Little, Brown & Co.

    b. Invasive interventions are of unclear value.
    c. Some severe cases may eventuate to use of chronic opioids where function may be improved. (See as follows, opioids for chronic non-malignant pain.)
F. Opioids: This class of medication remains the gold standard for severe or unremitting pain.
    1. Basic principles of opioid use (Table 33-4): Follow the WHO analgesic ladder (Fig. 33-3) and review expectations with patients. Explain that opioids are not curative, may be addictive, and have no prophylactic value. When used chronically, one should follow end-points of function, rather than pain.
    2. Efficacy: All opioids are equally efficacious when used in equianalgesic dosages; however, for unknown reasons individuals may respond better to one agent than to another.
    3. Synergy: The analgesia from opioids may be potentiated by other drugs (NSAIDs, antihistamines, clonidine, neuroleptics, and TCAs), allowing for an opioid-sparing maneuver.
    4. Administration: As needed (p.r.n.) dosing may reinforce the pain cycle, whereas long-acting agents may be preferable for long-term use.
    a. Oral, PR, SL, IM, IV, PCA, epidural, or spinal
    5. Adverse effects are common and often limit the use of drugs. Such effects are usually idiosyncratic; it is unclear why some patients react poorly and others do not. There are no predictors of which patients will experience which side effects and which

Table 33-4. Pharmacological Treatment of Acute Pain with Opioids

Drug	Approximate Equi-Analgesic Oral Dose	Approximate Equi-Analgesic Parenteral Dose	Recommended Starting Dose (adults more than 50 kg body weight)		Recommended Starting Dose (children and adults less than 50 kg body weight)[a]	
			Oral	Parenteral	Oral	Parenteral
Opioid agonist						
Morphine[b]	30 mg q3–4 hours (around-the-clock dosing) 60 mg q3–4 hours (single dose or intermittent dosing)	10 mg q3–4 hours	30 mg q3–4 hours	10 mg q3–4 hours	0.3 mg/kg q3–4 hours	0.1 mg/kg q3–4 hours
Codeine[c]	130 mg q 3–4 hours	75 mg q3–4 hours	60 mg q3–4 hours	60 mg q2 hours (intramuscular/subcutaneous)	1 mg/kg q3–4 hours[d]	Not recommended
Hydromorphone[b] (Dilaudid)	7.5 mg q3–4 hours	1.5 mg q3–4 hours	6 mg q3–4 hours	1.5 mg q3–4 hours	0.06 mg/kg q3–4 hours	0.015 mg/kg q3–4 hours
Levorphanol (Levo-Dromoran)	4 mg q6–8 hours	2 mg q6–8 hours	4 mg q6–8 hours	2 mg q6–8 hours	0.04 mg/kg q6–8 hours	0.02 mg/kg q6–8 hours
Meperidine (Demerol)	300 mg q2–3 hours	100 mg q3 hours	Not recommended	100 mg q3 hours	Not recommended	0.75 mg/kg q2–3 hours
Methadone (Dolophine, others)	20 mg q6–8 hours	10 mg q6–8 hours	20 mg q6–8 hours	10 mg q6–8 hours	0.2 mg/kg q6–8 hours	0.1 mg/kg q6–8 hours

(continued)

Table 33-4. (Continued)

Drug	Approximate Equi-Analgesic Oral Dose	Approximate Equi-Analgesic Parenteral Dose	Recommended Starting Dose (adults more than 50 kg body weight)		Recommended Starting Dose (children and adults less than 50 kg body weight)[a]	
			Oral	Parenteral	Oral	Parenteral
Oxycodone (Roxicodone, also in Percocet, Percodan, Tylox, others)	30 mg q3–4 hours	Not available	10 mg q3–4 hours	Not available	0.2 mg/kg q3–4 hours	Not available
Oxymorphone[b] (Numorphan)	Not available	1 mg q3–4 hours	Not available	1 mg q3–4 hours	Not recommended	Not recommended
Opioid agonist-antagonist and partial agonist						
Buprenorphine (Buprenex)	Not available	0.3–0.4 mg q6–8 hours	Not available	0.4 mg q6–8 hours	Not available	0.004 mg/kg q6–8 hours
Butorphanol (Stadol)	Not available	2 mg q3–4 hours	Not available	2 mg q3–4 hours	Not available	Not recommended
Nalbuphine (Nubain)	Not available	10 mg q3–4 hours	Not available	10 mg q3–4 hours	Not available	0.1 mg/kg q3–4 hours
Pentazocine (Talwin, others)	150 mg q3–4 hours	60 mg q3–4 hours	50 mg q4–6 hours	Not recommended	Not recommended	Not recommended

NOTE: Published tables vary in the suggested doses that are equi-analgesic to morphine. Clinical response is the criterion that must be applied for each patient; titration to clinical response is necessary. Because there is not complete cross-tolerance among these drugs, it is usually necessary to use a lower than equi-analgesic dose when changing drugs and to retitrate to response.
Caution: Recommended doses do not apply to patients with renal or hepatic insufficiency or other conditions affecting drug metabolism and kinetics.

[a]Caution: Doses listed for patients with body weight < 50 kg cannot be used as initial starting doses in babies < 6 months of age. Consult the Clinical Practice Guideline for Acute Pain Management: Operative or Medical Procedures and Trauma section on management of pain in neonates for recommendations.

[b]For morphine, hydromorphone, and oxymorphone, rectal administration is an alternate route for patients unable to take oral medications, but equi-analgesic doses may differ from oral and parenteral doses because of pharmacokinetic differences.

[c]Caution: Codeine doses > 65 mg often are not appropriate due to diminishing incremental analgesia with increasing doses but continually increasing constipation and other side effects.

[d]Caution: Doses of aspirin and acetaminophen in combination opioid/non-steroidal anti-inflammatory drug preparations must also be adjusted to the patient's body weight.

SOURCE: From Borsook, D., Lebel, A.A., & McPeek, B. (1995). *MGH handbook of pain management*. Boston: Little, Brown & Co.

Table 33-5. Anticonvulsants

Drug	Half-Life (hours)	Therapeutic Blood Levels, Seizures (mg/ml)	Toxic Concentration (mg/ml)	Maximum Daily Dose (mg/day)
Carbamazepine (Tegretol)	10–20	4–12	> 8–10	1,500
Clonazepam (Klonopin)	18–30	0.02–0.08	> 0.06	6
Phenytoin (Dilantin)	6–24	10–20	> 20	500
Valproic acid (Depakote)	12	50–100	>100–150	1,500–2,000 (60 mg/kg per day)

SOURCE: From Borsook, D., Lebel, A.A., & McPeek, B. (1995). *MGH handbook of pain management.* Boston: Little, Brown & Co.

narcotics will produce them. Thus, expect side effects and take preventive action. Tolerance to opioid's adverse effects, except constipation, occur.

a. Specific, but common, adverse effects that result from opioids include:

    i. Constipation: This is the most common side effect of opioids and it occurs with all opioids and persists over time. It may require use of a daily stimulating cathartic. If severe, oral dosages of naloxone can be used to treat this symptom.

Table 33-6. Treatment of Sympathetically Maintained Pain

Sympathetic blockade

    Local anesthetic applied to sympathetic chain

    IV Phenolamine

    IV Regional

        Guanethidine

        Ketanserin (serotonin atagonist)

        Oral medications

Sympathectomy

Spinal cord stimulation

Physical therapy

SOURCE: From Borsook, D., Lebel, A.A., & McPeek, B. (1995). *MGH handbook of pain management.* Boston: Little, Brown & Co.

      ii. Respiratory depression: This is a potentially serious complication. Tolerance occurs early in chronic therapy. Significant respiratory depression from opiates can also be managed with naloxone.

      iii. Nausea: Severe nausea and vomiting that is caused solely by opioids is rare and usually mild.

      iv. Pruritus: This symptom is rare with oral opiates and very common with spinal and epidural opioids; it probably occurs through a central mechanism. Tolerance occurs, responds to treatment with naloxone, antihistamines (except when caused by spinal opioids) and propofol (10 mg IVP q 10 minutes, 2 to 3 doses)

6. Tolerance to analgesia: When tolerance develops, use of increased dosing may be required. Changing agents may allow dosing at lower than equianalgesic dose, as cross-tolerance between opioids may not be complete. Tolerance impairs the ability to assess the appropriate opioid dose.

7. Opioids for chronic non-malignant pain: This pattern of use is highly controversial, but there is growing acceptance in well-chosen cases. Such management has been avoided owing to high abuse potential, tolerance, dependence, and other adverse effects. However, opioids may be a reasonable option for patients with chronic non-malignant pain who have failed all other reasonable conventional non-opioid interventions, and in whom opioids can improve function without substantial medication loss or aberrant dose escalations.

    a. **Guidelines for using opioids in chronic non-malignant pain** (derived from Portnoy, 1990) include:

      i. Try to individualize therapy; opioids can be tried if other analgesics fail.

      ii. Use a single opioid if possible.

      iii. Employ long-acting preparations.

      iv. Mix a single short-acting agent and a single long-acting agent.

      v. Use around-the-clock dosing rather than p.r.n., otherwise, limit the weekly amount if daily use is required.

      vi. Document the efficacy of opioid analgesia.

      vii. Monitor the analgesic and functional endpoints.

      viii. Focus on function rather than an analgesia.

      ix. Use an opioid contract and informed consent.

      x. Discuss side effects, addiction, dependence, tolerance, cognitive impairment, fetal dependency in pregnancy, rules of usage and prescribing, and the consequences of breaking the contract.

      xi. Designate a single prescriber for all opioids.

      xii. Designate a single pharmacy for all opioid prescriptions.

      xiii. Maintain a symptom diary.

      xiv. Do not provide over-the-phone prescriptions.

      xv. Maintain close follow-up.

      xvi. Maintain a high level of suspicion regarding toxicity and addictive tendencies. Watch for evidence of drug hoarding, acquisition of opioids by multiple physicians, uncontrolled dose escalations, or other aberrant behaviors.

      xvii. Consider tapering and discontinuing opioids.

      xviii. Hold strictly to usage guidelines.

      xix. Consult with an addictions specialist.

      xx. Periodically review the case with a multi-disciplinary team.

      xxi. Be aware of relative contraindications to opioid use: History of substance abuse (including ethanol), severe character disorder, inability to follow rules, use in substance abusers with pain that has proved resistant to all other therapeutic options; the relative nature of these contraindications must yield to compassionate use of narcotics.

G. Analgesic adjuvants (Tables 33-2, 33-5, 33-7)

1. Adjuvants, such as NSAIDs, antihistamines, clonidine, corticosteroids, neuroleptics, psychostimulants, and tricyclics, may increase the benefits of opioids.
2. Partial independent analgesic effects may be achieved with tricyclics, clonidine, baclofen, muscle relaxants, corticosteroids, antiarrythmics, and anticonvulsants (of these the TCAs are the most widely used and are discussed further later).
3. Antidepressants as analgesics (Table 33-7): TCAs but not SSRIs are well established to have independent analgesic properties.
   a. Specific TCAs supported as an analgesic by controlled studies include amitriptyline (Elavil), nortriptyline (Pamelor), desipramine (Norpramin), imipramine (Tofranil), and maprotiline (Ludiomil)
   b. Specific TCAs supported as an analgesic by anecdotal reports include doxepin, trazodone, and clomipramine
   c. TCA-associated analgesia: Complete analgesia is rare and side effects are common, so usually one must accept some mild side effects in exchange for analgesia. TCAs are particularly compelling when pain is accompanied by co-morbid depression or by insomnia. Reasonable goals of therapy include decreasing the pain intensity by 10–50% or decreasing pain from unbearable to bearable levels.
   d. Analgesic TCA dosages may be lower than antidepressant dosages; some patients may require higher dosages.
      i. Start at 10 or 25 mg
      ii. Increase the dosage upward slowly to minimize side effects and to avoid overshooting the minimal analgesic dose.
      iii. If intolerable side effects develop, change to desipramine or nortriptyline.
   e. Initial early analgesia may improve over 1 to 7 days to several weeks (it may require 2 to 4 weeks for maximal analgesia); analgesic effects persist over time.

H. Non-pharmacological approaches

1. Invasive techniques
   a. Nerve blocks and implantable devices: trigger point injections, epidural injections, selective nerve root injections, stellate ganglion and lumbar sympathetic nerve blockade
   b. Neurosurgery
      i. Augmentive
         (a) Intrathecal pump: typically it delivers an opioid but it may also be used for baclofen (spasticity) or for local anesthetic (less commonly)
         (b) Spinal cord stimulator (dorsal column stimulator): a catheter device that electrically stimulates the spinal cord placed in the epidural space—used in neuropathic pain and sympathetically maintained pain states
      ii. Ablative: Pain often recurs and can worsen.
         (a) Peripheral: radiofrequency lesions
            • efficacy for trigeminal and glossopharyngeal neuralgia
         (b) Spinal cord:
            • ganglionectomy: ablation of the dorsal gaglia
            • dorsal rhizotomy: sensory loss in lesioned distribution

Table 33-7. Antidepressants

Drug	Dosage (mg)	Usual Daily Dose (mg)	Anticholinergic Activity	Central Action	Hypotension	Sedation
Amitriptyline (Elavil)[a]	10–300	75–150	Strong	S(N)	Strong	Strong
Amoxapine (Asendin)	50–400	50–200	Minimal	N	Mild	Minimal
Bupropion (Wellbutrin)	50–100	50–300	Minimal	N/A	Minimal	Minimal
Clomipramine (Anafranil)[a]	25–250	20–150	Moderate	S(N)	Strong	Mild
Desipramine (Norpramin)[a]	75–300	50–150	Minimal	N	Mild	Minimal
Doxepin (Sinequan)	30–300	30–150	Moderate	S	Strong	Mild
Fluoxetine (Prozac)	5–80	20–40	Minimal	S	Minimal	Minimal
Imipramine (Tofranil)[a]	20–300	20–150	Moderate	N/S	Moderate	Moderate
Isocarboxazid (Marplan)	10–40	10–40	Minimal	MAOI	Mild	Moderate
Maprotiline (Ludiomil)	75–300	75–150	Mild	N	Mild	Mild
Nortriptyline (Pamelor)[a]	25–150	50–150	Mild	N/S	Moderate	Mild
Phenelzine (Nardil)	15–90	45–75	Mild	MAOI	Mild	Moderate
Protriptyline (Vivactil)	15–60	15–40	Moderate	N	Minimal	Mild
Sertraline (Zoloft)	50–200	50–100	Mild	S	Minimal	Mild
Tranylcypromine (Parnate)	10–45	10–20	Minimal	MAOI	Moderate	Mild
Trazodone (Desyrel)	50–600	150–300	Minimal	S	Moderate	Minimal
Trimipramine (Surmontil)	50–200	75–150	Moderate	S(N)	Strong	Mild

[a]Commonly used for neuropathic pain.

NOTE: S, serotonergic; N, noradrenergic; (N), weakly noradrenergic; MAOI, monoamine oxidase inhibitor.

SOURCE: From Borsook, D., Lebel, A.A., & McPeek, B. (1995). *MGH handbook of pain management*. Boston: Little, Brown & Co.

- dorsal root entry zone (DREZ): phantom limb pain
- midline myelotomy: for bilateral pain

(c) Central:

- mesencephalotomy: lesions of midbrain spinothalamic and secondary trigeminal tracts—for unilateral head and neck pain
- thalamotomy: sometimes with bilateral analgesia
- cingulotomy: for diffuse chronic pain associated with affective disorders

2. Non-invasive: physical therapy, transcutaneous electrical nerve stimulation (TENS), acupuncture (relatively non-invasive), massage, cognitive or behavioral therapy, distraction (e.g., hypnosis or biofeedback)

I. The multi-disciplinary approach
1. Goals of the multi-disciplinary approach include improved coping, a focus on function rather than analgesia, and decreased addictive behaviors. This approach offers alternatives to drugs, injections, or surgery for pain control and hopefully improvement in overall physical and psychological well-being. It strives to decrease behaviors that negatively impact on pain and function, to improve social supports, to decrease social isolation, and to decrease dependence on the health-care system
2. Somatic component
   a. Medical: neurology, internal medicine, pediatrics, physiatry, psychiatry
   b. Surgical: anesthesia, surgery, neurosurgery
   c. Rehabilitation: physiatry, physical therapy
3. Psychiatric component
   a. Medical: psychiatry
   b. Behavioral: behavioral medicine/cognitive therapy, individual and group psychotherapy
4. Alternative therapies: Unknown efficacy, but subsequent increased function as a result of moderate use of these activities may be beneficial. Examples include acupuncture, yoga, tai chi, massage, and herbal remedies.

Suggested Readings

Acute Pain Management Guideline Panel. (1992). *Acute pain management: Operative or medical procedures and trauma.* Clinical Practice Guideline. Rockville, Md.: Agency for Health Care Policy and Research, Public Health Service, U.S. Department of Health and Human Services. AHCPR Pub. No. 92-0032.

Bonica, J.J. (Ed.). (1990). *The management of pain* (2nd ed.). Philadelphia: Lea & Febiger.

Borsook, D., Lebel, A.A., & McPeek, B. (1995). *MGH handbook of pain management.* Boston: Little, Brown and Co.

Breitbart, W. (1989). Psychiatric management of cancer pain. *Cancer, 63,* 2336–2342.

Fields, H.L. (1987). *Pain.* New York: McGraw-Hill.

Foley, K.M. (1983). The practical use of narcotic analgesics. *Medical Clinics of North America, 66,* 1091–1104.

Hyman, S.H., & Cassem, N.H. (1989). Pain. In E. Rubenstein, & D.D. Fedeman (Eds.), *Scientific American medicine: Current topics in medicine. Subsection II.* New York: Scientific American, pp. 1–7.

NIH Concensus Development Conference. (1987). The integrated approach to the management of pain. *Journal of Pain and Symptom Management, 2,* 35–41.

Portnoy, R.Y. (1990). Chronic opioid therapy in nonmalignant pain. *Journal of Pain and Symptom Management, 5,* S46–S62.

Sternbach, R. (1974). *Pain patients: Traits and treatments.* New York: Academic Press.

Wall, P.D., & Melzack, R. (Eds.). (1995). *Textbook of pain* (3rd ed.). New York: Churchill-Livingstone.

CHAPTER 34
The Patient with Fatigue

Donna B. Greenberg

I. Introduction

Fatigue is multi-dimensional, a symptom with different meanings, causes, and physical manifestations. The complaint of fatigue may indicate specific impairments like poor concentration, inability to walk upstairs, or dyspnea on exertion. It may also convey the feeling of being overwhelmed, impotent, hopeless, or bored. It is one of the most common complaints in an ambulatory setting, seventh in one national ambulatory survey, unrelated to age, and more common in women than men. **Report of excessive fatigue is associated with higher rates of anxiety and depression.**

A. A clinician must distinguish whether fatigue has a medical cause, results from anxiety or depressive disorder, or has no clear etiology. Rational decisions regarding diagnosis depend on what patients mean when they say they are tired, on accompanying physical symptoms, on the time course and precipitants of fatigue, and on the level of daily physical and mental function.

B. Fatigue can become chronic (lasting longer than 6 months) and disabling; if so, it falls into the category of chronic fatigue, which will be discussed in Chapter 35.

C. Fatigue is multidimensional. It has affective components (anxious, sad, frustrated, angry); behavioral components (inability to initiate activity or to keep going, tendency to avoid social or challenging conditions); cognitive components (poor concentration, sleepiness, sense of greater effort required); and physical manifestations (dyspnea on exertion, palpitations with exertion, proximal muscle weakness [e.g., manifest by inability to climb stairs], and the need to sit or lie down).

D. Fatigue may be considered a normal response to effort or exercise.

E. Fatigue brings patients to the doctor (e.g., because of physically localized symptoms, an inability to meet expectations, fatigue that is out of proportion to the intensity or duration of activity, or fatigue that is amplified by anxiety or hypochondriasis).

II. Medical History

A. Pay attention to any known medical illness that has symptoms.

B. Direct the evaluation to the organ system most prominently affected.

C. Consider medical illnesses or conditions, like hypothyroidism, anemia, liver dysfunction, and general infection, that are associated with global fatigue.

D. Consider whether selected medical disorders associated with fatigue are possibilities. See Table 34-1.

Table 34-1. Medical Conditions Associated with Fatigue

Substance abuse	Alcohol, opiates, or cocaine
Medications	Anticholinergic, antihistamines, benzodiazepines, anticonvulsants, β sympathetic blockers
Sleep disorders	Sleep apnea, restless legs, or insomnia
Post-treatment	Surgery, chemotherapy, radiation therapy, or dialysis
Deconditioning	Bed rest, or less exercise
Cardiovascular	Angina or congestive heart failure
Pulmonary	Asthma, chronic obstructive lung disease, or pleural effusion
Rheumatologic	Systemic lupus erythematosus, or rheumatoid arthritis
Metabolic	Hypothyroidism, hypercalcemia, estrogen deficiency, hyperglycemia, hypoadrenalism, uremia, or pregnancy
Neurologic	Parkinson's disease, stroke, post-ictal states, multiple sclerosis dementia, or narcolepsy
Hematologic	Anemia
Hepatic	Hepatitis, or cirrhosis
Infection	HIV, acute Epstein-Barr virus, cytomegalovirus, subacute endocarditis, or with fever
Neoplastic	Malignancies and especially lymphoma (with sweats or pruritis)
Myopathy	Steroid-induced, thyroid disease, myositis, drug-induced, or paraneoplastic
Allergy	Recurrent allergic rhinitis

III. Interview

A. Clarify the meaning of fatigue to patients. Hear patients out. Let them put the symptom in context. Useful questions to ask include the following:

1. "What do you mean by tired?" This will help to distinguish physical from psychological meanings. The patient may feel sad, powerless, tense, or unable to walk down the street.
2. "What makes it worse?"
3. "What have you not been able to do?"
4. "Is there a time of day that it is worse?"
   a. Anxiety and dread of the day are worse in the morning and often improve as the day goes on in patients with melancholic depression.
   b. Dialysis patients who are fatigued in the morning are more apt to be depressed.
   c. Normal vigor is greater in the morning.
5. "Where do you sense it physically?"
   a. Dyspnea on exertion would direct attention to the lung, heart, or blood count.
   b. Difficulty getting up or climbing stairs would point to proximal myopathy.
   c. "Do you feel faint on rising?" This suggests postural hypotension.
6. "What made you come to the doctor now? What do you fear is causing fatigue?" These questions may lead to information on patients' worries.

7. "What do you wish that you could do, or do you have the desire to do things?"
   a. Loss of desire or interest (with dysphoria) occurs with depressive disorders.
   b. Loss of desire without dysphoria occurs with dementia and frontal lobe dysfunction. It may be a complaint of patients' relatives rather than of patients themselves.
   c. Boredom often reflects a situational loss of interest. The patient may have an inability to pay attention unless highly stimulated, so promient boredom may be the clue to attention deficit disorder.
   d. Fear (for instance, of failure) may prevent patients from initiating something they want. They may refer to the inhibition as fatigue.

B. Assess function. Determine the following:
   1. "What is a typical day like now?"
   2. "Are there things that you have been putting off or avoiding?"

C. Assess sleep. Ask the following:
   1. "Do you wake up rested?" as a clue to sleep disorder
   2. "Do you snore?" as a clue to sleep apnea
   3. "Are there periods of insomnia?"

D. Get a clear history of substance use.
   1. What is the pattern of alcohol, caffeine, and recreational drugs? All can disrupt sleep and energy.
   2. "Do you take over-the-counter medications?" Anticholinergic medications or antihistamines may be sedating.
   3. What are prescribed medications?

E. Assess other symptoms of mood disorder.
   1. Are sadness, loss, or guilt present?
   2. Do patients have an inability to feel pleasure for what is usually enjoyed?
   3. Can they concentrate on the newspaper or TV?
   4. Loss of appetite or increased eating may be evident by history or by weight change.
   5. Thoughts of death or suicide may be present.

F. Question the patient directly about panic attacks.
   1. Are there discrete episodes of intense anxiety with sudden onset and autonomic arousal, typically associated with fear of impending doom or loss of control, and a need to flee places where panic attacks occurred?
   2. Are there associated palpitations, pounding heart, trembling, sweating, smothering, dyspnea, chest pain, nausea, abdominal distress, dizziness, unsteadiness, derealization, depersonalization, numbness or tingling, hot flashes or chills?
   3. Are there other simple phobias like fear of heights or closed spaces?
   4. Is there a pattern of avoidance that fits with avoidance of places where previous panic attacks occurred or places where escape would be difficult?

G. Is there a history of many medically unexplained symptoms that suggests a pattern of chronicity?

IV. Examination of the Patient

A. The general physical examination searches for any abnormalities that might be a clue to occult causes of fatigue.

B. Pay special attention to vital signs.
   1. Fever
   2. Tachycardia

3. Increased respiratory rate

4. Postural blood pressure changes may be a result of deconditioning, blood or volume loss, or medications (like cisplatin, amitriptyline, or antihypertensives).

5. Weight loss or gain

C. Neurological examination

1. The presence of psychomotor retardation suggests Parkinson's disease or depression.

2. Signs of hyperventilation, like sighing or rapid breathing, specifically signify anxiety, depression, panic attacks, hypoxia, or dyspnea on exertion.

3. Depressed facies fits with depression.

4. Examination of muscle strength identifies myopathy.

D. In a general medical examination, special attention should focus on the following:

1. Lungs

2. Heart

3. Liver

4. Thyroid gland

5. Skin (pallor or jaundice)

6. Lymph nodes

E. Mental status examination

1. Assess cognition to rule out dementia.

2. Be cognizant of the pace of speech (for depression, anxiety, or hypomania).

3. Consider affective content to elucidate what emotions may be minimized by the patient.

F. Laboratory screening (if indicated)

1. Blood count

2. Erythrocyte sedimentation rate

3. Liver function tests: serum glutamic-oxacetic transaminase, alkaline phosphatase, total protein, and albumin

4. Calcium, bilirubin, and glucose

5. Blood urea nitrogen and creatinine

6. Electrolytes

7. Thyroid stimulating hormone

8. Urinalysis

V. Psychiatric Differential Diagnosis

A. Phase of life or stressful circumstance, for example, a job change, retirement, starting school, marriage, divorce, or birth of a child can be felt to be tiring especially when:

1. There is little conscious acknowledgment of the emotional energy required or the effort of adjustment.

2. Fatigue is amplified by situational anxiety.

3. Overwork is a chronic pattern associated with the feeling that one should be able to work harder.

4. Conflict is present, and the wish not to do something is not overtly acknowledged. Patients may be perfectionistic, fear failure, fear success, undervalue rewards, fear criticism, have limited frustration tolerance, tackle too much, or magnify the task (Burns, 1980).

5. The feeling of being coerced leads to fatigue as passive resistance.

    6. A situational rejection or humiliation occurs.

    7. There is often no acknowledgment that an energy budget may be overdrawn.

B. Grief is associated with fatigue and may be evident. Findings may include sighing, panic attacks, and a search for the missed person.

C. Panic disorder

    1. Fatigue is a central symptom of panic disorder. Neurocirculatory asthenia is an old name for the same disease.

    2. Exhaustion follows attacks.

    3. Avoidance may appear to be fatigue.

D. Major depressive disorder

    1. A subtype of depression, "atypical," is characterized by hypersomnia, by leaden feet, and by rejection sensitivity.

    2. Untreated depressive episodes may continue for more than a year in half of patients. Half of those with chronic fatigue syndrome had depression first.

    3. An increased sensation of effort is associated with depression.

    4. Impairment of effortful cognition is associated with depression.

    5. Dread of the day is typical of melancholia.

E. Bipolar or cyclothymia

    1. A normally hypomanic patient who returns to an emotional baseline feels an uncharacteristic lack of energy.

    2. Some patients have cyclothymia or mood cycles with energy alternating with apathy. The apathetic period may appear to be a state of fatigue.

F. Hypochondriasis is a condition of preoccupation and fear of having a serious disease. It is commonly associated with the fatiguing states of anxiety or depression.

G. Sleep apnea is associated with daytime sleepiness.

H. Alcohol abuse is associated with sedation and sleep disorder.

I. Loneliness—The feeling of abandonment or rejction may lead to a feeling of being overwhelmed, described as fatigue. Axis II diagnoses (e.g., narcissistic, borderline, and histrionic personality disorders) are a consideration.

VI. Treatment

A. Specific medical diagnoses lead to specific treatment.

B. Syndromal depression or panic disorder should lead to specific treatment (e.g., anti-depressant medications, anti-panic agents, or psychotherapy). Benzodiazepines may relieve fatigue if panic disorder caused fatigue.

C. Situational fatigue

    1. Hear the patient out.

    2. Rule out likely medical causes.

    3. Inform the patient that fatigue may be a symptom of stress, anxiety, sadness, or anger.

    4. Acknowledge the dominant emotion.

    5. Indicate the need for energy budgeting, rest, and recreation.

    6. Allow another evaluation if symptoms persist or check the following:

       a. Serial vital signs

       b. Serial weights

c. A diary for a longitudinal view

d. Descriptions from other family members

7. Psychotherapy may be appropriate to explore when conflict is persistent.

Suggested Readings

Buchwald, D., Pascualy, R., Bombardier, C., et al. (1994). Sleep disorders in patients with chronic fatigue. *Clinical Infectious Disease, 18*(suppl 1), S68–72.

Burns, D. (1980). *Feeling good.* New York: Penguin Books, pp. 75–86.

Cardenas, D.D., & Kutner, N.G. (1982). The problem of fatigue in dialysis patients. *Nephron, 30,* 336–340.

Cohen, M.E., White, P.D., & Johnson, R.E. (1948). Neurocirculatory asthenia, anxiety neuroses, or the effort syndrome. *Archives of Internal Medicine, 81,* 260–281.

Cohen, R.M., Weingartner, H., Smallberg, S.A., et al. (1982). Effort and cognition in depression. *Archives of General Psychiatry, 29,* 593–597.

Pukada, K., Straus, S., Hickie, I., et al. (1994). The chronic fatigue syndrome: A comprehensive approach to its definition and study. *Annals of Internal Medicine, 121,* 953–959.

Kellner, R. (1991). Chronic fatigue syndrome and fatigue. In *Psychosomatic syndromes and somatic symptoms.* Washington, DC: American Psychiatric Press, Inc., pp. 31–51.

Kroenke, K., Wood, D.R., Mangellsdorff, A.D., et al. (1988). Chronic fatigue in primary care. *Journal of the American Medical Association, 260,* 929–934.

Liebowitz, M.R., Quitkin, F.K., Stewart, J.W., et al. (1984). Psychopharmacologic validation of atypical depression. *Journal of Clinical Psychiatry, 45,* 22–25.

Manu, P., Matthews, D.A., Lane, T.J., et al. (1989). Depression among patients with a chief complaint of chronic fatigue. *Journal of Affective Disorders, 17,* 165–172.

National Ambulatory Medical Care Survey. (1978). *1975 Summary.* Hyattsville, MD: National Center for Health Statistics.

Rhoades, J.M. (1997). Overwork. *Journal of the American Medical Association, 237,* 2615–2618.

Roy-Byme, P.P., Weingartner, H., Bierer, L.M., et al. (1986). Effortful and automatic cognitive processes in depression. *Archives of General Psychiatry, 43,* 265–267.

Solberg, L.I. (1984). Lassitude: A primary care evaluation. *Journal of the American Medical Association, 251,* 3272–3276.

Wood, C., & Magnello, M.E. (1992). Diurnal changes in perceptions of energy and mood. *Journal of the Royal Society of Medicine, 85,* 191–194.

CHAPTER 35

The Patient with Chronic Fatigue Syndrome

DONNA B. GREENBERG

I. Introduction

A. Chronic fatigue syndrome (CFS) is a syndrome defined by consensus. Chronic fatigue is prominent and no etiology can be determined. Although research in the 1980s pursued a viral cause, no specific virus has been implicated. CFS is heterogeneous; it overlaps with many psychiatric and medical diagnoses (e.g., fibromyalgia, irritable bowel syndrome, multiple allergy syndrome, multiple chemical sensitivity syndrome). It is seen as a legitimate illness in contradistinction to the stigma of mental illness. **It has a social meaning with support from lobbies and support groups.**

1. Whereas acute mononucleosis is followed by fatigue, chronic mononucleosis does not account for the syndrome.
2. In primary care populations, 10% are fatigued 6 months after viral infection.
3. No link between laboratory and clinical parameters of the virus has been established.
4. Immune deficiency has been a feature of the syndrome (CFIDS) in some circles, but documentation of immune deficiency has been inconsistent and has never been as severe as in AIDS (Acquired Immune Deficiency Syndrome).

B. Medical syndromes by diagnostic criteria

1. **The criteria to diagnose CFS, revised in 1994, aim to define severe mental and physical exhaustion,** not somnolence or lack of motivation, a sensation that cannot be attributed to exertion or diagnosed disease (Fukada et al., 1994).
   a. **Chronic fatigue should be clinically evaluated as unexplained, persistent, or relapsing with a new or definite onset**
   b. **It should neither be caused by ongoing exertion nor substantially alleviated by rest.**
   c. **Substantial reduction in activities is a key feature.**
2. **Concurrent occurrence of four or more listed symptoms:**
   a. Self-reported impairment in short-term memory or concentration severe enough to cause substantial reduction in activities
   b. Sore throat
   c. Tender cervical or axillary lymph nodes
   d. Muscle pain
   e. Multi-joint pain without joint swelling or redness
   f. Headaches of a new type, pattern, or severity
   g. Unrefreshing sleep
   h. Post-exertional malaise of more than 24 hours
   i. Symptoms must have persisted or recurred during 6 or more consecutive months and did not predate fatigue.
3. **Idiopathic chronic fatigue**
   a. Clinically evaluated, unexplained chronic fatigue that fails to meet criteria for CFS
   b. The reason for failing to meet criteria is specified.

4. **Psychiatric exclusions**
   a. Current or within last 2 years: psychotic depression, bipolar disorder, schizophrenia, delusional disorder, anorexia nervosa, bulimia, substance abuse (within 2 years before the onset of chronic fatigue or afterward).
5. Current anxiety, anxiety disorder, or non-melancholic depression are not exclusions.

C. **Fibromyalgia—an overlapping condition, originally characterized by fatigue, sleep dysfunction, and myalgia. Revised criteria (Wolfe et al., 1990):**
   1. At least a 3-month history of diffuse musculoskeletal pain
   2. Tenderness identified by digital palpation at trigger points bilaterally.
      a. The standard is 11 of 18 tender points that are bilateral and above and below the diaphragm.
      b. Medial fat pad of the knee, prominence of the greater trochanter, 2 cm distal to lateral condyle, near the second costochondral junction, under the lower sternomastoid muscle, origin of the supraspinatus, insertion of the suboccipital muscle, mid-upper trapezius, and upper-outer quadrant of buttock

II. Evaluation of the Problem

A. **General Recommendations**
   1. **The diagnosis of CFS does not imply a single treatment**
   2. **The problem may be managed in a fashion similar to the management of somatoform disorders.**
      a. **Recognize that complete relief of the symptom is unlikely**
      b. **Treat co-morbid depression and anxiety aggressively.**
      c. **Choose treatments carefully because treatment is unlikely to change the patient's course**
   3. **A longitudinal relationship to one physician may be the most important aspect of management.**
   4. Remember that **gentle and firm management of requests,** hearing the patient but avoiding excess, is especially important. If the patient cannot go along with a cautious balance, anger will more likely end the relationship.

B. **Medical history**
   1. **Focus on associated symptoms** and medical history to clarify possible medical causes.
   2. **Obtain records** of all evaluations of symptoms of unclear etiology.
   3. **Look for a history of childhood illness** or a model for disability in the family.
   4. **Identify allergies.**
   5. **Clarify any history of substance abuse.**
   6. **Note treatments for previous medical disorder that may have left patients tired.**
   7. **Review all medications.**
   8. **Determine if there are any neurological impairments.**

C. **Interview**
   1. Allow the patient to tell the story of the illness.
   2. Validate the suffering state.
   3. Determine the functional level of the patient and establish what he or she cannot do.
   4. Assess the cost of disability and the losses.
   5. Question what supports would be lost if the patient's function began to improve.
   6. Determine if the patient is averse to consideration of a mix of physical and psychological causes of fatigue.

D. Examination of the patient
   1. Assess vital signs with postural blood pressure changes.
   2. Perform a thorough physical examination.
   3. Consider informal exercise testing.

E. Laboratory (Fukada et al., 1994)
   1. Blood count
   2. Erythrocyte sedimentation rate
   3. Liver function tests: serum glutamic-oxacetic transaminase, alkaline phosphatase, total protein, and albumin
   4. Calcium, bilirubin, and glucose
   5. Blood urea nitrogen and creatinine
   6. Electrolytes
   7. Thyroid stimulating hormone
   8. Urinalysis

F. Laboratory tests not generally recommended (Fukada et al., 1994):
   1. Creatine kinase, antinuclear antibody, and rheumatoid factor
   2. Chest x-ray
   3. Human immunodeficiency virus, hepatitis B or C antibody, Lyme serology, rapid plasma reagin test (RPR), toxoplasmosis serology, serum immunoglobulin levels, cytomegalovirus IgM serology, and Ebstein-Barr virus capsid antigen IgM serology.

G. Other laboratory tests as clinically indicated

H. Enlarging the work-up
   1. Acquire more data by obtaining a longitudinal record of function.
   2. Obtain additional data from friends or family.
   3. Document serial weights and temperature.

III. Psychiatric Differential Diagnosis

A. Acute situational fatigue—see previous section

B. Major depressive disorder: a common co-morbid diagnosis

C. Panic disorder: Symptoms of hyperventilation should not be overlooked. This is common with co-morbid depression.

D. Bipolar disorder may be a consideration in a patient whose hypomanic baseline or cyclothymia was not previously recognized.

E. Substance abuse not yet acknowledged to the physician

F. Somatization disorder
   1. **Accounts for 15% of CFS** patients in some studies.
   2. Patients have eight or more physical complaints with onset before age 30 leading to treatment over years; criteria require four pain symptoms, two GI symptoms, one sexual or reproductive symptom, and one symptom suggesting neurological disease.
   3. The diagnoses or CFS and somatization disorder depend in part on whether medical symptoms are attributed to psychiatric or physical categories.

G. Fatigue disorder by analogy to pain disorder
   1. Fatigue is analogous to pain in chronic pain disorder. The symptom is chronic, of unclear etiology, with an affective dimension, and with continuing question about an occult medical cause.

2. By analogy, fatigue can be colored by depression, anger, and anxiety.

3. Fatigue behavior, like pain behavior, reflects the ways a chronic symptom changes personal relationships. Patients may gain control by sustaining a role as a suffering disabled patient.

4. Like chronic pain patients, CFS patients have scores higher on scales of hypochondriasis, depression, and hysteria, but also have higher scores on scales of deviance.

H. Hypochondriasis

1. In this condition, the patient has such a fervent conviction of an illness that facts will not dissuade. This is a strong factor in a diagnosis that is supported by consensus criteria, support groups, anger, or the need to control the medical interaction.

2. The physician must find a balance between validating the patient's distress and dignity, while not accepting wholly the power of the label.

3. The physician's task is to give good care within honest boundaries, so that he or she does not feel coerced to hurt the patient.

I. Schizophrenia

1. A diagnosis of schizophrenia excludes patients from receiving the label of CFS. However, the prodrome of schizophrenia may include social withdrawal, inability to work, and preoccupation with delusions. When delusions or paranoia are not immediately apparent, these patients may appear to have CFS.

J. Neurasthenic neurosis or neurasthenia

1. This diagnostic category from the International Classification of Disease identifies some patients with CFS-like symptoms who do not meet criteria for any other psychiatric or medical diagnoses.

K. Character style or pathology

1. A sense of strength, not fatigue, is a basic somatic dimension of self-regard, so chronically low self-esteem may correlate with chronic fatigue (Horowitz, 1996).

2. **Loneliness is a predictor of chronic fatigue** (Kellner, 1991).

3. Patients who are easily humiliated or rejected may feel defeated, grief-stricken, and repeatedly fatigued.

4. Neurotic patients may complain of fatigue as a means of maintaining control over interpersonal interactions.

5. Patients who are socially isolated and more chronically vulnerable may not have skills to regulate personal demands and may express their sense of being overwhelmed as chronic fatigue.

IV. Treatment Strategies

A. Principles of medical evaluation

1. **Consider serious and treatable diagnoses** during the medical evaluation.

2. **Educate the patient about the role of inactivity in promoting fatigue.**

3. **Set improved function as the goal.**

4. **Defer requests for permanent disability.** This status will be counterproductive.

5. **Consider that psychotherapeutic and psychotropic interventions hold some promise.**

6. Prognosis is related to openness to treatment

B. Psychotropic medications

1. **Initiate an antidepressant trial** for those who have co-morbid depression, and titrate the dose slowly with consideration for side effects.

   a. Isolated reports note the benefit of nortriptyline, venlafaxine, or bupropion.

   b. Mixed results have been reported for fluoxetine in controlled studies, but fixed dose, tolerance of side effects, and heterogeneity of sample may be limiting methodological factors.

   c. Amitriptyline and cyclobenzaprine, which have been beneficial in fibromyalgia, have not had enduring benefit in one recent study, but the dosing strategy may have not been flexible enough (Carrette et al., 1994).

2. Benzodiazepines will benefit those with panic disorder in spite of initial sedation.

C. Cognitive treatment as developed by Wessely and Sharpe, 1995

1. **Be explicit about the goals of rehabilitation.**

2. **Discourage alternative evaluations or treatments.**

3. **Find factors that perpetuate symptoms.**

4. **Remember that treatment may temporarily increase fatigue.**

5. **Identify the harshness of the patient's all-or-none standards.**

6. **Replace responsibility for illness with responsibility for rehabilitation.**

7. **Structured sessions,** 5 to 20, every week or every other week

D. Behavioral treatment per Wessely and Sharpe, 1995

1. Increase activity by using realistic goals.

2. **Increase activity gradually regardless of symptoms.**

3. Grade tasks.

4. Restrict activity if the patient does too much too fast.

5. **Record baseline amounts of rest and build the same amount in divided doses into a concrete timetable.**

6. Remember that more control and predictable function is the goal.

7. **Emphasize function.**

V. Prognosis

A. Poor with patients with more than eight medically unexplained symptoms

B. Poor with lifetime dysthymia

C. Poor with high levels of disease conviction

D. Poor with greater duration of disease

Suggested Readings

Ablashi, D.V. (1994). Summary: Vital studies of chronic fatigue syndrome. *Clinical Infectious Diseases, 18*(suppl 1), S142–146.

Buchwald, D., Pascualy, R., Bombardier, C., et al. (1994). Sleep disorders in patients with chronic fatigue. *Clinical Infectious Diseases, 18*(suppl 1), S69–72.

Carette, S., Bell, M.J., Reynolds, J., et al. (1994). Comparison of amitriptyline, cyclobenzaprine, and placebo in the treatment of fibromyalgia. *Arthritis Rheumatology, 37,* 32–40.

Clark, M.R., Katon, W., Russo, J., et al. (1995). Chronic fatigue: Risk factors for symptom persistence in a 2.5 year followup study. *American Journal of Medicine, 98,* 187–195.

Deale, A., Husain, K., Chalder, T., & Wessely, S. (2001). Long-term outcome of cognitive behavior therapy versus relaxation therapy for chronic fatigue syndrome: A 5-year follow-up study. *American Journal of Psychiatry, 158,* 2038–2042.

Fiedler, N., Kipen, H.M., DeLuca, J., et al. (1996). A controlled comparison of multiple chemical sensitivities and chronic fatigue syndrome. *Psychosomatic Medicine, 58,* 38–49.

Fukada, K., Straus, S., Hickie, I., et al. (1994). The chronic fatigue syndrome: A comprehensive approach to its definition and study. *Annals of Internal Medicine, 121,* 953–959.

Goodnick, P.J. (1990). Buproprion in chronic fatigue syndrome. *American Journal of Psychiatry, 147,* 1091.

Gracious, B., & Wisner, K.L. (1991). Nortriptyline in chronic fatigue syndrome: A double-blind, placebo-controlled single case study. *Biological Psychiatry, 30,* 405–408.

Johnson, S.Y., DeLuca, J., Fiedler, N., et al. (1994). Cognitive functioning of patients with chronic fatigue syndrome. *Clinical Infectious Diseases, 18*(suppl 1), S84–85.

Kellner, R. (1991). Chronic fatigue syndrome and fatigue. In *Psychosomatic syndromes and somatic symptoms.* Washington, DC: American Psychiatric Press, Inc., pp. 31–51.

Kruesi, M.J.P., Dale, J., & Straus, S.E. (1989). Psychiatric diagnoses in patients who have chronic fatigue syndrome. *Journal of Clinical Psychiatry, 50,* 53–56.

Lynch, S., Seth, R., & Montgomery, S. (1991). Antidepressant therapy in the chronic fatigue syndrome. *British Journal of General Practice, 41,* 339–342.

Manu, P., Matthews, D.A., & Lane, T.J. (1988). The mental health of patients with a chief complaint of chronic fatigue. *Archives of Internal Medicine, 148,* 2213–2217.

Manu, P., Matthews, D.A., Lane, T.J., et al. (1989). Depression among patients with a chief complaint of chronic fatigue. *Journal of Affective Disorders, 17,* 165–172.

Parker, A.J.R., Wessely, S., & Cleare, A.J. (2001). The neuroendocrinology of chronic fatigue syndrome and fibromyalgia. *Psychological Medicine, 31,* 1331–1345.

Prins, J.B., Bleijenberg, G., Bazelmans, E., et al. (2001). Cognitive behavior therapy for chronic fatigue syndrome: A multicentre randomised controlled trial. *Lancet, 357,* 841–847.

Schweitzer, R., Robertson, D.L., Kelly, B., et al. (1994). Illness behavior of patients with chronic fatigue syndrome. *Journal of Psychosomatic Research, 1,* 41–49.

Sharpe, M.C., Johnson, B.A., & McCann, J. (1991). Mania and recovery from chronic fatigue syndrome. *Journal of the Royal Society of Medicine, 84,* 51–54.

Uhlenhuth, E.H., Turner, D.A., Purchatzke, G., et al. (1997). Intensive design in evaluating anxiolytic agents. *Psychopharmacology* (Berlin), *52,* 79–85.

Vercoulen, J.H.M.M., Swanink, C.M.A., Zinnan, F.G., et al. (1996). Randomized, double-blind, placebo controlled study of fluoxetine in chronic fatigue syndrome. *Lancet, 347,* 858–861.

Verhaest, S., & Pierloot, R. (1989). An attempt at an empirical delimitation of neurasthenic neurosis and its relation with some character traits. *Acta Psychiatry Scandinavia, 62,* 166–176.

Wessely, S., Chalder, T., Hirsch, S., et al. (1995). Postinfecticus fatigue—prospective cohort study in primary care. *Lancet, 345,* 1333–1338.

Wessely, S., & Sharpe, M. (1995). Chronic fatigue, chronic fatigue syndrome, and fibromyalgia. In R. Mayou, C. Bass, & M. Sharpe (Eds.), *Treatment of functional somatic symptoms.* Oxford, UK: Oxford University Press, pp. 285–312.

Wilson, A., Hickie, L., Lloyd, A., et al. (1994). Longitudinal study of outcome of chronic fatigue syndrome. *British Medical Journal, 308,* 756–759.

Wolfe, F., Smythe, H.A., Yunus, M.B., et al. (1990). The American College of Rheumatology 1990 criteria for classification of fibromyalgia: Report of the multi-center criteria committee. *Arthritis Rheumatology, 33,* 160–172.

CHAPTER 36

The Patient with Multiple Environmental Allergies/Idiopathic Environmental Intolerance

SUSAN ABBEY AND THEODORE A. STERN

I. Introduction

Multiple environmental allergies, multiple chemical sensitivity, environmental illness, environmental hypersensitivity disorder, chemical hypersensitivity syndrome, chemically-induced immune dysregulation syndrome, ecologic illness, total allergy syndrome, and twentieth-century disease have all been described in the medical literature. **It is unclear whether these disorders differ in more than name. Primary care management is the same for all these disorders.**

A. **The prevalence** of these processes is poorly defined. Women are overrepresented in most clinical settings. Recent studies have suggested that up to 20% of the population report hypersensitivity to at least one everyday chemical but less than 1% meet any of the diagnostic criteria that have been proposed.

B. **Intense controversy surrounds these diagnoses.** Clinical ecologists endorse them, while conventional medicine has concluded that they do not constitute distinct clinical syndromes. Clinical ecologists attribute them to low-level environmental exposure to chemicals that generally are considered safe and do not affect the rest of the population, resulting in multi-systemic symptoms. Conventional medicine does not support this view.

C. **Subjective symptoms are the hallmarks of these diagnoses.**

D. **Familiarity with the approach of clinical ecology and complementary or alternative environmental practitioners** to these disorders is important so that a primary care practitioner can build a therapeutic alliance with patients. Different mechanisms have been suggested for the development of these diagnoses. These mechanisms have different degrees of personal responsibility for symptom production; thus, perceived blame-worthiness is associated with some of them.

   1. **Clinical ecology proposes the following mechanisms:**
      a. Immunotoxicity of chemicals and foods
      b. Chemicals and foods that act via the olfactory nerve to activate the limbic system
      c. Impaired ability to detoxify environmental chemicals

   2. Conventional medicine proposes the following mechanisms:
      a. Learned response-conditioned responses that pair odors and autonomic symptoms of other origins
      b. Psychiatric disorders (e.g., somatoform disorder, mood and anxiety disorders)
      c. Social processes, including "mass hysteria"
      d. Iatrogenesis

E. **Misdiagnosis** of patients with well-defined toxic or allergic disease or irritant injuries as having one of these syndromes will preclude effective treatment by conventional medicine.

II. Evaluation of the Problem

A. General Recommendations

1. **Build an alliance** in order to work effectively with these patients. They often report unsatisfactory prior encounters with the medical profession.
   a. **Avoid debates about the validity of clinical ecology** and these diagnoses.
   b. **Focus on the potential for symptomatic relief** and improved quality of life which conventional medical approaches may offer.
   c. **Emphasize that rehabilitation is used successfully** for many chronic illnesses.
2. **Set achievable goals** for treatment. The goals should be specific, measurable, and relevant to the patient.
3. **Take a longer-term perspective.** Slow progress is better than setting overwhelming goals which cannot be met and which lead to abandonment of treatment.
4. **Consider referral to an occupational and environmental medicine specialist** to help make a diagnosis and to develop a management plan.
5. **Refer to experts in the area when compensation issues arise** so that the primary care practitioner is free to focus on working with the patient.

B. Medical History

1. **Review medical records** for evidence of past medical or psychiatric disorders which may have relevance to the patient's current problems.
2. **Review work and residential exposure information**, if relevant. Most primary care practitioners prefer to have this done by a specialist in occupational and environmental medicine as part of a consultation.

C. Interview

1. The basic interview may require several sessions to complete. Patients need to "feel heard" to engage in treatment.
2. **The basic interview should include a review** of the following:
   a. **Symptoms and their impact on quality of life.** Detail the frequency, severity, and impact on daily functioning and on quality of life of each symptom.
   b. **Avoided activities.** Specify situations and activities which the patient avoids.
   c. **Relationship between symptoms and exposure.** Review from the patient's perspective the exposure history at work and at home. Do symptoms always occur with exposure, or are there times when exposure produces no symptoms or when symptoms occur without exposure?
   d. **Review of systems** to rule out treatable medical disorders. Patients who present with these diagnoses may have undiagnosed medical disorders which can be treated. These patients have associated co-morbid contentious diagnoses, such as chronic fatigue syndrome or fibromyalgia.
   e. **Past personal and family history of medical and psychiatric disorders.** If the patient is resistant, explain that these are important "vulnerabilities" for slow recovery rather than being an implication that the patient's difficulties are "all in the head." Ask about earlier episodes of depression, anxiety disorders, and a history of trauma.
   f. **Current social situation and stressors.** These areas should be left until later in the interview or for subsequent interviews when the patient is more comfortable. Asking about the impact of an illness on a patient's life is better accepted than is asking directly about stressors, as stressors imply psychogenesis to most patients.

D. Examination of the Patient

1. **The mental status examination** is directed toward reviewing the symptoms and signs of psychiatric and neurologic disorders and should include assessment of the following:

   a. Mood and anxiety symptoms

   b. Suicidal ideation

   c. Thought form

   d. Thought content

   e. Cognitive functioning

2. **Physical examination** of the patient is typically normal but should focus on examination of the skin, eyes, and oropharynx for evidence of inflammation, as well as the lymph nodes, liver, and spleen.

3. **Laboratory examination** is used to rule out treatable medical disorders that contribute to the patient's presentation. Immunologic testing is not indicated and should be reserved for research settings.

   a. **Specific assessment of central nervous system function is not indicated unless it is needed to rule out other medical disorders.** Neuropsychological testing, neuroimaging (e.g., positron emission tomography [PET], single photon emission tomography [SPECT], and magnetic resonance imaging [MRI]) and neurophysiological techniques (e.g., electroencephalography [EEG], quantitative EEG, brain electrical activity mapping, and evoked potentials) are not useful in making these diagnoses and are appropriate only in research settings.

4. **Diagnostic tests** used by clinical ecologists which have not been validated by the standards of conventional medicine include exposure via sublingual drops and intradermal injections, the use of "neutralizing" substances to counteract the exposures, and the assessment of changes in pupil diameter and posture after exposure.

III. Psychiatric Differential Diagnosis

Psychiatric symptomatology is common but not universal in patients with these syndromes. No evidence of current psychological disturbance can be found in up to 25% of these patients. The increased prevalence of psychiatric symptomatology has led to an unhelpful debate about whether this constitutes evidence that psychiatric disorders are the causes or sequelae of these diagnoses. Identification of current psychiatric symptoms opens the door to treatments that may improve quality of life and functional status.

A. **The following psychiatric disorders should be considered** in the course of the interview and mental status examination.

1. **Somatoform Disorders**

   a. **A somatization disorder occurs before the onset of symptoms in up to 25%** of individuals with these syndromes, in contrast to a community prevalence of 0.1–2%.

   b. Hypochondriasis may form part of the presentation in some patients.

   c. Conversion disorder has been described in some sufferers.

2. **Mood Disorders**

   a. **Major depression has been diagnosed in up to 25% of these patients.**

   b. **Pre-existing major depression has been reported in nearly half of these sufferers.**

3. Anxiety Disorders

a. Many symptoms of these diagnoses are autonomic in origin and overlap with common symptoms of anxiety disorders (e.g., tachycardia, light-headedness, and breathlessness).

b. **Panic disorder is the most common anxiety disorder diagnosed in these patients and has been identified as a current problem in up to 25% of patients** and as an antecedent in up to 10%.

c. **Generalized anxiety (GAD) has been identified in up to 10% of patients** and found as a pre-existing problem in as many as 6%.

d. Two broad categories of post-traumatic stress disorder (PTSD) have been described in these patients.

　i. Industrial accidents or threatening exposures followed by the development of symptoms.

　ii. Adult sequelae of childhood physical and sexual abuse. The relationship between the abuse and the symptoms is poorly understood but may include psychophysiologic reactions which arose at the time of the initial abuse and are re-experienced and attributed to an environmental exposure and exposure as an adult to odors reminiscent of the offender, such as after-shave lotion, which precipitate panic reactions.

4. **Psychotic disorders.** Delusional disorder of the somatic subtype and schizophrenia have been described in a small number of these patients. The focus of the delusional material is related to themes of environmental exposure or contamination.

5. **Eating Disorders.** Anorexia nervosa may be misdiagnosed as multiple food hypersensitivity or may result from rotational diets.

6. **Malingering.** Malingering must always be considered in individuals who present with poorly understood physical symptoms and who are seeking compensation. Primary care practitioners are not in a position to make this diagnosis.

IV. Diagnostic Criteria

A. No specific symptom pattern defines these diagnoses.

B. No specific diagnostic criteria have been agreed on. There are at least four case definitions with a most recent 1999 consensus criteria. Attempts to develop research criteria for the diagnosis of multiple chemical sensitivity are the most highly developed. The 1999 consensus criteria include: (1) a chronic condition; (2) symptoms that recur reproducibly; (3) symptoms in response to low levels of exposure; (4) symptoms to multiple unrelated chemicals; (5) improvement or resolution when incitants are removed; (6) symptoms that occur in multiple organ symptoms.

C. No diagnostic laboratory tests exist.

V. Treatment Strategies

A. Treatment is directed toward improving function and providing relief of symptoms. Improved function may occur independently of symptom cessation; that is, the patient is able to maintain function and cope better with symptoms which continue to occur but that no longer disrupt occupational and social functioning.

B. Individualized treatment is targeted to the relevant aspects of a given patient's situation.

C. Successful treatment is based on a good working alliance with the patient. This requires that the primary care practitioner do the following:

1. **Convey interest and concern** about the patient.
2. **Do not debate the validity of the diagnosis.** Confrontation with these patients only increases their suffering and makes it less likely that they will accept treatment. Etiology is not always relevant to treatment; for example, treatments for depression are effective independent of its etiology.
3. **Defuse stigma** by not implying culpability for the symptoms.
4. **Avoid being judgmental about alternative therapies.** Encourage the patient to assess the potential risks of those therapies and educate the patient about the lack of evidence for their efficacy.
5. **Emphasize the "caring" of rehabilitation** rather than "curing" component.

D. **Encourage discontinuation of unnecessary** treatments which limit the patient's activity.
1. Many clinical ecology treatments unnecessarily limit the patient. Rehabilitation involves decreasing or eliminating the use of such treatments. Nasal oxygen is an example. Discontinuation of this treatment may require a graded decrease in oxygen use or monitoring via arterial blood gases to convince the patient of the safety of discontinuation. Examples of other treatments involving substantial alteration in lifestyle, significant avoidance behavior, social isolation, or other potential serious outcomes include the following:
   a. Nutritional treatments, including rotational diets which may lead to malnutrition
   b. Anti-*Candida* treatments, including dietary modifications, nutritional support, and antifungal medications (some of which are hepatotoxic)
   c. Detoxification, using dietary modifications and sauna chamber treatments
   d. Identification of substances associated with symptoms and then encouragement of avoidance or "immunotherapy" to reduce reactivity
   e. Implementation of major changes in the home environment: environmentally "safe" rooms or houses in which synthetic environmental contaminants which may "off-gas" are eliminated; steel, cotton, tiles, specially filtered air, and water delivery systems

E. **Encourage strategies aimed at reducing stress**
1. Stress is associated with worse functioning in a wide variety of medical and psychiatric disorders. Stress management can be facilitated through the development of skills related to the following:
   a. Decreasing the sources of stress (e.g., time management, effective communication, assertiveness training, and life skills training)
   b. Decreasing the psychophysiologic response to stress (e.g., relaxation techniques, meditation, yoga, and biofeedback)
2. Referral for professional help may be required if marital or family problems or financial stressors are significant.

F. **Treat identified psychiatric disorders**
1. **Facilitate acceptance of treatment** by explaining the following:
   a. **The use of psychiatric treatments does not mean that the cause of the symptoms is psychiatric.** Many patients will acknowledge psychiatric symptoms and attribute them to the neurotoxic effects of environmental chemicals.
   b. Psychiatric treatments are a concrete, practical step that can be undertaken to treat one part of the problem: "Let's treat what we can treat since there isn't a specific treatment for the syndrome."

2. **Pharmacotherapy is used when there are target symptoms,** such as depression, panic attacks, insomnia, generalized anxiety, and somatic manifestations of anxiety, such as palpitations or tremors.
   a. Facilitate treatment by doing the following:
      i. Explain that psychotropic medications have a variety of actions, including analgesia and sedation, and are used because of these actions in a number of "non-psychiatric conditions."
      ii. Deal directly with concerns about the use of "chemicals." Fears of further "damage" from "industrially-produced" medications are reasonable in the context of the patient's belief system and must be allayed.
      iii. Draw parallels with other medical disorders, such as the use of antidepressants in depressed cardiac or HIV-infected patients. While antidepressants may improve mood and level of functioning, no one would conclude that all of these disorders are due to depression.
      iv. Use a collaborative model that involves the patient and the physician to "explore the potential benefits of pharmacotherapy."
   b. Document target symptoms in terms of intensity, frequency, and impact on behavior. Monitor the effects of treatment against these target symptoms to determine whether the positive effects of treatment outweigh the associated side effects.
   c. Choose psychotropic medication on the basis of **target symptoms and clinician preference.**
      i. **Antidepressants** are used for depressive disorders and for other target symptoms, e.g., sleep disturbance. Antidepressants which have been used in this group include selective serotonin reuptake inhibitors (also effective for panic disorder and generalized anxiety disorder [GAD]), venlafaxine, nefazodone, bupropion, and tricyclic antidepressants, such as nortriptyline and desipramine.
      ii. **Benzodiazepines** are generally second- or third-line treatments. They play a role in the treatment of panic disorder and GAD, but must be used with care because of the possibility of the patients developing dependence and abuse problems.
      iii. **Antipsychotics** used in low to average doses may be helpful in patients with a psychotic component to their illnesses.
      iv. **Sedative-hypnotics** may be required for patients with insomnia. Depression should first be ruled out.
   d. **"Start really low and go really slow."** Treatment should be tailored to the patient's ability to tolerate the side effects. Keep in mind that the goal is an adequate trial. It is better to reach an effective dose over several months than never to reach an effective dose because of the side effects related to an overly rapid escalation in dose. Increased sensitivity to the side effects of drugs is common in this patient group.

3. **Behavioral treatments target avoidance and seek to increase activity and reduce disability.** Breaking the association between experiencing symptoms and discontinuing activity is important. There is no evidence that the symptoms worsen the long-term outcome. There is evidence from a number of studies of the chronically ill that avoidance or discontinuation of activity is associated with significant psychosocial morbidity.
   a. **Graded exposure is the key.** Behavioral desensitization may be compared with immunologic desensitization, that is, beginning with minimal "doses" and increasing slowly. Structured approaches are best. Keeping a written record of activities is helpful.
   b. **"Self-management" techniques,** such as relaxation techniques, including breath-control techniques, and imagery-based techniques are important adjuncts to behavioral desensitization.

    c. **Exercise** that is based on graded increases in activity can be very helpful. Exercise increases the level of physical conditioning, provides exposure to autonomic symptoms with a clear explanation different from "allergy," and assists in desensitizing the patient to physical sensations.

    d. **Encourage social activity.** Start with the level of activity which the patient can tolerate and increase it slowly.

4. **Psychotherapy** or counseling is indicated when specific interpersonal or intrapsychic issues maintain disability.

5. **Critical incident counseling** has been advocated to minimize post-traumatic symptomatology for workplace exposures where multiple workers are involved, however the efficacy of this technique is controversial.

G. Identify and minimize social contributors to disability.

1. Involve family members and friends when appropriate. Education may help them support the patient's rehabilitation program.

2. Scrutinize self-help groups. Does the group have a philosophy of encouraging activity and overcoming symptoms, or does it encourage withdrawal and inactivity?

H. Referral for Specialist Psychiatric Opinion

1. Indications for referral include clarification of diagnostic questions regarding Axis I or Axis II contribution to the level of dysfunction; management of treatment-resistant mood, anxiety, or psychotic disorders; and assistance in the management of suicidal ideation or behavior.

2. Supportive explanations regarding the consultation are essential for the patient. Tell patients how the consultation will be helpful to you in treating them. Reassure them that the consultation is not evidence that you do not take them seriously or are "dumping them."

Suggested Readings

AAAAI Board of Directors (1999). Idiopathic environmental intolerances. *Journal of Allergy and Clinical Immunology, 103,* 36–40.

Aaron, L.A., & Buchwald, D. (2001). A review of the evidence for overlap among unexplained clinical conditions. *Annals of Internal Medicine, 134,* 868–881.

American Medical Association Council on Scientific Affairs. (1991). *Clinical Ecology,* CSA Report K. Chicago: American Medical Association.

Black, D.W., Okiishi, C., & Schlosser, S. (2000). A nine-year follow-up of people diagnosed with multiple chemical sensitivities. *Psychosomatics, 41,* 253–261.

Black, D.W. (2000). The relationship of mental disorders and idiopathic environmental intolerance. *Occupational Medicine, 15,* 557–570.

Bornschein, S., Hausteiner, C., Zilker, T., & Forstl, H. (2002). Psychiatric and somatic disorders and multiple sensitivity (MCS) in 264 "environmental patients." *Psychological Medicine, 32*(8), 1387–1394.

Editorial. (1986). Clinical ecology position statement. *Journal of Allergy and Clinical Immunology, 78*(2), 269.

Engel, C.C. Jr., Adkins, J.A., & Cowan, D.N. (2002). Caring for medically unexplained physical symptoms after toxic environmental exposures: Effects of contested causation. *Environmental Health Perspectives, 110*(Suppl 4), 641–647.

Gilbert, M.E. (2001). Does the kindling model of epilepsy contribute to our understanding of multiple chemical sensitivity? *Annals of the New York Academy of Science, 933,* 69–91.

Graveling, R.A., Pilkington, A., George, J.P., et al. (1999). A review of multiple chemical sensitivity. *Occupational and Environmental Medicine, 56,* 73–85.

Howard, L.M., & Wessely, S. (1993). The psychology of multiple allergy. *British Medical Journal, 307,* 747–748.

Labarge, X.S., & McCaffrey, R.J. (2000). Multiple chemical sensitivity: A review of the theoretical and research literature. *Neuropsychology Review, 10,* 183–211.

Magill, M.K., & Suruda, A. (1998). Multiple chemical sensitivity syndrome. *American Family Physician, 58,* 721–728.

McKeown-Eyssen, G.E., Baines, C.J., Marshall, L.M., et al. (2001). Multiple chemical sensitivity: Discriminant validity of case definitions. *Archives of Environmental Health, 56,* 406–412.

Reid, S. (1999). Multiple chemical sensitivity—is the environment really to blame? *Journal of the Royal Society of Medicine, 92,* 616–619.

Rest, K.M. (1992). Advancing the understanding of multiple chemical sensitivity (MCS): Overview and recommendations from an AOEC workshop. In K.M. Rest (Ed.), *Advancing the understanding of multiple chemical sensitivity.* Princeton, N.J.: Princeton Scientific Publishing, pp. 1–14.

Salvaggio, J.E. (1991). Clinical and immunologic approach to patients with alleged environmental injury. *Annals of Allergy, 66,* 493–503.

Selner, J.C., & Staudenmayer, H. (1992). Psychological factors complicating the diagnosis of work-related chemical illness. *Immunology and Allergy Clinics of North America, 12*(4), 909–919.

Simon, O., Katon, W., & Sparks, P. (1990). Allergic to life: Psychological factors in environmental illness. *American Journal of Psychiatry, 140,* 901–906.

Simon, G., Daniell, W., Stockbridge, H., et al. (1993). Immunologic, psychological and neuropsychological factors in multiple chemical sensitivity: A controlled study. *Annals of Internal Medicine, 119,* 97–103.

Simon, G.E. (1992). Psychiatric treatments in multiple chemical sensitivity. In K.M. Rest (Ed.), *Advancing the understanding of multiple chemical sensitivity.* Princeton, N.J.: Princeton Scientific Publishing, pp. 67–72.

Sparks, P.J. (2000). Idiopathic environmental intolerances: Overview. *Occupational Medicine, 15*(3), 497–510.

Sparks, P.J. (2000). Diagnostic evaluation and treatment of the patient presenting with idiopathic environmental intolerance. *Occupational Medicine, 15*(3), 601–609.

Sparks, P.J., Daniell, W., Black, D.W., et al. (1994). Multiple chemical sensitivity: A clinical perspective: I. Case definition, theories of pathogenesis, and research needs. *Journal of Occupational Medicine, 36,* 731–737.

Sparks, P.J., Daniell, W., Black, D.W., et al. (1994). Multiple chemical sensitivity: A clinical perspective: II. Evaluation, diagnostic testing, treatment, and social considerations. *Journal of Occupational Medicine, 36,* 731–737.

Staudenmayer, H. (2000). Psychological treatment of psychogenic idiopathic environmental intolerance. *Journal of Occupational Medicine, 15*(3), 627–646.

Staudenmayer, H., Selner, M.E., & Selner, J.C. (1993). Adult sequelae of childhood abuse presenting as environmental illness. *Annals of Allergy, 71,* 538–546.

Terr, A.I. (1994). Multiple chemical sensitivities. *Journal of Allergy Clinical Immunology, 94,* 362–366.

Waddell, W.J. (1993). The science of toxicology and its relevance to MCS. *Regulation Toxicology Pharmacology, 18,* 13–22.

CHAPTER 37

The Patient with Irritable Bowel Syndrome

KEVIN W. OLDEN

I. Introduction

A. Definition

1. Irritable bowel syndrome (IBS) is a motor disorder of the bowel characterized by abdominal pain, altered stool form, altered stool consistency, and variable degrees of abdominal bloating, rectal urgency, perception of incomplete evacuation, and passage of stool mucus.

2. An international working team has developed standardized diagnostic criteria also known as the "Rome" criteria (Table 37-1). IBS almost always develops in adolescence and young adulthood.

B. Etiology

1. **IBS is not a psychiatric disorder. Although IBS is often associated with a variety of psychiatric conditions, particularly anxiety, mood and somatoform disorders, there is no evidence that IBS has a psychiatric etiology.**

2. IBS is not associated with any mucosal abnormality of the gut. Studies have demonstrated a wide variety of motor abnormalities involving not only the colon but also the esophagus, small bowel, and stomach. IBS can also be associated with a variety of extraintestinal symptoms including urinary urgency, headaches, and low back pain.

3. There are distinct differences between those **patients** with IBS who seek care and those who do not. **IBS** care seekers tend to have more psychological distress and poorer coping strategies than non-care seekers.

C. Epidemiology

1. Studies have shown that 10–22% of adults in Europe and North America meet the diagnostic criteria for IBS. The syndrome seems to have a similar prevalence in Asia, Africa, and South America.

Table 37-1. Diagnostic Criteria for Irritable Bowel Syndrome (Rome II Criteria)

At least 12 weeks or more, which need not be consecutive, in the preceding 12 months of abdominal discomfort or pain that has two out of three features:

(1) Relieved with defecation; and/or

(2) Onset associated with a change in frequency of stool; and/or

(3) Onset associated with a change in form (appearance) of stool.

---

2. IBS is more common in women. Most studies have demonstrated that 50–75% of patients with IBS who seek medical attention are women. In India, however, men are more likely to seek care for IBS.

3. IBS is common across ethnic groups. Studies have shown a prevalence of IBS between 10 and 30% among Africans, Europeans, East Indians, and Hispanics, and slightly lower in Southeast Asians.

D. Care-Seeking Behavior

1. **Despite being a common disorder, only 36% of men and 44% of women with IBS seek care. These later patients are more likely to show evidence of psychosocial distress.** Studies have shown that IBS care-seekers have elevated levels of anxiety, depression, and somatization as measured by standard psychological tests, including the Minnesota Multiphasic Personality Inventory (MMPI) and the Hopkins Symptom Checklist-90 (SCL-90).

2. IBS care-seekers are more likely to have a history of functional abdominal pain in childhood. IBS patients who seek care are more likely to somatize intra-familial conflicts.

E. Health Care Costs

1. It is estimated that productivity loss and allied health care costs caused by IBS exceed $20 billion annually in the United States.

2. IBS patients who seek care tend to be heavy users of health care services. They score higher on pain, illness-induced life disruption, and denial of psychological stressors on standardized scales, such as the Illness Behavior Questionnaire, and are more likely to have abnormal personality profiles on the MMPI.

3. In addition IBS patients enjoy poorer quality of life than do patients with other chronic medical conditions.

II. Evaluation of the Problem

A. General Recommendations

1. IBS can be a diagnosis of exclusion. **If the patient does not meet the Rome Criteria or if "alarm symptoms" are present, further work-up should be considered.** In this setting organic causes of diarrhea, abdominal pain, or constipation need to be evaluated in their own right. The clinician is cautioned, however, to avoid redundant or unnecessary work-up. Recent evidence has shown that absent "alarm symptoms" (see Table 37-2). The sensitivity and specificity of the Rome II Criteria is quite good.

2. Work-up of a functional complaint needs to be guided by specific findings obtained on history and physical examination. Symptoms suggestive of structural GI lesions (e.g., rectal bleeding, weight loss, or age of onset of symptoms in middle or late life) demand work-up on their own merit. Work-up should not be initiated for a complaint of "abdominal pain" *per se.*

3. The patient who meets the Rome criteria, has age-appropriate onset, and lacks abnormal findings on physical examination or routine screening laboratory studies can be safely diagnosed with IBS using the Rome Criteria. This is known as a "positive approach" to IBS diagnosis.

B. Medical History

1. Historical factors that suggest a diagnosis of IBS include absence of symptoms (particularly pain and diarrhea) when sleeping, age of onset under 40 years of age, and an alternating pattern of constipation and diarrhea.

Table 37-2. Clinical and Laboratory Findings Not Consistent with IBS

A. History Inconsistent with IBS

Diarrhea or pain that awakens the patient from sleep

Occult blood positivity

Painless diarrhea

Rapid onset of symptoms (as opposed to gradual onset)

Rectal bleeding

Weight loss

B. Laboratory Findings Inconsistent with IBS

Anemia

Elevated erythrocyte sedimentation rate (ESR)

Elevated liver studies

Qualitative stool fat positivity

Stool leukocytes on Wright stain

---

2. IBS can be confused with inflammatory bowel disease (IBD). There are a number of clinical and laboratory variables, however, that can differentiate the two disorders (Table 37-2).
3. A flexible sigmoidoscopy with rectal biopsy is mandatory in any diarrheal illness.
4. The differential diagnosis of constipation and diarrhea is extensive. In a patient with expected IBS, dietary history, particularly the use of non-absorbable sugars such as sorbitol or fructose, can often explain symptoms of diarrhea and bloating.
   a. Recent travel and medication usage can also direct the physician toward the need for specific work-up. Certainly, a history of travel to endemic areas warrants obtaining stool ova and parasite studies. Medication history should be taken to elicit use of medications that can cause bloating, constipation, or diarrhea. Any acute diarrhea should be evaluated with a stool culture and flexible sigmoidoscopy.
   b. The differential diagnosis of IBS-like symptoms is shown in Table 37-3.

Table 37-3. Conditions That Can Mimic IBS

Early HIV infection (chronic diarrhea)

Hyper- and hypothyroidism

Infectious diarrhea

Inflammatory bowel disease (IBD)

Ingestion of non-absorbable sugars (sorbitol, fructose, mannitol)

Lactose intolerance

Medication-induced bowel dymotility

Celiac disease

C. Interview

1. **IBS is often related to life stressors.** The clinician should make every effort to investigate for current and past stressors in the patient's life.

2. Sexual and physical abuse have been associated with IBS.

   a. Patients with a history of sexual and/or physical abuse have an increased prevalence of anxiety disorders, depression, somatoform disorders and post-traumatic stress disorder.

   b. The presence of a positive sexual or physical abuse history is often associated with poor health status, including more pain, number of surgeries, days spent in bed, and difficulty dealing with activities of daily living.

   c. Patients are unlikely to volunteer information about abuse. It is incumbent on the physician to inquire about these issues. This is particularly true with "refractory" patients who have not responded to conservative management.

   d. Other forms of trauma, including war survivor status, should also be investigated.

3. The physician should also investigate specific life symptoms that exacerbate the patient's symptoms. Work stressors, family difficulties, and social discord in any number of settings can all exacerbate IBS symptoms.

D. Examination of the Patient

1. IBS, being a motor disorder of the bowel, has no associated structural lesion and few findings on physical examination. There are certain findings that, although not diagnostic, certainly suggest IBS. **A firm, palpable sigmoid colon on physical examination can be suggestive of IBS.**

2. **The physical examination** should be directed at detecting other possible causes of IBS-like symptoms.

   a. HEENT: Goiter, proptosis (hyperthyroidism), thrush (AIDS), adenopathy (AIDS/lymphoma)

   b. Chest exam: Wheezing (carcinoid)

   c. Cardiac tricuspid murmur (carcinoid), mitral valve prolapse (possible concomitant panic disorder)

   d. Abdomen: Left lower quadrant tenderness (diverticulitis), masses, organomegaly, fistulae (Crohn's disease), mass or occult blood, or rectal bleeding

   e. Skin: Wasting, arthritis, or skin rashes (Pyoderma gangrenosum)

   f. Sigmoidoscopy: Ulcers, friability (IBD, infectious colitis), melanosis coli (laxative abuse), or masses (carcinoma)

3. **Laboratory studies:** In general, laboratory studies should be kept to the minimum required to rule out the most common causes of diarrhea and constipation. Invasive studies, like colonoscopy, ERCP, or laparoscopy, should only be performed if findings from initial blood work, physical exam, or sigmoidoscopy warrant them. The following laboratory studies are recommended:

   a. CBC: To rule out occult blood loss, IBD, and malabsorption

   b. ESR: Almost always elevated in IBD and other inflammatory diseases of the bowel. Normal in IBS.

   c. Stool Wright stain for fecal leukocytes: Can be seen with any inflammatory condition of the bowel

   d. Stool culture: For acute diarrhea

   e. Chemistry panel: To evaluate electrolytes (hypokalemia seen in a secretory diarrhea), phosphorus and calcium (elevated in hyperparathyroidism, which can give constipation). Liver enzymes (elevated in biliary tract disease). Obtaining serum amylase and lipase can screen for diarrhea caused by chronic pancreatitis.

      f. Thyroid function studies: To detect diarrhea or constipation induced by hyperthyroidism or hypothyroidism, respectively.

   4. Studies that are not recommended in the initial evaluation of IBS:

      a. Ova and parasite studies: Rarely positive in patients with IBS-like symptoms. An exception is the patient who gives a travel history to endemic areas, especially exposure to *Giardia lamblia,* which can cause symptoms of bloating and flatulence similar to IBS.

      b. Invasive studies to evaluate a patient's complaint of abdominal pain: The use of ERCP, laparoscopy, and CT scanning rarely yields positive results unless data from the initial level of evaluation generate an indication to perform more invasive studies. For example, a complaint of right upper quadrant pain should not lead to ERCP unless there are abnormal liver studies or abnormalities on biliary ultrasound.

III. Psychiatric Differential Diagnosis

A. Definition
   1. Patients with IBS have been found to have a 50–94% lifetime prevalence of Axis I psychiatric disorders. This is higher than the prevalence in normal controls and in patients with structural GI disorders. In addition, certain psychiatric diagnoses are particularly associated with IBS, including panic disorder, major depressive disorder, and somatization disorder.

B. Panic Disorder (See also Chapter 16)
   1. Forty-four percent of patients with panic disorder display GI symptoms and 25% meet the Rome criteria for IBS.

   2. The onset of GI symptoms frequently is concomitant with the panic symptoms. Treatment of panic disorder often leads to improvement in both the symptoms of IBS as well as the patient's panic symptoms.

C. Major Depressive Disorder (See also Chapter 14)
   1. Numerous studies have suggested that the prevalence of major depressive disorder in IBS is 8–50%. IBS patients have approximately twice the rate of depression as normal controls.

   2. There is some evidence to suggest that the constipation-predominant form of **IBS** may be more commonly associated with major depressive disorder.

   3. Identifying and treating the depressive illness can lessen GI symptoms, relieve the patients' level of distress about their bowel symptoms, and improve the symptoms of depression.

D. Post-Traumatic Stress Disorder (PTSD) (See also Chapter 56)
   1. The high prevalence of physical and sexual abuse in patients with IBS often leads to a concomitant diagnosis of PTSD. One study demonstrated a 36% prevalence of PTSD in IBS patients. Forty-eight percent identified physical or sexual abuse as the precipitant.

   2. It is important to note that many IBS patients can suffer PTSD without a history of abuse; therefore, history-taking should not be limited only to abuse.

E. Somatization Disorder (See also Chapter 29)
   1. One of the most challenging situations for the primary care physician (PCP) is managing the IBS patient with somatization disorder. These patients are intensely invested in a physical complaint, usually have other organ system complaints in

addition to their bowel complaint, and have a great deal of difficulty acknowledging emotional and social issues. Identification of somatization disorder is critical in that the management of these patients requires a more comprehensive approach.

F. Obsessive-Compulsive Disorder (OCD) (See also Chapter 19)

1. Many clinicians refer to patients who are focused on their bowels as having "bowel obsessions." This term lacks definition, however. Studies have suggested up to a 44% prevalence of IBS in obsessive-compulsive disorder (OCD) patients seeking treatment. Similar to IBS patients with panic disorder, patients with co-morbid OCD and IBS will have improvement of their IBS as well as OCD symptoms when the latter is identified and treated.

2. OCD can greatly complicate the care of IBS patients because of their unrelenting obsessive concerns about symptoms, drug side effects, and prognosis. Failure to diagnose OCD will often prevent amelioration of the patient's GI symptoms.

IV. Treatment Strategies

A. The Doctor-Patient Relationship

1. The most powerful therapeutic instrument in treating IBS is an effective doctor-patient relationship. The physician who listens to the patient and takes a careful psychosocial history will succeed over colleagues who attempt only medical management.

2. There is a 20–90% placebo-response rate induced in any medical intervention offered to IBS patients, and it can be enhanced by an attentive, empathic physician.

B. Approach to the Patient

1. Prognosis in IBS is positively impacted by a "positive" doctor-patient relationship, consisting of the following:
   a. Taking a psychosocial history
   b. Inquiring about what led the patient to seek care at this time
   c. Discussing the patient's symptoms and concerns in detail

C. Medical Management

1. **Serotonergic drugs.** In the last three years, increasing recognition of the role of serotonin subtypes has led to the development of new IBS specific drugs. Two of these are currently available. The first is Alosetron (Lotronex®) which is a 5-HT$_3$ *antagonist* specifically designed for the treatment of IBS with accompanying diarrhea. It acts to slow GI transit time, decreases rectal urgency, cramping, and pain and improves stool consistency in patients with diarrhea predominant irritable bowel syndrome. This agent is currently available in the United States under a restricted prescribing program. This is due to the fact that one in 700 patients who receive this drug will develop ischemic colitis. The exact mechanism of why ischemic colitis develops in a small number of patients is not clear. It is important to note that the restricted prescribing program for this drug is not restricted to gastroenterologists and is open to any physician who is willing to self attest comfort and skill in diagnosis and treatment of IBS.

A second drug which is currently available in the U.S. for the treatment of IBS with constipation is Tegaserod (Zelnorm®). Tegaserod is a 5-HT$_4$ *partial agonist*. This drug is a very different molecule from Alosetron and is not associated with ischemic colitis. It has been approved for the treatment of IBS with constipation in women. The recommended dose for Alosetron is 1 mg per day and for Tegaserod is 6 mg twice a day.

Cilansetron, a new 5-HT$_3$ *antagonist,* is currently in clinical trials for the treatment of IBS with diarrhea; however, this drug has not yet been approved for use in the United States.

Finally, Dexloxiglumide, a novel agent which is a CCK$_1$A *antagonist,* is also in clinical trials for the treatment of IBS with constipation. Again, this drug is not yet available in the United States.

These and other agents represent a new era for the treatment of irritable bowel syndrome using drugs specifically designed for the treatment of the global constellation of symptoms associated with IBS, i.e., pain, bloating and altered bowel habit, either diarrhea or constipation. We can look forward to an increasing number of disorder specific agents to be developed in the coming years.

2. **IBS patients are very sensitive to medication side effects and they need to be instructed on possible side effects in advance.** Alerting patients to potential medication side effects will preclude the abrupt termination of medications and loss of trust in the physician.

3. Anti-spasmodics
    a. These agents are somewhat helpful for abdominal cramping.
    b. Hyoscyamine p.o. or sublingual 0.125 mg every 4 hours or in the sustained release capsule (Levsin extend tabs 0.375 mg) p.o. b.i.d. are commonly used.

4. Pro-kinetic agents
    a. Metoclopramide (Reglan) has no role in IBS because it has no effect on the colon and has a 25% prevalence of neuropsychiatric side effects.

5. Antidepressants
    Antidepressants play an important role in the treatment of IBS for a variety of reasons:
    a. They can be used to treat co-morbid anxiety and mood disorders.
    b. They can also be used for their "neuromodulatory" effect on gut perception.
    c. The best studied of the antidepressants is desipramine (50 to 150 mg q.h.s.) for relief of IBS. The efficacy of desipramine treatment seems equally successful in constipation- and diarrhea-predominant IBS. Its effect in IBS is also independent from its anticholinergic effect.
    d. A number of recent studies have suggested a role for SSRIs in the treatment of IBS.
    e. Physicians should try any antidepressant until one is found that improves symptoms and can be tolerated by the patient. In IBS uncomplicated by psychiatric co-morbidity the dosage of antidepressant used is usually lower than the dose used to treat mood disorders (Tables 37-4 and 37-5).

D. Diet
1. A high-fiber diet is usually prescribed for IBS patients. The data on its benefits are conflicting, but the general health benefits of fiber supports its use.
2. The patient must be warned not to use excessive fiber, which can result in bloating and diarrhea.

E. Psychotherapy
1. Psychotherapy is a powerful tool in treating **IBS,** particularly in patients who have psychiatric co-morbidity, especially somatization, or depression, and in those who have failed to respond to purely medical interventions.

Table 37-4. Antidepressant Dosages Used for IBS

Antidepressant	Usual Dosage (mg/day)
Amitriptyline	10–200
Citalopram	10–20
Desipramine	10–150
Doxepin	10–100
Fluoxetine	10–20
Fluvoxamine	25–50
Imipramine	10–150
Escitalopram	10–20
Nefazodone	50–200
Paroxetine	10–20
Trazodone	25–200
Sertraline	25–50
Venlafaxine	37.5–75

Table 37-5. GI Side Effects of Antidepressants

Antidepressant	Decreases Lower Esophageal Sphincter Pressure	Nausea	Vomiting	Diarrhea	Constipation	Cramping
Amitriptyline	+				+	
Imipramine	+				+	
Fluoxetine		+	+	+		+
Fluvoxamine		+	+	+		+
Nefazodone		+				
Paroxetine		+	+	+		+
Trazodone	+				+	
Sertraline		+	+	+		+
Venlafaxine		+				+

2. The literature supporting the use of psychotherapy is quite positive. Cognitive-behavioral, interpersonal, and psychodynamic approaches have all been shown to be helpful.

3. Psychodynamic and cognitive-behavioral therapy (CBT) have been the most studied.

4. Psychotherapy can result in up to a 75% reduction in health care use, and improved mood and GI status as well as GI symptoms.

Suggested Readings

Boyce, P.M., Gilchrist, J., Talley, N.J., et al. (2000). Cognitive behavioral therapy as a treatment for irritable bowel syndrome. *Australian New Zealand Journal of Psychiatry, 34,* 461–469.

Budavari, A.I., & Olden, K.W. (2002). The use of antidepressants in irritable bowel syndrome. *Practical Gastroenterology, 26*(3), 13–27.

Drossman, D.A., Olden, K.W., Svedlund, J., et al. (2000). Psychosocial aspects of the functional gastrointestinal disorders. In D.A. Drossman, E. Corazziari, N.J. Talley, W.G. Thompson, & W.E. Whitehead (Eds.), *Rome II: The functional gastrointestinal disorders.* McLean: Degnon Associates, pp. 157–245.

Drossman, D.A., Talley, N.J., Leserman, J., et al. (1995). Sexual and physical abuse and gastrointestinal illness: Review and recommendations. *Annals of Internal Medicine, 123,* 782–794.

Drossman, D.A., & Thompson, W.G. (1992). The irritable bowel syndrome: Review and a graduated multicomponent treatment approach. *Annals of Internal Medicine, 116,* 1009–1016.

Francis, C.Y., & Whorwell, P.J. (1994). Bran and irritable bowel syndrome: Time for reappraisal. *Lancet, 344,* 39–40.

Greenbaum, D.S., Mayle, J.E., Vanegeren, L.E., et al. (1987). Effects of desipramine on irritable bowel syndrome compared with atropine and placebo. *Digestive Disease Science, 32,* 257–265.

Guthrie, E., Creed, F.H., Dawson, D., et al. (1993). A randomised controlled trial of psychotherapy in patients with refractory irritable bowel syndrome. *British Journal of Psychiatry, 163,* 315–321.

Herschbach, P., Henrich, G., & Von Rad, M. (1999). Psychological factors in functional gastrointestinal disorders: Characteristics of the disorder or the illness behavior? *Psychosomatic Medicine, 61,* 148–153.

Heymann-Monnikes, I., Arnold, R., Florin, I., et al. (2000). The combination of medical treatment plus multicomponent behavioral therapy is superior to medical treatment alone in the therapy of irritable bowel syndrome. *American Journal of Gastroenterology, 95,* 981–994.

Leserman, J., Drossman, D.A., Li, Z., et al. (1996). Sexual and physical abuse history in gastroenterology practice: How types of abuse impact health status. *Psychosomatic Medicine, 58,* 4–15.

Levy, R.L., Whitehead, W.E., Von Korff, M.R., et al. (2000). Intergenerational transmission of gastrointestinal illness behavior. *American Journal of Gastroenterology, 95*(2), 451–456.

North, C.S., & Alpers, D.H. (2000). Irritable bowel syndrome in a psychiatric patient population. *Comprehensive Psychiatry, 41*(2), 116–122.

Olden, K.W. (1996). *Handbook of functional gastrointestinal disorders.* New York: Marcel Dekker, Inc, pp. 1–402.

Olden, K.W., & Drossman, D.A. (2000). Psychological and psychiatric aspects of gastrointestinal disease. *Medical Clinics of North America, 84*(5), 1313–1327.

Owens, D.M., Nelson, D.K., & Talley, N.J. (1995). The irritable bowel syndrome: Long-term prognosis and the physician-patient interaction. *Annals of Internal Medicine, 122,* 107–112.

Smith, G.R., Rost, K., & Kashner, T.M. (1995). A trial of the effect of a standardized psychiatric consultation on health outcomes and costs in somatizing patients. *Archives of General Psychiatry, 52,* 238–243.

Stermer, E., Bar, H., & Levy, N. (1991). Chronic functional gastrointestinal symptoms in holocaust survivors. *American Journal of Gastroenterology, 86,* 417–422.

Tanum, L., & Malt, U.F. (2001). Personality and physical symptoms in nonpsychiatric patients with functional gastrointestinal disorders. *Journal of Psychosomatic Research, 50,* 139–146.

Vanner, S.J., Depew, W.T., Paterson, W.G., et al. (1999). Predictive value of the Rome criteria for diagnosing the irritable bowel syndrome. *American Journal of Gastroenterology, 94,* 2912–2917.

Walker, E.A., Katon, W.J., Hanscom, J., et al. (1995). Psychiatric diagnoses and serial victimization in women with chronic pelvic pain. *Psychosomatics, 36,* 531–540.

CHAPTER 38
The Patient with Cancer

MELISSA FRUMIN AND DONNA B. GREENBERG

I. Introduction

Cancer patients are living longer with their disease or are being completely cured. The psychiatric care of cancer patients can be important at all stages of the disease. Cancer and its treatment (e.g., chemotherapy and radiation therapy) can be toxic to the central nervous system (CNS) and can cause symptoms that mimic psychiatric illness. Adjustment reactions and co-morbid psychiatric syndromes can change a cancer patient's affect, behavior, and cognition.

A. Psychiatric syndromes in cancer patients
1. **Delirium, cognitive impairment, and changes in personality** can be caused by primary or metastatic disease to the brain. Pain medications, radiation treatment to the brain, and some chemotherapeutic agents can worsen cognition or cause delirium.
2. **Anxiety.** Fears of death, loss of control, abandonment, and changes in body image often accompany the diagnosis of cancer. Nausea and vomiting, initially associated with chemotherapy, can become a Pavlovian conditioned response to reminders of treatment. Claustrophobia may be a problem for a patient who needs magnetic resonance imaging or another type of imaging scan.
3. **Depression.** Major depressive disorders have a prevalence rate of 5–8% in the oncological population, as they do in patients with other medical illnesses. Chronic pain and a history of affective illness are risk factors for a depressive episode. Corticosteroids used in the treatment of cancer also predispose patients to depression.

II. Evaluation of the Problem

A. General approach
1. Cancer patients need to be evaluated in the context of the following factors:
    a. The phase and natural course of the cancer
    b. Present and past psychiatric illnesses
    c. Common complications of the treatment
    d. Adaptive and maladaptive responses to cancer

B. Medical history
1. **Review the medical record** to assess the stage of cancer, current treatments, likelihood of recurrence, toxicity of treatments, likelihood of CNS involvement, presence of emesis, and treatment consequences, such as loss of fertility.
2. **Review prior medical records,** which may give information about predisposing factors, such as previous treatments, substance abuse, or underlying medical conditions.

C. Interview
1. Cancer patients often seek medical attention at times of increased anxiety. **Begin by asking about the immediate concerns** of the patient. These concerns may include

physical symptoms which the patient fears could represent recurrent cancer. Any pain or lump is viewed as a possible sign of recurrent disease.

2. **Screen for past psychiatric illness.** Since major depression and anxiety syndromes are generally under-diagnosed, **the absence of a prior psychiatric diagnosis or treatment does not assure a healthy psychological history.** Screen for past depression, anxiety, and phobias. Persistent dysphoria, agitation, and insomnia may be mistakenly thought to indicate cancer symptoms rather than psychiatric illness, with a distinct natural history, that can be diagnosed and treated.

3. In **screening for depression** in a patient with cancer, it may be difficult to distinguish the neurovegetative symptoms of depression from the symptoms associated with cancer, since cancer and/or its treatment can cause lethargy, lack of appetite, poor sleep, and difficulty with concentration. To distinguish between the two, ask the following questions:

   a. How do you feel on a good day? How are your spirits when you have energy? Are you able to enjoy your customary activities?

   b. **Ask about suicidal thoughts.** Although relatively few patients with cancer attempt suicide, the risk of suicide is slightly increased compared with the general population. Some patients discuss suicide as a way to gain control over a situation in which they feel powerless or as an escape from an intolerable situation. Talking about suicide provides an opportunity to consider alternatives, to clarify fears, and to define the quality of life, the quality of care, and the limits of care a patient desires.

   c. Risk factors for suicide include advanced illness, poor prognosis, major depression, delirium, pain, loss of control, and a feeling of hopelessness. A personal history of a suicide attempt and/or a family history of suicide place a patient at increased risk.

   d. A patient who is actively suicidal should be placed in a secure environment and evaluated further.

4. **Screening for anxiety** is important in patients with cancer. Claustrophobia can interfere with obtaining imaging scans and radiation treatment. Patients can develop the conditioned response of anticipatory anxiety, nausea, and vomiting after emetic chemotherapy treatment. Risk factors for this conditioned anxiety include younger age, history of motion sickness, pre-morbid anxiety, and a greater number of emetic treatments.

5. **Cognitive impairment** can be tested initially with the Mini-Mental State Examination. If asked, patients may describe more subtle changes in thinking that disturb them and which may require more formal neuropsychological testing to clarify.

6. To assess **coping capacity** ask the patient and family the following questions:

   a. How did you cope with serious medical illness in the past?

   b. If this is a recurrence, how did you cope with the previous diagnosis and treatment?

   c. What are the stable relationships in your life?

   d. What additional resources can you draw on?

III. Adaptive versus Maladaptive Psychological Responses to Cancer

A. Pre-diagnosis

1. **Worrying enough** to seek medical advice about a physical symptom and the possibility of having cancer is adaptive.

2. **Hypervigilance** and an all-consuming preoccupation with the possible diagnosis, especially when that diagnosis is unlikely, constitute an abnormal response. Hypervigilance can also interfere with social and occupational functioning.

B. Diagnosis

1. **Patients may initially deny** or not believe the diagnosis, or minimize its severity. They may feel numb, frightened, or overwhelmed. A variably depressed mood in the first few months after the diagnosis can be a part of a normal response. Searching for hope in medical treatment can draw a patient's attention away from the trauma of diagnosis.

2. **Complete denial of the diagnosis prevents the patient from considering reasonable treatment choices. Hopelessness associated with a clinical depression can impair rational decision-making.**

C. Initial treatment

1. **Surgery. Grief reactions** to physical losses, such as an amputation or mastectomy, are common.

2. **Radiation.** A patient may fear radiation therapy and its toxicity to normal tissues. Uncontrolled pain or claustrophobia can make it difficult for a patient to remain calm, still, or isolated during treatment.

3. **Chemotherapy.** Fear of the side effects of nausea and vomiting may ensue. Loss of hair can be especially difficult for women. A host of commonly used drugs cause transient delirium (Table 38-1). Steroids, and some chemotherapeutic agents and biological treatments can cause delirium as well as depression, mania, and psychotic syndromes.

D. Post-treatment

1. After treatment, a patient will return to the pressures of life changed by the experience and anxious about the possibility of disease progression. Sometimes the emotional recognition of the trauma is delayed until the medical treatment has been completed. Anticipatory anxiety runs high before check-ups and imaging procedures, and worry often accompanies every ache or pain.

2. Depression or severe hypervigilance can prevent a patient from returning to their previous level of functioning.

E. Recurrence

1. Recurrence of a cancer is difficult and often devastating. Similar to the time of initial diagnosis, there is shock, anger, and disbelief, but the feelings at the time of recurrence are usually intensified. This is a time when unconventional treatments or second opinions are sought.

F. Terminal care/palliation

1. During the final stage, patients may fear abandonment, uncontrolled pain, indignity, and confusion. Expert palliative care focuses on symptom relief and care which reflects the patient's wishes. This is a time to take care of unfinished business and continue doing what is both valuable and possible each day.

IV. Psychiatric Symptoms with Medical Etiologies

A. Medical and neurologic illness in cancer patients can mimic primary psychiatric illnesses, such as anxiety, depression, and psychosis (see Table 38-1).

B. Medical conditions which mimic anxiety

1. **Akathisia.** Dopamine antagonists, such as perphenazine, prochlorphenazine, and droperidol, which are used commonly as anti-emetics, can cause restlessness and the

Table 38-1. Neuropsychiatric Side Effects of Drugs Used in Cancer

Drug	*Comments*
Hormones	
Corticosteroids	Insomnia, lability, depression, psychosis, and mania are dose-related
Tamoxifen	Exacerbation of menopausal symptoms
Anastrazole, letrozole	Hot flashes, asthenia, flu-like syndrome
Anticancer agents	
Procarbazine	Somnolence, psychosis, and delirium coincide with treatment
L-Asparaginase	Somnolence, lethargy, and delirium are common
Ifosfamide	Lethargy, seizures, and dysarthria are more common with renal impairment
Cytarabine	Delirium and cerebellar signs are related to dose and age
5-Fluorouracil	Delirium and cerebellar signs are uncommon
Methotrexate	Transient delirium is uncommon; white matter injury may be delayed
Vincristine, Vinblastine, Vinorelbine	Dysphoria, lethargy, and seizures
Paclitaxel	Used with steroids. Often causes fatigue associated with toxic sensory neuropathy
Gemcitabine	Flu-like syndrome with fatigue
Topotecan	Fatigue and asthenia
Biological agents	
Interferon	Initial flu syndrome, encephalopathy (dose-related), and organic affective and cognitive disorders with chronic use
Interleukin-2	Delirium is common

subjective feeling of needing to move one's legs. Akathisia must be distinguished from anxiety. To treat akathisia:

a. Stop the offending drug.
b. If the symptoms persist, treat with lorazepam (1 mg) or diphenhydramine (25 to 50 mg).

2. **Alcohol withdrawal.** Alcoholic patients often increase their alcohol intake after a cancer diagnosis or during the treatment phase. The tremulousness and agitation of alcohol withdrawal, especially in the inpatient setting, may mimic anxiety.
3. **Pulmonary emboli** are a complication of many cancers and can present as anxiety.
4. **Benzodiazepine withdrawal,** like alcohol withdrawal, can mimic anxiety. Replacement of the drug or a slow taper will decrease the likelihood of withdrawal symptoms.

C. Medical conditions which mimic depression

1. **Hypercalcemia** is a common metabolic complication of cancer. The clinical features of impaired concentration, lethargy, and anorexia can be confused with depression. A calcium level in the normal range may reflect elevated free calcium if a low albumin is also present.

2. **Hypothyroidism** resulting from thyroid or pituitary failure can occur after radiation to the neck or head.

D. Medical and neurological causes of delirium are common in patients with cancer, including:

1. Metastasis to the brain

2. Use of opiates and anticholinergic drugs

3. Electrolyte imbalance, including hyponatremia

4. Hypoxia

E. Paraneoplastic syndromes including **paraneoplastic limbic encephalitis,** may cause delirium from an autoimmune injury or from the **ectopic production of hormones.** Ectopic hormones include:

1. Increased anti-diuretic hormone causing hyponatremia

2. Increased parathyroid hormone causing hypercalcemia

3. Increased adrenocorticotropic hormone causing Cushing's syndrome, which often is associated with affective dysregulation.

V. Chemotherapy Treatments

A. Many chemotherapeutic agents have neuropsychiatric side effects. These agents include hormones, chemotherapy drugs, and biological agents. (Table 38-1).

1. **Hormones**

   a. **Corticosteroids.** Steroids are used for reduction of brain swelling during radiation treatment to the brain. They are adjuncts to treatment with paclitaxel and docetaxel. Dexamethasone, 10 mg (equivalent to more than 60 mg of prednisone) is also used to prevent nausea. Psychiatric symptoms can vary from mild hyperactivity and insomnia to emotional lability, agitation, mania, depression, and psychosis. The neuropsychiatric side effects of prednisone are prominent at doses above 60 mg/day or its equivalent. During repeated cycles of chemotherapy the response may vary. If the affective symptoms do not resolve immediately after steroids are stopped, the patient should be treated with psychotropic medications. To treat hyperactivity, neuroleptics, such as perphenazine and haloperidol may be used.

   b. **Tamoxifen.** Tamoxifen can cause menopausal symptoms, such as hot flashes, irritability, and interrupted sleep.

   c. **Anastrozole.** Hot flashes (12–26%); asthenia (16%); flu-like syndrome (14%); and depression (5%).

   d. **Letrozole.** Hot flashes (18%); fatigue (11%); insomnia (6%); and depression (5%).

2. **Chemotherapeutic agents**

   a. **Procarbazine** can cause somnolence, psychosis, and delirium with immediate onset and rapid resolution. It has a weak monoamine oxidase inhibitory effect. Tyramine restricted diets are not recommended, but serotonin reuptake inhibitors should not be prescribed concurrently. Because of a disulfiram (Antabuse) effect, alcohol should be avoided when procarbazine is administered.

b. **Cytarabine** at high doses can cause delirium with an onset of 2 to 3 days and a cluster of symptoms lasting a week. At high doses, a leukoencephalopathy can cause a syndrome of personality change, drowsiness, dementia, psychomotor retardation, and ataxia.

c. **5-Fluorouracil** can cause fatigue. Rare side effects include delirium, seizure, and a cerebellar syndrome.

d. **Methotrexate** can cause neurological toxicity when high doses are used or when it is administered intrathecally. A transient delirium can be seen on days 10 to 13.

e. **Vincristine, vinorelbine,** and **vinblastine** can cause side effects of dysphoria, lethargy, and, more rarely, inappropriate anti-diuretic hormone secretion, or seizures.

f. **Ifosfamide** can cause toxicity ranging from lethargy and dysarthria to seizures. Because of the increased risk of seizures, parenteral benzodiazepines, such as lorazepam, may be helpful. A delirium with hallucinations can occur soon after ifosfamide infusion.

g. **Gemcitabine** can cause a flu-like syndrome with fatigue (19%).

h. **Topotecan** can cause fatigue and asthenia (25%).

3. **Biologic agents**

a. **Interferon** can cause flu-like fatigue, poor concentration, psychomotor retardation, and lack of interest. Psychosis can be seen after administration of high doses. Affective symptoms and personality changes are both dose and duration of treatment-related. These symptoms are difficult to treat without adjusting the interferon dosing, but stimulants and serotonin reuptake inhibitors have been tried for this purpose.

b. **Interleukin-2 (IL-2)** and lymphokine-activated killer cells can cause a delirium that is dose-related and occurs predominantly at the end of treatment with IL-2 or several days after combined treatment. Recovery occurs in two to three days.

VI. Anti-emetic Treatments and Their Side Effects

A. **In the past, nausea and vomiting were overwhelming side effects of chemotherapy treatment. Through the use of drugs such as ondansetron, granisetron, dexamethasone, and benzodiazepines, the incidence of these side effects has greatly decreased.** However, a patient is more likely to develop conditioned anxiety and nausea to further treatment, as the number of previous episodes of nausea and vomiting increases.

1. The clinical presentation of conditioned anxiety includes insomnia, transient feelings of dread, increased overall anxiety, avoidance behaviors, dysphoria, and in some cases depression.

B. **Treatment for anticipatory nausea and vomiting.**

1. Medications. Minor tranquilizers, such as **alprazolam and lorazepam,** are effective and can be continued if nausea persists after chemotherapy treatment. The **addictive potential** is outweighed by the benefit if the use of the benzodiazepine is monitored and tapered after treatment.

2. Behavioral treatments (including hypnosis, distraction, and systemic desensitization) can also be effective.

C. **Prophylactic treatment for post-chemotherapy nausea and vomiting** given simultaneously with chemotherapeutic agents include:

1. **Ondansetron and granisetron,** serotonin (5-HT$_3$) antagonists, prevent chemotherapy-induced nausea and vomiting by blocking the serotonin released from the gut from chemotherapy. Migraine headache and diarrhea are also side effects.

2. **Dexamethasone,** which has an anti-emetic effect, is given adjunctively with the above agents. With dexamethasone, patients may have associated insomnia or agitation.

D. Post-chemotherapy treatment for nausea and vomiting
1. Both **minor and major tranquilizers** are effective. Antipsychotics are used in much lower doses to treat nausea and vomiting in the cancer population then they are used to treat psychosis. Major tranquilizers include the following:
   a. **Haloperidol and droperidol** are high-potency antipsychotics with the side effects of dystonia, akathisia, and oculogyric crises.
   b. **Perphenazine** is a high-potency antipsychotic with fewer extrapyramidal side effects than haloperidol and droperidol but is more sedating.
   c. **Olanzapine and other atypical antipsychotics** have anti-emetic effects, and are less apt to cause extrapyramidal side effects, but they are not yet available parenterally.
   d. **Prochlorperazine,** another neuroleptic, has a higher risk of agitation and extrapyramidal side effects than the other antipsychotics described above.
2. **Metoclopramide** is used to stimulate gastric emptying and to reduce nausea and vomiting. It is both a cholinergic and a dopamine antagonist. The risk of extrapyramidal side effects is dose-related.
3. **Anticholinergic agents** (scopolamine and diphenhydramine) can diminish nausea from organ distension or motion sickness but can also cause an anticholinergic delirium.

VII. Treatment Strategies

A. If all reversible causes of psychiatric illness from cancer or its treatment have been corrected and psychiatric symptoms still persist, the principles of treatment are the same as those used to treat the medically ill.
1. **Medications should be started at low doses and increased gradually.** This is especially true of the serotonin reuptake inhibitors, whose common gastrointestinal side effects can further debilitate a patient with cancer.
2. **The duration of treatment varies considerably** and depends on the response to treatment, the psychiatric history, and the stage of cancer.
3. **At every visit, review current medications.** Patients may self-medicate with drugs left over from another phase of treatment. For example, major tranquilizers prescribed for post-chemotherapy nausea may be used by a patient to treat anxiety, unnecessarily exposing the patient to the side effects of neuroleptics.
4. **Speak simply and repeat important points. Write down important points to improve communication.**

VIII. Psychosocial Interventions

A. Psychosocial interventions can help reduce anxiety about treatment, clarify medical information, decrease alienation through talking to others in a similar situation, and decrease feelings of isolation and helplessness. Whether psychological interventions can alter the course of the disease is controversial. The interventions commonly used include education, behavioral training, and individual or group therapy.
1. **Educational interventions** target technical and treatment issues.
2. **Behavioral training** has been used to reduce the psychological and physical stress from chemotherapy and radiation treatment. The techniques include relaxation,

hypnosis, meditation, biofeedback, and guided imagery. General distress and antici-patory side effects can be reduced with the use of these techniques.

3. **Individual and group therapy,** including supportive, psychoeducational, and inter-personal exploration, can help patients develop better coping strategies and reduce distress. Spiritual counseling can be helpful for those with strong religious beliefs.

4. **Many patients benefit from one or all of these treatments.** In general, a structured psychoeducational program combining these interventions and integrated into com-prehensive care is less stigmatizing for a newly diagnosed and treated patient. Weekly ongoing **group support programs** for patients with advanced disease who are dealing with pain and issues related to death and dying also can be helpful. These interventions, however, should be adjunctive to comprehensive medical care.

5. **Referral**. Most cancer centers offer some psychosocial interventions. The American Cancer Society can also be a source of referral for its own programs and for national self-help groups. All patients should know that these services are available even though they may not need to use them initially.

Suggested Readings

Derogatis, L.R., Morrow, R.G., Fetting, J., et al. (1983). The prevalence of psychiatric disorders among cancer patients. *Journal of the American Medical Association, 249,* 751–757.

Fawzy, F.I. (1999). Psychosocial intervention for patients with cancer: What works and what doesn't. *European Journal of Cancer, 35,* 1559–1564.

Fawzy, F.I., & Greenberg, D.B. (1996). Oncology. In J.R. Rundell, & M.C. Wise (Eds.), *Textbook of consultation-liaison psychiatry.* Washington, DC: American Psychiatric Press, pp. 672–694.

Holland, J.C. (Ed.). (1998). *Handbook of psychooncology.* New York: Oxford University Press.

Weisman, A.D. (1979). *Coping with cancer.* New York: McGraw-Hill.

CHAPTER 39
The Patient with HIV Infection

JOHN QUERQUES, JONATHAN L. WORTH, AND STEPHEN L. BOSWELL

I. Introduction

A. Human immunodeficiency virus type 1 (HIV-1) belongs to a family of RNA viruses, the lentiviruses, whose members typically cause both neurologic and immunologic disease in mammalian host species. **Infection with HIV-1 causes a range of clinical syndromes, the most advanced of which is the acquired immune deficiency syndrome (AIDS).**

B. More than two decades after its first appearance in 1981, **HIV infection in the United States has largely become a chronic, treatable illness.** However, its course is still frequently complicated by a host of neuropsychiatric conditions.

    1. **Many HIV high-risk groups are also at high risk for pre-morbid psychiatric disorders,** including substance-use and mood disorders, post-traumatic stress disorder, and personality disorders.

        a. In the HIV Cost and Services Utilization Study, nearly half of a nationally representative sample of 2,864 HIV-positive adults screened positive for major depression, dysthymia, generalized anxiety disorder (GAD), or panic attack during the preceding year; 12% screened positive for substance dependence.

    2. **Co-morbid HIV-related medical and neurologic diseases** and the medications used to treat patients with these illnesses can make the diagnosis of neuropsychiatric conditions difficult because of overlapping symptoms and signs.

    3. **A co-morbid substance-use disorder, if active, can result in poor treatment compliance, make identification of HIV-related conditions difficult because of diagnostic similarity, and can result in lower treatment effectiveness and increased side effects.** Moreover, efforts to keep a substance-use disorder in remission add substantially to the management needs of the patient.

    4. HIV infection can cause a subcortical dementing illness with significant neuropsychiatric symptoms.

C. Disposition planning for patients with HIV/AIDS can be difficult and complicated since many of these patients belong to groups that are typically disenfranchised, isolated, and marginalized and have poor social support systems: gay men, racial and ethnic minorities, indigents, and the addicted.

D. Some clinicians may have emotional difficulty in caring for patients with HIV/AIDS.

    1. Their social backgrounds may be very different from those of their patients (see item above).

    2. They may be close in age to a patient who has an incurable, life-threatening disease.

    3. The medical complications of HIV/AIDS can be severe and professionally challenging.

    4. The clinician may inappropriately undertreat a patient's pain syndrome if there is a known history of addiction or if such a history is assumed because the patient is from a racial or ethnic minority group.

II. Epidemiology

A. The Centers for Disease Control and Prevention (CDC) criteria for AIDS include both laboratory test criteria (CD4+ cell count below 200/μL or a percentage of total lymphocytes below 14) and clinical criteria (see Table 39-1). These criteria overlap with, but are not identical to, Medicare and Social Security Disability Insurance (SSDI) criteria, which also include functional impairment.

B. In the United States, HIV/AIDS high-risk groups principally consist of young adults and older adolescents but are otherwise demographically very diverse: men who have sex with men, including gay and bisexual men, male sex workers, and men and women who exchange sex for drugs; injection drug users and their sexual partners; heterosexuals in geographic areas with a high prevalence of HIV/AIDS; persons with chronic severe mental illness; and the children of these persons. Persons in these risk groups are disproportionately poor and/or belong to racial and ethnic minorities compared with the general U.S. population.

C. Due to the availability of highly active antiretroviral therapy (HAART) since 1996, new cases of and deaths due to AIDS have sharply declined, especially among men who have sex with men and injection drug users. However, AIDS is increasingly affecting racial and ethnic minorities and women.

D. As their HIV disease advances, persons with HIV/AIDS often relocate to their hometowns or counties of origin. Thus, clinicians may find themselves caring for new HIV/AIDS patients at advanced stages of disease who have just moved and are in the middle of a process of significant psychosocial adjustment.

Table 39-1. CDC Revised Classification System for HIV-1 Infection

Clinical Categories

CD4+ Lymphocyte Count	Asymptomatic; Primary HIV Infection or PGL[a]	Symptomatic; no A or C Conditions	AIDS Indicator Conditions[b]
≥ 500/μL	A1	B1	C1
200–499/μL	A2	B2	C2
< 200/μL	A3	B3	C3

[a]PGL = persistent generalized lymphadenopathy.

[b]AIDS Indicator conditions:
Candidiasis of the esophagus, trachea, bronchi, or lungs; coccidioidomycosis, disseminated or extrapulmonary; cryptococcosis, extrapulmonary; cryptosporidiosis with diarrhea persisting more than 1 month; cytomegalovirus disease of an organ other than liver, spleen, or lymph nodes; cytomegalovirus retinitis with a loss of vision; herpes simplex virus infection causing a mucocutaneous ulcer that persists longer than 1 month or bronchitis, pneumonitis, or esophagitis for any duration; HIV-associated dementia; histoplasmosis, disseminated or extrapulmonary; isosporiasis with diarrhea persisting more than 1 month; Kaposi's sarcoma; lymphoma of the brain (primary); other non-Hodgkin's lymphoma of B-cell or unknown immunologic phenotype; any mycobacterial disease caused by mycobacteria other than *Mycobacterium tuberculosis*, disseminated (at a site other than or in addition to lungs, skin, or cervical or hilar lymph nodes); disease caused by *M. tuberculosis*, disseminated or extrapulmonary (involving at least one site outside the lungs, regardless of whether there is concurrent pulmonary involvement); *Pneumocystis carinii* pneumonia; progressive multifocal leukoencephalopathy; *Salmonella* (non-typhoid) septicemia, recurrent; toxoplasmosis of the brain; HIV wasting syndrome

SOURCE: Centers for Disease Control and Prevention, 1993.

E. HIV/AIDS impoverishes patients economically and socially. As their disease progresses and renders them unable to work, patients who became infected when they had private and/or commercial health insurance find themselves uninsured or enrolled in government programs just as their medical needs increase.

III. Interaction between HIV/AIDS and Psychiatric Illness

A. Neuropsychiatric symptoms in a person with HIV/AIDS may be due to (see Table 39-2):
1. Primary psychiatric illness
2. Causes secondary to HIV/AIDS
   a. Toxic effects of HIV-1 directly within the central nervous system (CNS)
   b. Opportunistic infections
   c. Systemic complications of HIV infection
   d. HAART and other treatments (see Table 39-3)

B. When neuropsychiatric symptoms due to these secondary causes are treated with conventional psychiatric medications:
1. Therapeutic response and tolerance are poorer
2. Risk of side effects is greater

C. Optimum treatment of both systemic HIV disease and HIV CNS infection can improve the response to conventional psychiatric medications and lower the risk of side effects.

IV. Clinical Evaluation

A. General approach
1. **Attend to the patient's chief complaint.** Sometimes medical priorities do not match those of the patient. The problem list must incorporate both the patient's and the clinician's priorities.
2. **Corroborate information from third parties,** including other health care providers and the patient's caretakers.
3. **Ask about use of street drugs.** Substance abuse and dependence occur frequently among patients with HIV/AIDS and can be associated with significant neuropsychiatric complications.
4. **Assess the stage of systemic HIV disease** (CD4+ cell count, HIV RNA plasma level) and the presence of active illnesses.
5. **Assess the stage of HIV CNS infection.**
   a. The frequency and severity of clinically-important HIV CNS infection generally parallels systemic HIV disease.
   b. Screening for HIV CNS infection should be instituted. Ask patients if they have recent-onset problems with attention, concentration, short-term memory, word-finding, or clumsiness and if they think the "brain isn't working well." Computer-based tests of reaction time can be useful in screening large numbers of patients with HIV/AIDS.
6. **Determine current medications** and the timing of treatment initiation and discontinuation and dosage changes.
7. **Perform a psychosocial assessment**
   a. Realize that during the majority of the first two decades of the epidemic, patients faced the prospect of "dying with AIDS." With the advent of protease inhibitors in 1996, patients increasingly struggle with "living with HIV," that is, the hardships attendant to any chronic medical condition.

Table 39-2. Differential Diagnosis of Neuropsychiatric Symptoms in Patients with HIV/AIDS

1. Psychiatric disorders
2. Psychoactive substance intoxication/withdrawal
3. Primary HIV syndromes
   a. Seroconversion illness
   b. HIV CNS infection
   c. HIV-associated dementia
4. CNS opportunistic infections
   a. Fungi: *Cryptococcus neoformans, Coccidioides immitis, Candida albicans, Histoplasma capsulatum, Aspergillus fumigatus,* mucormycosis
   b. Protozoa/parasites: *Toxoplasma gondii,* amebas
   c. Viruses: JC virus (progressive multifocal leukoencephalopathy), cytomegalovirus (CMV), adenovirus type 2, herpes simplex virus, varicella zoster virus
   d. Bacteria: *Mycobacterium avium-intracellulare, M. tuberculosis, Listeria monocytogenes,* gram-negative organisms, *Treponema pallidum, Nocardia asteroides*
5. Neoplasms
   a. Primary CNS non-Hodgkin's lymphoma
   b. Metastatic Kaposi's sarcoma (rare)
   c. Burkitt's lymphoma
6. Medication side effects (see Table 39-3)
7. Endocrinopathies and nutrient deficiencies
   a. Addison's disease (CMV, *Cryptococcus,* HIV-1, ketaconazole)
   b. Hypothyroidism
   c. Vitamins A, B_6, B_{12}, and E deficiencies
   d. Hypogonadism
8. Anemia
9. Metabolic abnormalities: hypoxia; hepatic, renal, pulmonary, adrenal, and pancreatic insufficiency; hypomagnesemia; hypocalcemia; water intoxication, dehydration; hypernatremia; hyponatremia; alkalosis; acidosis
10. Hypotension
11. Complex partial seizures
12. Head trauma
13. Non-HIV-related conditions

SOURCE: Querques, J., Worth, J.L. (2000). HIV infection and AIDS. In T.A. Stern, & J.B. Herman (Eds.), *Psychiatry update and board preparation.* New York: McGraw-Hill, p. 208.

Table 39-3. Neuropsychiatric Side Effects of Medications Frequently Used in Patients with HIV/AIDS

Non-nucleoside reverse transcriptase inhibitors

Nevirapine	Headache
Delavirdine	Headache
Efavirenz	False-positive cannabinoid test, agitation, insomnia, euphoria, depression, somnolence, abnormal dreams, confusion, abnormal thinking, impaired concentration, amnesia, depersonalization, hallucinations
Tenofovir	Asthenia, anorexia

Protease inhibitors

Indinavir	Headache, asthenia, blurred vision, dizziness, insomnia
Ritonavir	Circumoral and peripheral paresthesias, asthenia, altered taste
Saquinavir	Headache
Nelfinavir	Headache, asthenia
Amprenavir	Headache
Lopinavir/ritonavir combination	Asthenia, headache, insomnia

Other antivirals

Acyclovir	Headache, agitation, insomnia, tearfulness, confusion, hyperesthesia, hyperacusis, depersonalization, hallucinations
Ganciclovir	Agitation, mania, psychosis, irritability, delirium

Antibacterials

Cotrimoxazole	Headache, insomnia, depression, anorexia, apathy
Trimethoprim-sulfamethoxazole	Headache, insomnia, depression, anorexia, apathy, delirium, mutism, neuritis
Isoniazid	Agitation, depression, hallucinations, paranoia, impaired memory
Dapsone	Agitation, insomnia, mania, hallucinations

Antiparasitics

Thiabendazole	Hallucinations, olfactory disturbance
Metronidazole	Agitation, depression, delirium, seizures (with IV administration)
Pentamidine	Hypoglycemia, hypotension, confusion, delirium, hallucinations

(continued)

Table 39-3. *Continued*

Antifungals

Amphotericin B	Headache, agitation, anorexia, delirium, diplopia, lethargy, peripheral neuropathy
Ketoconazole	Headache, dizziness, photosensitivity
Flucytosine	Headache, delirium, cognitive impairment

Others

Steroids	Euphoria, mania, depression, psychosis, confusion
Cytosine arabinoside	Delirium, cerebellar signs

SOURCE: Querques, J., & Worth, J.L. (2000). HIV infection and AIDS. In T.A. Stern, & J.B. Herman (Eds.), *Psychiatry update and board preparation.* New York: McGraw-Hill, p. 210.

---

     b. **Using a "marathon model" to cope with HIV/AIDS can be useful for both the clinician and the patient. Patients need to create four conditions "to run the HIV/AIDS marathon":**
        i. **Train.** Determine how the patient previously coped with adversity. How well has the patient coped? How well will these coping strategies work with HIV/AIDS?
        ii. **Establish a personal team.** When the patient is running down the raceway, are there faces in the crowd the patient recognizes? Who are the members of the patient's psychosocial support team?
        iii. **Take pit stops.** Can the patient "take a break" from HIV/AIDS?
        iv. **Develop corporate support.** Do employer, physician, other health care providers, and health care insurance and disability programs exist in the patient's case? How supportive and/or good are they?
     c. If any of these elements is absent or underdeveloped, poor psychosocial coping probably will result.
     d. The treatment plan should strengthen these requisite conditions.
     e. Using this model, the patient can be taught about coping mechanisms and may better understand psychosocial interventions.
   8. **Maintain confidentiality.** Know the state laws that pertain to HIV-related information. Consult with legal counsel regarding duty-to-warn cases (e.g., the appropriate response when a patient is knowingly placing others at risk for infection without their consent). If the patient is enrolled in clinical research trials, consult with the principal investigator about research-related information.
B. Major depression (see Chapter 14). Sad, demoralized, and frustrated moods are frequent and normal psychological reactions at many stages of HIV/AIDS. **While major depression is never a normal psychological reaction to HIV/AIDS, it is a common complication during the illness.** A pre-morbid major depressive disorder may recur as a result of the many stresses experienced during the course of HIV/AIDS. New-onset major depression also may result from the same stressors or occur secondarily as a result of the medical or neurologic complications of HIV/AIDS, medication side effects (see Table 39-3), or substance abuse.

1. **The evaluation is aimed at diagnosing the mood disorder accurately, characterizing its neurovegetative symptoms** (see Chapter 14), **and detecting underlying or co-morbid causes of major depression.** Determine the following:
   a. History of coincident medication changes or substance abuse
   b. History of coincident psychosocial stressors
   c. Cognitive testing if there are significant cognitive symptoms (see previous Section A.5)
   d. Complete blood count (CBC) if the patient is being treated with a nucleoside antiretroviral
   e. Thyroid function tests, free testosterone, and electrolytes if the patient is at risk for HIV-related endocrinopathy (CD4+ cell count below $100/\mu L$)
   f. Electrolytes, if the patient is experiencing active diarrheal illness
   g. Serum vitamin B_{12}, if there are any neuropsychiatric symptoms consistent with B_{12} deficiency
2. Pharmacotherapy is the first line of treatment.
   a. Tricyclic antidepressants (TCAs) and selective serotonin reuptake inhibitors (SSRIs) probably are equally effective and well tolerated.
   b. **Avoid agents that are sedating, highly anticholinergic, or anti-alpha-adrenergic** (e.g., amitriptyline, doxepin, and trazodone).
   c. Use geriatric dosing guidelines (see Chapter 49). Start at low doses and increase slowly; for example, start with 10 mg of nortriptyline, fluoxetine (Prozac), or paroxetine (Paxil).
   d. Bupropion (Wellbutrin, Wellbutrin XL, Wellbutrin SR) may be helpful if fatigue and decreased concentration are prominent neurovegetative symptoms.
3. Stimulants (e.g., dextroamphetamine [Dexedrine] and methylphenidate [Ritalin]) can be very useful in combination with traditional antidepressants (see Chapter 14).
4. Psychotherapy can be helpful, especially if there are clear precipitating psychosocial stressors.
   a. Strongly consider, in conjunction with pharmacotherapy, whether there is co-morbid unresolved bereavement or the patient is multiply bereaved.
   b. Consult with a clinician who has HIV/AIDS experience.

C. **HIV-associated dementia. HIV-associated dementia is a subcortical dementing illness caused by the toxic effects of HIV directly within the CNS.** Since the brain structures and neurotransmitters involved in the regulation of mood and neurovegetative functions are affected directly, it can include "psychiatric" symptoms.
   1. **HIV-associated dementia is now the preferred term for the conditions previously known as AIDS dementia complex (ADC),** HIV encephalopathy, and HIV-1-associated cognitive/motor complex. For the sake of brevity, we will use HIV dementia.
   2. **The incidence of HIV dementia parallels the progression of systemic HIV disease.** It affects less than 5% of patients with asymptomatic HIV infection but 15–66% of patients with AIDS-defining illnesses, depending on the effectiveness of CNS antiretroviral therapy and other factors. Its prevalence has decreased since the widespread use of HAART.
   3. The symptoms of HIV dementia include affective, behavioral, cognitive, and motor symptoms with a wide range of severity. The American Academy of Neurology's criteria for HIV dementia are outlined in Table 39-4. These symptoms generally have a low onset and are mild to moderate in severity, especially if the patient is on

---

Table 39-4. American Academy of Neurology Criteria for HIV-1-Associated Cognitive/Motor Complex

I. Acquired abnormality in at least two of the following cognitive abilities (present for 1 month): attention/concentration, abstraction/reasoning, memory learning, speed of processing, visuospatial skills, speech/language

    A. Decline verified by history and mental status examination. When possible, history should be obtained by an informant and examination should be supplemented by neuropsychological testing

    B. Cognitive dysfunction causing impairment of work or activities of daily living; impairment not attributable solely to severe systemic illness

II. At least one of the following:

    A. Acquired abnormality in motor function or performance verified by physical examination, neuropsychological tests, or both

    B. Decline in motivation or emotional control or change in social behavior characterized by any of the following: apathy, inertia, irritability, emotional lability, or new-onset impaired judgment characterized by socially inappropriate behavior or disinhibition

III. Absence of clouding of consciousness during a period long enough to establish the presence of I. above.

IV. Evidence for another etiology, including active CNS opportunistic infections or malignancy, psychiatric disorders (e.g., depressive disorders), active substance abuse, or acute or chronic substance withdrawal, must be ruled out by history, physical and psychiatric examination, and appropriate laboratory and radiologic tests.

SOURCE: American Academy of Neurology AIDS Task Force. (1991). Nomenclature and research case definitions for neurological manifestations of human immunodeficiency virus type-1 (HIV-1) infection. *Neurology, 41,* 778–785.

---

effective CNS antiretroviral therapy. Rarely, they can be abrupt in onset and/or severe, often when there is ineffective or no CNS antiretroviral therapy.

    a. **Cognitive** symptoms include problems with attention; concentration; short-term memory, including the forgetting of previously remembered names, phone numbers, and daily routines; and difficulty with activities requiring multiple steps or requiring that attention be paid in several different directions.

    b. **Behavioral** symptoms include change in social behavior, withdrawal, anergy, agitation, and, rarely, psychosis.

    c. **Motor** symptoms include gait disturbances, clumsiness, and changes in handwriting.

4. The evaluation has several goals: establishing the diagnosis, ruling out other causes, and obtaining objective measures of severity that can be used to judge treatment effectiveness and guide treatment planning for appropriate changes in activities of daily living, including work and self-care. The physician should perform or obtain the following:

    a. A neurologic evaluation

    b. A psychiatric evaluation

    c. Neuropsychological testing, using a test battery aimed at HIV dementia, which should take no longer than 1.5 hours to administer

    d. Brain magnetic resonance imaging (MRI)

e. Cerebrospinal fluid (CSF) examination if the symptoms are progressive or severe or if the CD4+ cell count is less than 100/μL

f. Blood tests for likely causes (e.g., anemia, an electrolyte or endocrine disorder, an opportunistic infection, syphilis)

g. Electroencephalography (EEG) (often it will not be helpful)

5. Treatment should be aimed at optimizing the antiretroviral regimen for viral CNS infection, controlling symptoms with psychiatric medications and supportive psychotherapy, and changing the patient's activities on the basis of cognitive strengths and overall level of function.

a. **Nucleoside antiretrovirals.** Zidovudine (AZT) achieves a higher CSF concentration than do the other agents in this group. AZT, if tolerated by the patient, should be given special consideration when one is choosing agents for combination antiretroviral therapy. Higher doses are probably more effective in reducing the symptoms of HIV dementia.

b. **Protease inhibitors.** None of the currently available agents achieves effective CSF concentrations, but their ability to decrease viral load may prevent or decrease symptoms of HIV dementia.

c. **Stimulants.** Dextroamphetamine and methylphenidate may reduce the symptoms of decreased attention and concentration and apathetic mood. Start with 10 mg every morning and assess effectiveness in two to three days and then increase the dose by 5-mg increments up to 20 to 30 mg; adverse side effects often develop at daily doses greater than 20–30 mg. If the positive effect wanes by the afternoon, add an afternoon dose—no later than 1 or 2 P.M.—that is one-half the effective morning dose. If the patient has difficulty remembering to take the afternoon dose, the use of a sustained-release preparation may be helpful.

d. For symptoms of depression, mania, or psychosis resulting from HIV dementia, see other sections in this chapter for symptomatic treatment.

e. **Insomnia.** Some patients with severe HIV dementia may experience near-delusional fear or terror during sleep initiation. A several-day trial of a low dose of a moderate-potency neuroleptic (the equivalent of haloperidol 0.5 to 1.0 mg) at bedtime—not on a p.r.n. basis—can be helpful. Also see the section on insomnia below.

f. **Delirium.** Some patients with severe HIV dementia worsen at night (i.e., they experience "sundowning"). Symptomatically, this is a delirium and can be treated with low doses of a moderate-potency neuroleptic (the equivalent of haloperidol 1 to 3 mg) at bedtime on a routine rather than p.r.n. basis.

D. **Mania** (see Chapter 21).

1. Unless the patient has a pre-morbid history of bipolar disorder, mania usually is a complication of advanced HIV disease or a side effect of HIV medication (Table 39-4).

2. New-onset mania should be considered a secondary mania until proved otherwise.

3. The evaluation is aimed at detecting underlying causes of mania.

a. History of coincident medication changes or substance abuse

b. Neurologic examination

c. Brain MRI

d. CSF examination if the patient is at risk for CNS opportunistic infection (CD4+ cell count below 100/μL)

4. Standard pharmacotherapy—a neuroleptic and lithium carbonate—often is poorly tolerated and/or is of low effectiveness. This is predicted by any MRI abnormality, including atrophy.

5. Valproate—use only the Depakote brand to minimize gastrointestinal (GI) side effects—is the treatment of choice; the dose should be determined by symptom control or by aiming for low therapeutic levels.

6. Clonazepam (Klonopin) can be helpful either alone or in addition to valproate; the usual dose is 1 to 3 mg daily.

E. **Anxiety and difficulty coping with illness** (see Chapters 16 and 32). HIV disease can be accompanied by multiple severe psychosocial stressors. Even patients who have a pre-morbid history that prepares them to cope with such adversity have difficulty (see IV.A.7.b).

1. Depending on their pre-morbid psychological coping skills, patients may present with a wide range of ineffective coping behaviors, including the following:

   a. New-onset acute stress reaction, panic attacks, adjustment disorders, grief reaction, complicated bereavement, minor and major depressions

   b. Recurrence of post-traumatic stress disorder-type syndromes, substance-use disorders, major mood disorders, and decompensation of severe personality disorders with chronic suicidal ideation

2. Frequently occurring HIV-related stressors include the following:

   a. **The diagnosis and medical management of HIV disease:** positive HIV serologic testing, determination of CD4+ cell counts and HIV RNA plasma levels, initiation of antiretroviral therapies, prophylactic therapy against opportunistic infections, first hospitalization, placement of indwelling IV catheters, initiation of IV therapies at home, and transfer to a hospice

   b. **The symptomatic experience of HIV disease:** first opportunistic infection, wasting syndrome, diarrheal illnesses, treatment-resistant pain and sleep disorders, vision-impairing disease, and cognitive and motor impairments

   c. **The psychosocial consequences of HIV disease:** loss of job and private health care insurance, loss of disability insurance, impoverishment, application for SSDI, application for welfare, and disclosure of HIV infection to sexual partners, family members, employers, and children.

3. The evaluation should determine the following:

   a. The patient's pre-morbid level of psychological coping skills and existing psychosocial support (see IV.A.7.b).

   b. An accurate psychiatric diagnosis

   c. The specific psychosocial stressor(s) underlying the onset or recurrence of the psychiatric disorder

   d. The development and implementation of a treatment plan using diagnostically appropriate symptomatic pharmacotherapy, supportive and psychoeducational psychotherapy, and community- and government-based psychosocial interventions

4. Pharmacotherapy

   a. **Benzodiazepines.** Short-term trials can be helpful in patients with acute or time-limited anxiety syndromes. Long-term trials are problematic due to physiologic accommodation and abuse and/or dependence and should be avoided. Refrain from starting even short-term trials in patients whose substance abuse disorder is in remission unless the trial is conducted in close consultation with the patient's addiction treatment team.

   b. **Antidepressants.** TCAs and SSRIs can be useful for chronic anxiety syndromes.

5. Psychotherapies

   a. **Supportive psychotherapy.** Short-term trials can be conducted effectively by primary-care physicians (PCPs), especially in patients with acute or time-limited syndromes.

However, when there are multiple severe psychosocial stressors or a co-morbid major mental disorder, a mental health professional can be more effective. Group psychotherapies, led by a mental health professional or peer-led, also can be very helpful, particularly if there is a specific group topic (e.g., coping with chronic illness, partners of patients, serologically discordant couples, or gay men, addicts, or Latino women with HIV disease).

b. **Cognitive-behavioral and psychoeducational psychotherapies** (see Chapters 9 and 10). These therapies encompass a wide range of therapies and interventions, many of which are aimed at the four components of the "marathon model" and moving the patient's locus of control back to himself or herself. They include self-relaxation and self-hypnosis training by audiocassette or a health care professional, provision of treatment choices, psychosocial support for domestic caretakers, and provision of instructions for self-administered therapies that rely on a patient's strongest cognitive domains (e.g., verbal versus visual information processing). Phone check-ins can be done by PCPs to determine medication effectiveness and side effects, to remind the patient of an upcoming office visit or laboratory test, or simply to "see if you're okay." Offering patients a "drug holiday" from medications (selected by the PCP) for a couple of days may give the patient a respite from taking 20 to 30 pills daily. However, patients must know the risks of intermittent dosing of protease inhibitors.

6. **Community- and/or government-based organizations.** Community and government organizations provide services that are aimed at the four components of the marathon model. In many cities with a high HIV prevalence, HIV/AIDS-specific community-based organizations have been developed to address many of the psychosocial, legal, financial, and housing problems faced by persons with HIV/AIDS. There are also government programs for persons who are disabled and/or impoverished as a result of HIV/AIDS. Access to such programs is essential, and an informed caseworker or social worker is invaluable in caring for HIV/AIDS patients.

F. **Insomnia** (see Chapter 27). Sleep disorders occur frequently in patients with HIV/AIDS and can be due to a wide range of causes, including neuropsychiatric disorders and symptoms (e.g., depression, anxiety, fear, and pain) and complications of systemic HIV disease, HIV CNS infection, and medication side effects (Table 39-3).

1. The evaluation is aimed at determining the cause(s) of insomnia, detecting co-morbid conditions that worsen a pre-existing sleep disorder, and assessing insomnia severity by using visual or numeric analogues or a sleep diary.
   a. A thorough clinical evaluation alone will determine the cause(s) of most HIV-related sleep disorders.
   b. A polysomnogram is useful in treatment-refractory sleep disorders.

2. Treatment options include both behavioral interventions and non-benzodiazepine pharmacotherapies.
   a. **Behavioral interventions.** Elements of good sleep hygiene include no daytime naps and no alcohol, caffeine, chocolate, tobacco, cigarettes, or other psychoactive substances.
   b. **TCAs.** Low doses of sedating TCAs (e.g., nortriptyline 10-25 mg qhs) can be useful. Avoid amitriptyline and doxepin because of their prominent side effects.
   c. **Serotonergic agents.** Low doses of trazodone (25-100 mg qhs) can be useful. Instruct patients that these medications may take a couple of days to have a full effect and must be taken routinely, not on a p.r.n. basis.
   d. **Antihistamines** (e.g., diphenhydramine).

3. **Benzodiazepine hypnotics** are advisable only for short-term use in acute causes of insomnia (e.g., adjustment disorder, acute stress reaction, exacerbations of a chronic sleep disorder).

   a. Some HIV-related sleep disorders are highly treatment-resistant and respond only to benzodiazepine hypnotics. To avoid physiologic accommodation to a specific benzodiazepine, a regimen of sequential one-month trials of different benzodiazepines can be useful (e.g., one month of lorazepam [Ativan] 1 mg, then one month of oxazepam [Serax] 15 mg, then one month of triazolam [Halcion] 0.25 mg, then back to lorazepam).

G. Pain (see Chapter 33). **Pain syndromes occur frequently during advanced stages of HIV disease. The most common syndromes are painful peripheral neuropathies** resulting from HIV infection and the neurotoxic side effects of nucleoside antiretroviral agents. Other common causes include herpes zoster and post-herpetic neuralgia.

1. The evaluation is aimed at determination of the cause(s) of the pain syndrome, detection of co-morbid conditions that amplify pain, and assessment of pain severity using visual or numeric analogues.

2. Therapeutic efforts should be targeted to:

   a. Attenuate or treat the underlying cause(s)

   b. Treat co-morbid conditions (e.g., depression, anxiety, fear)

   c. Plan treatment identically as for chronic pain syndromes (see Chapter 33)

   d. Instruct patients that non-opiate analgesics take several days to have an effect and must be taken routinely, not on a p.r.n. basis

3. **Opiates** are advisable only for short-term trials for acute pain syndromes, deafferentation pain syndromes, and exacerbations of chronic pain syndromes. For longer-term trials, use sustained-release preparations, either orally or transdermal.

   a. For patients on methadone maintenance, do not use an increased dose for analgesia. Use another opiate agent or the patient and the rest of the health care team will be confused about the treatment goals.

4. **Tricyclics.** Low doses of agents, such as nortriptyline and desipramine, can be useful. Use amitriptyline cautiously because of its side effects.

5. **Anticonvulsants.** Low doses of clonazepam can be useful, particularly for patients with hyperpathia. Use carbamazepine (Tegretol) cautiously and at low doses because of its dermatologic and hermatopoietic toxicity. Valproate may be helpful but is generally less effective than carbamazepine.

6. **Acupuncture** in conjunction with pharmacotherapy can be helpful.

7. **Lidocaine** 100 mg IV over 5 minutes can be very helpful for herpes zoster and post-herpetic neuralgia. Initial infusions must be done with electrocardiographic (ECG) monitoring. Infusion frequency can vary from every other week to twice weekly.

8. Transcutaneous electrical nerve stimulation (TENS) can reactive herpes zoster.

H. Substance abuse and dependence (see Chapters 52 and 53). Substance abuse and dependence occur with high frequency among all HIV risk groups and, when active, can play a role in HIV transmission, HIV risk behavior, viral replication, treatment noncompliance, and antisocial behavior.

1. Substance-use disorders need to be evaluated in all new patients and patients in follow-up who have a history of substance abuse.

   a. Directly question the patient about substance use.

   b. Include questions about the use of non-prescription pharmaceuticals (e.g., steroids).

    c. Use the CAGE questions as a quick and reliable screening test (see Chapter 52).

    d. Obtain third-party information.

2. Active addiction generally should be considered the first problem on a patient's problem list, surpassing HIV disease.

    a. Consider inpatient or outpatient detoxification.

    b. Refer to a 12-step program (e.g., Alcoholics Anonymous, Narcotics Anonymous).

    c. Refer to a substance abuse treatment program to plan and implement a comprehensive recovery program.

    d. Ask how the patient is paying for the drugs. The answer will often reveal the complex psychosocial aspects of addiction that need to be addressed in a successful recovery program.

3. As a stressor for an addiction in remission, HIV/AIDS can precipitate an addiction relapse. Thus, relapse prevention should be high on the problem list.

4. **Pharmacotherapeutic considerations**

    a. The following agents increase serum methadone concentrations: ritonavir and fluconazole.

    b. The following agents decrease serum methadone concentrations: nevirapine, efavirenz, ritonavir (mixed inducer-inhibitor), nelfinavir, lopinavir, and rifampin. Thus, initiation of these agents can precipitate acute opiate withdrawal.

    c. If the patient is using pharmaceuticals obtained on the street, do not prescribe them for the patient in the hope that you will be able to control the addiction or bring it into remission. Unfortunately, this is not the case.

I. Suicide (see Chapter 15). Patients with HIV/AIDS are at increased risk for suicide attempts and suicide. Accumulating evidence suggests that after AIDS, it may be the second leading cause of death among patients with HIV/AIDS. The reasons for this include pre-morbid psychiatric disorders and psychosocial stressors and neuropsychiatric and psychosocial complications of HIV/AIDS.

1. **Risk factors** include mood disorder (depression and mania), active substance-use disorders (including alcohol), coping with homosexuality as an adolescent, personality disorder, pain syndromes, illness-related problems at home or work, and the suffering aspects of illness (hopelessness, perceiving oneself as a burden to others, worthlessness, loss of independence, and loss of autonomy).

2. **Suicidal ideation** can be due to these factors as well as a manifestation of a psychological coping mechanism in patients with a severe personality disorder. Among patients at early stages of HIV infection, it can occur in response to fears of disease progression.

3. **Evaluation goals**

    a. Determine the severity of suicidal ideation and the safety of the patient.

    b. Diagnose the disorder or disorders, the components of psychological suffering, and the psychosocial stressors leading to thoughts of or attempts at suicide.

4. **Treatment goals**

    a. Ensure the safety of the patient until evaluation and treatment are possible. This may require a home visit, bringing the patient to an emergency room, or admitting the patient to an observation or inpatient psychiatric unit.

    b. Treat the etiologic disorder(s). For example, initiate antidepressant pharmacotherapy or optimize the analgesic regimen.

    c. Provide supportive psychotherapy as indicated by specific components of the patient's psychological suffering.

    d. Implement psychosocial interventions as indicated by the specific stressors.

V. Treatment

A. Pharmacotherapy (see Chapsters 66 to 68)

1. **Use geriatric dosing.** Start at low doses. Dose titration should be done slowly. Patients with HIV/AIDS have lower lean body mass and slowed drug metabolism.

2. **Avoid agents that block cholinergic, alpha-adrenergic, dopaminergic, and histaminergic receptors.** Patients with HIV/AIDS are very sensitive to drug side effects.

3. **Aim for low therapeutic drug levels when using nortriptyline, valproate, and lithium.** Standard levels for therapeutic serum drug levels do not account for HIV-related compromise of the blood-brain barrier. The brains of patients with HIV/AIDS probably "see" higher drug levels than do those of non-infected patients at a particular serum concentration.

4. **Consider the costs.** Medicare, the health care payer for many patients whose HIV disease has progressed to AIDS, does not pay for medications.

5. **Drug-drug interactions and antiretrovirals**

   a. **Clozaril (clozapine).** This antipsychotic frequently causes bone marrow toxicity, particularly within the first six months of treatment. Co-administration with AZT is relatively contraindicated. This poses a significant clinical dilemma, since some patients with schizophrenia respond only to clozapine. Close teamwork involving the PCP and the psychiatrist is needed to identify safe treatment options and coordinate changes in the treatment regimen. The use of clozapine and the protease inhibitor ritonavir is contraindicated.

   b. **Carbamazepine.** This agent—used frequently as a mood stabilizer, antimanic agent, and analgesic—can cause bone marrow toxicity. It must be co-administered cautiously. Substitution of valproate for carbamazepine should be considered.

   c. **Many antiretroviral agents** are metabolized by the hepatic cytochrome P-450 enzyme system; many also induce or inhibit its activity. All of the protease inhibitors inhibit the 3A4 isoform of cytochrome P-450. Ritonavir is the most potent inhibitor of 3A4 and it also inhibits the 2D6 isoform.

      i. **Agents that should not be co-administered with protease inhibitors:** ergots, midazolam (Versed), and triazolam

      ii. **Agents whose co-administration with ritonavir is contraindicated** include clozapine, pimozide (Orap), bupropion, alprazolam (Xanax), clorazepate (Tranxene), diazepam (Valium), estazolam (Prosom), flurazepam (Dalmane), triazolam, zolpidem (Ambien), meperidine (Demerol), and propoxyphene (Darvon).

      iii. **Agents whose co-administration with ritonavir requires low doses:** maprotiline (Ludiomil), nefazodone, trazodone, venlafaxine (Effexor, Effexor XR)

      iv. **Agents whose co-administration with other protease inhibitors requires the use of low doses and the testing of serum drug levels** include all of the agents listed in ii above, TCAs, SSRIs, clonazepam, diazepam, stimulants, neuroleptics, carbamazepine, methadone, oxycodone-containing products (Percocet, OxyContin), and hydrocodone-containing products (Vicodin).

      v. **Agents whose serum levels may be decreased** include alprazolam, ethinyl estradiol, lorazepam, oxazepam, temazepam (Restoril), codeine, hydromorphone (Dilaudid), and morphine.

      vi. Carbamazepine, phenobarbital, phenytoin, rifabutin, and rifampin can decrease levels of protease inhibitors.

B. Psychotherapy (see IV.E.5)

Useful Internet Resources

American Psychiatric Association AIDS Resource Center
www.psych.org/aids/

HIV/AIDS Treatment Information Service
www.aidsinfo.nih.gov

Joint United Nations Programme on HIV/AIDS
www.unaids.org

AEGIS (self-proclaimed largest HIV/AIDS Web site in the world)
www.aegis.com

Project Inform (HIV information for the lay public)
www.projectinform.org

Suggested Readings

American Academy of Neurology AIDS Task Force. (1991). Nomenclature and research case definitions for neurological manifestations of human immunodeficiency virus type-1 (HIV-1) infection. *Neurology, 41,* 778–785.

American Psychiatric Association. (2000). Practice guideline for the treatment of patients with HIV/AIDS. *American Journal of Psychiatry, 157,* 1–62.

Beckett, A., & Shenson, D. (1993). Suicide risk in patients with human immunodeficiency virus infection and acquired immunodeficiency syndrome. *Harvard Review of Psychiatry, 1,* 27–35.

Bing, E.G., Burnam, M.A., Longshore, D., et al. (2001). Psychiatric disorders and drug use among human immunodeficiency virus-infected adults in the United States. *Archives of General Psychiatry, 58,* 721–728.

Centers for Disease Control and Prevention. (1992). 1993 revised classification system for HIV infection and expanded surveillance case definition for AIDS among adolescents and adults. *Morbidity and Mortality Weekly Report,* (No. RR-17), 1–4, 15.

Chuang, H.T., Devins, G.M., Hunsley, J., et al. (1989). Psychosocial distress and well-being among gay and bisexual men with human immunodeficiency virus infection. *American Journal of Psychiatry, 146,* 876–880.

Clifford, D.B. (2000). Human immunodeficiency virus-associated dementia. *Archives of Neurology, 57,* 321–324.

Cournos, F., Empfield, M., Horwath, E., et al. (1991). HIV seroprevalence among patients admitted to two psychiatric hospitals. *American Journal of Psychiatry, 148,* 1225–1230.

Cournos, F., Forstein, M. (Eds.). (2000). What mental health practitioners need to know about HIV and AIDS. *New Directions for Mental Health Services, 87,* 1–136.

Empfield, M., Cournos, F., Meyer, I., et al. (1993). HIV seroprevalence among homeless patients admitted to a psychiatric inpatient unit. *American Journal of Psychiatry, 150,* 47–52.

Fernandez, F., & Levy, J.K. (1991). Psychopharmacotherapy of psychiatric syndromes in asymptomatic and symptomatic HIV infection. *Psychiatric Medicine, 9,* 377–394.

Fernandez, F., Adams, F., Levy, J.K., et al. (1988). Cognitive impairment due to AIDS-related complex and its response to psychostimulants. *Psychosomatics, 29,* 38–46.

Flexner, C. (1998). HIV-protease inhibitors. *New England Journal of Medicine, 338,* 1281–1292.

Grinspoon, S., & Bilezikian, J. (1992). AIDS and the endocrine system. *New England Journal of Medicine, 327,* 1360–1365.

Halman, M.H., Worth, J.K., Sanders, K.M., et al. (1993). Anticonvulsant use in the treatment of manic syndromes in patients with HIV-1 infection. *Journal of Neuropsychiatry and Clinical Neuroscience, 5,* 430–434.

Hays, R.B., McKusick, L., Pollack, L., et al. (1993). Disclosing HIV seropositivity to significant others. *AIDS, 7,* 425–431.

Hays, R.B., Turner, H., & Coates, T.J. (1992). Social support, AIDS-related symptoms, and depression among gay men. *Journal of Consulting and Clinical Psychology, 60,* 463–469.

Hintz, S., Kuck, J., Peterkin, J.J., et al. (1990). Depression in the context of human immunodeficiency virus infection: Implications for treatment. *Journal of Clinical Psychiatry, 51,* 497–501.

Holmes, V.F., Fernandez, F., & Levy, J.K. (1989). Psychostimulant response in AIDS-related complex patients. *Journal of Clinical Psychiatry, 30,* 5–8.

Hriso, E., Kuhn, T., Masdeu, J.C., & Grundman, M. (1991). Extrapyramidal symptoms due to dopamine-blocking agents in patients with AIDS encephalopathy. *American Journal of Psychiatry, 148,* 1558–1561.

Janssen, R.S., Saykin, A.J., Cannon, L., et al. (1989). Neurological and neuropsychological manifestations of HIV-1 infection: Association with AIDS-related complex but not asymptomatic HIV-1 infection. *Annals of Neurology, 26,* 592–600.

Kieburtz, K.D., Ketonen, L., Zettelmairer, N., et al. (1990). Magnetic resonance imaging findings in HIV cognitive impairment. *Archives of Neurology, 47,* 643–645.

Levy, J., & Fernandez, F. (1993). Memory rehabilitation in HIV encephalopathy. *Clinical Neuropathology, 12,* S27.

Lipton, S.A., Sucher, N.J., Kaiser, P.K., & Dreyer, E.B. (1991). Synergistic effects of HIV coat protein and NMDA receptor-mediated toxicity. *Neuron, 7,* 111–118.

Lyketsos, C.G., Hanson, A.L., Fishman, M., et al. (1993). Manic syndrome early and late in the course of HIV. *American Journal of Psychiatry, 150,* 326–327.

Maj, M., Satz, P., Janssen, R., et al. (1994). WHO neuropsychiatric AIDS study, cross-sectional phase II: Neuropsychological and neurological findings. *Archives of General Psychiatry, 51,* 51–61.

Marks, G., Richardson, J.L., & Maldonado, N. (1991). Self-disclosure of HIV infection to sexual partners. *American Journal of Public Health, 81,* 1321–1322.

McDonald, C.K., & Kuritzkes, D.R. (1997). Human immunodeficiency virus type 1 protease inhibitors. *Archives of Internal Medicine, 157,* 951–959.

Miller, E.N., Satz, P., & Visscher, B. (1991). Computerized and conventional neuropsychological assessment of HIV-1 infected homosexual men. *Neurology, 41,* 1608–1616.

Navia, B.A., Jordan, B.D., & Price, R.W. (1986). The AIDS dementia complex: I. Clinical features. *Annals of Neurology, 19,* 517–524.

Ostrow, D.G., Monjan, A., Joseph, J., et al. (1989). HIV-related symptoms and psychological functioning in a cohort of homosexual men. *American Journal of Psychiatry, 146,* 737–742.

Piscitelli, S.C., & Gallicano, K.D. (2001). Interactions among drugs for HIV and opportunistic infections. *New England Journal of Medicine, 344,* 984–996.

Portegies, P., Enting, R.H., de Gans, J., et al. (1993). Presentation and course of AIDS dementia complex. *AIDS, 7,* 669–675.

Praus, D.J., Brown, G.R., Rundell, J.R., & Paolucci, S.L. (1990). Associations between cerebrospinal fluid parameters and high degrees of anxiety or depression in United States Air Force personnel infected with human immunodeficiency virus. *Journal of Nervous Mental Disease, 78,* 392–395.

Price, R.W., & Brew, B.J. (1989). The AIDS dementia complex. *Journal of Infectious Disease, 158,* 1079–1083 (1992 revision).

Querques, J., & Worth, J.L. (2000). HIV infection and AIDS. In T.A. Stern, & J.B. Herman (Eds.), *Psychiatry update and board preparation.* New York: McGraw-Hill, pp. 207–218.

Rabkin, J.G. (1993). Psychostimulant medication for depression and lethargy in HIV illness: A pilot study. *Progress Notes, 4,* 1.

Remafedi, G., & Farrow, J.A. (1991). Risk factors for attempted suicide in gay and bisexual youth. *Pediatrics, 87,* 869–875.

Ronald, P.J.M., Robertson, J.R., & Elton, R.A. (1994). Continued drug use and other cofactors for progression to AIDS among injecting drug users. *AIDS, 8,* 339–343.

Rundell, J.R., Kyle, K.M., Brown, G.R., & Thomason, J.L. (1992). Risk factors for suicide attempts in a human immunodeficiency virus screening program. *Psychosomatics, 33,* 24–27.

Schmitt, F.A., Bigley, J.W., McKinnin, R., et al. (1988). Neuropsychological outcome of zidovudine (AZT) treatment of patients with AIDS and AIDS-related complex. *New England Journal of Medicine, 319,* 1573–1578.

Sidtis, J.J., Gatsonis, C., Price, R.W., et al. (1993). Zidovudine treatment of the AIDS dementia complex: Results of a placebo-controlled trial. *Annals of Neurology, 33,* 343–349.

So, Y.T., Holtzman, D.M., Abrams, D.I., & Olney, R.K. (1988). Peripheral neuropathy associated with acquired immunodeficiency syndrome. *Archives of Neurology, 45,* 945–948.

Todd, K.H., Samaroo, N., & Hoffman, J.R. (1993). Ethnicity as a risk factor for inadequate emergency department analgesia. *Journal of the American Medical Association, 269,* 1537–1539.

Tross, S., Price, R.W., Navia, B.A., et al. (1988). Neuropsychological characterization of the AIDS dementia complex: A preliminary report. *AIDS, 2,* 81–88.

Velentgas, P., Bynum, C., & Zierler, S. (1990). The buddy volunteer commitment in AIDS care. *American Journal of Public Health, 80,* 1378–1380.

Wong, M.C., Suite, N.D.A., & Labar, D.R. (1990). Seizures in human immunodeficiency virus infection. *Archives of Neurology, 7,* 640–642.

Worth, J.L., Savage, C., Baer, L., et al. (1993). Computer-based screening for AIDS dementia complex. *AIDS, 7,* 677–681.

Zierler, S., Feingold, L., Laufer, D., et al. (1991). Adult survivors of childhood sexual abuse and subsequent risk for HIV infection. *American Journal of Public Health, 81,* 572–575.

CHAPTER 40

The Patient Undergoing Organ Transplantation

LAURA M. PRAGER AND OWEN S. SURMAN

I. Introduction

Organ transplantation has become a reasonable and often successful intervention for patients with end-organ failure. Organs currently transplanted include the heart, lungs, liver, kidney, pancreas, and small intestine. Psychiatrists or other mental health professionals are involved in many stages of the transplantation process ranging from the pre-operative evaluation of candidates and, in some cases, living donors, to short- and long-term post-operative management of recipients and their families.

II. Overview of Transplantation

A. **All efforts at transplantation are limited by the potential for allograft rejection, by the side effects of the immunosuppressive medicines used to manage that rejection, and by the risks for infection inherent in any immunocompromised host.**

B. **Transplantation is also limited by:**
   1. **The mismatch between the number of patients who need transplantation and the availability of cadaveric organs.**
   2. **The financial cost of surgery.**

C. Scarcity of cadaveric organs has prompted participation of live donors including people who are related, those who may be emotionally but not biologically related, and some who are anonymous or previously unknown Good Samaritans.
   1. These options are currently available for kidney, liver, and lung transplantation candidates at some centers in the United States.
   2. These options are more common in other countries where religious or cultural ideology prohibits the use of cadaveric organs.
   3. **Living-organ donation has become widely accepted in the United States because of the increasing demand and limited supply for cadaver organs. Potential donors undergo a comprehensive psychological evaluation as well as medical work-up in order to ensure autonomy, informed consent, and absence of coercion.**
   4. Living-donor right lobe liver transplantation is a relatively new procedure and is associated with greater risk to the donor. As of April 2002, there have been two well-documented deaths from this procedure in the United States. The National Institutes of Health and the American College of Transplant Surgeons are currently studying this procedure and there are plans for a registry to more accurately track morbidity and mortality.

D. In the United States, the United Network for Organ Sharing (UNOS) is the non-profit corporation, endowed by Congress and reporting to the Department of Health and Human Services, that regulates the allocation of organs.

1. UNOS has the power to enforce its policies as Federal regulations.
2. It is divided into two branches:
    a. Organ Procurement and Transplant Network (OPTN)
    b. Scientific Registry
3. The OPTN divides the country into 11 distinct geographic regions and allocation of organs is done by local priority.
4. **The radius of distribution for each organ is dependent on the vulnerability of that organ to ischemic injury and the time required for air transport of the available organ.**
    a. Donor hearts are limited to a 500-mile radius.
    b. Lungs can live outside the body for only 6 hours.
5. Length of the waiting list for each organ can differ from region to region.
    a. Time spent waiting is the primary determining factor for kidney transplantation candidates and the only determining factor for lung candidates.
    b. Acuity of illness confers priority for heart and liver candidates.
    c. Pediatric recipients for kidneys and livers take precedence over adults.
    d. Full HLA compatability confers priority for kidney transplantation.
    e. Ventilatory support is a contraindication to transplantation for potential lung transplant recipients but confers priority listing to heart and liver candidates.
    f. Sepsis is a contraindication to transplantation for all solid organ candidates.

E. **Ethical/medicolegal considerations in recipient selection include:**
    1. **Rights-based approach,** which includes all candidates who wish to be included
    2. **Utilitarian-based approach** in which worth to society is a criterion for candidacy
    3. **Medically-based approach,** which offers candidacy to those who can benefit from transplantation
    4. **Potential candidates for transplantation are protected by the American with Disabilities Act (ADA) that prevents rejection of candidacy based on presence of a specific diagnosis,** such as schizophrenia or alcoholism.
    5. **The ADA does allow exclusion from candidacy based on risk-assessment and likelihood of benefit.**

III. Evaluation of the Patient

Psychiatric assessment and management of candidates for organ transplantation requires a thorough understanding of the unique problems faced by this population. Not all transplant teams have psychiatric consultants. Psychologists and/or social workers may do psychosocial assessments in some centers. However, all mental health professionals who work with transplant teams and who evaluate potential recipients and donors perform many different tasks.

A. **The Pre-Transplant Psychiatric Evaluation**
    1. Objectives:
        a. **Screen potential recipients for the presence of significant Axis I diagnoses** (mood, anxiety, psychotic disorders, and substance abuse), **Axis II diagnoses** (personality disorders), **and cognitive impairment** that might complicate management or interfere with ability to comply with treatment recommendations.
        b. **Determine whether or not a given candidate will be able to collaborate with the transplant team in a joint effort to optimize medical care** both pre- and post-transplant. This includes assessment of:

      i. Motivation for transplant

      ii. Compliance with previous recommendations by other caregivers

      iii. Availability of social supports and ease of access

      iv. Perseverance in the face of adversity

   c. Educate about risks and benefits of transplant

2. **Factors which complicate pre-transplant evaluation**

   a. Lack of reliable and predictive data re: "suitability for transplant"

   b. No uniformly accepted psychiatric guidelines for acceptance or rejection of transplant candidates

   c. Differences among transplant centers as to what degree of risk they are willing to assume

   d. Focus of psychosocial screening differs for each solid organ. Cardiac, liver, and lung programs have more stringent criteria than do kidney programs. Common exclusion criteria include:

      i. Current, active substance abuse (including tobacco use)

      ii. Poorly controlled schizophrenia with active psychotic symptoms

      iii. Suicidal ideation with plan or intent

      iv. History of multiple suicide attempts

      v. Dementia

      vi. Convicted felons

3. **Diagnosis**

Many psychiatric disorders are common in the transplant candidate population. Some arise due to the stress inherent in the patient's lengthy period of waiting for transplantation, others are more characteristic of patients with a particular type of end-organ failure.

   a. **Renal Failure**

      i. Depression is common among long-term dialysis patients

      ii. Organic mood disorders can occur secondary to endocrine abnormalities, such as hyperparathyroidism

      iii. Encephalopathy can be secondary to uremia and the so-called "dialysis disequilibrium"

      iv. Adjustment disorders often follow forced life-style changes

   b. **Cardiac Failure**

      i. Anxiety

      ii. Depression—particularly in patients who have prolonged stays in the ICU while awaiting transplant

      iii. Adjustment reaction

      iv. Delirium—particularly for patients in the ICU who require left ventricular assist devices or intra-aortic balloon pumps

      v. Encephalopathy secondary to decreased cerebral blood flow and/or medications

   c. **Hepatic Failure**

      i. Depression

      ii. Anxiety

      iii. Encephalopathy

   d. **Pulmonary Failure**

      i. Anxiety and panic are exceedingly common

      ii. Depression

      iii. Adjustment reaction in response to decreased ability to perform activities of daily living (ADLs) and the need to remain tethered to an oxygen tank

      iv. Delirium secondary to hypoxia or hypercapnia

4. **Treatment Strategies**

As in other areas of psychiatry, treatment plans are multi-faceted.

a. **Psychopharmacological agents** can and should be used when indicated. Choosing a medication regimen for potential transplant recipients with end-organ failure can be challenging. Many medicines, depending on their method of metabolism, will require dose adjustment based on presence of renal or hepatic failure. A good rule of thumb is to "start low and go slow."

  i. **Antidepressants**

  - Selective serotonin uptake inhibitors (SSRIs) (e.g., citalopram, fluoxetine, sertraline, paroxetine), are the first choice because of their benign side-effect profile and anxiolytic effects. Rarely, they may cause hyponatremia and SIADH.
  - Bupropion is more stimulating than other antidepressants but it also has a benign side-effect profile. It can also be helpful to patients who are struggling to remain abstinent from tobacco products.
  - Tricyclics are no longer a first-line choice because of their potential for cardiac (quinidine-like) effects.

  ii. **Anxiolytics**

  - Benzodiazepines can be invaluable in the management of anxiety, although some transplant teams are unwilling to use them because of their addictive potential. Shorter-acting agents are preferable (e.g. lorazepam and oxazepam). Alprazolam can be problematic because of its potential for rebound symptoms that are often indistinguishable from the anxiety symptoms themselves. Many long-acting agents have active metabolites that can accumulate, particularly in patients with hepatic dysfunction.

  iii. **Neuroleptics**

  - Patients with chronic psychotic disorders can and should be maintained on their existing antipsychotic regimen
  - Low-dose neuroleptics can be helpful in ameliorating anxiety, particularly in patients who cannot take benzodiazepines because of the risk for abuse.

  iv. **Mood Stabilizers**

  - Patients who require mood stabilizers such as lithium, valproic acid, or carbamazepine can be maintained on them prior to transplantation, with careful monitoring of dosing and blood levels. Lithium is customarily given after dialysis and levels will need to be adjusted in the patient with renal failure. Changes in protein binding affect levels obtained in standard monitoring of anticonvulsants (e.g., valproic acid)
  - Gabapentin can be particularly helpful in the management of steroid-induced mood lability.

  v. **Stimulants** can also be used as an adjunctive treatment for depression

b. **Psychotherapeutic interventions** are often extremely important, as candidates for transplant have a wide variation in their coping styles and the strength of their social support networks. Patients usually do best with supportive, cognitive, or behavioral approaches. Even the one-time psychiatric pre-transplant evaluation can serve as a good opportunity for listening and for validation of patients' hopes and concerns. Common issues raised include:

      i. Loss of occupational status with secondary financial pressures

      ii. Guilt over the lack of ability to perform at one's pre-morbid level of functioning

      iii. Change of role within the family system

      iv. Cognitive blunting or impairment

      v. Inability to perform sexually

      vi. Denial of the progressive nature of the disease

  c. **Substance abuse counseling** is essential for those who are struggling to remain abstinent. It is inappropriate for the transplant team to monitor the patient with urine toxicological screening, although many lung transplant programs do check cotinine levels. Such patients are better served by a referral to a substance abuse treatment program.

B. Care of the Post-transplant Patient

1. Short-term Care

Post-operatively, some patients recover rapidly and are able to leave the hospital within a few weeks. Others are less fortunate and can spend many weeks in an intensive care unit (ICU) before being transferred to the floor or to a rehabilitation facility. Patients can manifest the following:

a. **Organic Brain Syndromes**

      i. Etiologies of delirium include medication effect or medication withdrawal, metabolic changes, and infection

      ii. Cyclosporine, prednisone, and tacrolimus toxicity can produce a wide variety of neuropsychiatric symptoms that include seizures, sensorimotor changes, psychosis, delirium, and speech impairment. Liver transplant patients appear particularly vulnerable to such side effects. Central pontine myelinosis is a rare complication.

      iii. Heart transplant patients are at risk for intra-operative cerebral ischemia that can cause psychosis in the early post-operative period.

      iv. Management requires accurate assessment of the patient's mental status, hunt for etiology, and treatment of the underlying disorder, if possible. Judicious use of neuroleptics can ameliorate the symptoms.

b. **Depression** can result from:

      i. Medications, such as beta-blockers or benzodiazepines

      ii. Infection, particularly from cytomegalovirus (CMV)

      iii. Rejection

      iv. Recurrence of pre-morbid symptoms

c. **Anxiety** can follow:

      i. Medication effects—particularly from high-dose steroids

      ii. Withdrawal from sedative-hypnotics

      iii. Weaning from the ventilator

      iv. Pain, or anticipation of pain

d. **Post-traumatic Stress Disorder (PTSD)**

PTSD is uncommon but should be considered.

2. Long-term Follow-up

Transplant patients exchange one set of problems, those of end-organ failure, for another set of problems, those that attend the side effects of immunosuppressive medications, rejection of the allograft, and progression of systemic disease. Pre-morbid vulnerabilities can easily resurface in the setting of unmet expectations. **The presence of pre-transplant psychiatric symptoms appears to be the best predictor of post-transplant symptoms.**

    a. **Depression** may be related to

       i. Medication effects

      ii. Frequent medical setbacks

     iii. Bodily changes, such as weight gain, acne, and hirsutism, that are caused by steroids

     iv. Persistent weakness

      v. Reaction from family members who may either demand too much too soon or who are unable to see the patient as less dependent and/or more capable

    b. **Anxiety** can re-emerge in response to

       i. Side effects of medication

      ii. Anticipation and worry about allograft rejection

     iii. Concern regarding inability to live up to the expectations of self or others

     iv. Separation from caregivers (particularly members of the transplant team) and loss of other, tangible supports, such as dialysis or oxygen tanks

    c. **Substance Abuse** can also re-emerge even after the patient has had years of sobriety.

    d. **Non-compliance with medication regimens** deserves an assessment for depression and suicidality as well as an exploration of possible causes of anger at and disappointment in the treatment team.

3. **Treatment Strategies**

  Long-term care of the transplant patient can be guided by the same principles used pre-operatively. A combination of psychopharmacologic and psychotherapeutic intervention usually works best.

    a. **Psychopharmacologic treatment** is complicated by the neuropsychiatric side effects of the immunosuppressive medications and by the risk for multiple drug interactions.

       i. **Cyclosporine (CYA)** is a widely used immunosuppressive. Adverse effects include nephrotoxicity, hypertension, neurotoxicity, hypomagnesemia, hyperkalemia, hyperlipidemia, osteoporosis, and gastroparesis. It can increase lithium absorption leading to higher lithium levels. It is metabolized in the liver by the cytochrome P450 system. Carbamazepine and phenobarbital may decrease its levels through hepatic induction. SSRIs could increase its levels through inhibition of cytochrome P450 isoenzyme system, but that has not been demonstrated. Nefazodone (Serzone), however, is a source of very significant competitive inhibition.

      ii. **FK506 (tacrolimus)** is another immunosuppressive that is often used as a "salvage" therapy for patients who fail CYA. It can also cause neuropsychiatric symptoms, such as headache, insomnia, tremor, and visual hallucinations. It, too, is metabolized through the cytochrome P 450 isoenzyme system. Blood levels may be significantly affected by nefazodone. Combined use of ziprasidone (Geodon) is contraindicated because of potential QT interval prolongation.

     iii. **OKT3** is a monoclonal antibody that is used to treat organ rejection. It has neuropsychiatric side effects that include delirium, tremors, seizures, and sometimes, aseptic meningitis.

     iv. **Corticosteroids** continue to be a mainstay of immunosuppressive regimens and most transplant patients remain on them (at lower and lower doses) for the rest of their lives. They have numerous side effects (weight gain with fat distribution, easy bruising, osteoporosis, and hirsutism) including a tendency to cause emotional lability, hypomania or mania, as well as irritability and depression. Patients often manifest rapid cycling and can become psychotic. Benzodiazepines, such as clonazepam, or mood stabilizers, such as gabapentin, can be extremely helpful in ameliorating these uncomfortable symptoms.

b. **Psychotherapeutic Interventions**

The transplant patient can also benefit from supportive therapy. Pre-morbid issues, such as anxiety or depression, often thought to be a product of the end-organ failure, may not go away but may recur in a slightly different form. Other issues that may emerge include

  i. Curiosity about the donor and a wish to meet and thank the family
  ii. Fantasies about the donor organ causing personality changes within the recipient
  iii. Sadness over loss of the native organ and concerns about what might have happened to the missing body part
  iv. Worry that one is not taking full advantage of the "second chance" or "rebirth"
  v. Guilt over deriving benefit from someone else's loss

V. Conclusion

The patient with end-stage organ failure who is approaching transplant has few real options. Such patients are often desperate, sad, angry, and profoundly disabled. Prompt recognition and treatment of psychiatric symptoms can significantly impact quality of life for these patients. Post-transplant patients face different but equally daunting challenges. **Early recognition and treatment of psychiatric symptoms can often bolster compliance with medical regimens and prevent complications.**

Suggested References

Arnold, R.M., & Youngner, S.J. (1993). Back to the future: Obtaining organs from non-heart-beating cadavers. *Kennedy Institute Ethics Journal, 3,* 103–111.

Beresford, T.P., Turcotte, J.G., Meriond, R., et al. (1990). A rational approach to liver transplantation for the alcoholic patient. *Psychosomatics, 31,* 241–254.

Brown, T.M., & Brown, R.L.S. (1995). Neuropsychiatric consequences of renal failure. *Psychosomatics, 36,* 244–253.

Burdick, J.F., DeMeester, J., & Koyama, I. (1999). Understanding organ procurement and the transplant bureaucracy. In L.C. Ginns, A.B. Cosimi, & P.T. Morris (Eds.), *Transplantation.* Malden, Mass.: Blackwell Science, Inc., pp. 875–896.

Castelao, A.M., Sabate, J.M., Grino, S., et al. (1998). Cyclosporine-drug interactions. *Transplant Proceedings, 20*(suppl 6), 66–69.

Colon, E.A., Popkin, M.K., Matas, A., et al. (1991). Overview of noncompliance in renal transplantation. *Transplant Review, 5,* 175–180.

Cosimi, A.B. (1979). The donor and donor nephrectomy. In P.J. Morris (Ed), *Renal transplantation: Principle and practice.* New York: Grune & Stratton, pp. 69–87.

Dew, M.A., Roth, L.R., Schulberg, H.C., et al. (1996). Prevalence and predictors of depression and anxiety-related disorders during the year after heart transplantation. *General Hospital Psychiatry, 18*(suppl.), 48s–61s.

Hibberd, P.L., Surman, O.S., Bass, M., et al. (1995). Psychiatric disease and cytomegalovirus viremia in renal transplant recipients. *Psychosomatics, 36,* 561–563.

Levenson, J.L., & Olbrish, M.E. (1993). Psychosocial evaluation of organ transplant candidates: A comparative survey of process, criteria, and outcomes in heart, liver, and kidney transplantation. *Psychosomatics, 34,* 314–323.

Levenson, J.L., & Olbrisch, M.E. (2000). Psychosocial screening and selection of candidates for organ transplant. In P.T. Trzepacz, & A.F. DiMartini (Eds.), *The transplant patient.* Oxford, UK: Cambridge University Press, pp. 21–41.

Pizer, H., & Massachusetts General Hospital Transplant Unit. (1992). *Organ transplants: A patient's guide.* Boston: Harvard University Press.

Singer, P.A., Seigler, M., Whitington, P.F., et al. (1989). Ethics of liver transplantation with living donors. *New England Journal of Medicine, 3211,* 620–622.

Surman, O.S. (1989). Psychiatric aspects of organ transplantation. *American Journal of Psychiatry, 146,* 972–982.

Surman, O.S. (1999). Psychiatric considerations of organ transplantation. In L.C. Ginns, A.B. Cosimi, & P.T. Morris (Eds.), *Transplantation.* Malden, Mass.: Blackwell Science, Inc., pp. 709–724.

Surman, O.S. (2002). The ethics of partial liver donation. *New England Journal of Medicine, 346*(14), 1038.

Surman, O.S., & Cosimi, A.B. (1996). Ethical dichotomies in organ transplantation: A time for bridge building. *General Hospital Psychiatry, 18,* 135–185.

Surman, O.S., & Purilo, R. (1992). Reevaluation of organ transplantation criteria: Allocation of scarce resources to borderline candidates. *Psychosomatics, 33,* 202–212.

Trzepacz, P.T., DiMartini, A., & Tringali, R. (1993). Psychopharmacologic issues in organ transplantation: I. Pharmacokinetics in organ failure and psychiatric aspects of immunosuppressants and anti-infectious agents. *Psychosomatics, 34,* 199–207.

Trzepacz, P.T., DiMartini, A., & Tringali, R. (1993). Psychopharmacologic issues in organ transplantation: II. Psychopharmacologic medications. *Psychosomatics, 34,* 290–298.

Trzepacz, P.T., Gupta, B., & DiMartini, A.F. (2000). Pharmacologic issues in organ transplantation: Psychopharmacology and neuropsychiatric medication side effects. In P.T. Trzepacz, & A.F. DiMartini (Eds.), *The transplant patient.* Oxford, UK: Cambridge University Press, pp. 187–213.

CHAPTER 41
The Patient with Sexual Dysfunction

LINDA SHAFER

I. Introduction

A. Sexual Problems Occur Frequently and Cause Great Distress.
1. Fifty percent of American couples suffer from some type of sexual problem.
2. Twenty-four percent of Americans will experience a sexual dysfunction at some time in their lives.
3. Forty-three percent of women and 31% of men in the United States suffer from sexual dysfunction.
4. The primary care physician (PCP) is often the first to see the patient with sexual problems.
   a. Fifteen percent of medical outpatients present to their PCP with some kind of sexual complaint.
   b. The incidence of sexual problems in any medical practice is directly related to the frequency with which the clinician takes a sexual history.
   c. The PCP must be prepared to take a sexual history, assess the sexual problem, and initiate a therapeutic response.

II. Evaluation of the Problem

A. General Recommendations
1. **Sexual dysfunction is best understood by having knowledge of the stages of the normal sexual response, which vary with age and physical status.**
   a. Four-Step Model (Masters and Johnson)
      i. Excitement: arousal
      ii. Plateau: maximum arousal before orgasm
      iii. Orgasm: muscular contractions at 0.8-second intervals
      iv. Resolution: return to somatic baseline
      v. Refractory period: In men, it increases with age. In women, there is no refractory period.
   b. Triphasic Model (Helen Singer Kaplan)
      i. Desire
      ii. Excitement (arousal): vascular, innervated by the parasympathetic nervous system (2d, 3d, and 4th sacral segments of the spinal cord)
      iii. Orgasm: muscular, innervated by the sympathetic nervous system, whose reflex center is in the lumbar cord
   c. Aging Sexual Response
      i. Males are slower to achieve erections and need more direct stimulation to the penis to achieve erections.
      ii. Females have decreased levels of estrogen, which leads to decreased vaginal lubrication and narrowing of the vagina.

       d. Medications, diseases, injuries, and psychological conditions can affect the sexual response in any of its component phases, leading to different dysfunctional syndromes (Table 41-1).

         i. More than one sexual dysfunction can co-exist.

         ii. One sexual dysfunction can be the cause of another.

         iii. Primary sexual dysfunction: present since the onset of sexual activity

         iv. Secondary sexual dysfunction: occurs after a period of normal functioning

B. Medical History

1. Although most disorders were thought to have a psychological basis, newer diagnostic testing has identified more conditions having an organic etiology.
2. Most disorders share a mixed etiology.
3. Physical disorders, surgical disorders (Table 41-2), medications, and drug use or abuse (Table 41-3), can affect sexual functioning directly or cause secondary psychological reactions leading to a sexual problem.
4. Psychological causes are complex, ranging from superficial issues (fear of failure) to deep issues (profound depression).
   a. No direct correlation has been found between certain background factors and certain sexual dysfunctions.
   b. Predisposing, precipitating, and maintaining factors play a role in sexual problems (Table 41-4).

C. Sexual History

1. Be aware that patients are usually embarrassed to bring up and discuss a sexual problem.
2. Remember that physicians, too, are often uncomfortable discussing sexual issues because of fears of offending patients.
3. **Ask routine screening questions** as part of the medical history to give the patient a chance to talk about sexual problems:
   a. Is there anything you would like to change about your sex life?
   b. Have there been any changes in your sex life?
   c. Are you satisfied with your present sex life?

Table 41-1. Classification of Sexual Dysfunctions

Impaired Sexual Response Phase	Female	Male
Desire	Hypoactive sexual desire	Hypoactive sexual desire
	Sexual aversion	Sexual aversion
Excitement (Arousal) (Vascular)	Sexual arousal disorder	Erectile disorder
Orgasm (Muscular)	Orgasmic disorder	Orgasmic disorder
		Premature ejaculation
Sexual Pain	Dyspareunia	Dyspareunia
	Vaginismus	

Table 41-2. Medical and Surgical Conditions Causing Sexual Dysfunctions

Organic Disorder	*Sexual Impairment*
Endocrine	
Hypothyroidism, adrenal dysfunction, hypogonadism, diabetes mellitus	Low libido, impotence, decreased vaginal lubrication, early impotence
Vascular	
Hypertension, atherosclerosis, stroke, venous insufficiency, sickle cell disorder	Impotence, ejaculation and libido intact
Neurologic	
Spinal cord damage, diabetic neuropathy, herniated lumbar disc, alcoholic neuropathy, multiple sclerosis, temporal lobe epilepsy	Impotence, impaired orgasm Sexual disorder—early sign, low libido (or high libido)
Local Genital Disease	
Male: Priapism, Peyronie's disease, urethritis, prostatitis, hydrocele	Low libido, impotence
Female: Imperforate hymen, vaginitis, pelvic inflammatory disease, endometriosis	Vaginismus, dyspareunia, low libido, decreased arousal
Systemic Debilitating Disease	
Renal, pulmonary, hepatic diseases, advanced malignancies, infections	Low libido, impotence, decreased arousal
Surgical-Post-operative States	
Male: Prostatectomy (radical perineal), abdominal-perineal bowel resection	Impotence, no loss of libido, ejaculatory impairment
Female: Episiotomy, vaginal repair of prolapse, oophorectomy	Dyspareunia, vaginismus, decreased lubrication
Male and Female: Amputation (leg), colostomy and ileostomy	Mechanical difficulties in sex, low self-image, fear of odor

4. Additional routine questions to ask during the AIDS era include the following:
   a. Are you sexually active?
   b. Do you practice safe sex?
      i. Lack of knowledge of safe sex can contribute to the spread of AIDS.
      ii. Physicians should be prepared to discuss the benefits of safe sex techniques including the use of condoms and spermicides containing non-oxynol-9.
      iii. Failure to ask AIDS screening questions may result in allegation of inadequate treatment or even lead to a malpractice suit.
5. Interview Techniques
   a. Always **attempt to be sensitive and non-judgmental.**
   b. **Move from the more general to more specific topics** out of an appropriate context.
      i. Sexual issues can be easily integrated into the medical history when there is a review of systems, an introduction of a new medication, or the chief complaint involves a gynecological or urological problem.

Table 41-3. Drugs and Medicines Causing Sexual Dysfunction

Drug	Sexual Side Effects
Cardiovascular	
Methyldopa	Low libido, impotence, anorgasmia
Thiazide diuretics	Low libido, impotence, decreased lubrication
Clonidine	Impotence, anorgasmia
Propranolol	Low libido
Digoxin	Gynecomastia, low libido, impotence
Clofibrate	Low libido, impotence
Psychotropics	
Sedatives	
Alcohol	Higher doses cause sexual problems
Barbiturates	Impotence
Anxiolytics	
Diazepam	Low libido, delayed ejaculation
Alprazolam	
Antipsychotics	
Thioridazine	Retarded or retrograde ejaculation
Haloperidol	Low libido, impotence, anorgasmia
Antidepressants	
MAO inhibitors (Phenelzine)	Impotence, retarded ejaculation, anorgasmia
Tricyclics (Imipramine)	Low libido, impotence, retarded ejaculation
SSRI (fluoxetine, sertraline)	Low libido, impotence, retarded ejaculation
Atypical (trazodone)	Priapism, retarded or retrograde ejaculation
Lithium	Low libido, impotence
Hormones	
Estrogen	Low libido in men
Progesterone	Low libido, impotence
Gastrointestinal	
Cimetidine	Low libido, impotence
Methantheline bromide	Impotence
Opiates	Orgasmic dysfunction
Anticonvulsants	Low libido, impotence, priapism

    ii. Physicians should be aware of covert presentations of sexual problems (e.g., headache, insomnia, and low-back or generalized pelvic pain) that have no medical basis.

  c. Vary questions depending on the patient's age, social class or occupation, and the nature of the continuing relationship with you.

  d. Design the taking of the sexual history to fit the patient's needs and your time.

  e. If a sexual problem is uncovered, take a detailed history.

    i. Onset

    ii. Progression: How often? With all partners? On masturbation? With fantasy?

+--+

Table 41-4. Psychological Causes of Sexual Dysfunction

Predisposing Factors
   Lack of information and experience
   Unrealistic expectations
   Negative family attitude toward sex
   Sexual trauma—rape, incest

Precipitating Factors
   Childbirth
   Infidelity
   Dysfunction in the partner

Maintaining Factors
   Interpersonal issues
   Family stress
   Work stress
   Financial problems
   Depression
   Performance anxiety
   Gender identity conflicts

+--+

    iii. Assessment: Don't use "why" questions because this makes patients feel defensive. Use "what" questions, for example, "What do you think caused your problems?"

    iv. Attempts at resolution: Books, friends, clergy

    v. Patient's expectations and goals: Resolve the problem, save the marriage, an excuse for divorce

D. Examination of the Patient

  1. Physical Examination

    a. A thorough physical exam is indicated for every patient, with special attention paid to endocrine, neurologic, vascular, urologic, and gynecologic systems.

  2. Laboratory Examination

    a. Depends on the nature of the problem

    b. Depends on the index of suspicion (organic vs. psychological)

    c. Sexual history and physical exam often help determine the extent of the organic work-up, including what special laboratory studies and diagnostic procedures should be performed.

      i. Screening for unrecognized systemic disease includes complete blood count (CBC), urinalysis, creatinine, lipid profile, thyroid function studies, and fasting blood sugar (FBS).

      ii. Endocrine studies: testosterone, prolactin, luteinizing hormone (LH), and follicular stimulating hormone (FSH) for low libido and erectile dysfunction

      iii. Estrogen level and microscopic exam of vaginal smear for vaginal dryness

      iv. Sedimentation rate (rule out infection, inflammation, pelvic inflammatory disease), cervical culture, and pap smear for dyspareunia.

    d. Referral to urology, gynecology, endocrinology, neurology, or psychiatry is made on a case-by-case basis.

III. Psychiatric Differential Diagnosis

A. Depression (Major Depression or Dysthymic Disorder)
   1. Low libido, erectile dysfunction

B. Manic Phase (Bipolar Disorder)
   1. Increased libido

C. Generalized Anxiety Disorder, Panic Disorder, Post-traumatic Stress Disorder
   1. Low libido, erectile dysfunction, lack of vaginal lubrication, anorgasmia

D. Schizophrenia
   1. Low desire, bizarre sexual desire

E. Paraphilias
   1. Deviant sexual arousal

F. Gender Identity Disorder
   1. Dissatisfaction with one's own sex

G. Personality Disorder (Passive-Aggressive, Obsessive-Compulsive, Histrionic)
   1. Low libido, erectile dysfunction, premature ejaculation, anorgasmia

H. Marital Dysfunction-Interpersonal Problems

I. Fears of Intimacy/Commitment
   1. Deep, intrapsychic issues
   2. Range of sexual disorders including lack of vaginal lubrication

IV. Diagnostic Criteria

A. Disorders listed are not caused by organic factors (medical conditions, medication, or drugs of abuse) or by another (psychological) Axis I disorder. They all cause marked individual distress and interpersonal difficulties
   1. **Desire phase disorders**
      a. **Hypoactive Sexual Desire Disorder** (302.71 *DSM-IV*)
         i. Persistently deficient sexual fantasies and the desire for sexual activity
         ii. The number of couples presenting for sex therapy with desire disorders increased from 37% in the early 1970s to 55% in the early 1980s.
         iii. Overall 33% of women and 16% of men present with low libido.
         iv. Low desire is the most common female sexual disorder
      b. **Sexual Aversion Disorder** (302.79 *DSM-IV*)
         i. Persistent extreme aversion to, and avoidance of, all or almost all genital sexual contact with the sexual partner
         ii. Exact incidence is unknown; aversion is rare in men, higher in women
         iii. Primary sexual aversion is higher in men, secondary aversion higher in women.
         iv. The syndrome is associated with phobic avoidance of sexual activity or the thought of sexual activity.
         v. Twenty-five percent of these patients meet criteria for panic disorder.
         vi. Frequency of intercourse is once or twice a year.
         vii. Patients respond naturally to sex if they can get past their high anxiety and initial dread.
   2. **Arousal Phase Disorders**
      a. **Female Sexual Arousal Disorder** (302.72 *DSM-IV*)

        i. Persistent inability to attain or maintain the lubrication swelling response of sexual excitement until completion of the sexual act.

        ii. The incidence is approximately 21%

        iii. Linked to problems with sexual desire

        iv. Lack of vaginal lubrication may lead to dyspareunia.

    b. **Male Erectile Disorder** (302.72 *DSM-IV*—see Chapter 42)

3. **Orgasm Phase Disorders**

    a. **Female Orgasmic Disorder** (302.73)

        i. Persistent delay in, or absence of, orgasm following a normal excitement phase

        ii. Second most common category of female sexual dysfunctions: 5–8% totally anorgasmic, 26% unable to achieve orgasm without clitoral stimulation or during intercourse

        iii. The ability to have orgasm increases with sexual experience.

        iv. The diagnosis should not be made for women who can have orgasm with direct clitoral contact but find it difficult to reach orgasm during intercourse. This is a normal variant.

        v. Claims that stimulation of the Gräfenberg spot or G spot in a region in the anterior wall of the vagina will cause orgasm and female ejaculation have never been substantiated.

        vi. Look for the male sexual partner with premature ejaculation contributing to female orgasmic dysfunction.

    b. **Male Orgasmic Disorder** (302.74 *DSM-IV*)

        i. Persistent delay in, or absence of, orgasm following a normal sexual excitement phase

        ii. An infrequent disorder occurring in about 8% of men, who are usually sexually inexperienced.

        iii. Retarded ejaculation is usually restricted to failure to reach orgasm in the vagina during intercourse.

        iv. Orgasm can usually occur with masturbation or from a partner's manual or oral stimulation.

        v. The condition **must be differentiated from retrograde ejaculation,** where the bladder neck does not close off properly during orgasm, causing semen to spurt backward into the bladder.

        vi. Rule out retarded ejaculation in a couple presenting with infertility of unknown cause. The male may not have admitted his lack of ejaculation to his partner.

    c. **Premature Ejaculation** (302.75 *DSM-IV*)

        i. Persistent ejaculation with minimal stimulation before or after penetration and before the person wishes it.

        ii. Usually ejaculation occurs in less than 2 minutes with fewer than 10 thrusts.

        iii. Most common male sexual disorder, occurs in 31% of men.

        iv. Prolonged periods of no sexual activity make the problem worse.

        v. If the problem is chronic and untreated, secondary impotence often occurs.

4. **Sexual Pain Disorders**

    a. **Dyspareunia** (302.76 *DSM-1V*)

        i. Persistent genital pain before, during, or after sexual intercourse in either the male or the female.

        ii. Prevalence in females is 16%; prevalence in men is 3%.

        iii. Patients with persistent dyspareunia seek out medical treatment but the physical exam is often unremarkable, with no genital abnormalities.

      iv. In females, rule out vulvar vestibulitis.

      v. In post-menopausal females, rule out vaginal atrophy and dryness

      vi. If pain is caused solely by vaginismus or lack of lubrication, the diagnosis of dyspareunia is not made.

    b. **Vaginismus** (306.51 *DSM-IV*)

      i. Persistent involuntary spasm of the musculature of the outer third of the vagina that interferes with sexual intercourse

      ii. The frequency is unknown but vaginismus probably accounts for less than 10% of female disorders.

      iii. Diagnosis is often made on a routine gynecologic exam, when contraction of the vaginal outlet occurs as either the examining finger or a speculum is introduced.

      iv. High incidence of associated pelvic pathology

      v. Lifelong vaginismus has an abrupt onset, at first attempt of penetration, with a chronic course.

      vi. Acquired vaginismus may occur suddenly, following a sexual trauma or medical condition.

  5. **Sexual Dysfunction Not Otherwise Specified** (302.70 *DSM-IV*)

    a. No subjective erotic feelings despite otherwise normal arousal and orgasm (female analogue of premature ejaculation)

    b. It is unclear whether the sexual dysfunction is primary, caused by a medical condition, or substance-induced.

V. Treatment Strategies

A. Organically Based Sexual Disorders

  1. **Medical-Surgical Treatments—General**

    a. Treat pre-existing illnesses (e.g., diabetes, thyroid disorders).

    b. Stop or substitute for offending medications.

    c. Reduce alcohol consumption and smoking.

    d. Add medications for psychiatric conditions (e.g., depression).

    e. Consider the use of sildenafil for sexual side effects of antidepressants (SSRIs).

  2. Medical-Surgical Treatments—Male

    a. Correct hormone deficiencies (e.g., testosterone for hypogonadism).

    b. Initiate a pharmacologic erection treatment, for example, oral sildenafil, alprostadil injections (see Chapter 42).

    c. Initiate a trial of fluoxetine, sertraline, or clomipramine, for premature ejaculation.

    d. Consider an external penile suction device for erectile disorders (see Chapter 42).

    e. Perform surgery for vascular problems (e.g., endarterectomy).

    f. Implant a penile prosthetic device (see Chapter 42).

  3. Medical-Surgical Treatments—Female (Many new treatments under investigation)

    a. Correct hormone deficiency—to increase libido and decrease pain

      i. Estrogen replacement therapy in menopausal women.

      ii. Testosterone often used in combination with estrogen (Estratest) in menopausal women.

    b. Oral medication and vaginal creams under study to increase arousal, orgasm, libido.

      i. Sildenafil—Pilot studies; mixed results in post-menopausal women

      ii. Apomorphine—Pilot study for desire disorders

      iii. L-Arginine combined with Yohimbine—Pilot study

        iv. Phentolamine—Vaginal suppository (Vasofem)—under investigation

        v. Alprostadil—Vaginal suppository / topical cream (Femprox)—clinical trials.

    c. Consider FDA-approved external clitoral suction device (EROS-CTD)

B. Psychologically Based Sexual Disorders

1. General Principles

    a. If time is limited, schedule another appointment to take a detailed sexual history and initiate treatment.

    b. Conduct discussions about sex in the office, while the patient is fully clothed, not in the examining room.

    c. Use the pelvic exam to teach the female patient about sexual anatomy.

    d. Use the PLISSIT model—levels of treatment

        i. P-permission. Help reassure the patient regarding sexual activity. Alleviate guilt about activities that a patient feels are "bad" or "dirty." Use statistics to reinforce the range of normal activities.

        ii. LI-limited information. Provide information about anatomy and physiology. Correct myths and misconceptions.

        iii. SS-specific suggestions. Apply behavioral techniques used in sex therapy. There are general principles and specific techniques for each of the sexual dysfunctions.

        iv. IT-intensive therapy. Patients with chronic sexual problems or complex psychological issues may not respond to the first three levels and may benefit from consultation with a mental health professional skilled in dealing with sexual problems.

2. **Behavior Therapy (Sex Therapy)—General Principles**

    a. Improve communication between partners verbally and physically.

    b. Encourage experimentation.

    c. Decrease the pressure of performance by changing the goal of sexual activity away from erection or orgasm to feeling good about oneself.

    d. Relieve the pressure of the moment by suggesting there is always another day to try.

3. **Behavior Therapy (Sex Therapy)—Specific Suggestions**

    a. Hypoactive Sexual Disorder

        i. Initiate "sensate focus" exercises (non-demand pleasuring techniques) to enhance enjoyment without pressure. Help the individual or couple focus on "sensations," to feel and respond pleasurably to simple touching or massage, rather than on performance. Progress from non-genital to genital pleasuring.

        ii. Use erotic material.

        iii. Consider masturbation training with fantasy to help individuals become aware of conditions necessary for a positive sexual experience.

    b. Sexual Aversion Disorder

        i. Same as for hypoactive sexual desire

        ii. When the phobic/panic-type symptoms are displayed, the addition of antipanic medication (antianxiety or antidepressant) may be helpful.

    c. Female Sexual Arousal Disorder

        i. Usually requires referral.

        ii. Suggest the use of lubrication, such as saliva or KY jelly for vaginal dryness.

        iii. Post-menopausal women may benefit from topical estrogen cream given intermittently.

    d. Male Erectile Disorder (see Chapter 42).

    e. Female Orgasmic Disorder

        i. For women who have never had an orgasm, suggest self-stimulation, use of fantasy material, and Kegel vaginal exercises (contraction of pubococcygeus muscles).

    ii. Anorgasmic with partner. Use sensate focus exercises (from non-genital stimulation to genital stimulation). Use back protected position (male in seated position with female between his legs with back against his chest). Use controlled intercourse in the female-superior position (male lying on his back and female on top of him).

    iii. Anorgasmic during intercourse. Use the "bridge technique" in which the male stimulates the female's clitoris manually after insertion of the penis into the vagina.

  f. Male Orgasmic Disorder (During Intercourse)

    i. The female stimulates the male manually until orgasm becomes inevitable.

    ii. The penis is inserted into the vagina and thrusting begins.

    iii. Manual stimulation is repeated if there is no ejaculation.

  g. Premature Ejaculation

    i. Suggest an increase in frequency of sex.

    ii. Teach the "squeeze" technique in which the female (heterosexual couple) manually stimulates the penis. When ejaculation is approaching, as indicated by the male, the female squeezes the penis with her thumb on the frenulum. The pressure is applied until the male no longer feels the urge to ejaculate (15 to 60 seconds). Use the female superior position with gradual thrusting and the "squeeze" technique as excitement intensifies.

    iii. The "stop-start" method is an alternative to the "squeeze" technique. The female (heterosexual couple) stimulates the male to the point of ejaculation, then stops the stimulation. She resumes the stimulation for several stop-start procedures, until ejaculation is allowed to occur.

    iv. These techniques are applicable to the homosexual couple.

  h. Dyspareunia

    i. Treat any underlying gynecologic problem first.

    ii. Treat insufficient lubrication as described previously.

    iii. Treat accompanying vaginismus as described later.

  i. Vaginismus

    i. The female is encouraged to accept larger and larger objects into her vagina (e.g., her fingers, her partner's fingers, Hegar graduated vaginal dilators, syringe containers of different sizes).

    ii. Recommend use of the female superior position, allowing the female to gradually insert the erect penis into the vagina.

    iii. Use extra lubricant (KY jelly).

    iv. Practice Kegel vaginal exercises to develop a sense of control.

Suggested Readings

American Psychiatric Association. (1995). *Diagnostic and statistical manual of mental disorders* (4th ed., primary care version). Washington, DC: American Psychiatric Association.

Basson, R., Berman, J., Burnett, A., et al. (2000). Report of the international consensus conference on female sexual dysfunction: Definitions and classifications. *Journal of Urology, 163,* 888–893.

Basson, R., McInnes, R., Smith, M.D., et al. (2000). Efficacy and safety of sildenafil in estrogenized women with sexual dysfunction associated with female sexual arousal disorder. *Obstetrics Gynecology, 95*(4 Suppl 1), S54.

Crenshaw, T.L., & Goldberg, J.P. (1996). *Sexual pharmacology.* New York: W. W. Norton & Co.

Graziottin, A. (2001). Clinical approach to dyspareunia. *Journal of Sexual and Marital Therapy,* *27*(5), 489–501.

Laumann, E.O., Paik, A., & Rosen, R.C. (1999). Sexual dysfunction in the United States: Prevalence and predictors. *Journal of the American Medical Association, 281,* 537–544.

Marwick, C. (1999). Survey says patients expect little physician help on sex. *Journal of the American Medical Association, 281,* 2173–2174.

Maurice, W.L. (1999). *Sexual medicine in primary care.* New York: Mosby.

Metz, M.E., & Epstein, N. (2002). Assessing the role of relationship conflict in sexual dysfunction. *Journal of Sexual and Marital Therapy, 28*(2), 139–164.

Perlis, R.H., Fava, M., Nierenberg, A.A., et al. (2002). Strategies for treatment of SSRI-associated sexual dysfunction: A survey of an academic psychopharmacology practice. *Harvard Review of Psychiatry, 10*(2), 109–114.

Rosen, R.C. (2000). Prevalence and risk factors of sexual dysfunction in men and women. *Current Psychiatry Reports, 2*(3), 189–195.

Rosen, R.C. (2000). Sexual pharmacology in the 21st century. *Journal of Gender Specific Medicine, 3*(5), 45–52.

Rosen, R.C., & Leiblum, S.R. (1995). Treatment of sexual disorders in the 1990s: An integrated approach. *Journal of Consulting and Clinical Psychology, 63*(6), 877–890.

Shafer, L. (2000). Approach to the patient with sexual dysfunction. In A. Goroll, & A. Mulley (Eds.), *Primary care medicine.* Philadelphia: J. B. Lippincott Co., pp. 1178–1183.

Shafer, L. (1995). Sexual dysfunction. In K. Carlson, & S. Eisenstat (Eds.), *Primary care of women.* St. Louis: Mosby, pp. 270–274.

Shifren, J.L., Braunstein, G.D., Simon, J.A., et al. (2000). Transdermal testosterone treatment in women with impaired sexual function after oophorectomy. *New England Journal of Medicine, 343,* 682–688.

Simons, J.S. & Carey, M.P. (2001). Prevalence of sexual dysfunctions: Results from a decade of research. *Archives of Sexual Behavior, 30*(2), 177–219.

Steidle, C.P. (2002). Sexual dysfunction: Male and female issues. *International Journal of Fertility and Womens Medicine, 47*(1), 32–36.

CHAPTER 42
The Patient with Impotence

LINDA SHAFER

I. Introduction

A. Impotence or Erectile Dysfunction
Impotence is one of the most common problems affecting men. The primary care physician (PCP) is often the first doctor consulted about the problem.
1. Nearly all men have experienced erectile dysfunction at some time in their lives.
   a. Between 10 and 30% of men of all ages experience erectile dysfunction on a regular basis. In the United States, it is estimated that 30 million men have erectile dysfunction.
      i. The frequency of erectile dysfunction increases as men get older. By age 40, the estimated prevalence of erectile dysfunction is 39%. At age 70, the figure rises to 67%.
      ii. However aging by itself is not a cause of erectile dysfunction. The problem is more likely a result of medication use and medical problems that affect elderly men.

II. Evaluation of the Problem

A. General Recommendations
1. Although erectile dysfunction was once thought to be primarily owing to psychological causes, at least 50% of cases are now considered to have an organic basis. By using the most sophisticated erectile diagnostic techniques, such as infusion cavernosogram, an organic abnormality can be found in up to 85% of patients. In reality, erectile dysfunction is typically caused by a combination of physical and psychological factors.

B. General Medical History
1. Identify risk factors associated with, or accounting for, the erectile dysfunction (see Table 42-1).
2. Pay particular attention to the vascular, neurologic, and endocrine review of systems.
3. Review the medical history for medical and surgical conditions that cause erectile dysfunction (see Table 42-2).
4. Consider the possibility that medications, both prescribed and over-the-counter, and consumption of alcohol and illicit drugs are common, often unexpected, causes of erectile dysfunction (Table 42-3). It is estimated that 25% of cases of erectile dysfunction are caused by medications prescribed for another condition.

C. Sexual History
1. Obtain a detailed sexual history to help determine the etiology of the problem, as well as the direction and depth of treatment.
   a. **Use a non-judgmental style of interviewing,** while paying attention to the age, individual value system, and comfort level of the patient.
   b. **Characterize the nature of the problem.**

Table 42-1. Risk Factors Associated with Erectile Dysfunction

Hypertension	Pelvic trauma or surgery
Diabetes mellitus	Renal failure and dialysis
Smoking	Hypogonadism
Coronary artery disease	Alcoholism
Peripheral vascular disorders	Depression
Blood lipid abnormalities	Lack of sexual knowledge
Peyronie's disease	Poor sexual technique
Priapism	Interpersonal problems

    i. Onset-abrupt or gradual
    ii. Persistence
    iii. Progression or stability
    iv. Understand whether the problem varies with different partners, positions, or sexual settings.

c. **Question the patient about masturbation,** since it can help differentiate between a predominantly physical or psychological problem. Many patients are uncomfortable

Table 42-2. Medical and Surgical Conditions Causing Erectile Dysfunction

Systems	Medical and Surgical Condition(s)
Endocrine	Diabetes, thyroid disorder, pituitary adenoma, hypogonadism
Vascular	Atherosclerosis, angina, sickle-cell anemia, congestive heart failure
Neurologic	Multiple sclerosis, spinal cord disorder, polyneuropathy
Penile	Peyronie's disease, priapism, microphallus, phimosis
Renal	Renal failure (on dialysis)
Musculoskeletal	Arthritis
Pulmonary	Chronic obstructive lung disease
Surgical	Prostatectomy, radical prostatectomy, abdominal-perineal resection, renal transplantation, radical cystectomy, lumbar sympathectomy

Table 42-3. Drugs and Medication Causing Erectile Dysfunction	
Classifications	*Drug*
Antihypertensives	Methyldopa, clonidine, spironolactone, reserpine, propranolol, thiazides
Psychotropics	
Sedatives	Alcohol, barbituates
Anxiolytics	Diazepam, alprazolam
Antipsychotics	Thioridazine, chlorpromazine, haloperidol
Antidepressants	Monoamine oxidase inhibitors (phenelzine)
	Tricyclics (imipramine, clomipramine)
	Selective serotonin reuptake inhibitors (fluoxetine, sertraline)
Lithium	
Opiates	Morphine, heroin, methadone
Hormones	Estrogens, hydroxyprogesterone, steroids
Anticholinergics	Methantheline, propantheline
Miscellaneous	Cimetidine, metoclopramide, digitalis, clofibrate, disopyramide, baclofen

discussing masturbation and it is best to ask questions with the underlying assumption that most people masturbate.

    i. Ask the patient "How often do you masturbate?" rather than "Do you masturbate?"

  d. **Ask about morning or nocturnal erections,** as this too may help in the differential diagnosis.

  e. **Be aware that a history of occasionally adequate erections or sporadic successful intercourse does not rule out an organic etiology.**

  f. Remember that there may or may not be **associated problems with libido or ejaculation.**

  g. **Ask about the presence of psychological factors** that contribute to erectile dysfunction.

    i. Depression

    ii. Anxiety

    iii. Low self-esteem

    iv. Interpersonal problems

    v. Unrealistic expectations

    vi. Psychological complications of an organic problem

D. Examination of the Patient

  1. **Physical Examination**

    a. Examine the genitalia and prostate; evaluate the size and consistency of the testes, palpate the shaft of the penis to determine the presence of plaques, and perform a digital rectal exam of the prostate.

    b. Assess for signs of an endocrinopathy by examining male secondary sex characteristics and looking for other cutaneous manifestations (e.g., excessive dryness and hyperpigmentation).

    c. Assess the perineal region neurologically; check perianal sensation, anal sphincter tone, and the bulbocavemosus reflex (BC reflex).

        i. The BC reflex is elicited by squeezing the glans of the penis and noting reflex contraction of the external anal sphincter around the examining finger.

        ii. Test the integrity of the 2d, 3d, and 4th sacral segments of the spinal cord.

2. Laboratory Examination

a. Blood chemistry

    i. Testosterone and prolactin levels. If the screening testosterone level is low, repeat the exam and measure luteinizing hormone (LH), follicle stimulating hormone (FSH), and prolactin.

    ii. To exclude unrecognized systemic disease, check a complete blood count (CBC), urinalysis, creatinine (renal/urologic disease), lipid profile (atherosclerosis/vascular disease), thyroid function studies (hypothyroidism), and fasting blood sugar (FBS). If blood sugar results are equivocal, check a 2-hour post-prandial serum glucose (diabetes).

b. Non-invasive studies—Nocturnal Penile Tumescence (NPT)

    i. NPT confirms the total absence of erections, including erections that occur on awakening from sleep.

    ii. Physiological basis for testing-NPT episodes occur approximately every 90 minutes during REM (rapid eye movement) sleep (roughly three to five erections per sleep); the frequency decreases with age.

    iii. The absence of NPT suggests an organic disease.

    iv. Formal testing in a sleep lab measures penile tumescence while monitoring the EEG and eye movements (expensive).

    v. Inexpensive screening for NPT employs the "postage stamp" test. The patient is instructed to wrap a ring of postage stamps around the flaccid penis before going to bed at night. A positive test is finding that the stamps are separated at the perforations upon awakening.

    vi. Portable at-home monitoring is available to evaluate tumescence data (Rigiscan). A snap-gauge device is equipped with wires that break at different tensile strengths to measure rigidity.

c. Non-invasive vascular testing

    i. A penile brachial index (PBI) is obtained to determine arteriologic impotence by determining the ratio between the systolic penile blood pressure and the brachial systolic blood pressure (normal PBI > .75; abnormal PBI < .6)

    ii. Use of Doppler ultrasonography measures the diameter of arteries and rate of blood flow.

d. Invasive penile vascular testing requires consultation with urology.

    i. Papaverine (a smooth muscle relaxant) alone or in combination with phentolamine (an α-blocker) can be used for direct penile injection.

    ii. Normal penile vascularity is assumed if a firm erection is obtained 5 to 10 minutes after injection (age and dose-related).

    iii. Inability to attain full erection in 5 to 10 minutes or erection that lasts less than an hour suggests vascular disease.

e. Other invasive vascular testing used in selected cases in consultation with a specialist (persistent inability to achieve or maintain an erection)

      i. Cavernosometry—contrast media are injected into one corpora to identify abnormalities of drainage when vessels of the glans penis are visualized by fluoroscopy with spot x-ray capabilities.

      ii. Pelvic angiography

  f. **Neurological testing**—Extensive, requires consultation with neurology

      i. Dorsal nerve conduction latencies, evoked potentials, and cavernosal electromyography should be reserved for patients with a pre-existing neurologic disease.

III. Psychiatric Differential Diagnosis

A. Depression (Major Depression or Dysthymic Disorder)

B. Anxiety (performance anxiety) or Guilt

C. Obsessive "Anti-Fantasies" Focusing on the Negative Aspects of a Partner

D. Sexual Avoidance of Erotic Fantasies or Stimulation

E. Fears of Intimacy/Commitment-Intrapsychic Issues

F. Interpersonal Issues—Anger at Partner

IV. Diagnostic Criteria

A. Erectile Disorder (302.72 *DSM-IV*)

  1. The condition is defined as the inability to attain or maintain a satisfactory erection until completion of sexual activity, causing marked distress or interpersonal difficulty. The condition is not caused by the effects of a substance (drugs of abuse or medication), a general medical condition, or another (psychological) Axis I disorder.

  2. Primary (life-long)

    The male has never had successful intercourse.

    a. Occurs in 1% of men under age 35.

  3. Secondary (acquired)

    The dysfunction develops after a period of normal functioning.

    a. Inability to achieve successful intercourse occurs in 25% of attempts.

  4. Generalized (in all circumstances)

  5. Situational (limited to certain types of stimulation, situations, and partners).

V. Treatment Strategies

A. Organically Based Erectile Dysfunction

  1. **Medical therapies—non-operative**

    a. **Stop, or substitute for, offending medicines.**

    b. **Reduce alcohol consumption and smoking.**

    c. **Treat hormone deficiency states and abnormalities.**

      i. Use testosterone injections for hypogonadism.

      ii. Administer thyroid hormone for hypothyroidism.

      iii. Prescribe bromocriptine when elevated prolactin levels are present, after neuroimaging of sellar region of pituitary and obtain an endocrine consult.

    d. **Consider use of yohimbine,** an α-2 blocker, that blocks the outflow of blood from corporal tissues.

      i. Unfortunately, this is of limited usefulness.

    e. **Consider the use of sildenafil (Viagra).**

      i. It is taken 1 hour before sexual activity.

      ii. It blocks the activity of an enzyme (phosphodiesterase type 5) involved in relaxation of smooth muscle within the penis.

  f. **Consider new pharmacologic agents presently in clinical trials.**

      i. Transdermal testosterone gel

      ii. Topical Alprostadil gel—Prostaglandin E1 relaxes the smooth muscles of penis

      iii. Sublingual apomorphine (Uprima)— Dopamine agonist

      iv. Oral vardenafil (Nuviva)— Phosphodiesterase type 5 inhibitor

      v. Oral tadalafil (Cialis)— Phosphodiesterase type 5 inhibitor

      vi. Oral phentolamine (Vasomax)—α-adrenergic blocker relaxes the smooth muscles

2. **Drug self-injection therapies**

  a. Papaverine (a smooth muscle relaxant). Used alone or with phentolamine (an α-adrenergic blocker). When injected into the corpora of the penis, it will dilate blood vessels in the penis and block the outflow through the veins causing erection in 5 to 10 minutes in normal patients.

      i. Response is age-dependent and related to the absence of vascular disease.

      ii. Side effects—priapism, fibrosis.

  b. Prostaglandin El (PGE-1), also called Alprostadil. It is an FDA-approved drug under the brand name Caverject.

      i. A vasodilating substance used in penile self-injections.

      ii. Side effects—pain at injection site; associated with less priapism than papaverine and no fibrosis.

3. Transurethral delivery of Alprostadil

  a. Medicated urethral system for erection (MUSE)

      i. A thin plastic tube with a button on top is self-inserted into the urethra.

      ii. When the button is pressed, a pellet containing Alprostadil is released causing erection within 10 minutes, which lasts an hour.

      iii. Side effects—pain and urethral burning for 5 to 15 minutes.

4. Surgical therapies

  a. Vascular surgery to treat arterial insufficiency or excessive venous outflow are options but they have had limited success.

      i. Selection of patients follows adherence to strict criteria.

  b. Penile prostheses

      i. Useful for men who fail to respond to, or refuse, other forms of treatment.

      ii. Operative placement of implants are common in the United States.

      iii. The best candidate is in reasonable health with normal libido, sensation, and ejaculation, with approval/acceptance of the procedure by the sexual partner.

      iv. Types—semi-rigid rods malleable, inflatable.

      v. Complications—mechanical failure, infections, erosions.

      vi. Implants are made primarily of silicone. Silicone particle-shedding has been recorded, including migration to regional lymph nodes. No identifiable problems have been attributed to silicone particles.

5. External devices—vacuum constriction device.

  a. Traps blood in the penis by way of a constriction band after vacuum-assisted penile engorgement.

  b. A constriction band may remain in place for up to 30 minutes without any problem.

  c. Useful for those who are poor surgical risks or who desire non-surgical treatment.

B. Psychologically Based Erectile Dysfunction

1. General principles
   a. Give the patient permission to discuss the situation and provide reassurance by re-labeling sexual activities that are felt to be bad or sinful.
   b. Educate the patient by correcting myths and misconceptions.
2. Behavior therapy for erectile dysfunction.
   a. Goal—to decrease performance anxiety
   b. Educate the patient about ways to satisfy his partner without penile-vaginal intercourse.
   c. Prescribe "sensate focus" exercises.
      i. Non-demand pleasuring to help the couple focus on "sensations" rather than performance.
      ii. Progressing from non-genital massage to genital massage.
   d. Prohibit intercourse, even if erection occurs.
   e. Prescribe the female-superior position (female on top of male) to attempt non-demanding intercourse (heterosexual couple).
      i. The female manually stimulates the penis and if erection is obtained she inserts the penis into her vagina and gradual movement is begun.
      ii. This exercise may be done with a partial erection.
      iii. Emphasis is on pleasure of vaginal containment, not on getting an erection or reaching orgasm.
3. Hypnosis—selected cases
4. Psychotherapy and marital therapy-selected cases
5. Drug injection therapy can be beneficial to restore confidence while exploring psychological issues.

Suggested Readings

American Psychiatric Association. (1995). *Diagnostic and statistical manual of mental disorders* (4th ed., primary care version). Washington, DC: American Psychiatric Association.

Andersson, K.E., & Hedlund, P. (2002). New directions for erectile dysfunction therapies. *International Journal of Impotence Research, 14*(suppl 1), S82–S92.

Carson, C.C. (2002). Erectile dysfunction in the 21st century: Whom we can treat, whom we cannot treat and patient education. *International Journal of Impotence Research, 14*(suppl 1), S29–S34.

Feldman, H.A., Goldstein, B., & Rubinstein, D. (1994). Impotence and its medical and psychosocial correlates: Results of the Massachusetts male aging study. *Journal of Urology, 151,* 54–61.

Goldstein, I., Lue, T.F., Padma-Nathan, H., et al. (1998). Oral sildenafil in the treatment of erectile dysfunction. *New England Journal of Medicine, 338,* 1397–1404.

Johannes, C.B., Araujo, A.B., Feldman, H.A., et al. (2000). Incidence of erectile dysfunction in men 40 to 69 years old: Longitudinal results from the Massachusetts Male Aging Study. *Journal of Urology, 163,* 460–463.

Lue, T.F. (2000). Erectile dysfunction. *New England Journal of Medicine, 342,* 1802–1813.

Mulley, A.G., & Goroll, A.H. (2000). Medical evaluation and management of erectile dysfunction. In A. Goroll, & A. Mulley (Eds.), *Primary care medicine.* Philadelphia: J. B. Lippincott Co., pp. 761–770.

NIH Consensus Development Panel on Impotence. (1993). *Journal of the American Medical Association, 270*(t), 83–90.

Padma-Nathan, H., & Giuliano, F. (2001). Oral drug therapy for erectile dysfunction. *Urologic Clinics of North America, 28,* 321–334.

Rhoden, E.L., Teloken, C., Sogari, P.R., & Souto, C.A. (2002). The relationship of serum testosterone to erectile function in normal aging men. *Journal of Urology, 167*(4), 1745–1748.

Sadovsky, R. (2000). Integrating erectile dysfunction treatment into primary care practice. *American Journal of Medicine, 109*(Suppl 9A), 22S–30S.

Shafer, L. (2000). Approach to the patient with sexual dysfunction. In A. Goroll, & A. Mulley (Eds.), *Primary care medicine.* Philadelphia: J. B. Lippincott Co., pp. 1178–1183.

CHAPTER 43

The Patient with Infertility

RUTA NONACS AND LEE S. COHEN

I. Introduction

A. Definition. Infertility is defined as the failure to conceive after one year of regular sexual intercourse or the inability to carry a pregnancy to live birth.

B. Prevalence. Infertility is diagnosed in **approximately one of every six couples of child-bearing age.** Infertility rates rise with maternal age. About 10% of women under the age of 25 years suffer from infertility; this rate increases to 25% in women between 35 and 40 years of age. As more people choose to postpone childbearing, a growing number of couples are pursuing infertility treatment. Fortunately, successful conception occurs in 50–60% of couples who receive the appropriate treatment. However, the diagnosis of infertility and its evaluation and treatment are commonly perceived as emotionally stressful and may have a profound impact on both members of the couple.

II. Impact of Infertility on the Couple

A. Infertility as a source of emotional distress. While infertility does not necessarily lead to psychiatric illness, it does cause **significant emotional distress** for both members of the couple.
  1. **Sixty to ninety percent of infertile patients report significant psychological distress** related to this condition.
  2. Distress typically is manifested as feelings of sadness, anxiety, and irritability.
  3. Fifty percent of infertile patients report that the stress associated with infertility adversely affects their occupational and/or social functioning.
  4. Women in general report higher levels of distress than do men.

B. Infertility experienced as a loss. Having a child carries many different meanings for those who attempt to conceive. Those meanings determine the impact of infertility on a couple. In the broadest sense, infertility represents a loss. In response to this loss, an infertile patient experiences a pattern of responses similar to those described for bereavement.
  1. **Denial.** A patient may be unable to accept the diagnosis of infertility and as a result may avoid further evaluation and treatment.
  2. **Anger.** A patient may direct anger toward his or her partner or toward the physician. Anger often is related to a perceived loss of control.
  3. **Withdrawal and isolation.** Infertility may be viewed as socially or personally unacceptable. A patient may be reluctant to discuss this issue with friends or family members and avoid social situations where children are present.
  4. **Guilt and self-blame.** A patient may feel responsible for his or her inability to conceive and may dwell incessantly on it. He or she may believe that infertility is a punishment for a real or imagined transgression.

5. **Grief.** The patient may feel a profound sadness related to the inability to have children. The patient may feel that it is impossible to reach his or her full potential and may have a sense of being forced to abandon the most important dreams for the future.

6. **Acceptance.** Resignation or acceptance of infertility allows the patient to carry on with life.

C. **Infertility as a physical deficit.** To some patients, infertility also represents a **physical deficit.** It is a prolonged and sometimes chronic condition. Previously healthy men and women who undergo evaluation for, and treatment of, infertility become patients and are subjected to tests and procedures that can extend over several years. In many respects, these patients face many of the same issues faced by patients with a chronic medical illness.

1. The patient may experience a **loss of confidence and self-esteem.** He or she may feel unable to accomplish certain tasks and to attain certain goals.

2. **Feelings of inadequacy and helplessness** are common.

3. The patient may become **preoccupied with his or her physical well-being** and may present with **multiple somatic concerns.**

D. **The capacity to cope with infertility.** The ability to manage the intense feelings that often are associated with infertility depends on the coping strategies and emotional resources both members of a couple bring to the situation. Some couples perceive the diagnosis of infertility as a crisis that threatens the integrity of the relationship. In other cases, this experience may help the couple strengthen the interpersonal bond.

III. Evaluation and Treatment of Infertility

A. **Impact of psychiatric illness on infertility.** Although the early literature in this field suggested a **psychogenic basis for many cases of infertility,** there is little evidence to suggest a causal relationship between mood or anxiety disorders and infertility.

1. However, psychiatric disorders (e.g., major depressive disorder, post-traumatic stress disorder) may result in diminished frequency of sexual intercourse and can have an adverse effect on fertility.

2. Women with severe **bulimia or anorexia nervosa often** experience menstrual irregularities or amenorrhea and may present with reduced fertility.

3. **Stress may have a significant impact on the hypothalamic-pituitary axis** and on estrogen and progesterone function. In this manner, stress may adversely affect fertility, as the hormonal changes associated with stress may lead to abnormal menstrual cycles and impaired spermatogenesis.

4. Lower success rates for infertility treatment have been observed in female patients experiencing higher levels of depression and anxiety.

B. **Impact of psychotropic medications on fertility.** A variety of psychotropic medications may affect sexual function and fertility.

1. **Antidepressants frequently diminish libido and cause anorgasmia** or delayed orgasm. Several classes of antidepressants have been associated with these sexual side effects (see Chapter 66), including the following:

   a. Selective serotonin reuptake inhibitors (SSRIs), which produce sexual dysfunction in 30–50% of patients

   b. Tricyclic antidepressants (TCAs), particularly clomipramine and imipramine

        c. Monoamine oxidase inhibitors (MAOIs)

        d. Atypical antidepressants (e.g., nefazodone and bupropion), which are less commonly associated with sexual side affects

    2. **Dopamine antagonists, used as antipsychotic agents, can cause hyperpro-lactinemia,** which is associated with diminished libido, erectile dysfunction, and amenorrhea.

        a. Typical neuroleptics, particularly low-potency agents (e.g., chlorpromazine, and thiori-dazine), may cause hyperprolactinemia.

        b. Risperidone frequently elevates prolactin levels.

        c. Atypical neuroleptics (e.g., clozapine, olanzapine, and quetiapine) have not been associated with hyperprolactinemia and infrequently produce sexual side effects.

C. Diagnosis. Infertility specialists use a team approach in which a patient interacts with various doctors, nurses, and mental health specialists. The couple undergoes a variety of tests and procedures as part of this evaluation.

    1. For women, the evaluation typically includes an assessment of hormone levels, basal body temperature charting, hysterosalpingography, endometrial biopsy, laparoscopy, and hysteroscopy.

    2. For men, the evaluation includes an assessment of hormone levels, semen analysis, and, on rare occasions, testicular biopsy.

    3. In about 10% of cases no specific cause of infertility can be determined.

D. Medical treatment of infertility. Since the 1970s, **assisted reproductive technology** (ART) has provided infertile couples with a variety of options for treatment (Table 43-1). The choice of technique depends on the cause of the infertility, personal prefer-ence, and financial considerations.

    1. **Artificial or intrauterine insemination (IUI)** involves the transvaginal introduction of sperm into the uterus. **Therapeutic donor insemination (TDI)** utilizes donor sperm for this procedure.

    2. For *in vitro* **fertilization (IVF)**, harvested ova and sperm are incubated in a culture dish, with subsequent transfer of the fertilized egg or embryo to the uterus.

    3. **Gamete intrafallopian transfer (GIFT)** involves the introduction of a mixture of unfertilized ova and sperm into the fallopian tube.

    4. **Zygote intrafallopian transfer (ZIFT)** is a combination of IVF and GIFT, in which an egg fertilized *in vitro* is transferred to the fallopian tube.

    5. **Intracytoplasmic sperm injection (ICSI)** is a relatively new technique in which the genetic material from sperm is injected directly into the ovum. The fertilized egg is implanted using IVF techniques.

    6. IVF, GIFT, ZIFT, and ICSI also may be performed using donor eggs fertilized by the partner's sperm or donated sperm.

E. Psychological evaluation. Mental health specialists, typically psychologists and social workers, are an integral part of the infertility treatment program. **Psychological assess-ment and follow-up are an important part of the process.**

    1. In some clinics, a **psychological assessment** is a routine part of every infertility con-sultation. In most clinics, only patients undergoing ART or gamete donation are re-ferred for psychological evaluation.

    2. The majority of patients endorse a **need for emotional support** during infertility treatment, yet only a small fraction (10–20%) take advantage of available mental health services.

Table 43-1. Infertility: Causes, Treatments, Costs, and Success Rates

Cause of Infertility	Procedure	Cost of Procedure	Success Rate of Procedure (%)
Male Factors			
Low sperm count	Hormone treatment	$1,500-3,000	N.A.
Poor sperm motility	IUI	$100-250	10–15
Poor sperm morphology	TDI	$150-450	25
	IVF	$10,000-12,000	15
	ICSI + IVF/ZIIFT	$12,000-17,000	30–40
Varicocele	Surgery	$5,000-8,000	N.A.
Female Factors			
Functional factors	Hormone treatment	$1,500-3,000	N.A.
(endometriosis)	Surgery	$10,000-15,000	N.A.
Ovulation factors	Hormone treatment	$1,500-3,000	N.A.
	Egg donation plus IVF	$20,000-50,000	30
Tubal factors	IVF	$10,000-12,000	8-20
	GIFT	$10,000-15,000	12-25
	ZIFT	$10,000-15,000	30
Cervical factors	Hormone treatment	$1,500-3,000	N.A.
	IUI	$100-250	N.A.
Uterine factors	Surgery	$5,000-8,000	N.A.
	Surrogacy	$20,000-50,000	N.A.

NOTE: NA, data regarding success rates not available; IUI, intrauterine insemination; TDI, therapeutic donor insemination; IVF, *in vitro* fertilization; ICSI, intracytoplasmic sperm injection; ZIFT, zygote intrafallopian transfer.

SOURCE: Adapted from Meyers, M., Diamond, R., Kezur, D., et al. (1995). An infertility primer for family therapists: Medical, social, and psychological dimensions. *Family Practice, 34,* 219–228.

3. In addition to providing information on infertility treatment and facilitating decision-making, mental health professionals attempt to identify patients who need further psychological evaluation and treatment.

4. Psychological assessment often is used to decide who is inappropriate for certain types of infertility treatment. Although there are no standardized guidelines for making this type of decision, reasons for exclusion typically include severe marital strife, physical abuse, and any major mental illness which would impair the ability of either parent to care for a child.

IV. Psychiatric Consequences of Infertility Treatment

A. **Infertility treatment as a source of distress.** Although infertility treatment brings the hope of a "cure" and successful conception, it may place additional stress on the couple.

1. **Treatment is extremely time-consuming.** Frequent medical appointments are required, and treatment typically extends over several years.

2. Treatment presents a significant **financial burden** for most couples. Insurance companies vary widely in their willingness to reimburse patients for infertility treatment.

3. Patients are forced to engage in sexual activity on a predetermined schedule, which is later scrutinized by the treatment team.

4. The treatment of infertility is associated with **high failure rates;** 30–50% of those in treatment will be unable to conceive.

B. **Emotional distress as a consequence of treatment.** As the duration of evaluation and treatment increases and the couple repeatedly fails to conceive, the degree of emotional distress intensifies.

1. **Particularly stressful points in the evaluation and treatment process include the initial visit, the time of diagnosis, each failed attempt, and the termination phase of treatment.**

2. Women in general report higher levels of distress than do men.

3. Men experience greater levels of distress when it is discovered that infertility is related to a male factor (i.e., low sperm count, poor sperm quality).

4. **Sexual dysfunction occurs in up to one-half of women** who receive treatment for infertility. Women typically report less interest in sexual relations and diminished pleasure. Up to 30% of men experience transient erectile dysfunction in this setting.

5. **Marital discord is relatively common,** particularly when only one member of the couple is responsible for the infertility problem.

6. Feelings of depression and anxiety are given frequently as reasons for discontinuing infertility treatment.

C. **Psychiatric illness in an infertile patient.** Although most couples report feelings of depression and anxiety, only a small proportion of infertile patients develop symptoms severe enough to meet criteria for a major depressive episode or a formal anxiety disorder

1. Major depression occurs at a rate of about 10% in women during the treatment of infertility.

2. **Patients with a history of depression or anxiety disorder are at risk for relapse** in this setting, particularly if psychotropic medications were discontinued before attempts to conceive.

D. **Impact of fertility medications on psychiatric illness. Many of the medications used to treat infertility affect mood.** The individuals at highest risk are those with a history of mood or anxiety disorders.

1. **Clomiphene citrate** is associated with emotional lability, irritability, and insomnia.

2. **Progesterone** may cause depression and anxiety.

3. **Estrogens** may be associated with depression and fatigue.

4. **Gonadotropin-releasing hormone agonists** (e.g., leuprolide monoacetate) may cause anxiety, depressive symptoms, and mood instability.

5. **Bromocriptine** may on rare occasions precipitate psychotic symptoms.

V. Pregnancy in an Infertile Couple

A. **Psychological response to pregnancy.** Although pregnancy is obviously the desired outcome of infertility treatment, it often is associated with increased levels of anxiety.

1. Women with a history of infertility are particularly attentive to any physical changes that take place during pregnancy and are more likely to interpret them as negative.

2. Pregnancies in the infertile population are often treated as high risk and may require more intensive monitoring, which may cause significant distress for the couple.

B. Multiple gestations. In women who receive hormonal treatment and ART, multiple gestations are common.

1. **There is a significant increase in the rate of miscarriage and perinatal complications in women with multiple gestations.**

2. Mothers of triplets and quadruplets are at greater risk for the onset of a major depressive episode during the first post-partum year than are mothers of single infants or twins.

3. Children born into high-order multiple sets are more likely to suffer from neglect and developmental delay.

C. Impact of pregnancy loss. Approximately 10–20% of all pregnancies end in miscarriage. **After conception, infertile women have a significantly higher risk of miscarriage** than do women with no history of infertility. In addition, miscarriage is more common in older women.

1. Pregnancy loss is experienced as a devastating outcome. Spontaneous abortion is associated with high levels of depressive symptoms and anxiety.

2. Although estimates vary widely, 10–50% of women suffer an episode of major depression during the first 6 months after a spontaneous abortion.

3. Women at the greatest risk for developing an episode of major depression include those with a history of major depression and those who are childless.

4. The symptoms of major depression typically present during the first month after the loss and may persist for as long as a year.

5. **There is an increased rate of separation and divorce** among couples who experience a pregnancy loss.

VI. Management of a Patient with Infertility

A. Conceptualization of the problem. Although only one member of the couple may have an infertility problem, it is essential to treat infertility as a problem belonging to the couple.

1. **Meet with both members of the couple** at the initial visit and during subsequent visits as often as is deemed appropriate.

2. Arrange for individual visits to obtain thorough medical, social, and sexual histories.

3. Particularly when only one partner in the couple is responsible for the infertility problem, it is important to include the other partner to minimize feelings of blame and resentment.

B. Develop a plan of investigation and treatment with the couple.

1. **Present detailed information on the procedures available to the couple.**

2. Provide clear **information regarding the success rates** of the various procedures.

3. Supplement the material presented during the interview with written literature (e.g., a series of patient information brochures published by the American Society of Reproductive Medicine).

4. **Present the couple with multiple options and let the couple make the final decision.**

5. **Choose a termination date** for the treatment so that the process does not continue indefinitely.

6. **Discuss the viability of adoption** early in the process. It may take several years to make the necessary arrangements for adoption.

C. Coping with Infertility

1. During the course of treatment patients will be forced to make many difficult decisions and will benefit from **reassurance and empathic support.**
2. **Review common responses** to the condition of infertility (e.g., anger, grief, and marital tension).
3. **Ensure the availability of the medical staff** to discuss procedures, decisions, and the results of tests.
4. Mental health professionals familiar with infertility treatment can provide information and facilitate decision-making.
5. Patients may benefit from **peer support groups.** Resolve, Inc. (Somerville, MA), is a non-profit national organization which offers referrals, literature, and support groups for infertile couples.

D. Screen for signs of marital discord.

1. Encourage the couple to **discuss the quality of the relationship,** including sexual satisfaction.
2. If relationship difficulties are significantly affecting either partner's capacity to function at work or at home, refer the couple for **couples counseling.**

E. Assess for signs of depression and anxiety.

1. **Explore the patient's complaint of "depression"** to distinguish between an appropriate response and a disorder (e.g., major depression) which requires a specific treatment.
2. **Assess the impact of the depressive symptoms or anxiety** on the patient's ability to function at work and at home.
3. **Screen for** symptoms associated with **major depressive disorder** (see Chapter 14).
4. **Screen for** symptoms associated with **generalized anxiety disorder or panic disorder** (see Chapter 16).
5. If the symptoms interfere with the ability of a couple to function or participate in infertility treatment, there is a need for **additional support and treatment.**
   a. **Supportive or insight-oriented psychotherapy** may be helpful.
   b. **Cognitive-behavioral techniques** may be useful in minimizing the symptoms of anxiety and depression.
   c. **Pharmacologic management** of these symptoms may be required. In treating affected women, an attempt should be made to choose medications which can be continued during pregnancy if necessary. These pharmacologic options are outlined in Chapter 46.
6. There is evidence that counseling and support groups not only decrease levels of anxiety and depression but may also enhance quality of life and improve success rates of infertility treatment.

VII. Conclusion

A. Recognition of the problem. Infertility, as well as its evaluation and treatment, is perceived by most people as emotionally stressful. A patient with infertility requires close monitoring for signs of emotional distress and psychiatric illness.

1. Prolonged treatment for infertility is associated with high levels of distress.
2. Patients with a history of mood or anxiety disorders are at high risk for relapse in this setting.

3. Marital discord is common.

4. Even patients who do conceive experience heightened levels of emotional distress.

B. Psychiatric Treatment. While most patients benefit from reassurance and support, a small proportion of patients require more intensive treatment for depression or anxiety.

Suggested Readings

Berg, B.J., & Wilson, J.F. (1990). Psychiatric morbidity in the infertile population: A reconceptualization. *Fertility & Sterility, 53,* 654–661.

Eugster, A., & Vingerhoets, A.J.J.M. (1999). Psychological aspects of in vitro fertilization: A review. *Social Science Medicine, 48,* 575–589.

Klock, S.C., & Greenfeld, D.A. (2000). Psychological status of in vitro fertilization patients during pregnancy: A longitudinal study. *Fertility & Sterility, 73*(6), 1159–64.

Menning, B.E. (1980). The emotional needs of infertile couples. *Fertility & Sterility, 34,* 313–319.

Meyers, M., Diamond, R., Kezur, D., et al. (1995). An infertility primer for family therapists: Medical, social, and psychological dimensions. *Family Practice, 34,* 219–228.

Neugebauer, R., Kline, J., Shrout, P., et al. (1997). Major depressive disorder in the six months after miscarriage. *Journal of the American Medical Association, 227,* 393–398.

CHAPTER 44

The Patient with Premenstrual Syndrome

CLAUDIO N. SOARES, MAURIZIO FAVA, AND LEE S. COHEN

I. Introduction

A. Definition

Premenstrual syndrome (PMS) is a constellation of physical and psychological symptoms (see Table 44-1), related to the hormonal fluctuations of the menstrual cycle, that presents during the end of the luteal phase. Typically, these symptoms disappear shortly after the onset of menstruation. The *DSM-IV* has established strict research criteria for classification of this syndrome, which is called premenstrual dysphoric disorder, and has focused on the psychological and affective components of this syndrome (see Table 44-2). The concept of premenstrual dysphoric disorder differs from that of PMS in the greater severity of symptoms and the resulting impairment. Whereas PMS is likely to affect a significant number of women of child-bearing potential, a smaller percentage of women meet *DSM-IV* criteria for premenstrual dysphoric disorder.

Table 44-1. Physical and Psychological Symptoms of Premenstrual Syndrome

• Insomnia	• Lack of motivation or interest
• Weight gain	• Headaches
• Fatigue	• Backache
• Stomach ache	• Crying spells
• Affective instability	• Hot flashes
• Cold sweats	• Numbness or tingling in extremities
• Hypersomnia	• Breast swelling and soreness
• Fluid retention	• Restlessness
• Diminished concentration	• Clumsiness
• Hyperphagia	• Irritability
• Aggressive behavior	• Distractibility
• Carbohydrate craving	• Anxiety, nervousness
• Muscle pain	• Muscle tension
• Heart palpitations	• Chest pain
• Dizziness	• Agitation

Table 44-2. DSM-IV Research Criteria for Premenstrual Dysphoric Disorder

A. In most menstrual cycles during the past year, five (or more) of the following symptoms were present for most of the time during the last week of the luteal phase, began to remit within a few days after the onset of the follicular phase, and were absent in the week post-menses with at least one of the symptoms being either (1), (2), (3), or (4):

1. Markedly depressed mood, feelings of hopelessness, or self-deprecating thoughts
2. Marked anxiety, tension, feelings of being "keyed up" or "on edge"
3. Marked affective lability (e.g., feeling suddenly sad or tearful, or increased sensitivity to rejection)
4. Persistent and marked anger or irritability, or increased interpersonal conflicts
5. Decreased interest in usual activities (e.g., work, school, friends, hobbies)
6. Subjective sense of difficulty in concentrating
7. Lethargy, easy fatigability, or marked lack of energy
8. Marked change in appetite, overeating, or specific food cravings
9. Hypersomnia or insomnia
10. Subjective sense of being overwhelmed or out of control
11. Other physical symptoms, such as breast tenderness or swelling, headaches, joint or muscle pain, a sensation of "bloating," weight gain

B. The disturbance markedly interferes with work or school or with usual social activities and relationships with others (e.g., avoidance of social activities, decreased productivity and efficiency at work or school).

C. The disturbance is not merely an exacerbation of the symptoms of another disorder, such as major depressive disorder, panic disorder, dysthymic disorder, or a personality disorder (although it may be superimposed on any of these disorders).

D. Criteria A, B, and C must be confirmed by prospective daily rating during at least two consecutive symptomatic cycles. (The diagnosis may be made provisionally before this confirmation.)

SOURCE: *Diagnostic and statistical manual of mental disorders* (4th ed.). (1994). Washington, DC: American Psychiatric Association.

II. Epidemiology

A. PMS is quite prevalent in the general population and has been reported in women of all ages from menarche to menopause. It is not clear whether PMS intensifies as women age; in spite of anecdotal reports of gradual worsening of symptoms with age, one study found that the severity of symptoms actually decreased with age and was not associated with the duration of symptoms. There is also only anecdotal evidence linking PMS with pelvic surgery, initiation or discontinuation of oral contraceptives, or childbirth. Depending on the definition of PMS, and on the strictness of the criteria used, the estimated prevalence of this syndrome among cycling women ranges from 3–10%.

B. Premenstrual dysphoric disorder is thought to affect a relatively smaller number of women, with a prevalence rate of approximately 4% among menstruating women.

C. **The etiology** of PMS and premenstrual dysphoric disorder is unknown; many believe that these syndromes are the result of interactions of gonadal steroids with the central nervous system (e.g., neurotransmitters, neuromodulators, and neuronal gene expression) and with circadian systems affecting mood, behavior, and cognition.

III. Evaluation of the Problem

A. General Recommendations

1. The **evaluation** of the PMS patient should include the following determinations:
   a. **Physical and psychological symptoms** occurring during the premenstrual phase
   b. **Onset and course** of these symptoms (e.g., how many menstrual cycles in the past year have been affected)
   c. **Current and past psychiatric history,** in particular mood and anxiety disorders, which are quite common among patients seeking treatment for PMS. In fact, a study by Fava and co-workers (1992) found that **66% of women with prospectively confirmed premenstrual dysphoric disorder were diagnosed with mood or anxiety disorders.**
2. Be aware that many patients are convinced that they suffer from PMS; when they are carefully monitored for two or more cycles, however, they do not show signs of a cyclical pattern. Before making the diagnosis, it is imperative to obtain responses to **daily self-rated psychological and physical symptom questionnaires** for a minimum of two (possibly consecutive) symptomatic cycles. The use of these daily forms provides an objective assessment of this syndrome.
3. It is actually advantageous to assess patients not only **during the luteal phase,** that is, when women are expected to be symptomatic, but **during the follicular phase** of their menstrual cycle as well. This can ensure that the patient's symptoms present a cyclical nature and are not present throughout the menstrual cycle.
4. When evaluating a patient with PMS or premenstrual dysphoric disorder, the clinician must address the following questions:
   a. Are the symptoms reported during the luteal phase a mere exacerbation of an underlying mood or anxiety disorder? Do these symptoms emerge in the absence of a psychiatric disorder?
   b. Do the symptoms **recur** during most menstrual cycles, or is this a rare occurrence?
   c. What is the **impact** of these symptoms?
      i. Does the patient have difficulties in functioning at work and in the home?
      ii. Are interpersonal relationships affected by these premenstrual symptoms (i.e., is there social impairment as result of these symptoms)?

B. Medical History

1. **The evaluation** of the patient with PMS should also include a determination of:
   a. **Medical history and medications** currently being used. Several medical conditions (e.g., migraines, asthma, genital herpes, endometriosis, seizures, and allergies) may worsen during the premenstrual phase; others (e.g., thyroid disease, hypoglycemia) may mimic some of the symptoms of PMS.
   b. **Assess** the patient's use of **psychotropic drugs, alcohol, caffeine, and other dietary habits (including salt and carbohydrate intake). Psychoactive substances may mimic some of the symptoms of PMS.** In addition, the use of these substances may increase during the luteal phase, perhaps as an attempt to obtain relief from the PMS. Patients with premenstrual syndrome may also report carbohydrate craving during the luteal phase, and an increase in salt intake may be accompanied by increased fluid retention.

     c. **Gynecological history.** In particular, endometriosis and polycystic ovarian disease may present with symptoms mimicking PMS. The presence of dysmenorrhea should also be recorded, along with the history of previous pelvic surgeries.

C. Examination of the Patient

  1. In addition to obtaining psychiatric and medical history, the examination of the patient should include a mental status examination, a physical examination, and laboratory tests, when indicated.

    a. **The mental status examination** of the patient with PMS is often unremarkable, in particular if the patient is first examined in the follicular phase. During the premenstrual phase, patients may present with **anxious or depressed mood, accompanied by irritability and affective lability. Decreased concentration and attention** may affect the patient's performance in the Mini-Mental State Examination. **Suicidal ideation** has been reported during the premenstrual phase **in up to 10%** of cycling women in the general population. The presence of psychotic symptoms suggests a diagnosis other than premenstrual syndrome.

    b. The thorough **physical examination** of the patient with possible PMS should be performed to rule out other medical or gynecological conditions.

    c. **Laboratory tests** should be obtained only when there is a specific concern about an underlying medical condition mimicking the symptoms of PMS. Many studies have failed to document significant abnormalities in the hypothalamic-pituitary-gonadal axis in women with PMS or premenstrual dysphoric disorder. For this reason, there is no need to obtain laboratory tests of ovarian (i.e., estrogen and progesterone) or pituitary (i.e., follicle-stimulating hormone and luteinizing hormone) functioning.

IV. Psychiatric Differential Diagnosis

A. All mood and anxiety disorders fluctuate in severity. Some of these fluctuations may be the result of premenstrual worsening, others are caused by interaction with external factors, and some may be a response to seasonal variations. It is also important to distinguish between mere premenstrual worsening of mood and anxiety disorders and true PMS, as well as between these that two clinical entities and other sources of symptomatic fluctuation that are unrelated to the menstrual cycle. This can be determined by prospective administration of daily ratings completed by the patient throughout the month for at least two cycles.

B. Premenstrual exacerbation of mental disorders other than mood or anxiety disorders must also be considered before making the diagnosis. **Somatoform disorders, bulimia nervosa, substance use disorders, and personality disorders** may show a premenstrual worsening of symptoms during the luteal phase. Premenstrual dysphoric disorder or PMS could be considered an additional diagnosis if the symptoms are different from those symptoms usually experienced with the primary disorder.

C. Women with **general medical conditions** may also present with symptoms that mimic premenstrual dysphoric disorder. Conditions (e.g., seizure disorders, thyroid and other endocrine disorders, cancer, and endometriosis) should be distinguished from premenstrual dysphoric disorder by history, physical examination, and laboratory testing.

V. Treatment Strategies

A. Nutritional Supplements

  1. **Vitamin B$_6$** has been used over the past few years as a treatment for women with PMS. The rationale for its use is based on the observation that estrogen may increase

serotonin metabolism through a metabolic pathway involving vitamin B_6. The efficacy studies of vitamin B_6 have yielded mixed results, however, with improvement reported with doses as low as 50 mg/day.

2. The intake of carbohydrates has been found to increase the synthesis of brain serotonin by an insulin-mediated reduction in plasma levels of large neutral amino acids naturally competing with tryptophan, a serotonin precursor, for receptor-mediated transport across the blood-brain barrier. For this reason, **specially formulated, carbohydrate-rich beverages** (e.g., PMS Escape) have become available for the treatment of PMS. One of these beverages, known to increase the serum ratio of tryptophan to other large neutral amino acids, has been shown to be significantly more effective than an isocaloric placebo intervention in reducing symptoms of PMS.

3. **Vitamin E** has also been used to treat PMS, but the **evidence for its efficacy is still lacking**. Some studies have suggested the efficacy of magnesium and calcium supplements in the treatment of PMS, but larger controlled studies are needed to confirm the preliminary impression of their usefulness.

B. Psychotherapy and Physical Exercise

1. **Relaxation techniques** appear to be somewhat helpful, as are **cognitive-behavior therapy** and other forms of brief therapy. Very few studies have been conducted in this area; however, the evidence for the efficacy of these strategies in women with PMS is still lacking.

2. Women who engage in regular physical exercise report that exercise often helps with premenstrual symptoms. At least one study found that women engaging in aerobic exercise showed a greater improvement in premenstrual symptoms than did women engaging in non-aerobic exercise.

C. Hormones

1. **Oral contraceptives are commonly used** for the treatment of PMS, **despite the lack of consistent evidence for their efficacy,** particularly with regard to premenstrual mood and anxiety symptoms.

2. Similarly, **progesterone and synthetic progestins** have failed to show consistently a superiority to placebo in the treatment of PMS.

3. **Gonadotropin-releasing hormone agonist** (GnRH), which down-regulates pituitary gonadotropin secretion with chronic administration, **may be useful** in the treatment of PMS, but more controlled studies are necessary to establish its efficacy. Some researchers have successfully used a combination of GnRH and conjugated estrogen and progesterone to prevent the risks of osteoporosis and coronary artery disease that are reported with prolonged suppression of ovulation.

4. **Danazol,** a synthetic androgenic derivative of ethisterone with antigonadotropic activity, has been used in three double-blind, placebo-controlled studies in doses up to 400 mg/day. These studies suggest its efficacy in the treatment of PMS. However, significant side effects (e.g., nausea and breast pain), and the possibility of inducing mild hirsutism make this agent reasonable only for resistant cases.

D. Antidepressants

1. Several small, double-blind clinical trials, and a large, multi-center study have demonstrated that the selective serotonin reuptake inhibitor (SSRI) **fluoxetine,** at doses ranging from 20 to 60 mg/day **given throughout the menstrual cycle, was significantly more effective than placebo** in treating premenstrual dysphoria or

premenstrual symptoms. A recent report suggests that fluoxetine's efficacy may be maintained in the long term. There are anecdotal reports of the usefulness of fluoxetine when given only during the luteal phase, but no controlled studies of this specific approach are available at this time.

2. One open trial and a large placebo-controlled study showed that the SSRI, **sertraline**, in doses ranging from 50 to 150 mg/day throughout the cycle, **was effective in treating premenstrual dysphoria.** A double-blind study suggests the efficacy of another SSRI, paroxetine, although large, placebo-controlled studies are necessary to confirm these preliminary findings.

3. **Clomipramine,** a tricyclic antidepressant (TCA) with potent serotonin reuptake inhibitor effects, **has been found to be more effective than placebo** at doses ranging from 25 to 75 mg/day, **when given either for the full cycle or for the half-cycle.**

4. **Possible efficacy** in the treatment of PMS has been suggested for antidepressants, such as the cyclic antidepressant **nefazodone**, other TCAs (**desipramine, imipramine, nortriptyline**), and a monoamine oxidase inhibitor (MAOI), **phenelzine.**

E. Antianxiety Drugs

1. Although one small, crossover study failed to show a difference from placebo, a recent study has found **greater efficacy of alprazolam** (0.25 mg q.i.d. from day 18 of the menstrual cycle through day 2 of the next cycle), **compared to oral micronized progesterone and placebo.**

2. **Buspirone,** a 5-HT-$_{1A}$ serotonin receptor partial agonist with antianxiety properties, has shown, in mean doses of 25 mg/day, **efficacy in a small, placebo-controlled, double-blind study in the treatment of PMS,** although larger controlled studies are necessary to confirm its usefulness.

F. Other Drugs

1. Other drug treatments whose efficacy has been suggested by small studies or case reports are **lithium, fenfluramine** (a serotonergic appetite suppressant), **naltrexone** (an opiate antagonist), **bromocriptine** (a dopaminergic agonist), **atenolol** (a β-blocker), **mefenamic acid** (a prostaglandin synthesis inhibitor), and **doxycycline** (a tetracycline antibiotic).

2. **Non-steroidal anti-inflammatory agents** are used for the management of pain and headaches during the premenstrual phase, and **diuretics and spirolactone** are used for the management of edema and water retention.

VI. Conclusion

To effectively treat the patient who suffers from symptoms of PMS or premenstrual dysphoric disorder, it is crucial for the clinician to assess physical and psychological symptoms and their temporal relationship to the luteal phase. Once a diagnosis is established prospectively, there are many pharmacological treatment strategies available for women suffering from these disorders (see Table 44-3); **through their** use some of the more **debilitating symptoms may be lessened or may disappear.** Nutritional supplements, physical exercise, **and psychotherapy represent alternative approaches that can be considered, particularly when a patient suffers from milder** forms of PMS.

Table 44-3. Possible Treatment Strategies for Premenstrual Syndrome

- Nutritional supplements (e.g., vitamin B_6, carbohydrate-rich beverages, magnesium, and vitamin E)
- Psychotherapy (e.g., cognitive and behavioral therapy)
- Physical exercise (e.g., aerobic exercise)
- Hormones (e.g., oral contraceptives and progesterone/progestins)
- Antidepressants (e.g., fluoxetine, sertraline, and clomipramine)
- Antianxiety drugs (e.g., alprazolam and buspirone)
- Other drugs (e.g., fenfluramine and bromocriptine)

Suggested Readings

Altshuler, L.L., Cohen, L.S., Moline, M.L., et al. (2001). The expert consensus panel for depression in women. The expert consensus guideline series. Treatment of depression in women. *Postgraduate Medicine,* (SPRCM), 1–107.

Christensen, A.P., & Oei, T.P.S. (1995). The efficacy of cognitive behaviour therapy in treating premenstrual dysphoric changes. *Journal of Affective Disorders, 33,* 57–63.

Cohen, L.S., Soares, C.N., Otto, M.W., et al. (2002). Prevalence and predictors of premenstrual dysphoric disorder (PMDD) in older premenopausal women. *Journal of Affective Disorders, 70*(2), 227–234.

Fava, M., Pedrazzi, F., Guaraldi, G.P., et al. (1992). Comorbid anxiety and depression among patients with late luteal phase dysphoric disorder. *Journal of Anxiety Research, 6,* 325–335.

Freeman, E.W., Rickels, K., Sondheimer, S.J., et al. (1995). A double-blind trial of oral progesterone, alprazolam, and placebo in treatment of severe premenstrual syndrome. *Journal of the American Medical Association, 274*(l), 51–57.

Graham, C.A., & Sherwin, B.B. (1992). A prospective treatment study of premenstrual symptoms using a triphasic oral contraceptive. *Journal of Psychosomatic Research, 36*(3), 257–266.

Hahn, P.M., Van Vugt, D.A., & Reid, R.L. (1995). A randomized, placebo-controlled, crossover trial of danazol for the treatment of premenstrual syndrome. *Psychoneuroendocrinology, 20*(2), 193–209.

Johnson, S.R., McChesney, C., & Bean, J.A. (1988). Epidemiology of premenstrual symptoms in a nonclinical sample. I: prevalence, natural history and help-seeking behavior. *Journal of Reproductive Medicine, 33,* 340–346.

Pearlstein, T.B. (1995). Hormones and depression: What are the facts about premenstrual syndrome, menopause, and hormone replacement therapy? *American Journal of Obstetrics & Gynecology, 173*(2), 646–653.

Pearlstein, T.B., Halbreich, V., Batzar, L.D., et al. (2000). Psychosocial functioning in women with premenstrual dysphoric disorder before and after treatment with sertraline or placebo. *Journal of Clinical Psychiatry, 61*(2), 101–109.

Rausch, J.L., & Parry, B.L. (1993). Treatment of premenstrual mood symptoms. *Psychiatric Clinics of North America, 16*(4), 829–839.

Soares, C.N., Cohen, L.S., Otto, M.W., & Harlow, B.L. (2001). Characteristics of women with pre-menstrual dysphoric disorder (PMDD) who did or did not report history of depression. *Journal of Womens Health & Gender Based Medicine, 10*(9), 873–878.

Steiner, M., Steinberg, S., Stewart, D., et al. (1995). Fluoxetine in the treatment of premenstrual dysphoria. *New England Journal of Medicine, 332*(23), 1529–1534.

Sundblad, C., Modigh, K., Andersch, B., et al. (1992). Clomipramine effectively reduces premen-strual irritability and dysphoria: A placebo-controlled trial. *Acta Psychiatric Scandanavia, 85,* 39–47.

Yonkers, K.A., Halbreich, U., Freeman, E.W., et al. (1995). Efficacy of sertaline for treatment of premenstrual dysphoric disorder. Presented at the 148th Annual Meeting of the American Psy-chiatric Association. Abstract.

CHAPTER 45

The Patient Entering Menopause

ADELE C. VIGUERA, CLAUDIO N. SOARES, AND LEE S. COHEN

I. Introduction

A. Definitions

1. **Menopause is defined as the cessation of menses for 12 consecutive months.** It generally occurs at about age 50, with an age range of 41 to 59 years. Menopause occurs naturally with advancing age, but it may be secondary to oophorectomy (surgical menopause).

2. **The perimenopause is defined as the time of transition from regular menstrual functioning to the complete cessation of menses.** The median age at the onset of perimenopause is approximately 47.5 years. This phase may last from 5 to 10 years, and generally is accompanied by clinical and endocrinologic changes.

3. **The post-menopausal phase refers to the period after 12 months of amenorrhea.** During the menopausal transition a patient frequently experiences a variety of psychological, cognitive, and physical symptoms. Around 1,300,000 women reach menopause each year in the United States. With an average life expectancy of approximately 80 years, most women spend more than one-third of their lives after the onset of menopause.

B. Menopause and Mood Disorders

1. There have been some misconceptions associated with menopause. One of the most commonly cited myths is that the menopausal **"change of life" is** invariably associated with wide mood swings, anxiety, and depressive illness. Terms such as *menopausal syndrome* and *involutional melancholia* have been used loosely to refer to the emotional and physical symptoms of estrogen deficiency.

2. Although no specific mood disorder has been associated with the menopause per se, it is possible that changes in reproductive endocrine functioning observed during the perimenopause affect a woman's vulnerability to psychiatric disorders.

3. Studies have clearly demonstrated that **certain subgroups of women are more vulnerable to mood disorders** during specific reproductive phases, such as the premenstrual phase, the post-partum period, and the peri-menopause. The latter observation seems to be **particularly true for some women with history of earlier age at menarche, and a previous history of mood or anxiety disorders.**

II. Epidemiology

A. Prevalence of Depression

1. In general, women are at greater risk for depression than are men, with the highest prevalence of depression noted during the reproductive years, i.e., when women are

exposed to hormonal fluctuations. However, there is less of a consensus regarding the prevalence of menopause-related mood disturbances.

a. **Depressive symptoms seem to increase during the peri-menopause.**

b. **Women with a history of major depression appear to be at the greatest risk for depression during peri-menopause.**

c. Other factors, such as **menstrual and reproductive characteristics** (e.g., earlier age at menarche), **poor physical health, changes in social circumstances (marital disruption), and interpersonal stress, may also influence the prevalence of depression in this sub-population.**

d. It is therefore expected that the occurrence of these two conditions—a menopause-related depression—may lead to a significant compounded burden of illness with considerable public health implications.

III. Etiology

A. Neurobiologic Theories

1. **Neurobiologic theories** suggest that mood symptoms are secondary to changes in reproductive hormones

2. **Estrogen** has been shown to stimulate serotonergic and noradrenergic functions in the brain, and may play an important and complex role in **neuromodulation.** It has been hypothesized that a hypo-estrogenic state may promote mood changes.

3. Although the vast majority of menopausal women do not experience major depression, most experience uncomfortable vasomotor symptoms. The "domino hypothesis" suggests that these unpleasant somatic complaints and associated-insomnia have secondary effects on a woman's psychological well-being, leading to changes in mood.

B. Psychological Theories

1. Psychosocial stressors, including changing family roles, aging, a changing social support network, interpersonal losses, the onset of physical illness, and retirement, may play a role in a patient's mood disturbance.

IV. Evaluation of the Problem

A. General Recommendations

1. **Evaluation** of a patient entering menopause should include the following:

a. Assess the patient for the physical and psychological symptoms associated with menopause (Table 45-1).

b. **Determine the onset and course** of symptoms relative to the current hormonal status; evaluate whether the patient is peri-menopasual, menopausal, or post-menopausal as defined by clinical and menstrual history, corroborated by follicle-stimulating hormone (FSH) and estradiol levels. **Monitor symptoms on a daily basis** to provide information about the severity, stability, and pattern of symptoms.

c. **Obtain a thorough psychiatric history;** this is the most important part of the evaluation of a menopausal patient who presents with mood and anxiety symptoms. The psychiatric history (including a history of psychiatric treatments) is perhaps the best predictor of relapse in the menopausal period.

d. **Rule out current psychiatric illness.** Depression is a term that often is used imprecisely; transient mood swings often are confused with more serious major depressive

Table 45-1. Physical and Psychological Symptoms Associated with Menopause
Vasomotor symptoms: hot flashes, night sweats, palpitations *Affective symptoms:* depressed mood, anxiety, mood swings *Cognitive symptoms:* poor memory, lack of concentration, forgetfulness *Somatic complaints:* dizziness, fatigue, headache, insomnia, joint pain, paresthesias *Physical signs:* urogenital atrophy, dyspareunia, osteoporosis, cardiovascular disease

syndromes. Specifically, attempt to distinguish whether the patient is simply responding to physical discomfort and having difficulty adjusting psychologically to a phase of life (e.g., an adjustment disorder) or is experiencing a full-blown major depression (see Chapter 14).

e. **Assess the patient's ability to function.** Determine how much the reported symptoms—whether physical or emotional—interfere with the patient's ability to function.

f. **Inquire about specific sexual problems.** Determine whether a major mood disorder is contributing to decreased libido or whether physical discomfort (e.g., vaginal dryness) is secondary to a low-estrogen state.

g. **Inquire about the patient's general attitude about menopause.** A patient who has negative notions or is unaware about changes that occur during menopause may interpret the experience negatively. You may ask how the patient's mother handled the menopausal transition or this stage of development to get an idea of the patient's cultural and individual attitudes toward menopause, and learn about her family menstrual history.

h. **Assess the quality of the patient's relationships.** Ask about current relationships and changes in the perception of her role in the household, at work, and in society.

i. **Carefully assess for risk factors which may predispose a patient to peri-menopausal and menopausal mood disorders**, including history of depression, history of premenstrual syndrome (PMS) or post-partum depression, history of depression related to oral contraceptive use, premature menopause, and psychosocial factors, such as stress and negative expectations about menopause.

B. Medical History

Data gathering from the patient should include the following:

1. **Medical history and list of current medications**

   a. A low-estrogen state can precipitate cardiovascular disease, urogenital atrophy (causing stress incontinence and prolapse), and osteoporosis.

   b. Cigarette smokers and women who had menarche at earlier age may reach menopause earlier.

   c. The hormonal changes in menopause include a decrease in estrogen with subsequent elevations of luteinizing hormone (LH) and FSH. The endocrine profile of menopause is typically defined as an FSH level above 40 IU/L and an estradiol level below 25 pg/ml.

   d. A typical endocrine profile of a peri-menopausal patient consists of FSH above 25 IU/L and an estradiol level below 40 pg/ml. However, there may be a significant cycle-to-cycle variation, so the diagnosis of a menopausal status should not be made based solely on hormone levels.

e. In addition, it is important to rule out underlying medical conditions that can present with anxiety and/or depression (e.g., thyroid disturbances and arrhythmia).

2. **A history of alcohol use, prescription drug abuse, or use of illicit drugs** (which may mimic or exacerbate a mood disorder) should be obtained.

3. **Gynecologic history.** Inquire whether a patient has a naturally occurring menopause or one that is chemically or surgically-induced by oophorectomy. A patient who has had a surgical oophorectomy tends to experience more difficulties with mood and anxiety. Determine whether the patient still has her uterus. Unopposed estrogen replacement therapy may increase the risk for endometrial hyperplasia.

V. Examination of the Patient

In addition to a thorough psychiatric and medical history, **the examination of the patient should include a physical examination, a mental status examination, and laboratory tests when indicated.**

A. **The physical examination of a patient entering menopause should include an assessment of cardiovascular functioning, an inquiry about bone fractures or loss of height, and an analysis of urogenital difficulties, including dyspareunia, incontinence, prolapse, and vaginal dryness.**

B. **The mental status examination** of a patient entering menopause may be remarkable for anxiety, irritability, depressed mood, and affective lability.

C. **Laboratory tests**, such as thyroid function, FSH, and estradiol levels may be indicated.

VI. Psychiatric Differential Diagnosis

A. Since the existence of a specific menopause-related mood disorder has not been well established, **it is important to consider whether a patient's mood disturbance represents a pre-existing mood and/or anxiety disorder** which has intensified.

B. Other psychiatric disorders, such as substance abuse, bipolar disorder, eating disorders, somatoform disorders, and personality disorders, should be considered. Each of these disorders may worsen during the menopausal transition because of complex interactions with hormonal changes and external factors (including psychosocial stressors).

C. Women with general medical conditions may present with symptoms that mimic depression or anxiety; these conditions include diabetes, seizure disorders, cancer, and thyroid disease and should be ruled out by appropriate testing.

VII. Treatment Strategies

A. **Pharmacologic Strategies**

1. **Hormone replacement therapy (HRT) with estrogen is the cornerstone of the treatment** of menopausal patients who present with physical, somatic, or cognitive complaints. However, prescribing HRT depends on a careful risk-benefit analysis since some menopausal women may be at increased risk for breast and/or uterine cancer. Antidepressants, mood stabilizers, ECT, and psychotherapy are the treatments of choice for major mood or anxiety disorders. HRT is the treatment of choice for the management of physiologic symptoms (especially vasomotor symptoms and

vaginal dryness) and cognitive functioning. HRT also reduces the risk of heart disease and osteoporosis.

2. Recent data suggest that estrogen therapy may be effective to treat mood disturbances during the peri-menopause, along with well-established benefits observed for vasomotor symptoms, interrupted sleep, decreased libido, and dyspareunia resulting from vaginal dryness or atrophy. The clinician should clarify the temporal relationship between the onset of symptoms and the initiation of HRT. Mood and behavioral symptoms may result from inadequate estrogen and can remit after appropriate adjustment of the dose and regimen of HRT. At times, a change to an alternative form of estrogen replacement (e.g., transdermal or oral estradiol, or oral conjugated estrogens) may induce a remission of symptoms. **In general, it is recommended that HRT be adjusted before adjunctive psychopharmacotherapy is considered.** One must keep in mind, however, that cyclical mood and behavioral symptoms may be a direct consequence of HRT. **If there is no response in the patient's mental status after two to four weeks, re-evaluate for a primary psychiatric condition and consider the use of standard antidepressant treatments.** If the patient has a complicated psychiatric history, consider a referral or consultation with a psychiatrist.

3. **The addition of progestogens** decreases the risk of endometrial cancer; however, some forms of progestogens may worsen the patient's mood. By switching to a different progestogen preparation, or promoting a higher estrogen/progestogen ratio you may attenuate the mood-dampening effect of progestogens.

4. Although not typically considered a first-line treatment, **androgen replacement** may be used to enhance a patient's libido and sexual function, particularly in surgically-induced post-menopausal women.

5. If the diagnosis of major depression has been established, the treatment of choice for a peri-menopausal or menopausal woman is antidepressant treatment (see Chapter 14). All antidepressants are equally effective. If, however, a patient had a good response in the past to an antidepressant, this should guide antidepressant selection. Treatment should include a full therapeutic trial with adequate doses. If the patient presents with a complicated psychiatric history or a history of manic-depressive illness, a referral to a psychiatrist is advisable.

B. Psychotherapeutic Options

1. **Cognitive-behavioral therapy** may be used alone or in addition to pharmacotherapy to treat depression or anxiety. If the symptoms are severe, pharmacotherapy should be a mainstay of treatment.

2. **Supportive psychotherapy** may help a patient articulate her concerns and anxieties regarding perceived losses, adapt to changing roles in the family, and cope with other issues associated with aging (e.g., expectations about menopause).

C. Patient Education

Given the myriad negative myths surrounding menopause, most patients will benefit from learning what physiologic and psychological changes can be anticipated during the peri-menopausal-menopausal phase. Excellent resources on menopause, with suggestions on diet, exercise of mind and body, and healthy sexuality, are available in bookstores. Reassuring the patient that menopause is not a disease but a natural stage of a woman's development may help shatter pre-existing negative connotations of menopause. Suggesting to the patient that this transition may be full of opportunities for growth rather than being a period of stagnation may facilitate a more realistic and positive perspective on the "change of life."

VIII. Conclusions

Although there is no clearly defined menopause-related affective disorder, perimenopausal women describe a diminished sense of well-being. Certain subgroups of women (those with a history of mood and anxiety disorders) may be particularly vulnerable to mood and anxiety disorders during this phase. Differentation between the presence of depressive symptoms and a full-blown major depressive disorder is critical. **Estrogen may be helpful in the treatment of depressive symptoms but is not recommended as monotherapy for the treatment of major depression.** Estrogen may significantly enhance the quality of life and prevent serious degenerative diseases. Education of a patient about the normal physiologic and psychological signs and symptoms associated with menopause may demystify this natural developmental phase of life.

Suggested Readings

Ballinger, C.B. (1990). Psychiatric aspects of the menopause. *British Journal of Psychiatry, 156,* 773–787.

Halbreich, U., & Kahn, L.S. (2001). Role of estrogen in the aetiology and treatment of mood disorders. *CNS Drugs, 15*(10), 797–817.

Harlow, B.L., Wise, L.A., Otto, M.W., et al. (2003). Depression and its influence on reproductive endocrine and menstrual cycle markers associated with the perimenopause—The Harvard Study of Moods and Cycles. *Archives of General Psychiatry, 60*(1), 29–36.

Jensvold, M.F., Halbreich, U., & Hamilton, J.A. (1996). *Psychopharmacology and women: Sex, gender and hormones.* Washington, D.C.: American Psychiatric Press.

Schmidt, P.J., Neiman, L., Danaceau, M.A., et al. (2000). Estrogen replacement in perimenopause-related depression: A preliminary report. *American Journal of Obstetrics & Gynecology, 183*(2), 414–420.

Schmidt, P., & Rubinow, D. (1991). Menopause-related affective disorders: A justification for further study. *American Journal of Psychiatry, 148,* 844–852.

Soares, C.N., & Cohen, L.S. (2001). The perimenopause and mood disturbance: An update. *CNS Spectrums, 6*(2), 167–174.

Soares, C.N., Almeida, O.P., Joffe, H., & Cohen, L.S. (2001). Efficacy of estradiol for the treatment of depressive disorders in perimenopausal women: A randomized, double-blind, placebo-controlled trial. *Archives of General Psychiatry, 58,* 529–534.

CHAPTER 46
The Pregnant Patient

LEE S. COHEN

I. Introduction

Pregnancy typically is described as a time of emotional well-being for women, providing them with "protection" against the onset of, or the worsening of, psychiatric disorders. However, **systematic data regarding the course of psychiatric disorders during pregnancy are sparse.** Given the concerns about the known and unknown risks of pre-natal drug exposure as well as the risks of untreated psychiatric disorders during pregnancy, **clinicians who care for psychiatrically ill women during pregnancy frequently are caught between "a teratologic rock and a clinical hard place."**

II. Course of Psychiatric Disorder during Pregnancy

A. Mood Disorders

1. While earlier reports suggested that pregnancy is a time of decreased risk for the onset of mood disorders, a growing body of literature supports the clinical observation that **the prevalence of major and minor depression during pregnancy approximates 10%.**
2. It may be difficult to distinguish the symptoms of depression during pregnancy from the normative symptoms associated with pregnancy, including impaired sleep, fluctuating appetite, lower energy, and changes in libido.
3. However, these symptoms of depression should not be dismissed, since depression that develops during pregnancy may place both the mother and the fetus at risk.
4. New-onset major depression during pregnancy in particular should not be dismissed. It demands the same differential diagnostic evaluation offered to other patients with an emerging affective illness (appropriate ruling out organic causes of depression such as metabolic and endocrine abnormalities, drug-drug interactions, and substance abuse) (see Chapter 14).
5. Depression during pregnancy is clinically important, as **there is no stronger predictor of post-partum depression than affective disturbance during pregnancy.**

B. Anxiety Disorders

1. **An anecdotal literature supports the observations that new-onset panic attacks are less common and that panic symptoms in women with pre-existing gravid histories of panic disorder are less severe.** A more systematic review of patients with a history of panic disorder suggests heterogeneity in the clinical course.
2. Many women with severe pre-gravid histories of panic disorder continue to demonstrate symptoms of panic during pregnancy.
3. **Panic attacks during pregnancy are strongly predictive of post-partum worsening of anxiety;** they should not be clinically dismissed as a "normal anxiety reaction" associated with pregnancy.

    4. As in the case of mood disorders, new-onset panic symptoms or panic symptoms during pregnancy require a thoughtful diagnostic evaluation to rule out medical causes of anxiety (see Chapter 16).

C. Psychotic Illness

    1. While some investigators have suggested that patients with psychotic illnesses, such as schizophrenia, improve during pregnancy, **many chronically ill psychiatric patients appear to relapse quickly when antipsychotic medications are withdrawn, especially if the medications are withdrawn abruptly.**

    2. **Poor pre-natal care associated with evolving or worsening psychosis during pregnancy** (frequently seen after the discontinuation of antipsychotics) **is associated with a poor peri-natal outcome.** Thus, decisions regarding the appropriate management of patients with psychosis who become pregnant must be made carefully, with attention to the risks for potential harm to the fetus associated with untreated maternal psychosis versus those associated with pharmacologic interventions.

III. Relative Risk Assessment in Pregnancy: Pharmacologic Intervention versus Risk of Untreated Psychiatric Disorder

A. Risks of pharmacotherapy. Risks associated with pre-natal exposure to psychotropic agents include the following:

    1. **Teratogenic Risk or Risk of Gross Organ Malformation**

      a. Organ malformation occurs during the first trimester of gestation.

      b. When the frequency of congenital malformations after pre-natal exposure to a medication is increased compared with the baseline incidence of congenital malformations without such drug exposure, a drug is labeled a **teratogen.**

    2. **Risk of Peri-natal Toxicity**

      a. A broad range of syndromes of neonatal toxicity during the acute neonatal period have been reported in women who delivered while using any number of psychotropics. These symptoms have been and frequently are attributed to drug exposure at or near the time of birth.

      b. Such syndromes have been described across different classes (antidepressants, antipsychotics, and benzodiazepines) of psychotropic drugs.

      c. **The incidence of peri-natal toxicity is, however, in all probability extremely low.** The risk for peri-natal toxicity may be increased by decreased levels of plasma protein and protein-binding affinity as well as by diminished hepatic microsomal activity seen in the newborn.

    3. **Behavioral Teratogenesis**

    Behavioral teratogenesis **refers to the potential risk for longer-term neurobehavioral sequelae associated with fetal exposure to a particular drug.**

      a. An abundant animal literature supports the presence of changes in a broad range of neuromodulating systems, including noradrenergic, dopaminergic, cholinergic, and serotonergic-mediated neuronal pathways, after peri-natal exposure to psychotropics.

      b. The extent to which these findings can be extrapolated to humans is not clear.

      c. Small case series have attempted to delineate behavioral outcomes after pre-natal exposure to a spectrum of psychotropics, including antidepressants, benzodiazepines, lithium, and antipsychotics. However, reliable and definitive data regarding the risk of enduring neurobehavioral dysfunction after pre-natal exposure to any of the psychotropic medications are lacking.

IV. Risk of Untreated Maternal Psychiatric Disorders

A. The impact of untreated depression during pregnancy should not be discounted.

B. Aside from the obvious sequelae associated with untreated depression during pregnancy (diminished food intake, potential suicidal ideation, poor pre-natal care), **untreated depression has been associated with a poor neonatal outcome (higher rates of neonatal complications, lower Apgar scores).**

C. **Untreated anxiety during pregnancy also has been associated with poor neonatal outcomes.** An increased risk for **premature labor and other obstetric complications** (e.g., placental abruption and lower Apgar scores in newborns) has been described in the setting of severe, untreated anxiety during pregnancy.

D. It is an error to dismiss the real and potential impact of untreated maternal psychiatric illness while weighing the treatment options, including pharmacotherapy, for women who have a psychiatric illness during pregnancy.

E. Given the risk for recurrent affective disorder and chronicity after a relapse of a psychiatric illness, **failure to treat psychiatric disorders in gravid women may increase the likelihood of a patient's becoming more refractory to treatment over time.**

V. Psychotropic Drugs in Pregnancy (See Table 46-1)

A. Antipsychotics
   1. High-potency antipsychotics have not been shown to increase the risk for organ dysgenesis even after first-trimester exposure to this class of agents.
   2. **Low-potency antipsychotics (e.g., chlorpromazine, thiothixene) should be avoided because of potential adverse effects associated with fetal exposure to anticholinergic compounds.**
   3. While extrapyramidal symptoms have been noted in newborns whose mothers used antipsychotics during pregnancy, the incidence of these treatment-emergent symptoms is extremely low.
   4. Information regarding the potential teratogenic risk associated with a first exposure to newer antipsychotics, such as clozapine, risperidone, and olanzapine, is lacking. Thus, these agents typically are avoided during pregnancy. However, in treatment-resistant patients their use is not absolutely contraindicated.
   5. **The use of antipsychotics during pregnancy is not contraindicated.** High-potency neuroleptics are the treatment of choice, and discontinuation of these drugs in chronic mentally ill women may place these patients at significant risk for relapse.

B. Antidepressants
   1. **The putative safety of tricyclic antidepressants (TCAs) during pregnancy is well established.** Pre-natal exposure to these agents is not associated with an increased risk of organ dysgenesis after first-trimester exposure.
   2. **Fluoxetine is not associated with an increased risk of congenital malformations after first-trimester exposure.** There are more data supporting the reproductive safety of fluoxetine than there are for any other antidepressant. **There are also considerable data supporting the reproductive safety of citalopram.**
   3. Information regarding the reproductive safety of other, newer antidepressants, such as sertraline, paroxetine, venlafaxine, nefazodone, and fluvoxamine, is more limited than for fluoxetine.

Table 46-1. Guide to Psychotropic Drug Use in Pregnancy

Psychosis

1. Consider maintenance of low-dose antipsychotic therapy for chronically ill patients, which may offset the risk of relapse and the need for higher doses.
2. Remember to create a medical differential diagnosis for and work-up new-onset psychotic states.
3. Consider that high-potency neuroleptics (e.g., haloperidol, thiothixene) may be safer; data are lacking on the use of atypical antipsychotics (e.g., risperidone, clozapine, olanzapine).

Mania

1. Remember to create a medical differential diagnosis for and work-up new-onset manic symptoms.
2. Be aware that valproic acid and carbamazepine are associated with significant increases in the rate of congenital malformations (5% and 1%, respectively).
3. Remember to evaluate the need for prophylaxis.

Trimester I

1. Avoid lithium carbonate if possible, depending on the severity of the illness.
2. If the patient has been exposed to lithium before week 12, consider cardiac ultrasound at week 20.
3. If there is a clear need for anti-manic prophylaxis, discontinue lithium after documentation of pregnancy or consider the use of prophylactic lithium in a brittle bipolar woman, given the small absolute risk for Ebstein's anomaly (0.05%).

Trimesters II and III

1. After week 12 and with the need for treatment, lithium carbonate may be reintroduced.
2. Administer lithium in divided doses when lithium is indicated.
3. Maintain use of lithium across labor and delivery to minimize risk of post-partum relapse of illness.
4. Monitor plasma levels of lithium carefully during the acute puerperium given maternal fluid shifts.

Mania in pregnancy

1. Hospitalization of a manic, pregnant woman often is required.
2. Consider the use of neuroleptics, adjunctive clonazepam, and /or electroconvulsive therapy (ECT).

Depression

1. Remember to create a medical differential diagnosis for depression.
2. Withhold antidepressant medication in the first trimester if possible.
3. Be aware that an inability to care for oneself or to provide pre-natal care generally indicates the need for somatic therapy.
4. Secondary amines (nortriptyline, desipramine) are preferable to tertiary amine tricyclics.

Anxiety

1. Remember to create a medical differential of disorders.
2. Tricyclic antidepressants and fluoxetine (a selective serotonin reuptake inhibitor [SSRI]) are the treatments of choice.
3. Benzodiazepines are not contraindicated during pregnancy and during labor and delivery.

4. Although reproductive safety may be demonstrated with one member of a family of antidepressants, such as fluoxetine, it is a significant error to assume that drugs with a similar mechanism of action, such as sertraline and paroxetine, have equal reproductive safety in the absence of supportive data.

5. While perinatal toxicity has been described in newborns whose mothers delivered while on antidepressants, including TCAs and fluoxetine, the incidence of such perinatal syndromes is extremely low.

6. **Premature discontinuation of antidepressants during the peri-partum period** is an error, as depression during pregnancy strongly **predicts a risk for puerperal worsening of mood.** Thus, discontinuation of the medication at the precise time when a woman enters a period of risk, such as the post-partum period, is best avoided.

7. **TCAs and fluoxetine are the safest antidepressants to use during pregnancy.** Considerable data regarding the reproductive safety of these agents are available. **Extreme caution must be exhibited with respect to the premature discontinuation of antidepressants in women who have major depression during pregnancy.**

C. **Mood Stabilizers: Lithium, Valproic Acid, and Carbamazepine**
   1. **Lithium**
      a. Lithium carbonate typically has been avoided during pregnancy because of concerns regarding an increased risk for Ebstein's anomaly.
      b. However, **the risk for Ebstein's anomaly after pre-natal exposure to lithium carbonate during the first 12 weeks of gestation is estimated at 0.05% (1 in 2000) of cases.** Though this represents a ten-fold increase in the relative risk for congenital malformations compared with the frequency of malformations in the general population (1 in 20,000), the absolute risk is relatively small.
      c. **Given the risk of relapse, which has been estimated at 50–60% within 6 months of lithium discontinuation, severely ill women who require a mood stabilizer may benefit from maintenance treatment with lithium even during pregnancy.**
      d. However, **lithium discontinuation may be appropriate in patients with more modest illness.** For these women, lithium may be discontinued with re-introduction of the drug during the latter two trimesters of pregnancy or during the acute post-partum period.
      e. Post-partum prophylaxis with lithium is advised in women who have a bipolar disorder, as these patients have a 50–60% risk of relapse in the acute post-partum period. Prophylaxis with mood stabilizers, such as lithium, appears to reduce this risk to less than 10%.
   2. **Valproic Acid**
      a. Valproic acid is a mood stabilizer that is marketed as an anticonvulsant with **a well-established risk of neural defects approximating 5% after first-trimester exposure to this medication.**
      b. **Given the growing use of valproic acid in psychiatry, its use in women who are potentially childbearing should be scrutinized carefully** in the context of both attention to contraceptive practices in women who use the drug and consideration of switching to alternative mood stabilizers, such as lithium, in patients who are dependent on anti-manic agents for the preservation of affective stability.
      c. Given the **hundred-fold increase in the risk for congenital malformations after first-trimester exposure to valproic acid** compared to lithium carbonate, women who require treatment with anti-manic agents during pregnancy should consider a switch to lithium if they are maintained on valproic acid without a previous trial of lithium.

   3. **Carbamazepine**
      a. Carbamazepine **has been associated with a 1% risk of spina bifida after pre-natal exposure to this agent during the first 12 weeks of gestation.**
      b. While carbamazepine remains a common treatment during pregnancy for women who have seizure disorders, **its use as a mood stabilizer typically is avoided during pregnancy.** An exception to this includes women who have been non-responsive to lithium though they have proved to be carbamazepine-dependent with respect to the preservation of affective well-being.

D. Benzodiazepines
   1. Benzodiazepines have been associated with an increased risk for oral clefts after first-trimester exposure to these medications.
   2. However, considerable controversy exists regarding the absolute risk of oral clefts after first-trimester exposure to benzodiazepines. If it is increased at all, the increase is on the order of 0.5%.
   3. Perinatal toxicity, including hypotonia, temperature dysregulation, and benzodiazepine discontinuation syndromes, is extremely rare and has not been noted in several series of cases in which monotherapy with low doses of benzodiazepines have been administered to patients suffering from panic disorder at or around the time of labor and delivery.

VI. Electroconvulsive Therapy during Pregnancy

A. Electroconvulsive therapy (ECT) has been used during pregnancy for almost 50 years. **The safety of ECT during pregnancy is noted throughout the literature,** and ECT is too often avoided because of misconceptions regarding its potential effects on the fetus.

B. ECT is most appropriate in clinical situations where expeditious treatment is imperative, such as psychotic depression and mania. Failure to treat aggressively increases the likelihood of potential harm to both the mother and the fetus.

C. Appropriate collaboration between the obstetrician, primary care physician (PCP), psychiatrist, and anesthesiologist can facilitate thoughtful treatment of pregnant women with ECT and can maximize the likelihood of a positive clinical outcome.

VII. Screening for Psychiatric Illness during Pregnancy

A. Although not routine practice in most hospitals, **screening for psychiatric illnesses, such as mood and anxiety disorders, can easily be integrated into standard antenatal practice.**

B. Self-rated measures with good sensitivity can be used in most ante-natal settings and can be completed by a simple, non-invasive clinical history which inquires about current, family, and past psychiatric history.

C. The presence of psychiatric illness during pregnancy is a strong predictor of post-partum worsening of the disorder and may have an adverse impact on maternal-infant attachment and on later cognitive function in children.

D. Identification of women at risk for post-partum depression, as in the case of women who have a psychiatric illness during pregnancy, can facilitate early intervention and may minimize long-term maternal morbidity.

VIII. Conclusion

A. Psychiatric well-being during pregnancy should not be assumed.

B. A growing body of literature supports a relatively high prevalence of psychiatric illness in women during the childbearing years.

C. Clinicians who care for women during the childbearing years must have a working knowledge of both the potential risks of pharmacologic intervention and the risks of untreated maternal psychiatric illness.

D. Weighing the relative risk of treatment versus the risk of untreated maternal psychiatric illness facilitates thoughtful treatment planning for women, as treatment plans are tailored to individual clinical situations.

Suggested Readings

Altshuler, L.L., Cohen, L.S., Moline, M.L., et al. (2001). The expert consensus guidelines. Treatment of depression in women. *Postgraduate Medicine,* 1–107.

Altshuler, L.L., Cohen, L.S., Szuba, M.P., et al. (1996). Pharmacologic management of psychiatric illness during pregnancy: Dilemmas and guidelines. *American Journal of Psychiatry, 153*(5), 592–606.

Cohen, L.S., & Rosenbaum, J.F. (1998). Psychotropic drug use during pregnancy: Weighing the risks. *Journal of Clinical Psychiatry, 59*(suppl 2), 18–28.

Cohen, L.S., Sichel, D.A., Robertson, L.M., et al. (1995). Post-partum prophylaxis for women with bipolar disorder. *American Journal of Psychiatry, 152,* 1641–1645.

Nulinan, I., Rovet, J., Stewart, D., et al. (1997). Neurodevelopment of children exposed in utero to antidepressant drugs. *New England Journal of Medicine, 336,* 258–262.

CHAPTER 47
The Patient with a Post-partum Mood Disorder

LEE S. COHEN

I. Introduction

Post-partum major depression is a common but frequently missed diagnosis. This is a disorder that can be diagnosed by obstetricians and pediatricians who have frequent contact with post-partum women. If left untreated, post-partum depression can have serious consequences for both the mother and the child.

II. Classification of Post-partum Mood Disorders

A. Post-partum "Blues"

1. Post-partum blues are a time-limited condition involving mood lability that occurs in approximately 50–75% of post-partum women.
2. While considered a normal reaction after childbirth, it may predict the risk for post-partum depression.
3. **Symptoms develop within 2 to 3 days of delivery and last up to 2 weeks.**
4. Alterations in mood include lability, unexplained sadness, tearfulness, irritability, and anxiety.

B. Post-partum Depression

1. Post-partum depression is strictly **defined as major depression that develops within 4 weeks of delivery.** However, a more gradual onset of depression in post-partum women is common.
2. Post-partum depression is **observed following 5–10% of deliveries.**
3. Similar prevalence rates of puerperal and non-puerperal depression have been observed. The question whether post-partum mood disturbance is a unique entity or an episode of major depression that coincides with the post-partum period has been raised.
4. As with non-puerperal depression, the diagnosis of post-partum major depression cannot be made unless a woman has at least 2 weeks of either depressed mood or anhedonia and four other neurovegetative symptoms (see Chapter 14).

C. Puerperal Psychosis

1. Puerperal or post-partum psychosis **is a rare condition that occurs in 1 to 2 of every 1000 post-partum women.**
2. It is **acute in onset,** and symptoms typically arise within the first 2 to 3 days after delivery.
3. As with post-partum depression, it is unclear whether post-partum psychosis represents a discrete diagnostic entity.
4. Follow-up of women with puerperal psychosis reveals that **the majority eventually are diagnosed as having bipolar disorder or major depression** with psychotic features.

III. Predictors of Post-partum Mood Disorders

Factors which are consistently associated with post-partum major depression include:

A. Depression during Pregnancy

B. Psychiatric History

1. Women with a history of major depression or bipolar disorder have a 30–50% risk for developing a post-partum mood disorder; women with a history of post-partum psychosis have a 70–90% risk for recurrent puerperal psychosis.

C. A family history of mood disorders, including a post-partum mood disorder, may exist.

D. Psychosocial distress, for example, high levels of marital conflict and/or dissatisfaction, stress associated with child care, low levels of social and spousal support, and an increased number of stressful life events during pregnancy, may occur.

E. There may be **sensitivity to shifts in the hormonal milieu at other times in the life cycle,** for example premenstrual mood changes and possibly sensitivity to oral contraceptive pills.

F. Post-partum thyroiditis

IV. Etiology of Post-partum Mood Disorders

A. Hormonal Shifts

1. **Estrogen.** The post-partum period is associated with rapid shifts in the reproductive hormonal environment. Plasma levels of estrogen decline to pre-follicular levels within the first 48 hours post-partum. Since estrogen appears to exert both direct and indirect effects on neuromodulating systems that are presumed to be involved in the pathogenesis of mood disorders, investigators have considered whether hormonal dysregulation might catalyze onset of post-partum mood disorders.

2. **Progesterone.** Plasma levels of progesterone also change dramatically (i.e., with a decrease to non-pregnant levels) during the acute puerperium.

3. Despite the rapid fluctuations in hormonal environment associated with the puerperium, no studies suggest a direct association between such changes and onset of post-partum depression.

B. Psychosocial factors. Women with a history of mood disorders may be more vulnerable to the stresses, such as significant sleep deprivation, change in lifestyle, and social isolation, of new parenthood.

V. Screening for Post-partum Mood Disorders

A. Obstacles to making the diagnosis of post-partum mood disorders. The treatment of post-partum mood disorders often is delayed because an inquiry regarding the presence of symptoms is not made. Alternatively, if symptoms are noted, they frequently are discounted as part of "normal post-partum adjustment."

B. Post-partum screening. Obstetricians **at the 6-week post-partum visit and pediatricians at well-baby or immunization visits** have an opportunity to screen for post-partum mood disorders. Screening provides an opportunity to evaluate women who previously were identified as being "at risk" for a post-partum mood disturbance and allows the identification of an evolving mood disturbance in those without a history of prior depressive episodes.

C. **Rating scales.** Unfortunately, most of the scales used to screen for or diagnose depression have not been validated in puerperal women. However, **the Edinburgh Post-natal Depression Scale is a 10-item self-report scale that has been validated in post-partum women.** A score greater than 12 is a matter for concern and should be followed up on by a clinician (Table 47-1). Any patient who screens positive on question 10 (the thought of harming oneself) should be evaluated immediately.

Table 47-1. Edinburgh Postnatal Depression Scale

Today's date _____   Baby's age _____

Baby's date of birth _____   Birth weight _____

Triplets/twins/single _____   Male/female _____

Mother's age _____

Number of other children: 0 1 2 3 4 5 5+

HOW ARE YOU FEELING?

As you have recently had a baby, we would like to know how you are feeling now. Please underline the answer which comes closest to how you have felt in the past 7 days, not just how you feel today.

Here is an example, already completed:

I have felt happy:

　　Yes, most of the time
　　Yes, some of the time
　　No, not very often
　　No, not at all

This would mean: "I have felt happy some of the time" during the past week. Please complete the other questions in the same way.

IN THE PAST SEVEN DAYS

1. I have been able to laugh and see the funny side of things:
　　As much as I always could
　　Not quite so much now
　　Definitely not so much now
　　Not at all

2. I have looked forward with enjoyment to things:
　　As much as I ever did
　　Rather less than I used to
　　Definitely less than I used to
　　Hardly at all

3. I have blamed myself unnecessarily when things went wrong:
　　Yes, most of the time
　　Yes, some of the time
　　Not very often
　　No, never

(continued)

Table 47-1. *(Continued)*

4. I have felt worried and anxious for no very good reason:
   No, not at all
   Hardly ever
   Yes, sometimes
   Yes, very often

5. I have felt scared or panicky for no very good reason:
   Yes, quite a lot
   Yes, sometimes
   No, not much
   No, not at all

6. Things have been getting on top of me:
   Yes, most of the time I haven't been able to cope at all
   Yes, sometimes I haven't been coping as well as usual
   No, most of the time I have coped quite well
   No, I have been coping as well as ever

7. I have been so unhappy that I have had difficulty sleeping:
   Yes, most of the time
   Yes, sometimes
   Not very often
   No, not at all

8. I have felt sad or miserable:
   Yes, most of the time
   Yes, quite often
   Not very often
   No, not at all

9. I have been so unhappy that I have been crying:
   Yes, most of the time
   Yes, quite often
   Only occasionally
   No, never

10. The thought of harming myself has occurred to me:
    Yes, quite often
    Sometimes
    Hardly ever
    Never

Edinburgh Postnatal Depression Scale: Scoring Sheet

1. I have been able to laugh and see the funny side of things:
   As much as I always could   0
   Not quite so much now   1
   Definitely not so much now   2
   Not at all   3

2. I have looked forward with enjoyment to things:
   As much as I ever did   0
   Rather less than I used to   1

Definitely less than I used to	2
Hardly at all	3

3. I have blamed myself unnecessarily when things went wrong:

Yes, most of the time	3
Yes, some of the time	2
Not very often	1
No, never	0

4. I have felt worried and anxious for no very good reason:

No, not at all	0
Hardly ever	1
Yes, sometimes	2
Yes, very often	3

5. I have felt scared or panicky for no very good reason:

Yes, quite a lot	3
Yes, sometimes	2
No, not much	1
No, not at all	0

6. Things have been getting on top of me:

Yes, most of the time I haven't been able to cope at all	3
Yes, sometimes I haven't been coping as well as usual	2
No, most of the time I have coped quite well	1
No, I have been coping as well as ever	0

7. I have been so unhappy that I have had difficulty sleeping:

Yes, most of the time	3
Yes, sometimes	2
Not very often	1
No, not at all	0

8. I have felt sad or miserable:

Yes, most of the time	3
Yes, quite often	2
Not very often	1
No, not at all	0

9. I have been so unhappy that I have been crying:

Yes, most of the time	3
Yes, quite often	2
Only occasionally	1
No, never	0

10. The thought of harming myself has occurred to me:

Yes, quite often	3
Sometimes	2
Hardly ever	1
Never	0

SOURCE: Cox, J.L., Holden, J.M., & Sagovsky, R. (1987). Detection of postnatal depression: Development of the 10-item Edinburgh Postnatal Depression Scale. *British Journal of Psychiatry, 150,* 782–786.

VI. Diagnostic Criteria

A thorough history should be obtained from women who screen positive for a possible post-partum mood disorder. This should include an inquiry about possible predictive factors. Medical conditions (e.g., anemia of pregnancy, post-partum thyroiditis, Sheehan's syndrome) that mimic depression should be considered.

A. **Post-partum depression.** As is the case for non-puerperal depression, women must have five of nine symptoms, including depressed mood or diminished interest or pleasure, for more than two weeks (see Chapter 14).

   1. **Depressed mood most of the day.** A patient's mood can be very labile throughout the course of a day.
   2. **Markedly diminished interest or pleasure in all activities;** for example, the patient may be unable to enjoy playing with her baby. It is important to distinguish between the lack of opportunity to enjoy activities and the lack of pleasure in activities that previously were enjoyable.
   3. **Significant weight loss** (when not dieting) **or weight gain** with an accompanying decrease or increase in appetite. A disturbance in appetite must be distinguished from the desire to lose weight through dieting and from weight loss secondary to a lack of time to eat.
   4. **Insomnia or hypersomnia.** Most post-partum women have disrupted sleep. It is helpful to inquire whether waking up at night is due to the baby crying or to feeding schedules. An inquiry should also be made about whether the mother can fall back to sleep after tending to the baby and if, given the opportunity, can nap during the day.
   5. **Psychomotor agitation or retardation.**
   6. **Fatigue or loss of energy.** While fatigue is common immediately after delivery, persistent fatigue may herald a depressive disorder.
   7. **Feelings of worthlessness or excessive or inappropriate guilt.** Women who anticipated feeling joyful may feel guilty about being depressed. Women may question their ability as a mother and may feel shame about a lack of positive feeling towards the baby.
   8. **Decreased concentration ability or indecisiveness** may present as multiple calls and visits to the pediatrician for minor matters.
   9. **Recurrent thoughts of death, including thoughts of harming the baby.** Thoughts of infanticide can be frightening and can be a source of shame. Such thoughts are unlikely to be volunteered; they must be asked about directly.

B. **Puerperal psychosis.** Puerperal psychosis **is defined by the presence of at least two of the five symptoms listed below.** It can be confused with an acute delirium.
   1. **Delusions**
   2. **Hallucinations** that may occur in any sensory modality
   3. **Disorganized speech**
   4. **Grossly disorganized and usually agitated or catatonic behavior**
   5. **Negative symptoms,** such as thought blocking and interpersonal withdrawal

VII. Treatment

A. **Post-partum blues.** Post-partum blues are time-limited. **For the majority of women with this condition, reassurance is sufficient.** However, some women go on to develop post-partum depression. **Women with a persistently dysphoric mood should receive further evaluation.**

B. Post-partum depression. As is the case with non-puerperal depressive illness, the severity of post-partum depression occurs along a continuum.

1. **Self-help groups.** Self-help and other supportive groups, such as Depression after Delivery (DAD), provide support for women with a post-partum mood disorder and help decrease the isolation and stigma some women experience. DAD can be reached via a national telephone access number (1-800-944-4PPD).

2. **Interpersonal therapy.** Women with mild to moderate depressive symptoms have been shown to respond to interpersonal therapy. The treatment may be helpful in patients with more severe symptoms and who do not wish to take antidepressants.

3. **Hormonal therapy.** Hormonal therapies, including the use of estrogen and progesterone, have been suggested for the treatment of post-partum depression, but they have not been shown to be effective in sufficient numbers of studies to support their use.

    a. **Progesterone.** One open study has shown favorable results from progesterone therapy. However, this study has not been replicated successfully. Since progesterone may exacerbate the symptoms of depression in some women, its use is not widely recommended.

    b. **Estrogen.** Estrogen, used alone or as an adjunct, may effectively treat post-partum major depression. However, further evaluation is required.

4. **Antidepressants.** While few studies of pharmacologic treatment of post-partum major depression have been reported, antidepressants **have been shown to be effective.** The limited data point to a need for further systematic study to delineate which aspects of puerperal mood disturbance may be more responsive to certain antidepressants. **Post-partum major depression demands the same treatment offered to patients who suffer from major depression at other times.** Women who have post-partum major depression should be treated for similar periods of time and with doses comparable to those prescribed for patients with non-puerperal illness. Inadequate treatment may lead to the chronic morbidity noted in patients with untreated depression.

C. Post-partum psychosis. Given the strong association between puerperal psychosis and bipolar disorder, **the initial treatment may include the use of a mood stabilizer, a neuroleptic, and a benzodiazepine. Electroconvulsive therapy (ECT) is a rapidly effective treatment** that often works when psychopharmacologic treatment fails or when expeditious treatment is imperative. **Puerperal psychosis is a psychiatric emergency that typically requires treatment in an inpatient setting. Failure to provide such treatment may increase the risk of harm to the mother and the baby.**

VIII. Prophylaxis

A. Attention to risk factors. Women with a history of major depressive disorder, bipolar disorder, post-partum major depression, or puerperal psychosis are at increased risk for the puerperal onset or worsening of the disorder. Pharmacologic prophylaxis may protect them against this.

1. **Lithium.** Women with a history of bipolar disorder or puerperal psychosis have been shown to benefit from prophylactic lithium therapy instituted either a few weeks before delivery or no later than 2 days afterward.

2. **Antidepressants.** One non-controlled study of women with a history of post-partum depression showed a benefit from prophylactic treatment with tricyclic antidepressants (TCAs). However, a more recent placebo controlled study of nortriptyline in this population did not support efficacy of prophylaxis at least with this antidepres-

sant. Whether prophylaxis with an SSRI would afford greater protection against post-partum mood disturbance has yet to be determined.

IX. Breast-Feeding

A. **Use of psychotropics.** Many women who require pharmacologic treatment during the puerperium may wish to breast-feed the infant. Breast milk has well-described nutritional and health benefits for infants, and those benefits must be weighed against the risks of the presence of medication in breast milk. **All psychotropics are present to varying degrees in breast milk.**

   1. **Antidepressants.** There is no consensus about whether a particular antidepressant is safer for an infant during lactation. While infants older than 10 weeks are less likely to accumulate antidepressants, serum levels from the infant should be obtained to confirm this. **While little is known about the developmental effects of low levels of antidepressants in an infant's serum, it is recommended that breast-feeding be discontinued if levels are detected.**

   2. **Lithium.** Lithium concentrations equal to 50% of that found in maternal serum have been noted in breastmilk of newborns whose mothers are taking this medicine. **Breast-feeding while the mother is taking lithium is typically not recommended.**

   3. **Anticonvulsants.** Valproic acid and carbamazepine have been used by breast-feeding mothers. If they are used by the mother, serum levels are best be monitored in the infant.

X. Conclusions

Undiagnosed and untreated post-partum mood disorders can significantly affect the well-being of women and their families. Primary care providers are ideally situated to identify these disorders and initiate treatment and/or referral.

Suggested Readings

Altshuler, L.L., Cohen, L.S., Moline, M.L., et al. (2001). The expert consensus panel for depression in women. The expert consensus guideline series. Treatment of depression in women. *Postgraduate Medicine,* (SPEC NO), 1–107.

Cohen, L., & Altshuler, L. (1997). Psychopharmacologic management of psychiatric illness during pregnancy and the postpartum period. In D. Dunner, & J. Rosenbaum (Eds.), *Psychiatric Clinics of North America Annual of Drug Therapy.* Philadelphia: Saunders, p. 21-0.

Cohen, L., Viguera, A.C., et al. (2001). Venlafaxine in the treatment of postpartum depression. *Journal of Clinical Psychiatry, 62*(8), 592–596.

Cox, J.L., Holden, J.M., & Sagovsky, R. (1987). Detection of postnatal depression: Development of the 10-item Edinburgh Postnatal Depression Scale. *British Journal of Psychiatry, 150,* 782–786.

O'Hara, M.W. (1995). *Postpartum depression: Causes and consequences.* New York: Springer-Verlag.

Stowe, Z.M., & Nemeroff, C.B. (1995). Women at risk for postpartum-onset major depression. *American Journal of Obstetrics & Gynecology, 173,* 639–645.

Wisner, K.L., et al. (1994). Prevention of recurrent postpartum major depression. *Hospital and Community Psychiatry, 45*(12), 1191–1196.

Wisner, K., Perel, J., & Findling, R. (1996). Antidepressant treatment during breastfeeding. *American Journal of Psychiatry, 9,* 1132–1137.

CHAPTER 48

The Obese Patient

ANNE E. BECKER AND LEE M. KAPLAN

I. Obesity Is a Chronic Disease with a Multi-factorial Etiology

With recent research advances in understanding causes of and developing treatments for obesity, it is likely that increasing numbers of patients will present with a request for medical treatment of obesity. Because treatment of obesity poses medical and psychological risks as well as benefits to the prospective patient, it is essential to individualize the approach to the patient seeking treatment for weight control.

A. **Obesity is defined as a Body Mass Index (BMI) of 30 kg/m² or greater and is characterized by excess adipose tissue. Overweight is defined as a BMI between 25 and 30 kg/m². [BMI (kg/m²) = weight in pounds x 703 / (height in inches)²]**

B. It is estimated that **more than 30% of adult Americans are obese.** More than $45 billion per year is spent by consumers in the United States on weight loss services and products, and more than $100 billion is spent annually on associated health care costs. Obesity is associated with 300,000 excess deaths annually in the United States, second only to tobacco use (at approximately 450,000). Recent estimates indicate that obesity is the most expensive preventable disorder, however, outstripping even tobacco use.

C. **Obesity is associated with multiple medical complications.**
   1. **Mortality increases with increasing BMI above 23 kg/m², and even modest weight loss has been shown to reduce overall mortality and morbidity from diabetes, obstructive sleep apnea, hypertension, hyperlipidemia and multiple other disorders.**
   2. Despite the initial success of many weight loss therapies, subsequent return of lost weight is common; long-term maintenance of weight losses of at least 10% of initial body weight occurs in fewer than 5% of patients.

D. **The etiology of obesity is multi-factorial** and includes genetic susceptibility and dietary behaviors that may be elicited or exacerbated by environmental and psychosocial factors. Among individuals with obesity, personality types and psychological function vary widely; psychological functioning in this group does not differ significantly from other clinical populations.

II. Evaluation of Obesity

A. **General Recommendations.** Because medical and behavioral therapies for obesity are typically characterized by only modest control of weight and a very high rate of eventual weight regain, **it is essential that the patient be educated about realistic goals and expectations**. The clinician should educate the patient about the potential risks of obesity. Eliciting the patient's goals for seeking treatment and understanding of the likely outcomes is essential to establishing a reasonable and appropriate treatment plan.

1. Patients motivated by cosmetic more than health concerns should be evaluated carefully because treatments with substantial medical risks (e.g., pharmacotherapy or surgery) are not recommended for strictly cosmetic reasons. These patients should be screened for eating disorders and for an excessive concern with body shape.

2. **Countertransferential feelings should be carefully monitored** in treating the patient with obesity. Cultural attitudes inappropriately holding that obesity is primarily the result of poor self-control, laziness, or moral deficiencies continue to persist among the general public as well as the medical profession; obese patients often experience medical evaluations (especially history-taking) as humiliating. **The clinician should attempt to evaluate the patient in an empathic, nonjudgmental manner and engage the patient to participate actively in his or her treatment.**

B. **Medical and Psychiatric History**

A major goal of the medical and psychiatric history is to establish medical and psychosocial factors that cause, exacerbate, result from, are made more likely by, or complicate the management of obesity. **All patients seeking weight management should be screened for psychiatric illness and the psychosocial context of their obesity should be examined carefully.**

1. **The general medical history aims to identify complications of obesity and conditions that may contribute to it.**

   a. Obesity-associated complications can be classified as metabolic, anatomic, degenerative, neoplastic and psychological (see Table 48-1).

   b. Medical history should aim to identify medical disease that may contribute to obesity including hypothyroidism, Cushing's disease, polycystic ovary syndrome, or previous hypothalamic injury. Medications that may contribute to obesity should also be identified (see Table 48-2).

   c. Tobacco, alcohol, and other substance abuse should be carefully assessed, to assess the patient's susceptibility to addictive behavior, ability to participate in treatment programs, and whether he or she uses drugs (e.g., nicotine or cocaine) to facilitate weight control. Ongoing or previous substance abuse is a potential contraindication for treatment with anorexiant medications.

   d. Family history should elicit information about obesity and eating disorders, disorders that cause or complicate obesity, and history of addictions to alcohol, drugs, gambling or other activities.

2. **Psychiatric history should assess psychiatric illness that may contribute to obesity or pose special considerations for weight management.**

   a. History of illnesses that potentially cause or contribute to obesity (e.g., binge-eating disorder [BED], atypical depression, post-traumatic stress disorder [PTSD] or mental retardation) should be assessed.

   b. History of psychiatric conditions that may complicate or contraindicate weight loss therapies, including anorexia nervosa, bulimia nervosa, BED, poorly controlled psychosis, bipolar disorder, depression, and substance abuse.

   c. Psychotropic medications should be reviewed in detail for those causing weight gain (see Table 48-2). Most act by stimulating appetite.

      i. Atypical antipsychotic medications (e.g., olanzapine, clozapine) frequently cause significant weight gain.

      ii. Low-potency conventional antipsychotic medications (e.g., chlorpromazine, thioridazine) are also associated with weight gain.

Table 48-1. Medical Complications of Obesity

A. Metabolic
Diabetes mellitus, type 2
Hypertriglyceridemia
Hypercholesterolemia
Hypertension
Gallstones
Fatty liver disease
Pancreatitis
Obesity hypoventilation syndrome
Platelet dysfunction (hyper-
  coagulability)
Gout

B. Anatomic
Obstructive sleep apnea
Gastroesophageal reflux disease (GERD)
Asthma
Stress incontinence
Pseudotumor cerebri
Venous stasis
Stasis-associated cellulitis
Deep venous thrombosis
Pulmonary embolism from DVT
Fungal skin infections (intertrigo)
Decubitus ulcers
Accidental injuries

C. Degenerative
Atherosclerotic cardiovascular disease
Complications of diabetes (neuro-
  logical, ophthalmological, renal)
Heart failure
Pulmonary hypertension
Degenerative joint disease
Vertebral disc disease
Non-alcoholic steato hepatitis–related
  cirrhosis

D. Neoplastic
Breast carcinoma
Ovarian carcinoma
Endometrial carcinoma
Prostate carcinoma
Colorectal carcinoma
Gallbladder carcinoma
Pancreatic adenocarcinoma
Esophageal adenocarcinoma
Renal cell carcinoma

E. Psychological
Anxiety disorders
Depression
Binge-eating disorder

Table 48-2. Medications Commonly Associated with Weight Gain

Corticosteroids

Estrogens

Hormone-replacement therapy

Atypical antipsychotics

Low-potency conventional antipsychotics

Valproic acid (Depakote and others)

Monoamine oxidase inhibitors (MAOIs)

Cyclic antidepressants

Selective serotonin re-uptake inhibitors (SSRIs)

Lithium

Insulin

Sulfonylureas

Thiazolidinediones

          iii. All MAOIs can cause weight gain in susceptible patients, although tranyl-cypromine has also been reported to cause weight loss.

          iv. Lithium, when used long-term, has been associated with more than a 10 kg weight gain in 20% of patients.

          v. Valproic acid can cause significant weight gain.

          vi. Cyclic antidepressants can cause significant weight gain; mirtazapine (Remeron) is associated with significant appetite increase and weight gain.

          vii. SSRIs and bupropion are less commonly associated with weight gain. Of the commonly prescribed SSRIs, citalopram and paroxetine are most likely to cause weight gain. Fluoxetine and sertraline have been shown to cause significant, though generally transient weight loss in a small number of patients; however, many other patients gain weight with these therapies.

    d. Note that patients on MAOIs should not be treated concurrently with centrally-acting agents often used for weight control (e.g., sibutramine, phentermine, diethylpropion, bupropion, ephedrine, SSRIs). MAOIs are not a contraindication for using orlistat, an inhibitor of intestinal fat absorption.

3. **The psychosocial context of the patient's obesity and past efforts at weight management should be carefully assessed.**

    a. **Psychiatric disorders,** psychological symptoms, characterologic traits, or coping styles (e.g., body disparagement, low self-esteem, hopelessness or helplessness around weight control) that may affect an individual's ability to engage successfully in weight loss therapies should be identified.

    b. History of patient discomfort with or **resistance to previous attempts at weight loss** should be noted because they may reveal potential adverse effects or limitations of this therapy.

    c. **Psychosocial stressors** should be noted, as stressful life events are commonly associated with weight gain in susceptible patients.

    d. **Potential secondary gains of maintaining a high weight** should be identified (e.g., a sense of relative safety as a result of obesity; family or other social dynamics that may reinforce obesity or discourage addressing it).

    e. **The emotional impact of obesity** on the individual's life should be examined.

        i. Obesity is heavily stigmatized in contemporary U.S. culture, resulting in discrimination against the overweight in numerous social, educational, occupational, commercial and even medical environments. Patients with obesity are frequently caused to experience a sense of shame during the course of their medical care as a result of their failure to control their weight adequately.

        ii. There is a small, positive association between body mass index and symptoms of depression and anxiety disorders, which are particularly prevalent in patients with severe obesity (BMI > 40).

    f. **Sociocultural values** relating to ethnicity, gender, socioeconomic status, and educational background about dietary, weight, or body image issues may motivate or complicate weight management and should be explored. In the U.S., obesity is more prevalent among women, certain ethnic (e.g., African-Americans, Mexican-Americans, and Pacific Islanders) and socioeconomically disadvantaged groups. The higher rates are likely to reflect cultural values and lifestyles that facilitate or tolerate weight gain and social and economic barriers to health care and means of preventing overweight, as well as variations in genetic predisposition.

    g. Social history should assess the patient's use of physical activity and whether **occupational, medical or other personal circumstances** might interfere with increased activity or other interventions to induce weight loss.

C. Interview

The interview serves the dual purpose of gathering information and developing an alliance with the patient.

1. **Clarify the chief complaint and patient goals to determine the agenda and motivation for the patient; this clarification may suggest a primary etiology for the obesity.**

   a. A chief complaint focused on physical disability or discomfort caused by obesity will guide physical examination and suggest specific strategies for weight loss.

   b. A chief complaint focused on dissatisfaction with appearance should lead to an assessment of body image distortion or excessive concern with body weight or shape (e.g., as seen with bulimia or anorexia nervosa). Dissatisfaction with appearance is common in patients with moderate to severe obesity, however, and may provide motivation to pursue weight loss therapies necessary for control of medical complications.

2. **Obtain a weight and exercise history.** Where possible, the assistance of a dietician can be very helpful in obtaining a detailed weight history.

   a. **Determine the age of onset of obesity** (childhood, adolescence, or adulthood) and potential precipitants (e.g., pregnancy, injury, medications, smoking cessation, change in activity level, intercurrent illness, personal or family crisis, depression).

   b. **Establish whether there is a history of weight cycling or fluctuation.** Determine maximum and minimum weights during adulthood and the patient's perceptions of his or her desired and achievable weights. This provides an opportunity to identify unrealistic or inappropriate expectations and to help set healthy and realistic goals.

   c. **Review the history of interventions.** Prior attempts to lose weight should be chronicled, with special attention to successes, failures, and complications. A patient should be asked about professional (e.g., dietician or physician-supervised), self-help (e.g., Overeater's Anonymous), and lay interventions (e.g., dieting, exercise, fasting, purging).

   d. **Note the patient's dietary behaviors and exercise patterns.**

      i. Determine the general nutritional adequacy of the diet, calories consumed, and amount of dietary fat.

      ii. Determine the patterns of food consumption (e.g., desocialized patterns that include eating alone, binge eating, or overeating in the evening following a restrictive pattern of eating throughout the day, "grazing" versus sitting down for a scheduled meal); these can suggest useful interventions.

      iii. Determine the amount, type, and patterns of exercise, which can provide clues to patient motivation and suggest specific therapeutic interventions.

3. **All patients who present with obesity should be screened for psychiatric illness and psychological factors potentially contributing to, resulting from, or exacerbated by obesity.**

   a. **Ask about patterns of overeating or weight gain** associated with a depressed or anhedonic mood.

   b. **Assess potential preoccupation or excessive concern with weight or body shape** suggestive of bulimia nervosa, anorexia nervosa, or an atypical eating disorder.

   c. **Ask about binge-pattern eating** (clinically defined as episodic consumption of an unusually large amount of food within a discrete time period and associated with feeling diminished control over the eating) and emotions associated with the onset of and the period immediately after a binge (e.g., tension, relief, self-reproach). Specific foods, events, activities, or other environmental factors that trigger binge eating behavior should be determined.

   d. **Identify any inappropriate compensatory behaviors for overeating,** such as self-induced vomiting; laxative, diuretic, or diet pill use; fasting or restrictive eating; or excessive or compulsive exercise (e.g., exercise that exceeds conventional recommendations for fitness or a coach's program for competition, follows a rigid routine, or is compulsively pursued even in the presence of an injury or other adverse effects on health or well-being). Determine the frequency, duration, and precipitants of each of these behaviors, as well as their effects and complications. If a patient induces vomiting, he or she should be asked about a history of syrup of ipecac use—given that its chronic use can be associated with cardiomyopathy, myopathy, and death—so that immediate intervention can be made if necessary.

 e. **Ask about emotional precipitants and responses to overeating.** Assess the relative contributions of hunger and satiety and environmental or emotional cues to eating behavior.

 f. **Assess motivation to engage in weight loss** and ask whether the individual is aware of any sense of security, safety, or other advantages from being overweight. If the patient brings up a history of sexual or other trauma the primary care clinician should communicate concern and empathy without being intrusive. These patients should be referred to a mental health professional for further evaluation of this problem and its potential contribution to the individual's obesity.

D. Examination of the Patient

 1. **A physical examination should be performed to assess potential medical contributions to obesity,** such as Cushing's syndrome, hypothalamic or pituitary dysfunction, hypothyroidism, hyperinsulinemia, polycystic ovarian syndrome, or other genetic obesity syndromes, as well as medical complications of obesity (Table 48-1). Signs of bulimia nervosa should also be noted, if present, e.g., **Russell's sign** (scarring on the dorsal hand over the first metacarpal joints), dental caries, perimolysis, altered bowel sounds (associated with laxative abuse), and parotid gland enlargement.

 2. **Laboratory analysis** should be directed toward investigation of any suspected medical condition and identification of risk factors for embarking on a treatment program. Routinely, serum electrolytes, glucose, renal and liver function tests, uric acid, thyroid stimulating hormone, a serum lipid profile, and an ECG should be obtained. For a patient with significant cardiac risk, an exercise tolerance test (ETT) may be indicated before initiation of a program that includes increased physical activity. Hypokalemia, as well as other electrolyte abnormalities, may suggest purging by vomiting, laxatives, or diuretics.

 3. **Obesity assessment involves determination of the relationship of body weight to height, and an assessment of the size and distribution of body fat stores.**

  a. Adjustment of weight for height is best done by calculation of BMI by the formula BMI = weight (in kg) / (height in meters)^2 or [(weight in pounds) x 703 / (height in inches)^2]. It can also be determined from published tables or nomograms, such as the one shown in Figure 48-1. BMI is a useful benchmark for adult men or women of all heights or weights. Normal BMI values vary for children or adolescents, depending on their age and gender. Standard BMI curves for this population are available from the U.S. Centers for Disease Control and Prevention (www.cdc.gov).

   i. There are a variety of standards for categorizing weight by BMI. Figure 48-1 reflects World Health Organization standards as follows:

	BMI
Underweight	< 19
Healthy weight	19 to 25
Overweight	25 to 30
Obesity	> 30

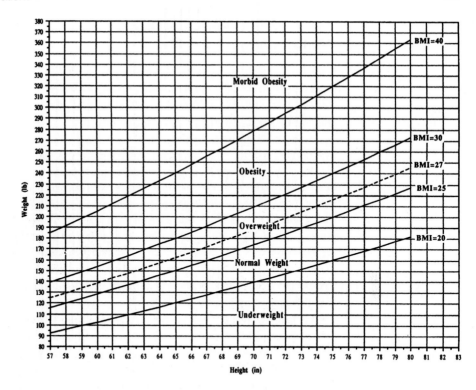

Figure 48-1.   Assessment of weight category based on Body Mass Index (BMI).*
*For use in men and women at least 18 years of age. [Adapted with permission from Body Weight Assessment Tool, Harvard Eating Disorders Center, Copyright 1995]

Obesity is further divided into three classes: Class I (BMI 30–35), class II (BMI 35–40), and class III (BMI > 40), which is often termed severe obesity.

    ii. The "ideal body weights" (IBW) listed in earlier Metropolitan Life Insurance Height-Weight Tables correspond to BMIs of approximately 19-21 kg/m^2. These weights are no longer considered appropriate therapeutic targets. IBW increases with age, and morbidity and mortality improve with modest weight loss (e.g., 10% of initial body weight) that may not even approach a return to IBW.

  b. **Fat distribution can be estimated by several methods.** The easiest and most useful parameter in general practice is waist circumference (the smallest circumference between the umbilicus and the pelvic crest) Regardless of BMI, waist circumferences that are > 35 inches for women and > 40 inches for men are associated with substantially elevated morbidity from metabolic syndrome (type 2 diabetes mellitus, hyperlipidemia, hypertension, platelet dysfunction, and associated cardiovascular disease).

  c. **Other methods for estimating body composition and fat stores include skin-fold thickness measures, bioimpedence analysis, and underwater weighing**, although these measures are used primarily as part of structured research protocols.

4. **The mental status examination will often be unremarkable.** The clinician should conduct it chiefly to assess mood and neurovegetative symptoms of depression, and to exclude any symptoms of severe psychiatric disorder or abnormalities in thought content or processing that may contribute to obesity or complicate its treatment.

III. Psychiatric Differential Diagnosis of Factors Contributing to Obesity

A major challenge to the primary care physician (PCP) in the evaluation and treatment of obesity is determining the degree to which psychological factors and psychiatric symptoms are contributors to, or sequelae of, the obesity.

A. **Binge-eating disorder (BED)** (see Chapter 20) is characterized by a binge pattern of overeating with episodic consumption of an unusually large quantity of food within a discrete period of time and associated with a feeling of diminished control over the eating. Binge-eating occurs on at least two days for a duration of at least 6 months to meet criteria for diagnosis of BED. Unlike patients with bulimia nervosa, persons with BED do not routinely engage in inappropriate compensatory behaviors to purge calories after such a binge. Other BED-associated symptoms may include eating rapidly, eating to the point of discomfort, eating without hunger cues, eating alone, and self-reproachful or depressed feelings after a binge. Patients routinely experience marked emotional distress in conjunction with their binge-eating behavior.

1. BED has a prevalence of 0.7–4% in the general population, and up to 29% among participants in weight loss programs.

2. BED is more prevalent among women than men, with a ratio of approximately 1.5:1; nonetheless, BED represents the most common eating disorder seen in men.

3. Onset of BED is generally in late adolescence or early 20s; the course is thought to be chronic. BED is associated with a history of severe obesity, frequent dieting, and significant weight cycling. Binge-eating may first develop after an individual is obese or may develop during treatment for obesity.

4. There is a strong relationship between binge-eating and psychiatric symptomatology, including higher rates of self-loathing, disgust about body size, depression, anxiety, and somatic concern. There appears to be a higher lifetime prevalence of major depression, substance abuse, panic disorder, and personality disorders in this population. Patients with BED may have difficulties with low self-esteem and in handling conflict.

B. **Bulimia nervosa and atypical eating disorders** may also be associated with binge pattern eating and abnormal weight gain.

1. Bulimia nervosa is less prevalent than BED, occurring in 1–3% of young adult women. Women are affected far more often than men, with a ratio of 9:1.

2. The diagnosis of bulimia nervosa is made in patients who exhibit both recurrent binge-eating and inappropriate compensatory behaviors to purge calories or prevent weight gain at least twice weekly for a duration of at least 3 months. The most common methods of purging are self-induced vomiting and laxative use, although excessive use of diuretics, diet pills stimulants, or exercise are seen as well. Patients may also alternate binge-eating with restrictive-eating or fasting to compensate for calories ingested during a binge. There is often a preoccupation with weight and food, and self-image is excessively or inappropriately influenced by body shape and weight. The diagnosis of bulimia nervosa is excluded in an individual with concurrent anorexia nervosa.

3. Symptoms are often covert and bulimia nervosa may be suggested by a history of weight preoccupation or fluctuations or characteristic findings on physical exam. Direct questioning in a non-judgmental way can often elicit disclosure of symptoms, although patients may be unwilling to admit to or discuss them. Patients are sometimes

reluctant to seek medical attention for fear that giving up their behaviors will result in further weight gain.

4. Eating disorders not otherwise specified (ED NOS), or atypical eating disorders, represent various combinations of symptoms that include restrictive-eating, binge-eating, and purging, as well as a preoccupation with or excessive concern with body shape and weight, but that do not meet specific criteria for anorexia, bulimia nervosa, or BED. Depending on the symptoms, these patients can present in a variety of weight ranges, including overweight and obesity.

C. **Major depressive disorder (MDD), with atypical features,** or atypical depression, can present with increased appetite that leads to excessive weight gain. Patients with atypical depression meet criteria for MDD, including depressed or anhedonic mood most of the day, every day for at least 2 weeks, but present with hypersomnia (instead of insomnia or early morning awakening) and hyperphagia (instead of poor appetite).

1. Overeating associated with atypical depression is distinguished from bulimia nervosa and BED by its relation to a mood disorder, characteristics of the eating, and the absence of excessive concern with weight and body shape.

D. **Anxiety disorders, adjustment disorders, and psychotic or mood disorders** are not necessarily associated with obesity but may potentially contribute to it through changes in appetite or dietary patterns. For example, some individuals with anxiety or mood symptoms eat in response to emotional cues rather than to hunger and satiety cues. In such individuals, eating or overeating may be experienced as soothing and thus may assist in affective regulation. Alternatively, chronically psychotic patients with poor ability to care for themselves may selectively eat readily available, high-calorie, high-fat foods, resulting in significant weight gain.

E. **Mental retardation** is associated with an increased prevalence of obesity, especially among those living in community settings.

F. **Psychological factors affecting obesity** are diverse. These factors exert their influence over obesity by alteration of appetite, eating patterns, or physical activity. Overeating in response to emotional cues (as opposed to physiologic hunger) is common. For some patients, secondary gains associated with obesity may cause resistance to treatment.

IV. Treatment Strategies for Obesity Complicated by Psychological Factors or Psychiatric Illness

Treatment for obesity should be guided by a thorough assessment of psychological factors and psychiatric symptoms that may contribute to, or result from, obesity, or may complicate the treatment process. If a primary cause of the obesity is an eating or mood disorder, the underlying disorder should be addressed along with the obesity. If obesity is perpetuated by maladaptive patterns of eating, then behavioral control of these symptoms is essential. If the psychosocial context contributes to the obesity (e.g., if an individual appears to associate secondary gains with obesity), psychotherapy may be helpful in addressing the underlying conflicts or other issues that likely will interfere with successful engagement with weight loss treatment. If obesity is associated with co-morbid psychiatric disease, a multi-disciplinary team including the primary care provider, a mental health professional, and a dietician can provide the most coordinated and effective treatment.

A. **Standard treatments for obesity should be individualized** based on the severity of the weight disorder, its medical complications, the patient's motivation, and the prior history and outcomes of weight loss therapy. The PCP can begin by monitoring and supervising self-help efforts, collaborating with a dietician to educate the patient about nutrition and realistic weight loss and maintenance goals, introducing tools to modify behavior, and assessing a patient's ability to pursue and tolerate an exercise regimen. If these interventions generate inadequate results, more aggressive approaches can be pursued in collaboration with specialists in nutrition or obesity.

1. **Diet, exercise, and behavior modification comprise the first-line approach to weight loss.** Although many patients are quite sophisticated about calorie and fat content of foods, they should nevertheless meet with a dietician for guidance on how to design and implement a balanced hypocaloric diet for initial weight loss and long-term weight maintenance. Behavior modification strategies can be introduced most easily in this setting.

   a. Moderate caloric restriction diets include more than 800 kcal/day *in toto* (generally 1,000 to 1,200 kcal/day) but less energy than is required for weight maintenance. Such diets should include an appropriate balance of calories from carbohydrates, fat and protein (generally 15–25% of calories from fat).

   b. Adequate exercise is critical for successful maintenance of weight loss. Inclusion of a vigorous exercise program protects against loss of lean body (i.e., muscle) mass that otherwise accompanies most acute weight loss. Maximal benefit will result from exercising at least 3 days a week for at least 20 minutes at an intensity level that expends approximately 300 kcal.

   c. Behavioral treatment of obesity is typically conducted in small groups meeting for one to two hours per week over the course of 12 to 20 weeks. Principles of behavioral therapy to facilitate lifestyle modification can be introduced in this setting by the group leader (usually a psychiatrist, psychologist or dietician). Table 48-3 summarizes the components of behavior modification treatment for weight control.

      i. **Self-monitoring** enhances the patient's awareness of patterns of eating and exercise that contribute to obesity. Patients should keep a daily log of their eating (time, foods, circumstances) that includes a description of emotions associated with the onset of eating; information should be entered soon after completion of the meal or episode of food intake. **Target behaviors are identified for change.**

      ii. **Stimulus control** helps an individual to change his or her environment by minimizing cues to eat or overeat. This approach may include encouraging the patient to avoid shopping while hungry, to store high-calorie foods in a place where they are relatively inaccessible, or to regulate the times and places of eating.

      iii. **Reinforcement of positive behaviors** can take the form of encouragement and support from peers, family, and health professionals or a tangible reward.

      iv. Patterns of thinking related to target behaviors are identified and modified.

   d. **Hypnosis** is a useful adjunct to behavioral treatment. Hypnosis is relatively contraindicated, however, in individuals with a history of dissociative disorders or episodes.

2. **Very low calorie diets** (VLCDs) typically consist of 400 to 800 kcal/day, often in the form of pre-mixed powdered formulas, re-constituted with water. They provide protein, some carbohydrates and micronutrients; they must be supplemented by fluids. Individuals must undergo careful medical evaluation before embarking on a VLCD and must be medically monitored during the process for electrolyte abnormalities, muscle wasting, cardiovascular dysfunction, and the possible need for the adjustment of medication dosages.

Table 48-3. Behavior Modification Treatment Components

Component	Description	Examples
Self-monitoring	Recording of target behaviors and factors associated with behaviors	Food and exercise records, moods and environment associated with overeating
Stimulus control	Restricting environmental factors associated with inappropriate behaviors	Keep away from high-fat foods; eat at specific times and places; set aside time and place for exercise
Contingency management	Rewarding appropriate behaviors	Prizes for achieving exercise goals
Changing behavior parameters	Directly altering target behavior topology	Slow down eating; self-regulate exercise
Cognitive-behavior modification	Changing thinking patterns related to target behaviors	Counter social pressure to be thin to reduce temptation to diet

SOURCE: Foreyt, J.P., & Goodrick, G.K. (1993). Evidence for success of behavior modification in weight loss and control. *Annals of Internal Medicine, 119*, 698–701.

    a. **VLCDs are generally reserved for individuals when BMI is > 40 after more conservative therapy has failed.** They are contraindicated in patients with a history of disordered eating, ECG or electrolyte abnormalities, or a need for frequent adjustment of medication doses.

    b. Although VLCDs are usually effective in inducing weight loss acutely, long-term outcome of VLCDs, used in combination with behavior modification, is generally no better than behavior therapy alone.

    c. VLCDs may precipitate binge-eating in susceptible individuals.

3. **Pharmacotherapy** has been effective in achieving weight loss, although results vary from patient to patient. **Agents currently approved by the FDA for weight loss include sibutramine, phentermine, diethylpropion, and orlistat. Other FDA agents that may be useful to treat obesity include bupropion, topiramate, fluoxetine, and sertraline, although FDA approved for other indications, their use for obesity is off-label.** In each case, the drug works well in a minority of patients, but there are currently no predictors of who will respond. To be maximally effective, medications should be used in combination with diet, exercise, and behavior modification. These agents should not be used for cosmetic purposes and should be restricted to use in individuals with clinically significant obesity (BMI > 30 or BMI > 27 in association with an obesity-related medical disorder). Patients must be screened for potential contraindications to use of these agents and monitored for potential medical and psychiatric complications. Realistic weight goals (e.g., a weight reduction of no more than 10–15%) should be reviewed with patients before initiating drug therapy. No weight-loss drugs are yet approved for use in children or pregnant women. All appetite suppressants should be stopped two weeks before any planned general anesthesia.

a. *Sibutramine* is a monoamine reuptake inhibitor that **acts as a serotonergic and adrenergic agent. It inhibits appetite and increases energy expenditure.** In the setting of behavioral therapy, it induces an average of 10% weight loss. Side effects may include hypertension, tachycardia, constipation, and insomnia. It is contraindicated in patients with uncontrolled hypertension or on MAOI therapy.

b. *Phentermine* is the safe component of the earlier "Phen-Fen" combination. It **is an adrenergic agent that induces modest weight loss.** Potential side effects include tachycardia, restlessness, insomnia, and hypertension. Phentermine is contraindicated in patients with heart disease, uncontrolled glaucoma, pregnancy, or on MAOI therapy.

c. *Diethylpropion* **is an adrenergic agent long-approved for weight loss therapy.** It induces modest weight loss but is limited by side effects that may include tachycardia, restlessness, insomnia, and mild hypertension. Diethylpropion is contraindicated in patients with ischemic heart disease, dysrhythmias, uncontrolled hypertension or glaucoma, or on MAOI therapy.

d. *Orlistat* **is a pancreatic lipase inhibitor that blocks absorption of up to 30% of ingested fat.** Weight loss is generally moderate and limited by substitution of fats with carbohydrates in the diet. Adverse effects include steatorrhea with high-fat diets, fat-soluble vitamin deficiencies. Patients on orlistat should supplement their diet with vitamins A, D, E, and K.

e. *Bupropion,* an antidepressant, has been **shown to exert moderate weight-loss effects in two short-term studies.** Bupropion is contraindicated in patients with seizure disorders or on MAOI therapy. Bupropion is also relatively contraindicated in patients with eating disorders due to their potentially higher risk of seizure while on this medication.

f. *Topiramate,* **an anticonvulsant and mood stabilizer,** can often counteract the weight gain-promoting effects of several psychotropic drugs, including olanzapine, clozapine, valproic acid, lithium, and other mood stabilizers. A high incidence of sedation and cognitive dysfunction limits its use as a general purpose weight loss agent, however.

g. **SSRIs can induce weight loss** in a small number of patients. Fluoxetine and sertraline are the SSRIs most likely to cause weight loss, and paroxetine and citalopram are least likely to do so. SSRIs are contraindicated in patients on MAOI therapy.

h. **Potential psychiatric contraindications to use of adrenergic or serotonergic appetite suppressant drugs include history of psychotic disorder, MDD, bipolar disorder, or history of substance abuse.** If anorexiant medications are deemed necessary in individuals with these disorders, they should be used with caution and close monitoring. Guidelines for safe use among individuals with eating disorders have not been established. They should not be used for patients with active bulimia nervosa and should never be used in an individual with anorexia nervosa.

i. **Anorexiant medications are contraindicated in patients taking MAOIs.** Anorexiants should not be started during or within 14 days of a patient's having taken an MAOI, and an appropriate drug washout period should elapse after discontinuing an anorexiant drug before beginning an MAOI.

j. Concurrent use of other antidepressant medications (including SSRIs) or lithium is a relative contraindication for use of anorexiant medications but has not been adequately studied. Patients treated with sibutramine and SSRIs must be monitored carefully for hypertension, tachyarrhythmias, other cardiovascular abnormalities, and new cognitive/behavioral changes.

k. In addition to their potential adverse medical effects, potential side effects of anorexiant medications include psychiatric symptoms (e.g., euphoria, dysphoria, agitation, and psychosis). Chronic intoxication with anorexiant drugs can manifest as irritability, insomnia, hyperactivity, personality changes, or psychosis. There is also some potential for abuse.

4. **Surgery is an alternative approach for severe obesity** (BMI > 40 or BMI > 35 in association with a complicating medical disorder). **Gastric bypass and vertical banded gastroplasty** are both highly effective in achieving weight loss (usually 50–65% of excess weight); controlled studies demonstrate somewhat greater efficacy with gastric bypass. Peri-operative complications (e.g., wound infection, hernia, venous thrombosis, pneumonia) are similar to other major abdominal procedures in this population; they must be weighed against the potential benefit for each patient.

   a. Post-operative non-compliance (e.g., binge-eating) can lead to pouch dilatation or staple line disruption, and patients should be evaluated for their ability to adhere to an appropriate post-operative regimen before being recommended for surgery.

   b. Weight-loss surgery is often associated with resolution of BED in the short-term, but the long-term impact of surgery on binge-eating is unclear. There are no clear-cut predictors of responses, however, and patients with BED must be evaluated carefully by a psychiatrist or psychologist experienced in the management of patients undergoing obesity surgery before such surgery is recommended.

   c. Gastric weight-loss surgery is contraindicated in patients with ongoing substance abuse, poorly controlled major psychiatric illness, and bulimia nervosa. If the patient is deemed at risk for post-operative non-compliance, psychiatric treatment and re-evaluation are indicated before surgery is recommended.

B. **Treatment of underlying psychiatric illness and psychological factors affecting appetite and ingestive behavior is an essential component of obesity treatment.**

   1. **Eating disorders** complicated by obesity are optimally treated by a team of health care professionals including the PCP, psychiatrist or other mental health professional, obesity specialist, and dietician, to address medical, psychological, and nutritional issues relevant to care. Individuals with anorexia nervosa should never be given treatment to facilitate weight loss. As a general rule, weight-loss treatment should also be avoided in individuals with bulimia nervosa since such treatment is likely to exacerbate symptoms. In such cases, the primary symptoms of bulimia nervosa should be addressed prior to initiation of weight-loss treatment in overweight individuals. For overweight patients with BED with a history of either weight cycling or early-onset binge-eating, it may be helpful to address the primary symptoms of BED prior to initiating weight-loss treatment.

      a. Binge-pattern eating associated with bulimia nervosa or BED can be treated with a combination of psychotherapy and psychotropic medication. Binge-eaters in behaviorally based weight-loss programs may be more refractory to treatment than non-binge eaters. Although some of these patients lose less weight initially, exhibit higher dropout rates, and more rapid return of lost weight, long-term weight loss results are statistically similar in binge-eating and non–binge-eating subgroups.

      b. **Cognitive-behavioral therapy (CBT) is the best established treatment for bulimia nervosa and BED.**

      c. Interpersonal therapy, psychodynamic psychotherapy, motivational enhancement therapy, dialectical behavioral therapy, guided imagery, and guided self-change are also useful treatment modalities for BED and bulimia nervosa depending on the patient's presentation, treatment goals, and capacities.

      d. Group and family-based therapies are useful in treating bulimia nervosa. Group CBT, group interpersonal therapy, and group dialectical behavior therapy are effective in treatment of BED.

    e. Pharmacotherapy has been shown to reduce symptoms associated with BED and is associated with a significantly greater rate of weight loss than placebo in this population. Fluvoxamine (50–300 mg/day in divided doses) and sertraline (50–200 mg/day) have been shown to reduce the frequency of binges in BED. Fluoxetine (20–80 mg/day) has been shown effective in treating BED in one controlled study but not in another at 60 mg/day. Topirimate (50–600 mg/day) and silbutramine (15 mg/day) have each been shown effective in reducing the symptoms of BED.

    f. **A variety of agents reduce binge frequency in bulimia nervosa;** these agents should be chosen according to their side-effect profiles. Dosing schedules should be adjusted to times when the drug is likely to be absorbed rather than lost by purging.

        i. **Fluoxetine, the only agent approved by the FDA for the treatment of bulimia nervosa,** is well tolerated and is not generally associated with weight gain. If fluoxetine is chosen, the dosage should be steadily increased to 60 mg daily as tolerated, because this dose has been associated with a more complete clinical response.

        ii. **Imipramine and desipramine** at standard antidepressant doses are effective but can cause significant weight gain and are less well tolerated in this population.

        iii. Although not associated with weight gain, **bupropion is contraindicated in patients with bulimia** because of reported higher incidence of drug-induced seizures in this population; the mechanism of this effect is unknown. MAOIs are also relatively contraindicated in patients with bulimia nervosa given reports of spontaneous hypertensive crisis in this population, risks associated with stimulant and diet pill use, and dietary indiscretion. These agents are also associated with weight gain in many patients.

    g. For severe bulimia in which purging symptoms pose a significant risk to medical health (e.g., frequent purging associated with dehydration or hypokalemia, or ipecac use) inpatient care or partial hospitalization may be indicated to stabilize the patient medically and control the purging symptoms.

    h. In more severely disturbed patients eating disorder symptoms (including binge-eating) often serve some essential organizing function. Therefore, great care should be taken in assessing whether a patient can tolerate rapid discontinuation of his or her symptoms. If the patient is medically stable and appears at risk of serious psychological decompensation, attempts to eradicate symptoms may need to be postponed until alternative coping strategies are established. If this is the case, the patient should be educated about the medical risks of the symptoms and enter psychotherapy while being closely medically monitored. In such cases, primary weight loss therapy may be a significant stressor for the patient and relatively contraindicated.

2. **Atypical depression** associated with hyperphagia and weight gain should be managed by evaluating and treating the underlying depression with an appropriate combination of pharmacotherapy and psychotherapy (see Chapter 14). Although the pharmacological therapy should be directed primarily at the mood symptoms, agents unlikely to exacerbate obesity (such as fluoxetine, sertraline or bupropion) should be chosen for the overweight patient whenever possible. The patient should also be introduced to behavioral techniques that will assist in controlling excessive eating.

3. **If anxiety, adjustment disorder, or psychotic or mood illness contribute to behaviors associated with obesity,** these underlying illnesses should be treated appropriately. Whenever possible, medications should be chosen that are least likely to exacerbate weight gain.

4. Management of **obesity in the mentally retarded patient** should include assessment of the environmental context, with particular attention to diet and opportunities for

physical activity. Caretakers should be enlisted in management to avoid the use of food for rewards, to modify the environmental stimuli that contribute to the overeating, and to encourage an increased level of physical activity by the patient when appropriate.

5. **Management of psychological factors** that contribute to obesity should begin with an assessment of whether the patient can tolerate successful weight loss or the elimination of the behaviors that contribute to obesity and a determination as to what factors may affect his or her engagement in treatment.

   a. Individual or group psychotherapy—cognitive-behavioral, interpersonal, or psychodynamic—can assist the patient in identifying the emotional precipitants to overeating and the potential secondary gains in resisting weight loss and remaining overweight. Some patients for whom obesity provides necessary social distancing may not tolerate weight loss. These patients should be treated for their underlying psychological distress; weight loss treatment may need to be modified or deferred with consultation by a mental health professional.

   b. Some patients requesting weight loss treatment will be normal weight or only marginally overweight. They may seek weight loss because of the social premium on slimness or because they suffer from various degrees of body disparagement.

      i. Patients in the former group should be educated about the medical risks of aggressive weight loss treatment modalities that may contraindicate their use for cosmetic goals. For marginally overweight patients, less aggressive approaches to weight loss and maintenance should be encouraged, including modification of exercise and eating behaviors.

      ii. Overweight patients who present with preoccupation with or overvaluation of body weight and shape, a distorted body image, or body disparagement should be treated with psychotherapy before or concomitantly with any weight loss therapy. For these patients, failure at initiation or maintenance of weight loss (e.g., weight cycling) may be particularly troublesome.

6. **The patient embarking on a weight-loss program should be prepared for the potential emotional sequelae of the weight loss, as well as the potential for regain of lost weight.** Patients who encounter or anticipate these difficulties should be referred for individual or group psychotherapy or couples therapy to assist them through this process.

   a. Weight loss in obese patients results in short-term reductions in depression and anxiety. Behavioral weight-loss treatments are associated in the short-term with decreased body dissatisfaction, increased self-esteem, and better interpersonal functioning. Similarly, surgical treatment of morbid obesity is associated with improvements in mood, self-esteem, and interpersonal functioning. Regaining lost weight is often associated with adverse psychological reactions, however.

   b. Dieting can be a stressor in itself, or it may enhance vulnerability to stress. Dieting also appears to increase the risk for developing an eating disorder; in susceptible patients, it can lead to a pattern of food restriction and binge-eating that can exacerbate obesity and body-image problems.

   c. Interpersonal relationships may be affected by successful weight loss, and patients may find themselves confronted with difficulties associated with the management of greater intimacy and increased socialization, as well as the destabilization of relationships that relied in part on the social and psychological consequences of the obesity itself.

Suggested Readings

Allison, D.B., Fontaine, K.R., Manson, J.E., et al. (1999). Annual deaths attributable to obesity in the United States. *Journal of the American Medical Association, 282,* 1530–1538.

Appolinario, J.C., Bacaltchuk, J., Sichieri, R., et al. (In press). A randomized, double-blind, placebo-controlled study of sibutramine in the treatment of binge eating disorder. *Archives of General Psychiatry.*

Arnold, L.M., McElroy, S.L., Hudson, J.L., et al. (2002). A placebo-controlled, randomized trial of fluoxetine in the treatment of binge-eating disorder. *Journal of Clinical Psychiatry, 63,* 1028–1033.

Atkinson, R.L., & Hubbard V.S. (1994). Report on the NIH workshop on pharmacologic treatment of obesity. *American Journal of Clinical Nutrition, 60,* 153–156.

Becker, A.E. (2003). Outpatient management of eating disorders in adults. *Current Women's Health Reports, 3,* 221–229.

Becker, A.E., Hamburg, P., & Herzog, D.B. (1998). The role of psychopharmacologic management in the treatment of eating disorders. *Psychiatric Clinics of North America, 5,* 17–51.

Becker, A.E., Grinspoon, S.K., Klibanski, A., & Herzog, D.B. (1999). Eating disorders. *New England Journal of Medicine, 340,* 1092–1098.

Bolocofsky, D.N., Spinler, D., & Coulthard-Morris, L. (1985). Effectiveness of hypnosis as an adjunct to behavioral weight management. *Journal of Clinical Psychology, 41,* 35–41.

Bruce, B. (1996). Binge eating among the overweight population: A serious and prevalent problem. *Journal of the American Dietetic Association, 96,* 58–61.

Diagnostic and statistical manual of mental disorders (4th ed.). Washington, DC: American Psychiatric Association, pp. 320–327, 339–344, 384–386, 539–550, 678, 729–731.

Foreyt, J.P., & Goodrick, G.K. (1993). Evidence for success if behavioral modification in weight loss and control. *Annals of Internal Medicine, 119,* 698–701.

Goldstein, L.T., Goldsmith, S.J., Anger, K., et al. (1996). Psychiatric symptoms in clients presenting for commercial weight reduction treatment. *International Journal of Eating Disorders, 20,* 191–197.

Grilo, C. (2002). A controlled study of cognitive behavioral therapy and fluoxetine for binge eating disorder (abstract). Eating Disorders Research Society Annual Meeting Scientific Program and Abstracts. Charleston, South Carolina.

Hudson, J.I., McElroy, S.L., Raymond, N.C., et al. (1998). Fluvoxamine in the treatment of binge-eating disorder: A multicenter placebo-controlled, double-blind trial. *American Journal of Psychiatry, 155,* 1756–1762.

Hyman, S.E., Arana, G.W., & Rosenbaum, J.F. (1995). *Handbook of psychiatric drug therapy* (3rd ed.). Boston: Little, Brown and Company, pp. 5–123.

Istvan, J., Zavela, K., & Weidner, G. (1992). Body weight and psychological distress in NHANES I. *International Journal of Obesity, 16,* 999–1003.

Jimerson, D.C., Herzog, D.B., & Brotman, A.W. (1993). Pharmacologic approaches in the treatment of eating disorders. *Harvard Review of Psychiatry, 1*(2), 82–93.

Kopelman, P.G. (2000). Obesity as a medical problem. *Nature, 404,* 635–643.

McElroy, S.L., Arnold, L.M., Shapira, N.A., et al. (2003). Topiramate in the treatment of binge eating disorder associated with obesity: A randomized, placebo-controlled trial. *American Journal of Psychiatry, 160,* 255–261.

McElroy, S.L., Casuto, L.S., & Nelson, E.B. (2000). Placebo-controlled trial of sertraline in the treatment of binge-eating disorder. *American Journal of Psychiatry, 157,* 1004–1006.

Must, A., Spadaro, J., Coakley, E.H., et al. (1999). The disease burden associated with overweight and obesity. *Journal of the American Medical Association, 282,* 1523–1529.

NIH Technology Assessment Conference Panel. (1983). Methods for voluntary weight loss and control. *Annals of Internal Medicine, 119,* 764–770.

Physician's desk reference. (1995). Montvale, NJ: Medical Economics Data Production Company.

Report of a WHO study group, Diet, nutrition, and the prevention of chronic diseases. (1990). *WHO Technical Reports Service, 797,* 1–204.

Rimmer, J.H., Braddock, D., & Fujiura, G. (1993). Prevalence of obesity in adults with mental retardation: Implications for health promotion and disease prevention. *Mental Retardation, 31*(2), 105–110.

Sarr, M.G., & Balsiger, B.M. (2001). Bariatric surgery in the 1990's. *Swiss Surgery, 7,* 11–15.

Spitzer, R.L., Yanovsky, S., Wadden, T., et al. (1993). Binge eating disorder: Its further validation in a multisite study. *International Journal of Eating Disorders, 13*(2), 137–153.

Stunkard, A.J., & Wadden, T.A. (1992). Psychological aspects of severe obesity. *American Journal of Clinical Nutrition, 55*(2 suppl), 524S–532S.

Stunkard, A., Berkowitz, R., Tarikut, C., et al. (1996). D-Fenfluramine treatment of binge eating disorder. *American Journal of Psychiatry, 153,* 1455–1459.

Sturm, R. (2002). The effects of obesity, smoking, and drinking on medical problems and costs. Obesity outranks both smoking and drinking in its deleterious effects on health and health costs. *Health Affairs, 21,* 245–253.

Telch, C.F., & Agras, W.S. (1994). Obesity, binge eating and psychopathology: Are they related? *International Journal of Eating Disorders, 15,* 53–61.

Wadden, T.A., & Foster, G.D. (2000). Behavioral treatment of obesity. *Medical Clinics of North America, 84,* 441–461.

Wadden, T.A., & Steen, S.N. (1996). Improving the maintenance of weight loss: The ten per cent solution. In H. Angel, H. Anderson, & C. Bouchard (Eds.), *Progress in obesity research: 7.* John Libbey & Company Ltd/7th International Congress on Obesity, pp. 745–750.

Williamson, D.F., Pamuk, E., Thun, M., et al. (1995). Prospective study of intentional weight loss and mortality in never-smoking overweight US white women aged 40–64 years. *American Journal of Epidemiology, 141,* 1128–1141.

Wilson, G.T. (1993). Relation of dieting and voluntary weight loss to psychological functioning and binge eating. *Annals of Internal Medicine, 119,* 727–730.

Wilson, G.T., Nonas, C.A., & Rosenblum, G.D. (1993). Assessment of binge eating in obese patients. *International Journal of Eating Disorders, 13,* 25–33.

Wing, R.R., & Greeno, C.G. (1994). Behavioural and psychosocial aspects of obesity and its treatment. *Bailliere's Clinical Endocrinology Metabolism, 8,* 689–703.

Wolf, A.M., & Colditz, G.A. Current estimates of the economic cost of obesity in the United States. *Obesity Research, 6,* 173–175.

Yanovski, S.Z., & Yanovski, J.A. (2002). Obesity. *New England Journal of Medicine, 346,* 591–602.

CHAPTER 49

The Geriatric Patient

M. Cornelia Cremens and Michael Langan

I. Introduction

In 1900, 3.1 million Americans were over the age of 65; today elderly Americans number approximately 35 million and **by 2030 one in five Americans will be 65 or older**. Clearly, the aging of America presents challenges for how we will provide much needed care. Taking a history from an elderly person does not require special skills but may require patience, close observation, and a systematic approach. **Elderly persons and their families tend to underreport their symptoms and blame those symptoms on advancing age. Altered physical responses in the elderly may result in less specific symptoms that interfere with the physician's ability to make a correct diagnosis.** For example, an infection, heart attack, or stroke may present as malaise, a decline in physical function, or impaired cognition. **Visual and auditory impairments, cognitive decline, a slowed response to questions, and vague complaints are other obstacles that can make an interview arduous and less informative.** The approach outlined below can be helpful in overcoming these difficulties.

II. Evaluation of the Patient

The purpose of the evaluation is to elicit medical, psychological, pharmacologic, and functional data to establish an organized and comprehensive care plan.

A. Identification of the Presenting Problem

Attempts to establish the chief complaint and history of a current illness can be frustrating. Many older patients are unable to formulate a single complaint or problem; the problem often is wrapped in a complex array of **vague complaints** and family issues.

1. The **chief complaint** relating to an acute illness may be buried among complaints relating to multiple organ systems and chronic conditions.

    a. **Acute medical or psychiatric illness often presents differently in older patients** compared with young adults. Illness in one system may manifest itself as symptoms in another system.

    i. Confusion, personality change, lack of interest, and fatigue may be the only complaints relating to an acute medical illness.

    ii. Alternatively, medical symptoms, such as malaise, constipation, chronic pain, and a decline in physical function, may present as somatic manifestations of psychiatric illness in the elderly. Depression, dementia, and psychosis can be overlooked when they are erroneously attributed to a medical condition.

    iii. Family members often are baffled by a geriatric patient's behavior. Directing questions to them rather than to the identified patient usually does not aid the history-taking and may distance the physician from the patient.

b. **Vague complaints** pose a difficult problem. The history may have to be taken over the course of several visits.

   i. Once a level of comfort is attained between the physician and the patient, each complaint can be evaluated better.

   ii. While **scheduling multiple visits** may appear to be inconvenient for the patient, repeated visits aid in the development of a comfortable rapport between the patient, the family, and the doctor.

2. **Discussions with family members** can be held in front of the patient or while the patient is otherwise occupied. Frequently, information is conveyed that makes the patient upset or uncomfortable. **The physician can to some degree allay the patient's suspicions or anxieties by explaining initially that he or she will meet with both the patient and the family member or caregiver individually and then together.** At times, patients may reveal valuable information to the physician only after confidentiality has been assured.

B. Medical History

Evaluate a patient's cognition and mood before taking the medical history. If prominent memory problems or confusion are seen, ask the patient's permission to speak with a family member. Medications usually are numerous and should be itemized carefully. Before the initial appointment, request that the patient bring in all prior, current, and over-the-counter medications from home. Questions regarding medical history, while similar to those asked of younger patients, also should include prior immunizations and other preventive interventions.

1. **Geriatric syndromes** are problem complexes that combine or cross over multiple organ systems (Table 49-1). In identifying geriatric syndromes, a more global approach to the care plan is initiated. Older patients usually have disturbances of multiple systems that lead to specific problems, such as falls, incontinence, and delirium.

2. Obtaining a **social history** is very important with an older patient. This may be initiated at the first visit and completed during a subsequent visit. The developmental history of the patient's birth, education, marriage, and employment is essential to a broad assessment of current function.

Table 49-1. Geriatric Syndromes

Altered mental status	Malnutrition
Delirium	Incontinence
Dementia	Urinary
Depression	Fecal
Incompetence	Constipation
Sensory impairments	Frailty
Loss of vision	Failure to thrive
Hearing loss	Immobility
Falls	

Table 49-2. Basic Activities of Daily Living	
Mobility	Hygiene
Dressing	Feeding
Bathing	Toileting

a. **Living Arrangements**
   i. Determine whether the patient continues to live independently in his or her own home or apartment and whether the patient and family want the patient to continue to live independently. Many older patients struggle to maintain a home without considering workable alternatives, such as assisted living and elder housing.
   ii. **Establish the patient's living preference** early in the evaluation process in order to help the patient maintain independence, if possible.

b. **Financial and Economic Status**
   i. **Most elderly patients live on a fixed income** and are careful with money. Therefore, expensive medications, food, housing, or transportation lead to poor compliance.
   ii. **Financial abuse of the elderly is common;** however, it is not easily discovered in the initial interview. Concerns and fears regarding financial security, factual or not, can lead to a significant deterioration in the patient's health.

c. **Dietary Assessment**
   i. A thorough dietary assessment of every older patient is essential.
   ii. Proper nutrition depends on multiple factors, including medical and psychiatric health, dentition, and financial status.
   iii. The use of over-the-counter dietary supplements should be included in the dietary assessment.

3. **Activities of daily living (ADLs) and instrumental activities of daily living (IADLs)** are essential in the assessment of an elderly person's ability to live independently.

   a. **ADLs** measure the functional independence of patients with regard to basic tasks (Table 49-2). Asking a patient what he or she does in a typical day can give a physician an idea of that patient's ADL or IADL ratings. If the patient is having difficulty managing basic personal care tasks, multiple services will be required to care for the patient adequately.

   b. **IADLs** measure more complex tasks that require a greater degree of cognitive and physical ability (Table 49-3). Some patients may be impaired in only one or two of these areas; having a family member or outside agency assist a patient with specific tasks alleviates the burden for that patient.

Table 49-3. Instrumental Activities of Daily	
Independent living	Doing laundry
Shopping	Taking medications
Cooking	Managing finances
Telephoning	Taking transportation
Housekeeping (light)	

4. **Pharmacotherapy**

Many illnesses in the elderly are misdiagnosed or dismissed as a normal process of aging because of the failure to recognize how diseases and drugs affect the older patient. Both overprescribing inappropriate or unnecessary drugs and underprescribing potentially beneficial drugs can create a problem. The greater the numbers of drugs prescribed the greater the risk of developing adverse drug events. Even though the elderly represent 13% of the population of the United States, they consume more than one-third of prescription drugs. An assessment of medications should be part of every visit and it should include over-the-counter medications, vitamins, and supplements. Multiple physicians may be concurrently prescribing medications. **Polypharmacy** also increases the risk of noncompliance. Estimates of non-compliance with prescription medications range from 40–75% in the ambulatory elderly. **Poor compliance** is often due to issues of memory loss, limited mobility, and poor vision. Whenever possible, medications should be dosed once or twice daily.

5. **The issue of an advance directive, durable power of attorney, and/or health care proxy should be addressed** with the patient during the initial or second visit.

   a. **Competent patients** are asked to express their wishes regarding treatment for a terminal illness or traumatic event. The reason for this discussion should be reiterated carefully. The goal is to be able to carry out the wishes of a patient when he or she is unable to speak for him or herself. Patients should be reassured that this will not adversely affect the level of care they receive.

C. Interview

An interview of an elderly patient can be simple or exceedingly frustrating, depending on the level of the patient's cognitive abilities or impairments. The physician should attempt to establish a relationship, however limited. If the doctor talks exclusively to the family, it prevents the doctor from getting to know the patient and the patient from getting to know and trust the doctor.

1. **Establish a rapport with the patient by sitting in a relaxed and calm manner** while the patient begins the history in his or her own words. If the physician is relaxed and unhurried, the patient's story will unfold easily.

   a. Discussion with the family is best conducted after an initial interview with the patient has been completed, no matter how brief that interview may be.

2. **Explain carefully any tests, procedures, or future testing** to the patient and family. **Repeat the instructions or write them down** so that the patient can refer to them after leaving the office.

D. Examination of the Patient

A psychiatric evaluation of an elderly patient proceeds in a manner similar to that of a younger patient: it involves an assessment of the patient's appearance, behavior, and ability to engage in a discussion with the physician. However, **good communication skills are more important in interviewing older patients.** Older patients may have visual and auditory impairments and choose not to tell the doctor about them. Stress the need to have eyeglasses on and hearing aids in place (check that the batteries are working) during the interview. The aim of the history and examination is to determine reversible or remediable problems while focusing on the geriatric syndromes of delirium, dementia, depression, sensory impairments, falls, incontinence, and malnutrition. During the initial appointment the

Table 49-4. Geriatric Depression Scale[a]

1. Are you basically satisfied with your life?

2. Have you dropped many of your activities and interests?

3. Do you feel your life is empty?

4. Do you often get bored?

5. Are you hopeful about the future?

6. Are you bothered by thoughts you cannot get out of your head?

7. Are you in good spirits most of the time?

8. Are you afraid something bad is going to happen to you?

9. Do you feel happy most of the time?

10. Do you often feel helpless?

11. Do you often get restless and fidgety?

12. Do you prefer to stay at home rather than going out and doing new things?

13. Do you frequently worry about the future?

14. Do you feel you have more problems with your memory than most?

15. Do you think it is wonderful to be alive now?

16. Do you often feel downhearted and blue?

17. Do you feel pretty worthless the way you are now?

18. Do you worry a lot about the past?

19. Do you find life very exciting?

20. Is it hard for you to get started on new projects?

21. Do you feel full of energy?

22. Do you feel that your situation is hopeless?

23. Do you think that most people are better off than you are?

24. Do you frequently get upset over little things?

25. Do you frequently feel like crying?

26. Do you have trouble concentrating?

27. Do you enjoy getting up in the morning?

28. Do you prefer to avoid social gatherings?

29. Is it easy for you to make decisions?

30. Is your mind as clear as it used to be?

[a]Answers indicative of major depression are answered no to 1, 5, 7, 9, 15, 19, 27 and yes to the remaining 20. A score of 11 of 30 is a positive screen for depression.

SOURCE: Yesavage, J.A., & Brink, T.L. (1983). Development and validation of a geriatric depression screening scale: A preliminary report. *Journal of Psychiatric Research, 17*, 37–49.

evaluation begins by observing the patient's gait, appearance, behavior, interaction with family members, and ability to communicate his or her history to the doctor.

1. **Speech and cognition** are easily noted during the initial stages of the interview.

   a. Impaired speech may be indicative of a depression, a dementia, a thought disorder, or a neurologic sequelae of a stroke.

   b. Cognitive impairment can be prominent or subtle (e.g., frontal lobe deficits), and further evaluation may be indicated.

2. **Evaluation of an older patient's mood is often difficult,** because the elderly are not likely to describe themselves as depressed or anxious. They focus instead on somatic complaints, such as vague aches and pains and strange feelings or tastes.

3. **Affect can be confusing** at times, as in patients with Parkinson's disease, in whom the lack of facial expression often is interpreted as depression. Similarly, emotional incontinence, in which the patient laughs or cries for periods of time without feeling sad or happy, often is seen in patients with organic states, such as dementia and post-stroke conditions, and may be inappropriately considered depressive behavior. Frontal lobe lesions can present as disinhibition or euphoria, in which patients may tell silly jokes (*witzelsucht*).

4. **Psychosis** can be a manifestation of a primary psychiatric problem or can be from an underlying organic illness. Delusions associated with dementia are common and are usually simple, involving impaired memory, paranoia, and persecution without concomitant hallucinations. Schizophrenia (life-long or late-onset) consists of bizarre persecutory delusions and auditory hallucinations and has a chronic course. Visual hallucinations typically have an organic etiology.

III. Diagnostic Criteria

The formulation of a diagnosis involves multiple factors. The complex nature of both medical illness and psychiatric illness in an older patient requires a full assessment of medical, functional, nutritional, cognitive, and affective symptoms. Scales can be useful adjuncts to a thorough examination and can be used to track the progress of improvement or impairment; they should not be relied on to make the diagnosis in an older patient.

IV. Scales and Questionnaires in the Evaluation of Psychiatric Diagnoses

A. **The Geriatric Depression Scale (GDS)** was developed and validated by Yesavage and Brink (1983); it has been widely used in primary care settings and is valuable in patients without cognitive impairment (Table 49-4). If cognitive impairment is present, combining this scale with the Mini-Mental State Examination may be helpful. However, **the GDS is not valid in patients with cognitive impairment.**

B. **The Beck Depression Inventory (BDI)** is another excellent tool for assessing depression. Both the GDS, and the BDI are self-rating scales and may be mailed to the patient before the first appointment.

C. **The Mini-Mental State Examination (MMSE)** is the most frequently used scale for testing cognitive impairment (Table 49-5). It is most useful as a screening test to indi-

Table 49-5. Mini-Mental State Examination

	Maximum Score
Orientation	
1. What is the (year) (season) (date) (day) (month)?	(5)
2. Where are we: (state) (county) (town) (hospital) (floor)?	(5)
Registration	
3. Name three objects	(3)
Attention and calculation	
4. Serial 7s	(5)
Recall	
5. Ask for three objects repeated above	(3)
Language	
6. Name a pencil and a watch	(2)
7. Repeat the following: "No ifs ands or buts"	(1)
8. Follow a three-stage command	(3)
9. Read and obey the following: "Close your eyes"	(1)
10. Write a sentence	(1)
11. Copy design	(1)
	Total score (30)

SOURCE: Folstein, M.F., Folstein, S.E., & McHugh, P.R. (1975). Mini-mental state: A practical method for grading the cognitive state of patients for the clinician. *Journal of Psychiatric Research, 12,* 189–198.

cate whether more comprehensive neuropsychiatric testing is needed. The Short, Portable, Mental Status Questionnaire (SPMSQ) is similar to the MMSE but it does not address orientation, remote memory, writing, constructional praxis, or calculations.

D. **The Functional Dementia Scale (FDS)** covers a broad range of symptoms, allowing the physician to broaden the scope of the evaluation when the caregiver focuses on only the most burdensome symptoms (Table 49-6). The FDS is scored by a family member or caregiver who is with the patient most of the time.

V. Conclusion

A thorough initial examination, although time-consuming, allows the physician to formulate comprehensive care and work with the patient and the patient's family to achieve the stated goals. Older patients appreciate the time, concern, and attention given to them. The trust and rapport established in the beginning are of substantial benefit to the future care (with regard to compliance and communication) of the elderly.

Table 49-6. Functional Dementia Scale

Scoring

None or little of the time	circle 1
Some of the time	circle 2
Good part of the time	circle 3
Most of the time	circle 4

1. Has difficulty in completing simple tasks	1 2 3 4
2. Spends time either sitting or in apparently purposeless activity	1 2 3 4
3. Wanders at night or needs to be restrained to prevent wandering	1 2 3 4
4. Hears things that are not there	1 2 3 4
5. Requires supervision or assistance eating	1 2 3 4
6. Loses things	1 2 3 4
7. Appearance is disorderly if left to own devices	1 2 3 4
8. Moans	1 2 3 4
9. Cannot control bowel function	1 2 3 4
10. Threatens to harm others	1 2 3 4
11. Cannot control bladder function	1 2 3 4
12. Needs to be watched so does not injure self	1 2 3 4
13. Destructive	1 2 3 4
14. Shouts or yells	1 2 3 4
15. Accuses others of doing him or her bodily harm or stealing his or her possessions when the accusations are not true	1 2 3 4
16. Is unaware of limitations imposed by illness	1 2 3 4
17. Becomes confused and does not know where he or she is	1 2 3 4
18. Has trouble remembering	1 2 3 4
19. Has sudden changes of mood	1 2 3 4
20. If left alone, wanders aimlessly during the day or needs to be restrained to prevent wandering	1 2 3 4

SOURCE: Moore, J.T., Bobula, J.A., Short, T.B., & Mischell, M. (1983). A functional dementia scale. *Journal of Family Practice, 16,* 499–503.

Suggested Readings

Avorn, J., & Gurwitz, J.H. (1995). Drug use in the nursing home. *Annals of Internal Medicine, 123,* 195–204.

Beyth, R.J., & Shorr, R.I. (2002). Principles of drug therapy in older patients: Rational drug prescribing. *Clinics in Geriatric Medicine, 18,* 577–592.

Brangman, S.A. (2002). Twenty common problems in geriatrics. *Journal of the American Geriatrics Society, 50,* 1904–1906.

Callahan, E.H., Thomas, D.C., Goldhirsch, S.L., & Leipzig, R.M. (2002). Geriatric hospital medicine. *Medical Clinics of North America, 86,* 707–729.

Coffey, C.E., & Cummings, X. (Eds.). (1994). *Textbook of geriatric neuropsychiatry.* Washington, DC: American Psychiatric Press.

Folstein, M.F., Folstein, S.E., & McHugh, P.R. (1975). Mini-mental state: A practical method for grading the cognitive state of patients for the clinician. *Journal of Psychiatric Research, 12,* 189–198.

Hazzard, W.R., Bierman, E.I., Blass, J.P., et al. (Eds.). (1994). *Principles of geriatric medicine and gerontology* (3rd ed.). New York: McGraw-Hill.

Mehta, R.N., & Potter, J.F. (2002). Essentials of clinical geriatrics. *Journal of the American Geriatrics Society, 50,* 1902–1903.

Moore, J.T., Bobula, J.A., Short, T.B., & Mischell, M. (1983). A functional dementia scale. *Journal of Family Practice, 16,* 499–503.

Reichel, W. (Ed.). (1995). *Care of the elderly: Clinical aspects of aging* (4th ed.). Baltimore: Williams & Wilkins.

Sadavoy, J., Lazarus, L.W., Jarvik, L.F., & Grossberg, G.T. (Eds.). (1996). *Comprehensive review of geriatric psychiatry,* vol. 11 (2nd ed.). Washington, DC: American Psychiatric Press.

Yesavage, J.A., & Brink, T.L. (1983). Development and validation of a geriatric depression screening scale: A preliminary report. *Journal of Psychiatric Research, 17,* 37–49.

Zubenko, G.S., & Sunderland, T. (2000). Geriatric psychopharmacology: Why does age matter? *Harvard Review of Psychiatry, 7,* 311–333.

CHAPTER 50

The Patient Requiring Rehabilitation

TERRY RABINOWITZ AND THEODORE A. STERN

I. Introduction

A. Although state-of-the-art health care is a reality for many in the United States, there is often pressure placed upon acute care facilities to discharge patients as quickly as possible. Many clinicians bemoan the fact that their patients are being discharged from the hospital "quicker and sicker" as lengths of stay plummet. At times, this leads to conditions that are unfavorable for independent living. **The need for appropriate aftercare following hospitalization for an acute illness is increasing and rehabilitative care for both inpatients and outpatients is becoming a common component of comprehensive care.**

B. **The patient with a chronic illness or disease is at greater risk for developing a psychiatric problem.**

    1. Rates for depression in amputees are reported to range from 35–58%; for those with stroke it is 25–30%; and for those with cancer, it is 6–25%.

    2. When compared to the general population, suicide is 15 to 20 times more common in cancer patients, as much as 15 times higher in those with spinal cord injuries, and 2 to 6 times greater in those with stroke.

C. **It is crucial to understand, to diagnose, to treat, or to refer for treatment, those patients who have, or who develop psychiatric problems during their rehabilitation.** Failure to do so will lead to longer and more costly treatment, increased morbidity, and poorer outcomes.

II. Range of Potential Problems That May be Experienced During Rehabilitation

A. Patients receive rehabilitative care in a rehabilitation hospital or as outpatients. In either case, this phase of treatment may continue for months or years and it may disrupt many areas of a patient's life. Patients may be exposed to scores of unfamiliar clinicians, and new or painful procedures. Moreover, they may be processing and accepting their losses with varying degrees of success. During this period, a myriad of psychiatric problems may challenge the diagnostic skills of care providers. Any organ system may be dysfunctional and require rehabilitative treatment. When rehabilitation is successful, a safe, productive, and meaningful life can be anticipated.

B. Expect to often encounter the "Eight Ds" (i.e., clinical manifestations of psychiatric problems in patients undergoing rehabilitation).

    1. **D**epression may develop in response to the loss of a limb and to the feeling that one is no longer productive, attractive, or desirable.

    2. **D**isruptive behaviors may impede successful rehabilitation, e.g., as occurs when a child is separated from his or her parents.

    3. **D**espondency in a terminally ill patient may lead to a loss of hope and to unnecessary suffering.

4. **Delirium** or acute confusion may be a complication of a variety of conditions, e.g., drug toxicity, head trauma, or metabolic disturbance.

5. **Dementia** may interfere with a patient's understanding of recommended exercises or recollection of medication schedules.

6. **Delusions** (or other psychotic symptoms) may be a consequence of head trauma or may have been present in someone with a pre-existing psychiatric disorder.

7. **Discomfort** (AKA: pain), one of the most common symptoms in hospitalized or ambulatory patients, is often inadequately treated; left untreated it typically leads to distress, that often complicates co-morbid psychiatric conditions.

8. **Disquiet** (i.e., anxiety) may make it virtually impossible for a patient to follow instructions, to cooperate with treatment, or to sleep.

C. In addition to the adjustments that a patient must make to his or her illness, incapacity, or disability, there are significant external changes that will be encountered.

1. **The patient may feel displaced, alone, abandoned, and forgotten when rehabilitation takes place far from his or her home.**

2. **Disturbances in school or work attendance, marriage, and parent-child relationships** caused by lengthy hospitalizations or treatments may cause patients to feel that they are a financial, emotional, or other burden to loved ones.

3. **A "state" of incapacity,** where the patient becomes accustomed to being disabled, may be a consequence of prolonged illness and treatment.
   a. This can progress to permanent disability.
   b. These behaviors may be unintentionally reinforced by others or by conscious or unconscious wishes of the patient to remain in the sick or disabled state.

4. **Travel to assorted outpatient appointments may be stressful,** may be financially challenging, may be difficult or impossible because of lack of appropriate transport vehicles, and may be so time-consuming or tiring that pleasurable activities will have to be sacrificed.

5. **Adaptation** to the styles, behaviors, sex, age, and unfamiliarity of multiple treaters during the rehabilitation phase can be problematic. See Table 50-1.

6. **Impaired communication** due to illness or disability can interfere with meaningful interactions with family, friends, and care providers.
   a. **Frustration** often ensues, e.g., in a patient with an expressive aphasia who appreciates their own communication difficulties.

Table 50-1. Some Potential Differences or Similarities Between Clinician and Patient that May Affect Data Collection and Clinical Care

Gender	Appearance
Race	Financial state
Sexual orientation	Health
Age	Personality
(Dis)ability	Profession
Education	Other . . .

D. The pre-existing mental state will have a profound effect on patient treatment and on prognosis.

  1. **Depression** in an alcoholic who, while intoxicated, crashes his car into and kills a pedestrian may lead to a belief that he is unworthy of medical treatment or of living.

  2. **Paranoid schizophrenia,** with auditory command hallucinations and poor medication compliance; may lead someone so affected to attempt suicide (by jumping out of a window, sustaining multiple fractures and head trauma). Later, suspicions and the belief that staff is trying to poison him may interfere with the patient's appropriate assessment and administration of psychotropics and narcotics.

  3. **Antisocial personality disorder** in an armed robber who shot a police officer and who in turn was shot and paralyzed; may lead to belligerence and refusal to participate in physical or occupational therapy. The patient may challenge you to discharge him in his current condition saying, "Then I will die and it will be on your conscience." Though it may be tempting to let him die, the challenge is to provide him with the best possible care.

III. Evaluation

A. Past behavior is a very reliable predictor of future behavior. Thus, it is imperative to derive as much data as possible about an individual's psychiatric history. Consider the biological (i.e., medical), psychological, and social functioning (i.e., the biopsychosocial health) of each patient when you ask the questions presented in Table 50-2.

Table 50-2. Essential Psychiatric Questions to be Answered by all Rehabilitation Patients

Have they ever been under the care of a psychiatrist or received psychiatric treatment?

Do they take any drugs for psychiatric problems?

Have they ever been suicidal or made a suicidal gesture or attempt?

Have they ever been violent in or out of hospital?

Have they ever received in- or outpatient treatment for alcohol or drug abuse or dependence?

     Is there any history of withdrawal symptoms or complications?

Are they now, or have they in the past, ever been in trouble with the law?

Have they ever received in- or outpatient rehabilitative treatment?

     How did it go?

     Were they cooperative, disruptive, or threatening?

Is there any history of delirium?

What is the level of the patient's intellectual functioning?

     Has it changed as a result of whatever occurred to necessitate this hospitalization?

What are the patient's social supports?

     Are they reliable?

     How have they performed in the past?

B. The basic structure of **the psychiatric clinical interview should not vary much from the format of a typical medical evaluation.** The questions from Table 50-2 can be incorporated into the interview, keeping in mind that the answers to these questions will help to shape the treatment plan. Thus, if the interview needs to be shortened for any reason, the most important questions should be answered first!

1. **The interview should begin with the chief complaint and should progress through the standard items** keeping in mind that the evaluation may require specific alterations depending upon the patient and the rehabilitation setting.

2. **Maintenance of patient confidentiality, dignity, and sensitivity may require use of a private place,** but this may not always be possible in the hospital.

3. **Interviews may need to be brief, performed at optimal times of the day** (e.g., because of fatigue, need to fit between essential studies/treatments), **and be conducted with the help of family members or hospital staff.**

4. **Communication problems,** due to head injury, metabolic disturbances, or speech, and hearing problems, may interfere with understanding or cooperation.

5. **Assumptions** will have to be made in some situations.

C. Once the general interview is completed, **specific questions pertinent to the rehabilitation setting must be answered;** these are presented in Table 50-3.

D. **Patients may withhold important information** or be so disabled, apathetic, or anergic that they cannot communicate effectively. In such cases, it is appropriate to glean essential information in non-traditional ways.

1. **Surreptitious observation** of the patient can help to confirm or to refute the inability to speak, to hear, or to move an extremity, or if there is less suffering than asserted. Compare your own observations with those of other staff members.

2. **Limbic probes** that bypass the modulatory effects of higher cortical centers may be particularly useful.
   a. A non-offensive joke or story, or an unexpected silly gesture may induce a broad smile in an otherwise stone-faced individual who complains of depression.
   b. In the patient who appears angry or indifferent following a catastrophic event, and who refuses to speak, a question like, "Do you feel like crying?" may produce copious tears confirming your suspicion that your patient is quite depressed despite their stoic countenance.

3. **Facilitating language** may be useful.
   a. Ask if they feel depressed, suicidal, despondent, hopeless, useless, or worthless. These words will not cause a problem that did not already exist and they will help to free the patient to express what is on his or her mind.

Table 50-3. Psychiatric Questions for a Rehabilitation Patient

What is the meaning of the injury or illness to the patient?

How does their situation or condition affect their self-image?

What does the patient think the effect of their state has on family or friends?

How do they feel about their change or loss of function (e.g., in work, sexual relations, academic endeavors, athletic pursuits)?

E. It is often helpful to assume that each patient existed in an equilibrium state with respect to their biopsychosocial function before their need for rehabilitation.

1. The diagram in Figure 50-1a illustrates the relative pre-morbid contributions of a patient's biological, psychological, and social strengths that contributed to this equilibrium. For any patient, the contribution of each of the three principle components should be estimated after all data collected has been synthesized.

2. Figure 50-1b shows how these values might change in response to the stress of an illness.

   a. Note how the circles representing the values for all three components have decreased in size.

   b. The circles have not all reduced uniformly showing that, in this particular patient, the biological "reserves" were less affected than were the social or psychological ones.

   c. Every patient will start off with a unique collection of relative strengths that will change in response to a specific stressor. Changes may be predicted from past responses but remember that other hidden factors may be operating that can influence these changes.

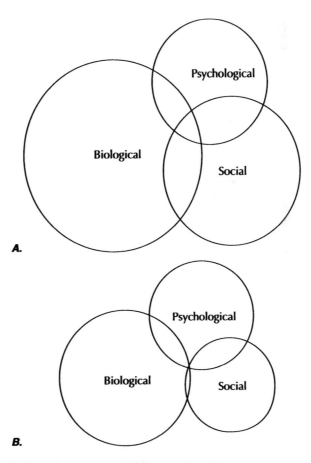

Figure 50-1. *A.* The relative premorbid strengths of the three principle components of a particular patient's biopsychosocial support system. Strength is proportional to circle size. *B.* A possible change that could occur in the relative strengths of a patient's biopsychosocial support system in response to a stressor. Strength is proportional to circle size.

IV. Treatment

A. The goal of psychiatric treatment in the rehabilitation setting is the same as that in any clinical milieu: **the restoration of optimum function.**

B. Treatments can be divided into two major categories: psychological and pharmacological; one or both types of treatment may be indicated in a patient based upon clinical findings.

C. Psychological treatment may have little relationship to what is generally understood to be outpatient psychotherapy. The purpose here is to help the patient get through an arduous period of their life as efficiently and with as little trauma as possible. It is not the time for deep exploration of the unconscious.

    1. The patient may be too weak or disabled to tolerate long or frequent sessions. This is a very clear instance where **"quality is better than quantity,"** and if the clinician effectively conveys to the patient that they are listening, that they care, and that they will try to help, the length of the therapeutic session will have less importance than will the intervention itself.

    2. **Sessions should be focused around the chief complaint.**

        a. Background information should be obtained only insofar as it is relevant to the current situation.

        b. As is done when obtaining the history, facilitating words and statements such as, "You look sad. How do you feel?" will be helpful.

    3. Consultation with the family will be more the rule than the exception. Permission to consult with others should *always* be obtained from the patient unless a life-threatening situation arises or the patient is incompetent.

D. Pharmacological treatment may be provided to a greater percentage of rehabilitation patients than it is to psychiatric patients in general.

    1. This may be due in part to the higher prevalence of some psychiatric disorders (e.g., depression or anxiety) accompanying prolonged hospitalizations, mood-altering side effects of essential non-psychotropic medication(s), or delirium, which may be due to multiple causes.

    2. **Keep the treatment streamlined.** This will help to avoid polypharmacy and its complications.

        a. Consider if multiple conditions (e.g., depression, anxiety, and agitation) can be treated with *one* medication.

        b. Consider if taking away one or more drugs may be as or more effective than adding others.

    3. Remember that **dosage adjustments may have to be made;** e.g., for patients on dialysis, with hepatic disease, with alterations in consciousness, and in the aged.

    4. Always consider the effects of the patient's disease and medications on **pharmacodynamics and pharmacokinetics.**

    5. If the response to a medication is sub-optimal, check serum levels of the drug *and* re-check your diagnosis.

    6. Always **consider drug interactions.**

    7. Remember that a depressed patient may not have the "luxury" of 3 to 4 weeks to respond to a typical antidepressant. **Consider if psychostimulants can be started** and then followed by standard antidepressant therapy.

    8. Electroconvulsive therapy (ECT) may be particularly useful for some of these patients.

    9. See Table 50-4.

Table 50-4. Psychotropic Drugs That May be Especially Useful in Rehabilitation Patients.[a]

Class	Drug	Features
Neuroleptic	Haloperidol	Excellent control of agitation and fear; generally little or no effect on cardiovascular or respiratory system; no dosage adjustments required in dialysis patients; may be given PO, IM, or IV.
Atypical neuroleptics	Aripiprazole, olanzapine, quetiapine, risperidone, ziprasidone	Reported to produce fewer or less severe extrapyramidal side effects (e.g., stiffness, bradykinesia, and parkinsonism) than typical neuroleptics, such as haloperidol. They are only available at present as PO medications (exception is ziprasidone, now available IM).
Benzodiazepines/anxiolytics	Lorazepam, oxazepam, and temazepam	Good anxiety control; no active metabolites; may be useful for short-term management of sleep disturbances.
Sympathomimetics/psychostimulants	Dextroamphetamine and methylphenidate	Potential rapid reversal of some depressive symptoms; short half-life. May be given PO, PR.
Selective serotonin reuptake inhibitors (SSRIs)/antidepressants	Citalopram, fluoxetine, fluvoxamine, paroxetine, and sertraline	As effective as heterocyclic antidepressants, but much safer; fewer fewer anticholinergic and cardiovascular effects than heterocyclics. Much safer than heterocyclics in overdose.
Other antidepressants	Bupropion, mirtazapine, nefazodone, and venlafaxine	See above for SSRIs

[a]This table is only a general guide; consider each patient individually and always know all drugs they are receiving and be aware of all potential drug interactions.

V. Conclusions

A. In general, patients receiving inpatient rehabilitative treatment will have psychiatric problems similar to those of other hospitalized patients.

B. Expect to encounter the "8 Ds" as described above.

C. The primary care physician can manage many psychiatric problems in rehabilitation patients without psychiatric consultation, but should consider consultation when:

1. There is a history of psychiatric disorder
2. The patient is receiving multiple (i.e., three or more) psychotropic medications
3. Before you get into trouble—if you think that you should probably consult a psychiatrist. . . YOU SHOULD!

Suggested References

Cassem, N.H., Stern, T.A., Rosenbaum, J.F., & Jellinek, M.S. (Eds.). (1997). *Massachusetts General Hospital handbook of general hospital psychiatry* (4th ed.). Boston: Mosby.

Rabinowitz, T. (2002). Delirium: An important (but often unrecognized) clinical syndrome. *Current Psychiatry Reports, 4,* 202–208.

Rundell, J.R., & Wise, M.G. (Eds.). (2002). *Textbook of consultation—liaison psychiatry* (2nd ed.). Washington, DC: American Psychiatric Press, Inc.

Sadock, B.J., & Sadock, V.A. (Eds.). (1999). *Comprehensive textbook of psychiatry* (7th ed.). Baltimore: Williams and Wilkins.

CHAPTER 51
The Patient Receiving Palliative Care

JOHN L. SHUSTER, GORMAN R. JONES III, AND THEODORE A. STERN

I. Introduction

Providing appropriate care at the end of a patient's life requires a qualitative shift in approach from the care usually provided in the primary care setting. There is much a physician can continue to do in the context of a palliative approach to care. **Care for a patient with a terminal illness should focus on maximizing the quality of life and minimizing suffering.** Provision of excellent symptom control, maintenance or repair of family and other interpersonal relationships, maintenance of the day-to-day activities necessary for sustaining a comforting home environment, attendance to spiritual and existential concerns, and the reaching of important life goals (or coming to terms with not reaching them) are important aspects of hospice and palliative care. A discussion of the issues related to palliative care requires a clear understanding of often imprecise terminology. A list of definitions of the terms used in this chapter is provided below.

A. **Quality of life is a subjective assessment of the degree to which needs perceived by the patient as essential are met.** Essential needs (physical, psychological, social, and spiritual) are unique to each patient. A patient's assessment of quality of life is largely dependent on the values which have the greatest meaning to that individual. While distress from physical symptoms has a powerful and obvious effect on quality of life, the elements of quality-of-life assessment are not limited to factors related to physical health or well-being. For example, healthy and supportive interpersonal relationships and deeply held spiritual beliefs may allow some patients to experience an excellent overall quality of life despite serious and persistent physical symptoms. By this definition, quality of life is difficult to measure with standardized instruments that are widely accepted as measures of this factor.

B. **Suffering is the distress caused when the needs perceived by the patient as essential to the quality of life are not met.**

C. **Terminal illness is the state of disease at which cure or survival is no longer a reasonable expectation.** Given the physician's duty to do no harm, continued aggressive treatment generally is neither clinically nor ethically appropriate for the terminally ill, since the potential benefits do not outweigh the potential risks and side effects. For purposes of eligibility for hospice admission, terminal illness generally is defined as expected survival below 6 months.

D. **Palliative care is treatment aimed primarily at reducing suffering and maximizing the quality of life.** Palliative care is usually, but not exclusively, provided to terminally ill patients. In the setting of terminal illness, palliation is usually the primary or only goal of treatment.

E. **Hospice is a multi-disciplinary approach which provides comprehensive palliative care to patients with terminal illnesses (expected survival of 6 months or less).** Hospice care differs from primary care in several ways.

 1. **A multi-disciplinary team approach is essential to hospice care.** The team includes physicians, nurses, social workers, chaplains, volunteers, and others involved in routine patient care.

 2. **The focus of care is shifted from cure or survival to quality of life.**

 3. **Much of the care (ideally, all the care) delivered by a hospice team is provided in the patient's home.** Hospice care can, however, be delivered in settings, such as general hospitals, nursing homes, and specialized hospice or palliative medicine units, when necessary.

 4. **Care is also provided for the family.** Assistance with psychosocial problems, help with the work of day-to-day home care of a dying patient, and follow-up care (including bereavement services) after the death of the patient are among the services typically offered.

F. **Supportive care is a treatment approach in which principles of palliative care are applied to the benefit of patients who may still be undergoing active treatment of disease.** Supportive care often is provided by a palliative medicine specialist in collaboration with the primary treating physician (e.g., the cancer pain clinic model).

II. Practical Problems in Entering Patients into Palliative Care

Most physicians understand and endorse hospice and palliative care as concepts, but there is ample evidence that American physicians' practice patterns do not approach the ideal for dying patients. **Ideally, patient and physician should have an ongoing dialogue which begins well in advance of the onset of terminal illness, resulting in a mutual understanding of the patient's preferences in regard to end-of-life care.** All too often, however, physicians provide aggressive care in the face of medical futility, leave patients' suffering undertreated, or simply proceed with a plan of treatment without awareness or acknowledgment of the patient's wishes concerning end-of-life care. **Certainly, reaching an agreement with a patient that the time has come to shift the focus of treatment to palliative care is one of the most challenging and delicate situations a physician can face.** However, these decisions represent one of the most important events in a patient's life and relationship with his or her physician. This part of the patient's care is too important to avoid, ignore, or leave to chance. A number of common obstacles to making appropriate referrals for hospice and palliative care can be anticipated and overcome.

A. **Awareness and utilization of palliative care resources.** The limited coverage of end-of-life issues in most medical school curricula and the generally poor integration of hospice services into the health care system leaves most physicians with a limited understanding of hospice and palliative care. Many physicians have misconceptions about the safety, efficacy, and addiction potential of effective and appropriate palliative treatments. However, most of the principles of palliative care are straightforward, and most palliative care and hospice services are enthusiastic about providing information and assistance to physicians and potential patients.

B. **Difficulty determining appropriateness for hospice and palliative care.** A practical difficulty in referring patients for palliative care consists of determining when such a referral is appropriate. Even in patients with cancer, estimation of survival is challenging and imprecise. Further complicating this problem, good palliative care tends to stabilize a terminally ill patient's clinical condition, altering prognostic estimates. The National Hospice Organization has published guidelines for estimating the prognosis in patients with non-malignant diseases. These guidelines provide a rational initial approach to estimating the prognosis in a patient with a terminal illness.

C. **Informing the patient and family of the need for, and appropriateness of, palliative care.** This is one of the most difficult clinical skills for a physician to master. Success in this interaction with a terminally ill patient requires skill in breaking bad news, the ability to dispel myths about hospice care, and the ability to educate family members about the dying process.

1. **Breaking bad news** is a skill that can be developed. Determining which family members the patient would like to have present and providing a private and comfortable physical setting help ensure a successful discussion of a patient's terminal prognosis. Start by determining what the patient already knows and understands about his or her condition and then provide accurate, jargon-free information to confirm what the patient understands correctly and fill gaps in his or her understanding. The amount and detail of information provided in the initial meeting should be consonant with the patient's response to general information. Empathetic silence from a caring physician is often more helpful than additional information when the patient feels overwhelmed by the impact of such bad news. Small increments of information provided over several sessions may be tolerated and remembered best.

2. **Dispelling myths about hospice and palliative care.** Many patients erroneously feel that a hospice referral means that the physician is giving up. Indeed, a shift to a palliative focus of treatment generally means that a decision has been made to give up on aggressive treatment aimed at a cure, but patients should be helped to understand that this does not mean that the physician is giving up on them. Many patients have unrealistic concerns about the addictive potential of narcotics, antidepressants, and anxiolytics. Additionally, most patients are not aware of the services offered by hospices. A discussion of the care and support available from a hospice can help soften the blow of first hearing about a terminal prognosis.

3. **Educate caregivers about the dying process.** Some aspects of the dying process may create significant emotional distress in terminally ill patients and their families, especially in the last days and hours of a patient's life. Education may be very helpful to caregivers. Some of the common problem areas include the following:

   a. **Loss of appetite and thirst.** These are normal parts of dying. Patients need not be forced to eat or drink but should be allowed to have food and drink *ad lib* for comfort.

   b. **Respiratory alterations.** Caregivers often are distressed after observing respiratory changes, such as Cheyne-Stokes respiration and agonal respirations. Caregivers should be reassured that unconscious patients with these breathing patterns are not suffering. Alert patients with dyspnea may get dramatic relief from narcotics.

   c. **"Death rattle"** is commonly seen in the last hours of life as a moribund patient fails to clear respiratory secretions.

D. **Collaboration with the hospice team.** Out of habit, preference, or necessity, many primary care physicians (PCPs) perform a wide variety of medical services and procedures without assistance. This part of the culture of primary care is highly valued by patients and is one of the chief appeals of a career in primary care practice but may make the shift to collaboration with a multi-disciplinary team of providers difficult. Clear communication and negotiation regarding roles and expectations (e.g., how much assistance the PCP wants or needs from the hospice physician, how the PCP can be contacted most efficiently when the hospice nurse needs to discuss a patient problem) allow the PCP to continue to guide and coordinate care with the assistance of the team, maintaining appropriate continuity of care to patients at the end of life.

III. A General Approach to Palliative Care

A. **Ask about suffering** in a general way before focusing on individual symptoms or symptom clusters. The experience of suffering is unique to each individual. An approach to palliative treatment that is based on preconceived assumptions about suffering may cause the physician to miss the opportunity to address the causes of suffering which are important to the patient. Beginning with an open-ended question, such as "What causes you to suffer the most?" can help keep the assessment and intervention focused on the patient's needs. While this approach to the discussion of suffering may require more time initially, it helps establish a helpful and effective treatment plan which ultimately will save time. Additionally, such empathic questioning is often helpful in relieving suffering.

B. **Tolerate the patient's preferences.** Asking about suffering is not enough. Effective palliative care requires one to adapt planned treatments and even the overall focus of treatment to the patient's answers to questions about suffering. This requires flexibility in treatment planning and the capacity to tolerate patient decisions that differ from medical recommendations.

C. **Be knowledgeable about the physical symptoms.** Although a full discussion of the physical symptoms which contribute to suffering in the setting of terminal illness is beyond the scope of this chapter, vigilance for the presence or emergence of symptoms, such as pain, nausea and vomiting, weakness, anorexia, and dyspnea, is a key component of palliative medicine. Persistent physical symptoms may contribute greatly to the emergence and persistence of psychological symptoms. For example, depressive symptoms are very difficult to relieve in the presence of undertreated pain.

D. **Screen for mental disorders and psychological symptoms** (especially depression, anxiety, and delirium) which are common complications of terminal illness. Screening for these common complications should be part of the routine assessment of patients entering palliative care.

E. **Appreciate that interpersonal (family) and role functioning has a powerful impact** on the quality of life in patients with a terminal illness. Dying patients commonly fear abandonment by caregivers, including family members and health care providers. This fear, combined with their dependence on those people for care, often leads to conflicted interactions even in the healthiest families. These pressures can cause major problems in families with a history of conflicted relationships. Similarly, changes in a patient's ability to function in a variety of roles (e.g., spouse, parent, sexual partner, employee, and caregiver) may cause suffering, depending on the value of those roles to the patient. Often the patients who are the most capable and successful in life suffer the most from these changes in role functioning. This apparent paradox may best be understood by assessing the degree of change from the patient's functional baseline (and the implicit loss of control associated with these changes) compared with others who may cope more effectively as a result of greater familiarity with suffering.

F. Deal with the patient's spiritual and existential concerns. The experience of dying stirs strong feelings in most terminally ill patients and their families. Many are troubled by lingering regrets, broken relationships, and unmet goals. Many are concerned about the nature or possibility of continued existence after death. Concerns about the future condition of the things which hold great personal meaning for the patient, such as the well-being of the family after death occurs and the continuation of an important life project, such as a family business, are also common. Recognizing their importance, hospice programs have integrated care for these common causes of suffering into the services they provide. PCPs can do much to relieve the suffering caused by spiritual and existential concerns by asking about them and by demonstrating an understanding of their importance. The hospice staff can be consulted regarding problems in these areas. Attending to these sources of suffering in a dying patient can be one of the most rewarding aspects of providing cam for the dying.

IV. Neuropsychiatric Complications of Terminal Illness

A. General issues. In deciding on the appropriate treatment for the neuropsychiatric complications of terminal illness, it is important to bear general guidelines in mind. Since relief of suffering as perceived and reported by the patient is a primary goal of palliative care, the principles which guide good general psychiatric diagnosis and treatment should be applied with flexibility. For example, **symptoms in a terminally ill patient which are subthreshold for a formal diagnosis of a mental disorder (such as depression) but cause substantial suffering should be treated aggressively.** Similarly, mental disorders are most appropriately left untreated in the setting of terminal illness when they do not cause substantial suffering or when the treatment might place the patient at risk for more suffering (e.g., quiet delirium in the terminal stages of disease).

1. **The neuropsychiatric complications of terminal illness are commonly unrecognized and undertreated.** Recognition may be hindered by the clinician's limited experience in diagnosing mental disorders in the setting of serious physical illness, difficulty interpreting clinical information in the setting of unremarkable pre-morbid psychiatric histories, and concerns about stigmatization if a diagnosis of a mental disorder is made. Many clinicians underestimate the prevalence and severity of these disorders at the end of life.

2. Additionally, **a mistaken understanding of problems, such as depression and anxiety, as a universal and even appropriate part of the experience of dying contributes to undertreatment.** Worry, fearfulness, discouragement, and sadness are seen in many (and possibly all) patients with terminal illness, at least transiently. These symptoms may flare up at times of predictable distress (e.g., diagnosis, notification of disease progression, family conflict). However, if such symptoms are manifestations of a mental disorder or otherwise cause persistent and substantial suffering, they should be treated. Like pain and other physical symptoms in a dying patient, mental disorders should be recognized as the complications they are and be treated aggressively to relieve suffering and maximize the quality of life. There is no reason for pessimism about the treatment of mental disorders at the end of life. With careful administration, treatments for the mental disorders which commonly complicate terminal illness are safe, well tolerated, and effective.

B. Depression (see Chapter 14)

1. **Depression rates** are positively correlated with the presence and severity of serious physical illness. Estimates vary, but as many as 77% of patients with a terminal illness may suffer from clinically significant depression.

2. **Evaluation** of depression in terminal illness
   a. The high prevalence of depression in terminal illness, the burden of suffering caused by depression, and the effectiveness of available treatments should lead the clinician to screen for depression in all terminally ill patients.
   b. A history of similar depressive symptoms should be elicited, particularly in regard to previously effective treatments.
   c. The diagnosis is made by using unmodified *DSM-1V* criteria, which include some symptoms which also can be caused by serious physical illness. Diagnostic confidence is increased if some of the psychological features of depression are prominent, such as anhedonia, guilty feelings, hopelessness, morbid ruminations, self-loathing, suicidal ideation, and easy tearfulness.
   d. An interview with the patient should balance data gathering with support and reassurance. Many patients find the topic of depression difficult to approach initially but are comforted to hear that there are treatments which offer effective relief from their suffering. A skillfully administered interview can be therapeutic.
   e. Examination of the patient should elicit the diagnostic criteria for a major depressive episode. Even though treatment may be initiated in the absence of a full major depressive episode, these symptoms provide a reliable means of monitoring the treatment response.
3. **The differential diagnosis** is listed in Table 51-1. Many of these items can mimic or exacerbate depression in terminally ill patients.
4. **Treatment strategies** include the provision of emotional support, concurrent aggressive treatment of other problems (e.g., pain and nausea) which can exacerbate depression, and individual or family psychotherapy in selected cases. Effective treatment for depression in the setting of terminal illness generally requires the use of antidepressant drugs (Table 51-2).

Table 51-1. Differential Diagnosis of Depression in Terminal Illness

Mood disorders (major depression, dysthymia, bipolar disorder)

Anger

Anxiety

Coping and personality style (avoidant, schizoid)

Delirium ("quiet" type)

Dementia

Emotional "numbing" (adjustment disorder)

Interpersonal problems

Narcissistic injury

Side effects of treatment

Spiritual and existential concerns

Strong feelings of loss of control or autonomy

Undertreated nausea and/or vomiting

Undertreated pain

Other undertreated physical complications

Table 51-2. Pharmacologic Treatments for Depression in Terminal Illness

Generic Name	Approximate Daily Dose Range, mg	Route	Comments
Psychostimulants			
Dextroamphetamine	2.5–20 daily	PO	Rapid onset of action and clearance if side effects emerge.
Methylphenidate	2.5–20 b.i.d.	PO	
Pemoline	37.5–75 b.i.d.	PO, SL	Pemoline comes in a chewable form which can be absorbed without swallowing. Tolerance may develop, requiring a dose increase. May precipitate agitation or delirium in susceptible patients. May be drugs of choice in terminal illness.
Serotonin reuptake inhibitors			
Citalopram	10–60 daily	PO	Mild headache, jitteriness, and GI upset are the most common adverse effects. May cause serotonin syndrome in combination with other serotonergic agents. May slow metabolism of other drugs cleared through the cytochrome P450 system.
Escitalopram	10–40 daily	PO	
Fluoxetine	20–80 daily	PO	
Fluvoxamine	50–300 daily	PO	
Paroxetine	10–60 daily	PO	
Sertraline	50–200 daily	PO	
Tricyclic antidepressants			
Amitriptyline	10–150 daily	PO, IM, PR	Anticholinergic effects, sedation, orthostasis, and dry mouth are troublesome side effects. Can worsen constipation caused by opiates. Can help treat pain, especially neuropathic pain. May stimulate appetite.
Clomipramine	10–150 daily	PO	
Desipramine	12.5–150 daily	PO, IM	
Doxepin	12.5–150 daily	PO, IM	
Imipramine	12.5–150 daily	PO, IM	
Nortriptyline	10–125 daily	PO	
Other medications			
Bupropion	75–450 daily	PO	A stimulating agent with a risk of seizures; t.i.d. dosing.
Mirtazapine	15–45 daily	PO	Sedating, promotes appetite.
Nefazodone	200–600 daily	PO	Risk of liver failure: b.i.d. dosing.
Trazodone	25–600 daily	PO	Sedating, can induce orthostasis; has some anticholinergic properties; risk of priapism.
Venlafaxine	75–375 daily	PO	New agent: b.i.d.–t.i.d. dosing.

NOTE: PO, per os; SL, sublingual; IM, intramuscular; PR, per rectum; b.i.d., twice a day; t.i.d., three times a day.

SOURCE: Adapted from Breitbart, W., Levenson, J.A., & Passik, S.D. (1993). Terminally ill cancer patients. In W. Breitbart, & J.C. Holland (Eds.), *Psychiatric aspects of symptom management in cancer patients.* Washington, DC: American Psychiatric Press, pp. 173–230.

C. Anxiety (see Chapter 16)

1. Anxiety **rates** are also positively correlated with the presence and severity of serious physical illness. Especially in illnesses which compromise the ease and comfort of respiration, anxiety can be a significant source of additional suffering.

2. **Evaluation of anxiety** in terminal illness

   a. Like depression, the high prevalence of anxiety in a patient with a terminal illness, the burden of suffering caused by anxiety, and the effectiveness of available treatments should lead the clinician to screen all terminally ill patients for anxiety. Clinically significant anxiety usually is easy to detect.

   b. A history of similar anxiety symptoms should be elicited, particularly in regard to previously effective treatments. The symptoms of post-traumatic stress disorder may re-emerge after years of remission in a dying patient, and so a history of traumatic life events should be explored.

   c. An interview with the patient should balance data-gathering with support and reassurance. Attempts should be made to detect specific fears (e.g., fear of dying, and the fear of abandonment) as well as the symptoms of anxiety disorders. Like depressed patients, anxious patients usually are comforted when they hear that there are treatments which offer effective relief from their suffering. A skillfully administered interview can be therapeutic.

   d. Examination of the patient should attempt to elicit the diagnostic criteria for panic attacks, anxiety symptoms related to physical symptoms (e.g., dyspnea, pain, and nausea), and the criteria of the formal anxiety disorders.

3. **The differential diagnosis** is listed in Table 51-3. Many of these items can mimic or exacerbate anxiety disorders in terminally ill patients.

4. **Treatment strategies** include the provision of emotional support, concurrent aggressive treatment of other problems (e.g., nausea, dyspnea) which can exacerbate anxiety, and individual or family psychotherapy in selected cases. Effective treatment for anxiety in the setting of terminal illness generally requires the use of anxiolytic drugs (Table 51-4). Benzodiazepines may suppress the respiratory drive and lower blood

---

Table 51-3. Differential Diagnosis of Anxiety in Terminal Illness

Anxiety disorders (panic disorder, generalized anxiety disorder, post-traumatic stress disorder)

Coping and personality style (avoidant, dependent)

Delirium

Fear

Side effects (akathisia from antiemetics)

Spiritual and/or existential concerns

Undertreated pain

Other undertreated physical complications (dyspnea or sepsis)

Withdrawal states (opiates and sedatives)

Table 51-4. Anxiolytic Medications Commonly Used in Terminal Illness

Generic Name	Approximate Daily Dosage Range, mg	Route
Benzodiazepines		
Very short-acting		
Midazolam	10–60 per 24 hours	IV, SC
Short-acting		
Alprazolam	0.25–2.0 t.i.d.-q.i.d.	PO, SL
Lorazepam	0.5–2.0 t.i.d.-q.i.d.	PO, SL, IV, IM
Oxazepam	10–15 t.i.d.-q.i.d.	PO
Intermediate-acting		
Chlordiazepoxide	10–50 t.i.d.-q.i.d.	PO, IM
Long-acting		
Clonazepam	0.5–2 b.i.d.-q.i.d.	PO
Clorazepate	7.5–15 b.i.d.-q.i.d.	PO
Diazepam	5–10 b.i.d.-q.i.d.	PO, IV, PR
Non-benzodiazepines		
Buspirone	5–20 t.i.d.	PO
Neuroleptics		
Chlorpromazine	12.5–50 q 4–12 hours	PO, IM, IV
Haloperidol	0.5–5 q 2–12 hours	SC, IV, PO, IM
Methotrimeprazine	10–20 q 4–8 hours	SC, PO, IM
Olanzapine	2.5–10 b.i.d.	PO
Quetiapine	12.5–50 q 4–12 hours	PO
Risperidone	0.5–4 q 8–12 hours	PO
Thioridazine	10–75 t.i.d.-q.i.d.	PO
Antihistamines		
Hydroxyzine	25–50 q 6 hours	PO, IV, SC

NOTE: PO, per os; IM, intramuscular; PR, per rectum; IV, intravenous; SC, subcutaneous; SL, sublingual; b.i.d., two times a day; t.i.d., three times a day; q.i.d., four times a day; q 4–8 hours, every 4 to 8 hours; hs, at bedtime. Parenteral doses are generally twice as potent as oral doses; intravenous bolus injections should be administered slowly.

SOURCE: Adapted from Breitbart, W., Levenson, J.A., & Passik, S.D. (1993). Terminally ill cancer patients. In W. Breitbart, & J.C. Holland (Eds.), *Psychiatric aspects of symptom management in cancer patients.* Washington, DC: American Psychiatric Press, pp. 173–230.

pressure, but caution with dosing and the use of shorter-acting agents minimize these risks. Concerns about these potential adverse effects should not interfere with the relief of suffering in a dying patient.

D. Confusion and delirium (see Chapter 23)

    1. Rates of delirium are correlated with the presence and severity of serious physical illness. Delirium has long been understood as a marker of serious systemic illness

affecting the central nervous system. As many as 95% of all patients may develop delirium near the end of life.

2. **Evaluation of delirium in terminal illness**

   a. Delirium, especially when accompanied by agitation, generally is easy to detect in the terminally ill. Since delirium impairs cognition and awareness, it often causes more apparent suffering in the family members than in the patient.

   b. A history of episodes of delirium should be elicited, particularly in regard to effective treatments and the duration and course of the recovery period. Withdrawal states should always be considered as possible causes of current or past episodes of delirium.

   c. An interview with the patient probably will be limited by the patient's cognitive impairment. Thus, the questions should be direct, simple, and focused. Informing the patient and family that these symptoms are a manifestation of the underlying physical illness, not the onset of a new set of problems (e.g., psychotic illness), can provide some comfort.

   d. Examination of the patient should focus on the neurocognitive status, including the use of a scale (such as the Mini-Mental State Examination) which can be administered serially to help monitor the response to treatment. Delirious patients exhibit impairments in higher cortical functioning as well as disturbances of consciousness and arousal. Evidence of cerebral dysfunction on neurologic examination (e.g., asterixis and myoclonus) is consistent with delirium.

3. **The spectrum of presentation** of delirium in terminal illness is listed in Table 51-5.

4. **Treatment strategies** generally focus on the pharmacologic management of symptoms (Table 51-6). A search for potentially reversible causes of the delirium may be conducted if the patient's overall condition and potentially salvageable quality of life warrant that. Laboratory investigation should be limited to minimally invasive studies which are likely to lead to specific interventions. Education and emotional support provided to patients and family members can help ease the suffering caused by delirium. Benzodiazepines appear to be most effective in terminal delirium when the goal of therapy is sedation of an agitated patient, rather than reverse of cognitive dysfunction. In a substantial minority of cases, heavy sedation (e.g., infusion of midazolam) may be required to control agitated delirium at the end of life.

Table 51-5. Spectrum of Presentation of Delirium in Terminal Illness

Quiet delirium

Agitated delirium

Terminal anguish

Terminal restlessness

Multifocal myoclonus

Generalized seizures

Coma

Table 51-6. Medications Commonly Used for Delirium in Patients with Terminal Illness

Generic Name	Approximate Daily Dosage Range, mg	Route
Neuroleptics		
Chlorpromazine	12.5–50 q 4–12 hours	PO, IV, IM
Haloperidol	0.5–5 q 2–12 hours	PO, IV, SC, IM
Olanzapine	2.5–5 q 4–12 hours	PO
Quetiapine	12.5–50 q 4–12 hours	PO
Risperidone	0.5–4 q 8–12 hours	PO
Thioridazine	10–75 q 4–8 hours	PO
Benzodiazepines		
Lorazepam	0.5–2.0 q 1–4 hours	PO, IV, IM
Midazolam	30–100 per 24 hours	IV, SC

NOTE: Parenteral doses are generally twice as potent as oral doses. IV, intravenous infusion or bolus injections should be administered slowly; IM, intramuscular injections should be avoided if repeated use becomes necessary; PO, oral forms of medication are preferred; SC, subcutaneous infusions are generally accepted modes of drug administration in the terminally ill.

SOURCE: Adapted from Breitbart, W., Levenson, J.A., & Passik, S.D. (1993). Terminally ill cancer patients. In W. Breitbart, & J.C. Holland (Eds.), *Psychiatric aspects of symptom management in cancer patients.* Washington, DC: American Psychiatric Press, pp. 173–230.

Suggested Readings

American Psychiatric Association. (1994). *Diagnostic and statistical manual of mental disorders* (4th ed.). Washington, DC: American Psychiatric Press.

Breitbart, W., Levenson, J.A., & Passik, S.D. (1993). Terminally ill cancer patients. In W. Breitbart, & J.C. Holland (Eds.), *Psychiatric aspects of symptom management in cancer patients.* Washington, DC: American Psychiatric Press, pp. 173–230.

Buckman, R. (1992). *How to break bad news: A guide for health care professionals.* Baltimore: Johns Hopkins University Press.

Cassell, E.J. (1991). *The nature of suffering and the goals of medicine.* New York: Oxford University Press.

Chochinov, H.M., Hack, T., Haggard, T., et al. (2002). Dignity in the terminally ill: A cross-sectional cohort study. *Lancet, 360*(9350), 2026–2030.

Doyle, D., Hands, G.W.C., & McDonald, N. (Eds.). (1993). *Oxford textbook of palliative medicine.* Oxford: Oxford University Press.

Folstein, M.F., Folstein, S.E., & McHugh, P.R. (1975). "Mini-Mental State": A practical method for grading the cognitive state of patients for the clinician. *Journal of Psychiatric Research, 12,* 189–198.

Hearn, J., & Higginson, I.J. (1998). Do specialist palliative care teams improve outcomes for cancer patients? A systematic literature review. *Palliative Medicine, 12*(5), 317–332.

Jaconsen, P.B., & Breitbart, W. (1996). Psychosocial aspects of palliative care. *Cancer Control, 3,* 214–222.

Lipowski, Z.J. (1990). *Delirium: Acute confusional states.* New York: Oxford University Press.

Lo, R.S., Woo, J., Zhoc, K.C., et al. (2002). Quality of life of palliative care patients in the last two weeks of life. *Journal of Pain & Symptom Management, 24*(4), 388–397.

Mitchell, G.K. (2002). How well do general practitioners deliver palliative care? A systematic review. *Palliative Medicine, 16*(6), 457–464.

National Hospice Organization Medical Guidelines Task Force. (1995). *Medical guidelines for determining prognosis in selected non-cancer diseases.* Arlington, VA: National Hospice Organization.

Reb, A.M. (2003). Palliative and end-of-life care: Policy analysis. *Oncology Nursing Forum, 30*(1), 35–50.

Rhymes, J.A. (1996). Barriers to palliative care. *Cancer Control, 3,* 230–235.

Rodin, G., Craven, J., & Littlefield, C. (1991). *Depression in the medically ill. An integrated approach.* New York: Mazel.

Shipman, C., Addington-Hall, J., Barclay, S., et al. (2001). Educational opportunities in palliative care: What do general practitioners want? *Palliative Medicine, 15*(3), 191–196.

Shipman, C., Addington-Hall, J., Barclay, S., et al. (2002). How and why do GPs use specialist palliative care services? *Palliative Medicine, 16*(3), 241–246.

Shuster, J.D., Stem, T.A., & Greenberg, D.B. (1992). Pros and cons of fluoxetine for the depressed cancer patient. *Oncology, 6,* 45–55.

Storey, P. (1994). *Primer of palliative care.* Gainesville, Fla.: Academy of Hospice Physicians.

The SUPPORT Study Principal Investigators. (1995). A controlled trial to improve care for seriously ill hospitalized patients. *Journal of the American Medical Association, 274,* 1591–1598.

CHAPTER 52
The Alcoholic Patient

JOHN A. RENNER, JR. AND MICHAEL F. BIERER

I. Introduction

A. **Alcohol abuse** spans the continuum from brief episodes of excessive drinking to chronic patterns that produce significant problems but never progress to psychological or physical dependence (Table 52-1).

B. **Alcohol dependence (alcoholism)** is defined as the excessive and recurrent use of alcohol despite medical, psychological, social, and/or economic problems. As classified in *DSM-IV* (Table 52-1), it usually includes tolerance and withdrawal symptoms, but these signs of physical dependence are not required for the diagnosis.

C. **Alcohol-related problems** affect more than 10% of drinkers and are the third leading cause of death in the United States. Alcoholism causes 80% of cases of hepatic cirrhosis, and patients injured under the influence of alcohol fill 50% of American trauma beds.

Table 52-1. DSM-IV Diagnostic Criteria

ALCOHOL ABUSE: One or more of the following present at any time during the same 12-month period.

1. Alcohol use results in failure to fulfill **major obligations.**
2. Recurrent use in **physically dangerous situations** (such as drunk driving).
3. Recurrent alcohol-related **legal problems.**
4. Continued use despite recurrent **social or interpersonal problems.**
5. Has never met criteria for Alcohol Dependence.

ALCOHOL DEPENDENCE: Three or more of the following present at any time during the same 12-month period.

1. Tolerance.
2. Withdrawal.
3. Use in larger amounts, or for longer periods, than intended.
4. Unsuccessful efforts to cut down or control use.
5. A great deal of time spent obtaining alcohol, using or recovering from alcohol use.
6. Important activities given up.
7. Continued use despite knowledge of problems.

SOURCE: Adapted from American Psychiatric Association. (1994). *DSM-IV* Criteria for Substance Abuse and Substance Dependence.

499

1. The primary care model provides an ideal approach for
   a. Early identification of problem drinking
   b. Building motivation to enter treatment
   c. Improved management for chronic patients
2. In 1994, the National Comorbidity Survey reported that the majority of U.S. patients with serious psychiatric disorders abused alcohol or other drugs. Individuals in this group accounted for more than half of all lifetime psychiatric disorders in the United States; they usually had a history of three or more disorders, one of which was a substance-abuse disorder.
   a. 37% of alcohol abusers have at least one other mental illness.
   b. 25–50% of suicides involve alcohol.
   c. 29% of mentally ill individuals abuse alcohol or other drugs.

D. **Effective treatment of drinking problems** requires more than familiarity with the medical aspects of alcoholism. Clinicians must also understand the following:
   1. The distinction between detoxification (the gradual elimination of alcohol from the body) and definitive treatment for alcohol dependence
   2. The stages of the recovery process and the way in which ambivalence impedes a patient's progress toward sobriety
   3. The types of psychiatric problems that commonly complicate the management of these patients

II. Evaluation of the Problem

A. **General recommendations.** Screening for alcohol-related problems should be routine for all patients who enter a primary care clinic (see section II.D below). Individuals with alcohol problems are at high risk for the abuse of other drugs and should be screened for other legal and illegal substances (see Chapters 53 and 60).

B. **Review of systems.** Any of the following medical problems heightens the probability of an alcohol use disorder:
   1. Gastrointestinal bleeding
   2. Pancreatitis
   3. Cirrhosis and hepatitis
   4. Cardiomyopathy
   5. Labile hypertension
   6. Electrolyte abnormalities
   7. Intracranial hemorrhage and/or a history of recurrent trauma
   8. Sleep disorders
   9. Peripheral neuropathy

C. **Psychiatric and Social Problems Associated with Alcoholism**
   1. **Mental disorders commonly co-morbid with alcohol abuse:** antisocial personality disorder, conduct disorder, mania, and schizophrenia
   2. **Mental disorders sometimes co-morbid with alcohol abuse:** major depressive disorder, anxiety disorders, attention deficit hyperactivity disorder, and post-traumatic stress disorder
   3. Erratic school or employment history
   4. Domestic violence
   5. Marital problems, especially multiple divorces

Table 52-2. The CAGE Questionnaire

"**C**"   Have you ever felt you should **Cut** down on your drinking?

"**A**"   Have people **Annoyed** you by criticizing your drinking?

"**G**"   Have you ever felt bad or **Guilty** about your drinking?

"**E**"   Have you ever had a drink first thing in the morning to steady your nerves or to get rid of a hangover (**Eye opener**)?

SCORING: Item responses on the CAGE are scored 0 or 1, with a higher score indicative of alcohol problems. A score of 2 or more is considered clinically significant.

SOURCE: Published in the *American Journal of Psychiatry*, 1974, the American Psychiatric Association.

D. **Alcoholism screening instruments.** In addition to questions regarding the quantity and frequency of drinking, several instruments are available for detecting less overt problems.
1. **CAGE** includes four simple questions that can be easily inserted into the medical interview (Table 52-2). Two or more positive responses correlate with significant alcohol-related problems. This is a quick and reliable screening tool even for patients who try to hide alcohol abuse and is a more reliable indicator than are elevated liver function tests.
2. The **Alcohol Use Disorders Identification Test (AUDIT)** is a 10-item questionnaire developed by the World Health Organization for the early detection of patients with alcohol problems in the primary care setting (Table 52-3).

Table 52-3. The Alcohol Use Disorders Identification Test (AUDIT)

Please circle the answer that is correct for you

1. How often do you have a drink containing alcohol?

Never	Monthly or less	Two to four times a month	Two to three times a week	Four or more times a week

2. How many drinks containing alcohol do you have on a typical day when you are drinking?

1 or 2	3 or 4	5 or 6	7 to 9	10 or more

3. How often do you have six or more drinks on one occasion?

Never	Less than monthly	Monthly	Weekly	Daily or almost daily

4. How often during the last year have you found that you were not able to stop drinking once you had started?

Never	Less than monthly	Monthly	Weekly	Daily or almost daily

5. How often during the last year have you failed to do what was normally expected from you because of drinking?

Never	Less than monthly	Monthly	Weekly	Daily or almost daily

(continued)

Table 52-3. *(Continued)*

6. How often during the last year have you needed a first drink in the morning to get yourself going after a heavy drinking session?

| Never | Less than monthly | Monthly | Weekly | Daily or almost daily |

7. How often during the last year have you had a feeling of guilt or remorse after drinking?

| Never | Less than monthly | Monthly | Weekly | Daily or almost daily |

8. How often during the last year have you been unable to remember what happened the night before because you had been drinking?

| Never | Less than monthly | Monthly | Weekly | Daily or almost daily |

9. Have you or someone else been injured as a result of your drinking?

| No | Yes, but not in the last year | Yes, during the last year |

10. Has a relative or friend or a doctor or other health worker been concerned about your drinking or suggested that you cut down?

| No | Yes, but not in the last year | Yes, during the last year |

Procedure for Scoring AUDIT Questions 1-8 are scored 0, 1, 2, 3, or 4; Questions 9 and 10 are scored 0, 2, or 4 only; the response coding is as follows:

	0	1	2	3	4
Question 1	Never	Monthly or less	Two to four times per month	Two to three times	Four or more times per week
Question 2	1 or 2	3 or 4	5 or 6	7 to 9	10 or more
Questions 3–8	Never	Less than monthly	Monthly	Weekly	Daily or almost daily
Questions 9–10	No		Yes, but not in the last year		Yes, during the last year

The minimum score (for non-drinkers) is 0, and the maximum possible score is 40. A score of 8 or more indicates a strong likelihood of hazardous or harmful alcohol consumption.

   3. **The Michigan Alcoholism Screening Test (MAST)** is a 25-question instrument that takes longer to administer but is a more accurate screening tool than CAGE, especially for women and the elderly (Table 52-4).

   E. **Interviewing the patient.** Suspected substance-abuse patients should be approached in a respectful and non-judgmental manner. A confrontational approach on the part of the clinician has been shown to decrease the rate of successful referral to alcohol

Table 52-4. Michigan Alcoholism Screening Test (MAST)

Clinical utility of instrument	To screen for alcoholism with a variety of populations
Research applicability	Useful in assessing extent of lifetime alcohol-related consequences
Copyright, cost, and source issues	No copyright
	Cost: $5 for copy, no fee for use
	Source:
	Melvin L. Selzer, M.D.
	6967 Paseo Laredo
	La Jolla, CA 92037

Points		YES	NO
( )	0. Do you enjoy a drink now and then?	___	___
(2)	1. Do you feel you are a normal drinker? (By normal we mean you drink less than or as much as most other people.	___	___
(2)	2. Have you ever awakened the morning after some drinking the night before and found that you could not remember a part of the evening?	___	___
(1)	3. Does your wife, husband, a parent, or another near relative ever worry or complain about your drinking?	___	___
(2)	4. Can you stop drinking without a struggle after one or two drinks?[a]	___	___
(1)	5. Do you ever feel guilty about your drinking?	___	___
(2)	6. Do friends or relatives think you are a normal drinker?[a]	___	___
(2)	7. Are you able to stop drinking when you want to?[a]	___	___
(5)	8. Have you ever attended a meeting of Alcoholics Anonymous (AA)?	___	___
(1)	9. Have you gotten into physical fights when drinking?	___	___
(2)	10. Has your drinking ever created problems between you and your wife, husband, parent, or other relative?	___	___
(2)	11. Has your wife, husband (or other family members) ever gone to anyone for help about your drinking?	___	___
(2)	12. Have you ever lost friends because of your drinking?	___	___
(2)	13. Have you ever gotten into trouble at work or school because of drinking?	___	___
(2)	14. Have you ever lost a job because of drinking?	___	___
(2)	15. Have you ever neglected your obligations, your family, or your work for 2 or more days in a row because you were drinking?	___	___

(continued)

Table 52-4. *(Continued)*

(1)	16. Do you drink before noon fairly often?	___	___
(2)	17. Have you ever been told you have liver trouble? Cirrhosis?	___	___
(2)	18. After heavy drinking have you ever had delirium tremens (DTs) or severe shaking, or heard voices or seen things that really weren't there?[b]	___	___
(5)	19. Have you ever gone to anyone for help about your drinking?	___	___
(5)	20. Have you ever been in a hospital because of drinking?	___	___
(2)	21. Have you ever been a patient in a psychiatric hospital or on a psychiatric ward of a general hospital where drinking was part of the problem that resulted in hospitalization?	___	___
(2)	22. Have you ever been seen at a psychiatric or mental health clinic or gone to any doctor, social worker, or clergyperson for help with any emotional problem where drinking was part of the problem?	___	___
(2)	23. Have you ever been arrested for drunk driving, driving while intoxicated, or driving under the influence of alcoholic beverages (IF YES, How many times?[c])	___	___
(2)	24. Have you ever been arrested, or taken into custody, even for a few hours, because of other drunk behavior? (IF YES, How many times?[c])	___	___

[a]Alcoholic response is negative.

[b]5 points for each Delirium Tremens

[c]2 points for each arrest.

SCORING SYSTEM: In general, five points or more would place the subject in an "alcoholic" category. Four points would be suggestive of alcoholism, and three points or less would indicate the subject was not alcoholic.

Programs using the above scoring system find it very sensitive at the five-point level, and it tends to find more people alcoholic than anticipated. However, it is a screening test and should be sensitive at its lower levels.

SOURCE: Selzer, M.L. (1975). The Michigan Alcoholism Screening Test: The quest for a new diagnostic instrument. *American Journal of Psychiatry, 127,* 1653–1658.

SUPPORTING REFERENCES

Hedlund, J.L., & Vieweg, B.W. (1984). The Michigan Alcoholism Screening Test (MAST): A comprehensive review. *Journal of Operational Psychiatry, 15,* 554.

Skinner, H.A. (1979). A multivariate evaluation of the MAST. *Journal of Studies on Alcohol, 40,* 831–844.

Skinner, H.A., & Sheu, W.J. (1982). Reliability of alcohol use indices: The Lifetime Drinking History and the MAST. *Journal of Studies on Alcohol, 43,* 1157–1170.

Zung, B.J. (1980). Factor structure of the Michigan Alcoholism Screening Test in a psychiatric outpatient population. *Journal of Clinical Psychology, 36,* 1024–1030.

Zung, B.J., & Charalampous, K.D. (1975). Item analysis of the Michigan Alcoholism Screening Test. *Journal of Studies on Alcohol, 36,* 127–132.

treatment. A moralistic approach is never helpful, is likely to alienate and demoralize patients, and may increase denial and diminish the motivation for treatment (see section IV.B below).

III. Differential Diagnosis

Many disorders may mimic alcoholism and complicate the diagnostic process.

A. Medical Problems
1. Mild alcohol intoxication is marked by disinhibition, and more severe intoxication is marked by delirium, ataxia, or even coma. The clinician needs to rule out life-threatening conditions, such as head injuries and neurologic and metabolic problems, such as hypoglycemia.
2. Alcohol use disorders may mimic insomnia and can cause any of the problems listed in section II.B above.

B. Psychiatric problems. The presence of a non-alcohol-induced psychiatric disorder is suggested by psychiatric symptoms that precede alcohol use, are greater than what would be expected given the amount and duration of drinking, and last longer than 4 weeks after detoxification. In practice, it can be difficult to distinguish primary from secondary psychiatric disorders.
1. **Dysthymia and major depressive disorder,** with or without suicidality, can be difficult to distinguish from the depression induced by chronic alcohol consumption. More than 60% of alcoholics are clinically depressed when admitted for detoxification, and many complain of dysthymia during the early months of sobriety. Any alcoholic or intoxicated individual who expresses suicidal ideation should be managed carefully as a serious suicide risk regardless of the presence or absence of major depressive disorder.
2. **Anxiety** is a common symptom during alcohol withdrawal but it usually clears within a few days. Some alcoholics also complain of generalized anxiety and/or panic attacks lasting up to 12 months after detoxification. These symptoms are difficult to distinguish from a co-morbid anxiety disorder and they require a full psychiatric evaluation.
3. **Schizophrenia** and other psychotic disorders may be confused with delirium tremens or alcoholic hallucinosis because of the presence of hallucinations.

IV. Treatment Strategies

While a brief office intervention may be sufficient for people with minor alcohol problems, referral to specialized treatment usually is required for individuals who are alcohol-dependent. As demonstrated in the NIAAA-funded Project Match, Cognitive-Behavioral Therapy, 12-step facilitation therapy, and motivation-enhancement therapy are almost equally effective in reducing the amount and frequency of drinking in patients willing to accept treatment. However, successful referral of some alcoholics can be a long-term process during which treatment interventions must be matched to the needs of the individual patient. Clinicians must understand the stages alcoholics usually pass through during the recovery process, the importance of using intervention skills, and the need to identify and treat co-morbid psychiatric conditions. The critical treatment question is: Which treatment for which patient at which time?

Table 52-5. The Stages of Behavioral Change

1. **Precontemplation**	Drinker is unaware that alcohol use is a problem, or has no interest in changing drinking pattern.
2. **Contemplation**	Drinker becomes aware of problems, but is still drinking and is usually ambivalent about stopping.
3. **Preparation**	Previous pattern continues, but drinker now makes decision to change. May initiate small changes.
4. **Action**	Behavioral change begins; is typically a trial and error process with several initial relapses.
5. **Maintenance**	New behavior pattern is consolidated; relapse prevention techniques help to maintain change.
6. **Relapse**	Efforts to change are abandoned. Cycle may be repeated until permanent sobriety is established.

SOURCE: Adapted from Prochaska, J., DiClemente, C., & Norcross, J. (1992). In search of how people change: Applications to addictive behaviors. *American Psychologist, 47,* 1102–1114.

A. The stages of behavioral change. The work of Prochaska and associates (1992) has provided a paradigm for the process of behavioral change, including change in patients with addictive disorders. Individuals commonly move through a series of specific stages on the road from abusive drinking to stable sobriety. Successful treatment involves helping the alcoholic move from one stage to the next through the use of those intervention techniques which are most effective at each stage. Typically, patients cycle through this process several times before achieving stable sobriety. This approach works best when the clinician recognizes the importance of a gradual stepwise progression through the stages of change rather than demanding instant recovery (Table 52-5 and Fig. 52-1).

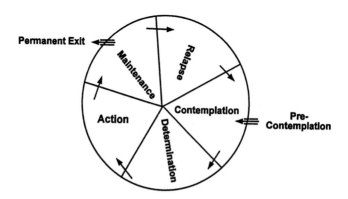

Figure 52-1.   Stages of behavioral change. [Adapted from Miller, W.R., & Rollnick, S. (1991). *Motivational interviewing: Preparing people to change addictive behavior.* New York: Guilford Press.]

Again, note the importance of a longitudinal relationship in the primary care provider wherein behavioral change can be reinforced continuously over time.

B. Motivational interviewing techniques. Basing their work on the stages of change model, Miller and Rollnick (1991) elaborated a counseling style designed to avoid patient resistance, to resolve ambivalence about drinking, and to induce change. The basic concepts of this approach are as follows:

1. The therapist's style is a powerful determinant of a patient's resistance and change.
2. Confrontation of the problem is a goal, not an intervention style.
3. Argumentation is a poor tool with which to induce change.
4. When resistance is evoked, patients tend not to change.
5. Motivation can be increased by specific treatment techniques.
6. Motivation emerges from the interaction between the patient and the therapist.
7. Ambivalence is normal, not pathologic.
8. **Helping patients resolve ambivalence is the key to change.**
9. This interviewing technique suggests the following approaches for use during each stage in the recovery process.

C. Moving patients from precontemplation to contemplation. Many primary care patients may be unaware that their drinking is a problem. Thus, the physician should do the following:

1. **Provide feedback and explore the patient's perspective on alcohol and its effects;** do not confront or argue.
   a. Perform a physical examination and obtain laboratory data, including liver function tests, blood alcohol concentration, and mean corpuscular volume
   b. Administer an assessment instrument (CAGE, AUDIT, or MAST)
   c. Review the quantity and frequency of the patient's drinking
2. **Summarize your findings and connect drinking to identified problems.**
3. **Involve the patient's family** in this process whenever possible.
4. If the patient refuses to accept your conclusions, maintain medical follow-up, listen sympathetically to the patient's complaints, and encourage the patient to agree to an "evaluation" of his or her problems.
5. The goal here is to help patients connect their problems to their drinking.

D. Moving Patients from Contemplation to Preparation

1. **Explore the patient's ambivalence about drinking.** Start with the positive side:
   a. Positive: What do you like about your drinking?
   b. Negative: What problems does your drinking create?
2. **Help the patient internalize this conflict;** do not become part of the conflict.
3. Help the patient discuss his or her anger, humiliation, guilt, and resentment.
4. Search out the patient's wish to control and/or stop drinking.
5. The goal here is to help the patient resolve his or her ambivalence; do not recommend action until the patient has made the decision to stop.

E. Moving Patients from Preparation to Action

1. **Clarify the patient's goal: to stop drinking, to control drinking, or to explore problems.**
2. **Recommend treatment options** if the patient wishes to stop drinking.
3. Recommend substance abuse counseling if the patient wishes to "control" alcohol use or remains highly ambivalent about drinking.

Table 52-6. Sample Menu of Treatment Options

1. Inpatient detoxification
2. Outpatient detoxification
3. Substance abuse counseling / "alcohol clinic"
4. Self-help programs
5. Family counseling
6. Supportive medical counseling (primary care follow-up)
7. Medications: disulfiram, naltrexone
8. Intensive rehabilitation (partial hospitalization, inpatient rehab)
9. "Dual-diagnosis counseling" (skilled psychotherapy)
10. Long-term residential (alcohol half-way houses)

---

4. Support the patient's self-efficacy: "You can do it!"
5. The goal here is to develop an action plan. Let the patient choose from a menu of treatment options (Table 52-6).

F. Action/Active Quitting Begins
   1. **Focus on directive behaviorally-based therapy. Give the patient specific prescriptions for gaining and maintaining sobriety;** for example, go to Alcoholics Anonymous (AA), stop socializing with other drinkers, see a counselor.
   2. Avoid passive non-directive forms of psychotherapy.
   3. Anticipate a trial-and-error process to refine treatment needs.
   4. **Provide ongoing optimism and support.**
   5. **Work with self-help programs.**
      a. **Alcoholics Anonymous** is the primary treatment resource for most alcoholics. It relies on group support to guide alcoholics through a process of spiritual renewal and characterologic change. An emphasis on "one day at a time," reliance on one's "higher power," and spirituality are central to the AA philosophy.
      b. Substance abuse professionals rely on AA to complement other types of interventions. Its immediate accessibility, the connection to a strong social network of sober individuals, and the provision of free, unlimited 24-hour-a-day support make it an invaluable resource.
      c. Schizoid individuals or loners and persons with more severe psychopathology may be uncomfortable in a self-help group. Professionally run groups and individual counseling are the preferred options for such patients.
      d. Non-religious persons may find Rational Recovery and similar self-help programs effective alternatives to AA.
      e. **Clinicians sometimes need to reassure patients that AA does not discourage the use of appropriately prescribed medication for the treatment of medical and psychiatric conditions.**
      f. **Successful referral to self-help programs requires familiarity with the resources available in the local community.**
         i. Try to match the program to the patient's age, race, social or professional status, and religious or sexual orientation if the patient wishes.

      ii. Insist that the patient initially attend four or five different groups to "shop around."

      iii. Most programs provide a volunteer to escort a newcomer to the first meeting. This greatly facilitates referral.

G. **Maintenance. Relapse prevention** is a specialized form of cognitive-behavioral therapy that was developed to help alcoholic patients maintain sobriety.

    1. Alcoholics are taught to identify high-risk situations and predictors of relapse. Feelings, thoughts, and behaviors that trigger craving and relapse are explored, and the patient is taught to modify them.

    2. Making the distinction between lapses (brief slips) and full relapses helps patients terminate drinking episodes promptly before they experience a complete loss of control. Re-defining such events as opportunities for learning reduces guilt and demoralization and enhances the likelihood of a successful outcome.

    3. These techniques are most helpful after a patient has achieved an initial period of sobriety.

V. Medications in the Treatment of Alcoholism

In addition to the drugs used to treat alcohol withdrawal, medications are now available that significantly enhance the long-term management of alcoholism.

A. **Detoxification**

    1. **Benzodiazepines are the preferred medications for detoxification** because of their excellent side effect profile.

      a. Long-acting benzodiazepines, such as **chlordiazepoxide and diazepam,** are the standards for uncomplicated detoxification. When high enough initial doses (> 60 mg diazepam over 24 to 36 hours) are used, these drugs are self-tapering.

      b. The short-acting benzodiazepine, **lorazepam,** is recommended only for an individual with significant liver disease, cognitive impairment, unstable medical problems, or age greater than 65 years. This drug has to be tapered over 4 to 8 days, but it is metabolized to the glucuronide form and rapidly is excreted by the kidney, giving the clinician more flexibility in managing an unstable patient.

    2. Symptom-triggered dosing based on withdrawal scales, such as the Clinical Institute Withdrawal Assessment (CIWA-Ar), works best but requires frequent monitoring. This approach provides adequate control of symptoms, avoids overmedication, and shortens the period of detoxification treatment.

B. **Medications for Long-Term Treatment**

    1. Naltrexone is an opiate antagonist that has been found to reduce craving and relapse in alcoholics. Given in doses of 50 mg orally per day, it is well tolerated and seems to work best in patients who describe intense craving. There is some data to suggest that naltrexone is not effective in men with more chronic and severe alcoholism. Additional research is being conducted to evaluate higher doses, alternate dosing schedules and subgroups of alcoholics that may respond best to this drug. It is contraindicated in a patient taking opiates or one with acute hepatitis or liver failure.

    2. Disulfiram inhibits alcohol metabolism, leading to elevated levels of acetaldehyde. Doses of 250 mg orally per day can produce tachycardia, dyspnea, nausea, and vomiting if the patient drinks.

      a. In controlled trials, disulfiram has been no better than placebo in producing continuous abstinence, but it does reduce the number of days on which the patient drinks and the severity of concurrent medical problems.

    b. Disulfiram works best in a stable, motivated patient who is followed closely by his or her physician.

    c. Liver function tests must be monitored periodically for signs of disulfiram-induced hepatitis.

    d. Disulfiram also inhibits dopamine beta-hydroxylase and may exacerbate psychosis in some schizophrenics. Reducing the daily dose to 125 mg and adding a high-potency dopamine-blocking agent, such as haloperidol, may resolve the problem.

  3. Ondansetron, a selective 5-HT_3 antagonist, has reduced alcohol consumption in early-onset alcoholics, suggesting that subtypes of alcoholics may have differential responses to pharmacotherapy. Late-onset alcoholics have not been responsive to this medication.

  4. Acamprosate, a derivative of the amino acid taurine, acts as the glutamate receptor and has been found to increase abstinence in a number of recent medication trials. It is available in Europe and is in the final stage of FDA review. Used alone or in combination with other anticraving drugs, such as naltrexone, these medications represent a significant advance in our options for the treatment of alcohol dependence.

C. Treating associated symptoms. After detoxification, alcoholics may experience various distressing symptoms and may pressure their physicians to provide medication for those complaints. After a careful evaluation to rule out co-morbid psychiatric conditions, patients should be reassured that these symptoms are common in early recovery and usually resolve with extended sobriety. Avoiding prescribed medications helps patients learn that they are moving beyond dependency on exogenous chemicals.

  1. **Anxiety.** Relaxation techniques and cognitive-behavioral interventions can be utilized. Avoid the prescription of benzodiazepines because of their abuse potential in this population.

  2. **Depression.** Psychotherapy often is helpful in managing the guilt and depression experienced by some recovering alcoholics. Antidepressant drugs have not been proved effective in the treatment of low levels of dysphoria in this population.

  3. **Insomnia.** If appropriate sleep hygiene does not resolve the problem, use the sedating antidepressant trazodone (25 to 100 mg PO q.h.s.). It has no significant abuse potential and is effective for long-term use. Sedative-hypnotic drugs should be avoided because of their abuse potential.

VI. Managing Dual-Diagnosis Patients

Psychiatric diagnoses made during periods of active drinking are highly unreliable. The patient should be observed after a minimum of 2 weeks of sobriety to confirm any diagnoses. Once it is clear that the symptoms are not secondary to the patient's alcoholism, any co-morbid psychiatric disorder must be treated. **Failure to adequately diagnose and treat co-morbid psychiatric disorders is the most common cause of failure of alcoholism treatment.**

A. Anxiety Disorders

  1. **Panic disorder** may precede the development of alcoholism and usually becomes more severe after extended drinking. Behavioral psychotherapy and antidepressants, such as paroxetine and imipramine, have proven to be effective treatments.

  2. **Generalized anxiety disorder** should be treated with buspirone 5 mg t.i.d., building up slowly to 10 to 20 mg PO t.i.d. If no response, paroxetine or other selective-serotonin reuptake inhibitors (SSRIs) may be used.

3. **Attention deficit hyperactivity disorder (ADHD)** can be treated with methyl-phenidate 10 to 20 mg PO t.i.d., though these patients must be followed carefully for signs of stimulant abuse.

4. **Post-traumatic stress disorder (PTSD)** and co-morbid alcohol abuse are very difficult to treat. Such patients should be referred to specialized treatment programs.

B. Major depressive disorder. Various tricyclic antidepressants (TCAs) and the SSRIs have been used with some success in depressed alcoholics, though there have been few adequately controlled clinical trials. For patients who have not responded to other antidepressants, nefazodone can be considered. It is effective for reducing anxiety and improving sleep; however, patients on nefazodone must be monitored for signs of hepatic failure. The use of this medication is contraindicated in patients with a history of hepatitis.

C. Bipolar disorder. Mood-stabilizing drugs can have dramatic benefits in these cases. Adequate control of manic episodes often eliminates excessive drinking.

1. Bipolar I: Lithium in the standard dose range is most effective.

2. Bipolar II: Valproic acid (and possibly gabapentin) may have some advantage in this patient group.

D. Schizophrenia. Intensive long-term counseling for substance abuse must be provided in conjunction with comprehensive psychiatric management. Schizophrenic patients do poorly in most AA groups and may be highly ambivalent about sobriety, since they often use alcohol to moderate psychotic symptoms or reduce the side effects of antipsychotic medications. In patients where insight or intentionality is impaired, influencing external contingencies, which in turn reward or discourage behaviors, may be an effective intervention.

VII. Criteria for Referral for Inpatient Detoxification

A. A history of failure in outpatient detoxification or multiple relapses

B. Active suicidal ideation or acute psychosis

C. A history of delirium tremens or alcohol withdrawal seizure(s).

D. Co-morbid medical problems that require frequent daily monitoring during detoxification

E. Severe withdrawal symptoms that have not responded adequately to initial oral doses of benzodiazepines.

F. Lack of a sober and safe environment for outpatient detoxification.

VIII. Criteria for Referral for Specialized Long-Term Alcoholism Treatment

A. A history of multiple treatment failures

B. Alcoholics with a serious co-morbid psychiatric condition, especially if they have not responded to initial efforts at psychiatric management

C. Alcoholics who also abuse other drugs **(polysubstance abuse)**

D. Homeless persons or alcoholics living in very unstable environments

Suggested Readings

Ait-Daoud, N., Johnson, B.A., Prihoda, T.J., et al. (2001). Combining ondansetron and naltrexone reduces craving among biologically predisposed alcoholics: Preliminary clinical evidence. *Psychopharmacology* (Berl), *154*(1), 23–27.

American Psychiatric Association. (1995). *Diagnostic and statistical manual of mental disorders* (4th ed., Primary Care Version). Washington, DC: American Psychiatric Press.

Anton, R.F. (2001). Pharmacologic approaches in the management of alcoholism. *Journal of Clinical Psychiatry, 62*(suppl 20), 11–17.

Bein, T.H., Miller, W.R., & Tonigan, J.S. (1993). Brief intervention for alcohol problems: A review. *Addiction, 88,* 315–335.

Ciraulo, D.A., & Renner, J.A. (1991). Alcoholism. In D.A. Ciraulo, R.I. Shader (Eds.). *Clinical manual of chemical dependence.* Washington, DC: American Psychiatric Press.

Clark, W. (1995). Alcohol problems. In J. Noble (Ed.), *Textbook of primary care medicine.* St. Louis: Mosby.

Clark, W. (1995). Effective interviewing and intervention for alcohol problems. In M. Lipkin, S. Putman, & A. Lazare (Eds.), *The medical interview.* New York: Springer Verlag.

Friedman, L., Fleeting, N.F., Roberts, D.H., & Hyman, S.E. (Eds.). *Source book of substance abuse and addiction.* Baltimore: Williams & Wilkins.

Johnson, B.A., Roache, J.D., Javors, M.A., et al. (2000). Ondansetron for reduction of drinking among biologically predisposed alcoholic patients: A randomized controlled trial. *Journal of the American Medical Association, 284*(8), 963–971.

Kessler, R.C., McGonagle, K.A., Zhao, S., et al. (1994). Lifetime and 12-month prevalence of *DSM-III-R* psychiatric disorders in the United States. *Archives of General Psychiatry, 51,* 8–19.

Krystal, J.H., Cramer, J.A., Krol, W.F., et al. (2001). Naltrexone in the treatment of alcohol dependence. *New England Journal of Medicine, 345*(24), 1734–1739.

Mayfield, D., McLeod, G., & Hall, P. (1974). The CAGE questionnaire: Validation of a new alcoholism instrument. *American Journal of Psychiatry, 131,* 1121–1123.

Miller, W.R., & Rollnick, S. (1991). *Motivational interviewing: Preparing people to change addictive behavior.* New York: Guilford Press.

O'Malley, S.S., Jaffe, A.J., Chang, G., et al. (1992). Naltrexone and coping skills therapy for alcohol dependence. *Archives of General Psychiatry, 49,* 881–887.

Prochaska, J., DiClemente, C., & Norcross, J. (1992). In search of how people change: Applications to addictive behaviors. *American Psychologist, 47,* 1102–1114.

Project MATCH Research Group. (1998). Matching alcoholism treatments to client heterogeneity: Project MATCH three-year drinking outcomes. *Alcoholism Clinical and Experimental Research, 22*(6), 1300–1311.

Rollnick, N., Heather, N., & Bell, A. (1992). Negotiating behavior change in medical settings: The development of brief motivational interviewing. *Journal of Merit Health, 1,* 25–37.

Saitz, R., Mayo-Smith, M.F., Roberts, M.S., et al. (1994). Individualized treatment for alcohol withdrawal. *Journal of the American Medical Association, 272,* 519–523.

Sandberg, G.G., & Marlatt, G.A. (1991). Relapse prevention. In D.A. Ciraulo, & R.I. Shader (Eds.), *Clinical manual of chemical dependence.* Washington, DC: American Psychiatric Press.

Saunders, J.B., Aasland, O.G., Babor, T.F., et al. (1993). Development of the Alcohol Use Disorders Identification Test (AUDIT): WHO collaborative project on early detection of persons with harmful alcohol consumption III. *Addiction, 88,* 791–804.

Selzer, M.L. (1971). The Michigan Alcoholism Screening Test: The quest for a new diagnostic instrument. *American Journal of Psychiatry, 127,* 1653–1658.

Sullivan, X.T., Sykora, K., Schneiderman, J., et al. (1989). Assessment of alcohol withdrawal: The revised Clinical Institute Withdrawal Assessment for alcohol scale (CIWA-Ar). *British Journal of Addiction, 84,* 1353–1357.

CHAPTER 53

The Cocaine or Opiate-Abusing Patient

DAVID R. GASTFRIEND AND JAMES J. O'CONNELL

I. Introduction

Cocaine and opiate abuse are major public health problems that lead to increased use of emergency departments and physicians' offices for diverse reasons.

A. The United States has an estimated 6 million hardcore drug users, a number that has been stable since the mid-1990s.

B. Drug use patterns occur in waves that reflect drug supply, social mores, and economic conditions.

1. Public awareness of the United States cocaine epidemic and its connection to HIV-transmission has reduced cocaine's popularity among non-dependent users. In its place, intranasal heroin abuse (smoked and snorted) has emerged owing to increased purity and decreased cost. Since intravenous (IV) use is not required, users assume this to be risk-free. Patients need warnings of this erroneous assumption; heroin promotes sexual risk-taking and severe drug dependence (to the point of requiring methadone maintenance treatment even in the absence of needle use) and it can progress to needle use.

2. **Drug-seeking behavior is common with cocaine and heroin users.** Primary care physicians (PCPs) and emergency departments are prime targets for dependent individuals seeking prescriptions for mood-altering controlled substances, including benzodiazepines, particularly alprazolam (Xanax), but long-acting agents, such as clonazepam (Klonopin) have street value as well; opiate analgesics, including propoxyphene (Darvon) and sustained-release oxycodone (OxyContin); and barbiturates. The complaints are often legitimate signs and symptoms of an anxiety disorder, injury, or migraine headache. If the patient presents with only vague symptoms, specifically insists on a specific agent, or blocks contact with prior providers or significant others, fulfillment of the request may risk further harm to the patient.

3. **The cost-benefit analysis shows that inpatient treatment saves four dollars for every dollar spent and outpatient care saves 12 dollars for each dollar spent, primarily in decreased crime and health care costs.**

4. The physician's intervention can have lasting impact, even on seemingly unmotivated patients, through the use of the Stages of Change Model: promote the patient's *Contemplation* of substance consequences, foster *Determination* to change, help to specify a lifestyle *Action* plan, and then sustain ongoing *Maintenance* recovery efforts (such as mutual-help meeting participation, e.g., Alcoholics Anonymous).

II. Evaluation of the Problem

A. The clinician has three tasks when addressing possible heroin and cocaine abuse:

1. **Screen all patients for drug use and problems:** "What substances or drugs have you ever tried? Have you had any problems? Has anyone had any concerns about your substance use?"

2. Diagnose an abuse or dependence disorder

3. Intervene to promote the patient's action to change pathologic substance use. Of these factors, intervention is the most important. The message is: "How can we help you become safer and healthier?"

B. A covert medical history for cocaine or heroin use is common among addicted individuals. Over 50% of callers to a national hotline visited an emergency department at least once for cocaine complications without revealing that cocaine was the cause. Initially, the clinician must rely on historical and circumstantial clues to cocaine or heroin etiologies. Interview of a family member or significant other, separately from the patient, may be pivotal.

C. Complications of Cocaine Abuse and Dependence

1. Psychiatric: Panic, depression, and mania in susceptible individuals

2. Cardiovascular: Hypertension, acute myocardial infarction, arrhythmia, and rupture of the ascending aorta

3. Pulmonary: Bronchitis, pulmonary edema, spontaneous pneumomediastinum, and respiratory arrest

4. Central nervous system (CNS): CVA, generalized seizure, and fungal cerebritis

5. Obstetrical: Abruptio placentae, placental vasoconstriction, and spontaneous abortion

6. Miscellaneous: Anosmia, nasal septum perforation, sexual dysfunction, hyperpyrexia, ischemic bowel, hepatitis, and abscess

D. Interview

Determine the route, pattern, and links to drug access and the presence of abstinence symptoms. Review the history of impulse control problems and assess the degree of ego or psychological strength. Assume that the individual is using other substances, either for self-treatment of the acute effects of cocaine, or as a separate dependency.

E. Examination

1. **Physical signs** may include weight loss, anorexia, needle tracks (flat, with ecchymoses, in contrast to raised with heroin), a solitary long fingernail, evidence of skin popping (pock-size "insect bites" secondary to intradermal injection), fresh or scarred bite marks on lips or tongue, worn teeth, nosebleeds, and nasal septum ulceration.

2. **Urine toxicology** (Figure 53-1)

III. Diagnostic Criteria for Psychoactive Substance Use Syndromes (See Table 53-1)

A. Substance-induced organic disorders are always listed in addition to the abuse or dependence diagnosis.

B. Criteria for diagnosis of substance abuse (only one required): Role failure, hazardous use, recurrent legal or social problems.

C. Criteria for substance dependence (≥ 3 in a 12-month period, maladaptive, with distress and impairment):

1. Tolerance-absolute (i.e., consumes increasing quantity of substance over time) or relative (i.e., over time, notes decreasing subjective euphoria with same amount of substance)

2. Withdrawal-characteristic symptoms (or symptoms are avoided through continued substance use)

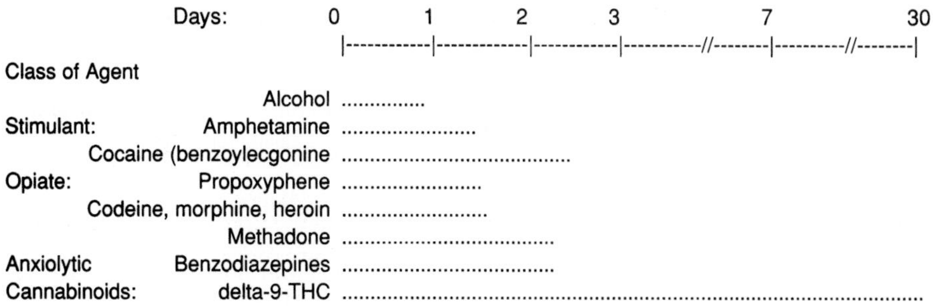

```
Days:           0      1      2      3          7          30
                |----------|------------|----------|----------//--------|----------//--------|
Class of Agent
                     Alcohol  ...............
Stimulant:           Amphetamine  ........................
          Cocaine (benzoylecgonine  ...........................................
Opiate:              Propoxyphene  ........................
          Codeine, morphine, heroin  ..........................
                     Methadone  .....................................
Anxiolytic           Benzodiazepines  .....................................
Cannabinoids:        delta-9-THC  ....................................................................................................
```

Fig. 53-1. Maximal duration of detection in urine. [American Academy of Pediatrics. (1988). *Substance abuse: A guide for health professionals.* Elk Grove Village, IL.] **Hair testing detects amphetamines, cocaine, marijuana, opiates, and phencyclidine for ~90 days.**

3. Larger amounts or periods of use than intended
4. Persistent desire or unsuccessful efforts to cut down
5. Excessive time spent obtaining, using, or recovering from a substance
6. Activities given up because of substance use
7. Continued use despite knowledge of problem

- Remission: early or sustained, full or partial, on agonist (e.g., methadone), on antagonist (e.g., disulfiram) or in controlled environment (e.g., halfway house, hospital, or prison)

Table 53-1. Substance-Induced Disorders and Their Associated States

Substance-Induced Disorder	*Causal Agents and Associated State(s)*
1. Delusional	Alcohol, amphetamines, cannabis, cocaine, hallucinogens, phencyclidine (PCP) intoxication
2. Delirium and hallucinosis	All intoxicants, except for caffeine and nicotine
3. Withdrawal delirium	Alcohol and sedative anxiolytics (includes relative withdrawal)
4. Hallucinogen persisting perception disorder	Post-hallucinogen flashbacks
5. Mood disorder	Intoxication with all, except caffeine, cannabis, and nicotine
6. Anxiety disorder	With either intoxication or withdrawal, except with nicotine and opioids
7. Sleep disorder	Intoxication or withdrawal, with alcohol, sedatives, stimulants, or opioids.

IV. Treatment Strategies for Cocaine Abuse and Dependence

A. Management of Acute Cocaine Intoxication

1. Onset: within seconds when administered IV or via inhalation
2. Duration: 30 to 60 minutes intranasal; lethal doses metabolized in 1 hour; recovery ≤ 48 hours
3. Course: euphoria yields to a "crash" within hours: dysphoria, anxiety, irritability, agitation
   a. Cocaine delirium-disorientation with violence within 1 to 6 hours. Delirium subsides as the pharmacologic effects wear off.
   b. Cocaine delusional disorder-rapid: Persecution, jealousy, homicidality. Delusional disorder may produce formication (i.e., "bugs crawling on my skin") with excoriations. May last longer than 1 week, rarely longer than 1 year.
4. Differential diagnosis: Mania, amphetamine, or PCP intoxication. Distinguished only on the basis of urine toxicology.
5. Treatment: usually resolves with hypersomnolence; provide security if homicidal. Overdose (OD) requires life support: airway, O_2, and occasionally ventilation. Usually not required in occasional use except in life-threatening OD or *psychosis*.
   a. Hyperpyrexia—ice baths.
6. Rx: diazepam 5 to 10 mg PO for mild agitation; IV for seizure (5 mg/minute)
   a. For severe β-adrenergic state: propranolol (Inderal) 1 mg IV q minute up to 8 minutes or labetolol (Normodyne or Trandate) 2 mg IV q minute an α- and β-blocker with less risk of unopposed alpha stimulation and high blood pressure exacerbation than propranolol.

B. Disrupting Binge Cycle: Requires 2 to 7 treatment contacts per week, initially, in a drug-focused multi-modal program including:

1. Individual, family/couples, and group therapy.
2. Peer support groups (12 step—Alcoholics Anonymous or Narcotics Anonymous or Cocaine Anonymous or Rational Recovery)
3. Educational sessions—must include family
4. Behavioral techniques: Urine testing with contingencies; restricting money, access, and social activity; monitoring by significant other; frequent, immediate contact with support p.r.n. for cravings

C. Relapse Prevention

1. Initial abstinence: Enforce isolation from drug use, strict avoidance of cues
2. Cues (e.g., cashing paycheck) can be partially reintroduced as mental images while developing coping strategies
3. Gradual re-entry to cue-rich environment
4. Continuous, then periodic maintenance therapies. Strengthen memories of negative consequences (e.g., hear and then present "drug-a-log" talks at 12-step fellowship meetings), decrease and/or learn to manage external stress.

D. Pharmacotherapy of Cocaine Craving and Withdrawal

1. Tricyclic antidepressants (TCAs) reverse intracranial self-stimulation (ICSS) changes in animals, promote receptor downregulation, and correct cocaine's chronic effect. Desipramine (Norpramin): More than five controlled trials indicate efficacy for cocaine dependence, even in the absence of a major depressive disorder (Note: hepatic enzyme induction is common, so assure that serum levels have reached usual therapeutic range for antidepressant efficacy).

2. Dopamine (DA) agonists: Bromocriptine (Parlodel), amantadine (Symmetrel): rapid onset; acute use decreases craving. Bromocriptine: Controlled trials show mixed efficacy; side effects are frequent: gradual initiation is required to prevent headache, nausea, dizziness, or psychosis. Dose: 0.625 mg t.i.d., increased to 7.5 to 12.5 mg/day as tolerated. Amantadine: unclear efficacy but better tolerated. Dose: 200 mg/day the first 2 weeks, then b.i.d.

V. Opiate Abuse and Dependence

A. Initial Effects: Individuals dependent on opiates have usually initiated drug use to achieve analgesia, a "rush," a state of well-being, or euphoria.

B. Chronic Use: Results in a loss of most of the positive effects, leaving adverse signs or symptoms, such as apathy, lethargy, drowsiness, mental clouding, motor retardation, smooth muscle inhibition (constipation, urinary hesitation, miosis), orthostatic hypotension, nausea, or vomiting.

C. Heroin Overdose

1. Signs: Needle tracks, miosis, bradycardia, depressed respirations, cyanosis, stupor/coma, hypothermia, and non-cardiogenic pulmonary edema
2. Treatment: Naloxone (Narcan): A pure opiate antagonist, 0.4 mg (1 mL), repeated q 5 minutes p.r.n. or IV drip-4 mg/L D5W @ 100 mL/hour. Overdose may last 1 to 4 hours, requiring antagonist to be repeated p.r.n., especially for methadone overdose (24 to 28 hours). It is important to note that after reversing respiratory depression, naloxone may precipitate withdrawal; therefore, careful monitoring is necessary, and naloxone should be terminated as consciousness is restored.

D. Opiate Withdrawal

1. Onset: The patient generally admits to the need for drugs but may exaggerate symptoms—avoid overdose by monitoring signs:
   a. Mild signs: Sweating, yawning, lacrimation, tremor, rhinorrhea, marked irritability, dilated pupils, and increased respiratory rate
   b. Severe signs: 48 to 72 hours after last dose-insomnia, tachycardia, hypertension, nausea, vomiting, abdominal cramps, and diarrhea that may lead to dehydration
2. Duration: The onset of heroin withdrawal is within 8 to 12 hours and lasts 5 to 10 days; untreated. Methadone withdrawal begins at 30 to 48 hours and lasts 2 to 4 weeks.

E. Treatments for Chronic Opiate Dependence

1. Abstinence model: This is the only choice if the patient has been dependent for less than 1 year. FDA regulations permit only an acute detoxification using methadone over 30 days or an extended detoxification using methadone for up to 180 days. The abstinence model is best for stable, employable, highly motivated patients, with support (e.g., drug-dependent health providers with licensure contingency contracts). The abstinence approach is a poor choice for the chronic recidivistic patient.
2. Methadone dosing: Methadone at $\geq$ 70 mg/day (in licensed clinics only or during medical or surgical hospitalization) is associated with decreased heroin use, HIV risk, and criminality. (See Table 53-2.) Withdrawal: Onset in 30 to 48 hours, over 2 to 4 weeks. Buprenorphine is another option for outpatient use.
3. Alternative Treatments
   a. Harm Reduction: Needle exchange in high-frequency injectors achieves relatively low rates of HIV incidence even in high seroprevalence areas such as New York City.

Table 53-2. Opiate Agents, Dose Equivalencies, and Sources

Agent	Dose (mg) Equivalent[a]	Source
Hydromorphone (Dilaudid)	0.5	Semi-synthetic
Methadone (Dolophine)	1	Synthetic
Diacetylmorphine (Heroin)	1–2	Semi-synthetic
Morphine	3–4	Natural opium poppy derivative
Oxycodone (Percodan)	3–4	Semi-synthetic
Paregoric	6–12	Natural opium poppy derivative
Meperidine (Demerol)	20	Synthetic
Codeine	30	Natural opium poppy derivative
Propoxyphene (Darvon)	45–60	Synthetic

[a]Dose equivalencies adapted from Jaffe and Martin, in Gilman and Goodman, *Pharmacologic Basis of Therapeutics,* 1985, and others.

    b. Rapid Detox (≤ 5 days): Uses a combination of clonidine 0.1 to 0.2 mg PO q.i.d. with p.r.n. doses for vital sign elevations, followed by naltrexone 12.5 mg PO on day 1 and increasing over 2 to 5 days to 50 mg/day. A more comfortable and rapid alternative is clonidine (same doses) with buprenorphine (Buprenex) 2 mg sublingual followed by naltrexone induction from 12.5 mg on the first day to 50 mg on day 2. Clonidine and buprenorphine are discontinued on day 3 (O'Connor, 1995).

VI. Concomitant Substance Abuse/Dependency

A. Cocaine use is commonly associated with benzodiazepines or alcohol to reduce cocaine-induced anxiety with sedation and reduce the post-cocaine crash.
    1. The lifetime prevalence of alcohol dependence among cocaine dependent individuals is 62%.
    2. In the United States, 12 million per year combine alcohol with cocaine.
    3. Therefore: Watch for alcohol withdrawal, which may require inpatient detoxification.

B. Cocaine IV use is often associated with heroin
    1. Multiple drug use is also an associated feature of antisocial personality disorder.
    2. Significant cocaine use persists during methadone maintenance—even after 5 years, 12.5% of the most motivated and successful patients in Beth Israel's Medical Maintenance cohort (New York City) were discharged because of chronic cocaine use.
    3. Health education reduces IV cocaine use in heroin addicts.
    4. Cocaine use is significantly associated with multiple needle-sharing.

C. Heroin with cocaine IV use ("speedball") adversely affects prognosis in methadone maintenance.

D. Alcoholism: prevalence in heroin addicts—50%
    1. Treat simultaneously: Relapse in one is associated with relapse in the other.

2. Opiates and alcohol: Maintain on methadone during detoxification, consider disulfiram (Antabuse) later.

3. Alcohol detoxification, rehabilitation, or pharmacotherapy, such as disulfiram, should not interfere with methadone prescribing.

Suggested Readings

Ball, J., & Ross, A. (1991). *The effectiveness of methadone maintenance treatment.* New York: Springer-Verlag.

Brust, J.C.M. (1993). *Neurological aspects of substance abuse.* Boston: Butterworth-Heinemann.

Cartwright, W.S. (2000). Cost-benefit analysis of drug treatment services: review of the literature. *Journal of Mental Health Policy Economics, 3*(1), 11–26.

Fingerhood, M.I., Thompson, M.R., & Jasinki, D.R. (2001). A comparison of clonidine and buprenorphine in the outpatient of opiate withdrawl. *Substance Abuse, 22*(3), 193–199.

Galanter, M., & Kleber, H.D. (1999). *Textbook of substance abuse treatment.* Washington, DC: American Psychiatric Press.

Gastfriend, D.R. (1998). Pharmacotherapy of substance abuse and dependence. *Psychiatric Clinics of North America Annual of Drug Therapy, 5,* 211– 229.

Gastfriend, D.R., Lu, S.H., & Sharon, E. (2000). Placement matching: Challenges and technical progress. *Substance Use & Misuse, 35*(12–14), 2191–2213.

Koesters, S.C., Rogers, P.D., & Rajasingham, C.R. (2002). MDMA ("ecstasy") and other "club drugs". The new epidemic. *Pediatric Clinics of North America, 49*(2), 415–433.

Koob, G.F. (2000). Neurobiology of addiction. Toward the development of new therapies. *Annals of the New York Academy of Sciences, 909,* 170–185.

Mee-Lee, D., Shulman, G.D., Fishman, M., Gastfriend, D.R., & Griffith, J.H. (Eds.). (2001). *ASAM patient placement criteria for the treatment of substance-related disorders* (2nd Ed-Revised [ASAM PPC-2R].). Chevy Chase, MD: American Society of Addiction Medicine, Inc.

Mendelson, J.H., & Mello, N.K. (1996). Management of cocaine abuse and dependence. *New England Journal of Medicine, 334,* 965–972.

O'Connor, P.G., & Kosten, T.R. (1998). Rapid and ultrarapid opioid detoxification techniques. *Journal of the American Medical Association, 279*(3), 229–234.

Simkin, D.R. (2002). Adolescent substance use disorders and comorbidity. *Pediatric Clinics of North America, 49*(2), 463–477.

Stimmel, B. (2002). *Alcoholism, drug addiction, and the road to recovery: Life on the edge.* Binghamton, NY: Haworth Press.

CHAPTER 54
The Patient Receiving Steroids

ISABEL T. LAGOMASINO AND THEODORE A. STERN

I. Steroid Use and Complications

Glucocorticoids play a prominent role in the treatment of a wide range of medical illnesses (Table 54-1). Available in a variety of preparations and doses (Table 54-2),

---

Table 54-1. Selected Indications for Glucocorticoid Use

Neurologic diseases	Neoplastic diseases
Multiple sclerosis	Leukemia
Spinal cord injuries	Lymphoma
Respiratory disorders	Rheumatic disorders
Symptomatic sarcoidosis	Psoriatic arthritis
Tuberculosis	Rheumatoid arthritis
Aspiration pneumonitis	Acute gouty arthritis
Gastrointestinal diseases	Collagen diseases
Ulcerative colitis	Systemic lupus erythematosus
Regional enteritis	Systemic dermatomyositis
Renal disorders	Acute rheumatic carditis
Nephrotic syndrome	Dermatologic diseases
Glomerulonephritis	Pemphigus
Endocrine disorders	Severe erythema multiforme
Adrenocortical insufficiency	Severe psoriasis
Hypercalcemia associated with cancer	Ophthalmic diseases
Non-suppurative thyroiditis	Herpes zoster ophthalmicus
Hematologic disorders	Diffuse uveitis and chorioretinitis
Idiopathic thrombocytopenic purpura	Optic neuritis
Secondary thrombocytopenia	Allergic states
Autoimmune hemolytic anemia	Bronchial asthma
	Contact dermatitis
	Drug hypersensitivity reactions

SOURCE: Adapted from *Physician's desk reference* (49th ed.). (1995). Montvale, NJ: Medical Economics Data Publication Company.

Table 54-2. Glucocorticoid Preparations

Generic Name	Approximate Equivalent Dose	Usual Starting Dose, mg/day	
		Moderate Illness	Severe Illness
Short-acting			
Cortisone[a]	25.0	100–200	
Hydrocortisone[a]	20.0	80–160	
Prednisone	5.0	20–40	60–100
Prednisolone[a]	5.0	20–40	60–100
Methylprednisolone[a]	4.0	16–32	48–80[b]
Intermediate-acting			
Triamcinolone[a]	4.0	16–32	48–80
Paramethasone	2.0	8–16	24–40
Long-acting			
Dexamethasone[a]	0.75	3–6	9–15
Betamethasone[a]	0.6	2.4–4.8	7.2–12.0

[a]Parenteral forms are available (oral and parenteral dosages are generally comparable).
[b]Higher-dose parenteral therapy may be used for severe illness.
SOURCE: Adapted from Kahl, L. (1992). Arthritis and rheumatologic diseases. In M. Woodley, & A. Whelan (Eds.), *Manual of medical therapeutics* (27th ed.). Boston: Little, Brown.

they are prescribed for their widespread beneficial effects despite their known adverse effects on multiple organ systems (Table 54-3). Neuropsychiatric complications from glucocorticoid use occur in approximately 5% of patients and may involve alterations in affect (depression or mania), behavior (psychosis), and cognition (delirium or dementia).

II. Neuropsychiatric Complications from Steroid Use

Although commonly grouped under the umbrella term, **steroid psychosis,** the psychiatric complications resulting from steroid therapy (Table 54-4) may include several different clinical presentations.

A. **Clinical symptoms. The psychiatric sequelae of glucocorticoid use lack a pathognomonic presentation;** individual patients may display different symptoms during the same course or different courses of steroid therapy. Several generalizations, however, may be made.

   1. **Mild euphoria** is common after the initiation of steroid treatment.
   2. **Depression and mania each account for roughly one-third of the resulting serious psychiatric syndromes, making mood disorders the most common psychiatric complication.**
   3. **Psychosis and delirium** each account for roughly one-sixth of the serious psychiatric syndromes; auditory and visual hallucinations, delusions, mutism, catatonia,

---

Table 54-3. Adverse Effects of Glucocorticoids

Neurologic effects	Musculoskeletal effects
Increased intracranial pressure	Muscle weakness
Convulsions	Steroid myopathy
Vertigo	Osteoporosis
Headache	Aseptic necrosis of femoral heads
Gastrointestinal disturbances	Dermatologic disturbances
Peptic ulcer	Thin fragile skin
Pancreatitis	Petechiae and ecchymoses
Abdominal distension	Facial erythema
Ulcerative esophagitis	Increased sweating
Renal effects	Ophthalmic effects
Sodium retention	Posterior subcapsular cataracts
Fluid retention	Increased intraocular pressure
Hypokalemic alkalosis	Glaucoma
Hypertension	Exophthalmos
Endocrine disturbances	Allergic difficulties
Menstrual irregularities	Urticaria
Development of cushingoid state	Anaphylactic reactions
Adrenocortical unresponsiveness	Allergic or hypersensitivity reactions
Manifestations of latent diabetes	Further localized effects

SOURCE: Adapted from *Physician's desk reference* (49th ed.). (1995). Montvale, NJ: Medical Economics Data Publication Company.

---

and alterations in sensory perception, attention, concentration, and memory commonly occur.

4. Specific symptoms such as **insomnia, irritability, anxiety,** and obsessive-compulsive behavior may be associated with a general syndrome or may occur independently.

B. **Incidence. Up to 30%** of patients who receive glucocorticoids develop some psychiatric symptoms; **roughly 5% develop more severe psychiatric syndromes,** including depression, mania, psychosis, and delirium.

Table 54-4. Neuropsychiatric Complications from Steroid Use

Syndromes include depression, mania, psychosis, and delirium

Symptoms include insomnia, irritability, anxiety, and obsessive-compulsive behavior

Serious psychiatric syndromes may occur in 5% of patients undergoing treatment

Complications usually begin within the first 1 or 2 weeks of treatment

Difficulties usually last 1 to 3 weeks and resolve completely

C. **Time of onset.** The latency from the initiation of steroid therapy to the onset of psychiatric complications is **quite variable;** symptoms may begin within hours of the start of treatment or after several months of ongoing therapy. Among the patients who develop psychiatric complications, an estimated 40% develop symptoms within the first week of therapy, 60% develop symptoms within the first 2 weeks, and 90% develop symptoms within the first 6 weeks.

D. **Duration of symptoms.** The duration of psychiatric symptoms resulting from glucocorticoid therapy is **quite variable.** A reduction in steroid dose or discontinuation of treatment may shorten the course of complications. In general, patients who develop delirium appear to recover within 1 week, while those with depression, mania, or psychosis appear to recover within 3 weeks. Most patients have full recoveries within 6 weeks; some, however, experience recurrent psychiatric symptoms or die from suicide.

1. Several patients have reportedly developed life-long cycling mood disorders after glucocorticoid exposure. Steroids thus may be capable of inducing chronic syndromes; more realistically, they may be capable of "unmasking" underlying disorders to which patients are already predisposed.

2. Patients who develop psychiatric difficulties from glucocorticoid use may be more likely to contemplate, attempt, or complete suicide than are patients with similar psychiatric symptoms resulting from other etiologies.

III. Risk Factors for Neuropsychiatric Complications from Steroid Use

Identification of the potential risk factors (Table 54-5) for the development of psychiatric syndromes from steroid use may allow for the prophylaxis, or early recognition and treatment of, such syndromes.

A. **Age.** Age does not appear to be a significant risk factor for steroid-induced psychiatric syndromes. Patients who develop psychiatric symptoms, like those who receive glucocorticoid therapy, are between 8 and 71 years old.

B. **Gender.** Women may be more likely than men to develop psychiatric sequelae from glucocorticoid use. Approximately 60% of the patients in the literature who have had psychiatric sequelae were women, even when patients with conditions, such as systemic

---

Table 54-5. Risk Factors for Neuropsychiatric Complications

Likely Risk Factors	*Unlikely Risk Factors*
Female gender	Age
Systemic lupus erythematosus or pemphigus	Prior psychiatric illness
Doses greater than 40 mg/day of prednisone	Family psychiatric history
	Prior steroid complications
	Specific steroid preparations
	Different dosing schedules
	Duration of treatment

lupus erythematosus (SLE) and rheumatoid arthritis (which occur much more frequently in women), were excluded. An estimated 15–20% of women who undergo steroid therapy will develop neuropsychiatric complications compared with 3% of men.

C. **Concurrent illness.** Patients with SLE and pemphigus may be predisposed to steroid-induced psychiatric symptoms. Up to 33% of patients with SLE and 20% of patients with pemphigus develop psychiatric sequelae from steroid treatment compared with 5% of patients with other conditions. The increased rate of complications in patients with SLE may be partly secondary to the high incidence of neuropsychiatric symptoms in SLE patients, even in the absence of steroid exposure.

D. **Psychiatric history.** A history of psychiatric illness is not a clear risk factor for the development of psychiatric difficulties from glucocorticoids. The vast majority of patients who develop difficulties secondary to steroids have no prior psychiatric illness, and the vast majority of patients with psychiatric disorders who receive glucocorticoid therapy have no complications.

E. **Family psychiatric history.** The presence of psychiatric illness in the family does not appear to be a predisposing factor for the development of steroid-related psychiatric complications.

F. **Steroid history.** The presence or absence of a psychiatric syndrome during a previous course of glucocorticoid treatment does not predict the reaction to a future course of treatment. Patients who develop complications during one course of steroids may be free of difficulties during subsequent courses, or may develop a very different psychiatric symptomatology. Those who remain free of complications during one course of steroids may develop significant problems during future courses.

G. **Preparation.** All steroid preparations may produce neuropsychiatric side effects. Even focal preparations, such as steroidal nasal sprays, have been reported to induce psychiatric symptoms.

H. **Dosage. The strongest predictor of steroid-related psychiatric syndromes is the use of 40 mg or more of prednisone or its equivalent per day.** Estimates, which are quite conservative, predict that 1% of patients receiving 40 mg or less of prednisone per day will develop neuropsychiatric complications, 5% of patients receiving 41 to 80 mg per day will develop complications, and 20% of patients receiving 81 mg or more per day will develop complications. Among patients with SLE or pemphigus who may be predisposed to steroid-related psychiatric difficulties, the risk for developing symptoms also appears to be dose-related.

I. **Dosing schedule.** Although both alternate-day dosing and divided daily dosage of glucocorticoids have been thought to reduce psychiatric adverse effects, neither schedule has proved beneficial.
   1. Alternate-day dosing of corticosteroid treatment, which has been found to reduce the incidence and severity of somatic side effects, may produce rapid mood cycling, with agitation, impulsivity, and irritability on "on" days and lethargy, withdrawal, depression, and forgetfulness on "off" days.
   2. Divided daily dosing of steroids, resulting in multiple daily doses of less than 40 mg of prednisone or its equivalent, may offer some protection against psychiatric symptomatology in patients on high-dose steroids.

J. **Duration of treatment.** The duration of glucocorticoid treatment does not appear to have a significant effect on the development of psychiatric sequelae. Some patients experience symptoms with a single steroid dose, while others remain without difficulties on extended maintenance doses.

IV. Related Neuropsychiatric Syndromes from Steroid Use

Patients who receive glucocorticoids may develop neuropsychiatric syndromes which are related to, but distinct from, the depression, mania, psychosis, or delirium induced by their use.

A. **Steroid withdrawal syndrome.** Steroid discontinuation may produce psychiatric symptoms similar to those produced by steroid administration. Depression, anhedonia, listlessness, fatigue, slowed mentation, confusion, disorientation, anorexia, agitation, and anxiety all may result from steroid withdrawal; fever, nausea, arthralgias, weakness, and desquamation of the skin also may occur. Most symptoms, which are thought to be secondary to varying degrees of hypothalamic-pituitary-adrenal (HPA)-axis suppression, physiologic and psychological dependence, and original disease recurrence, last 2 to 8 weeks and resolve spontaneously. More persistent symptoms may require steroid replacement followed by a slow taper.

B. **Steroid dependence.** Physical and psychological dependence on steroids may exist even in the absence of HPA-axis suppression. Some patients have been known to steadily increase their steroid doses in an attempt to overcome tolerance to their euphoric effects, even to the point of inducing a cushingoid status.

C. **Steroid dementia.** The acute or chronic use of corticosteroids may produce cognitive impairment (deficits in attention, concentration, memory retention, mental speed and efficiency, and occupational performance) which may be confused with dementia. Although cognitive changes usually resolve after the reduction or discontinuation of steroid use, recovery may take from 2 to 24 months.

V. Management of Neuropsychiatric Complications from Glucocorticoid Use

Proper management of psychiatric sequelae from steroid therapy involves prescribing steroid treatment as judiciously as possible, identifying potential risk factors for complications, considering prophylactic treatments, conducting serial mental status examinations, and employing different techniques to reduce emergent symptoms (Table 54-6).

A. **Steroid discontinuation.** Up to 90% of patients who develop psychiatric complications from glucocorticoid use and then have their steroids reduced or discontinued experience a full resolution of their symptoms. Patients who develop steroid withdrawal symptoms from a reduction in steroid dose usually can be managed with a temporary increase in the dose and a slower taper. Certain patients may be unable to undergo a steroid reduction secondary to severe medical disease and may require further intervention.

B. **Neuroleptics.** As many as 90% of patients with mania, psychosis, or delirium resulting from steroid use respond well to neuroleptics. Low doses of neuroleptics, equivalent to roughly 5 mg of haloperidol daily, have been reported to be effective.

C. **Electroconvulsive therapy.** Patients with severe mania or depression from glucocorticoid treatment, who often have psychotic features, respond well to electroconvulsive therapy.

Table 54-6. Treatment of Neuropsychiatric Complications	
Emergent Syndrome	*Possible Interventions*
Depression	Steroid reduction or discontinuation
	Lithium carbonate
	Antidepressants (with caution)
	Electroconvulsive therapy
Mania	Steroid reduction or discontinuation
	Lithium carbonate
	Neuroleptics
	Electroconvulsive therapy
Psychosis	Steroid reduction or discontinuation
	Neuroleptics
Delirium	Steroid reduction or discontinuation
	Neuroleptics

D. Antidepressants. Although antidepressants may be safe and effective in the treatment of depressive syndromes caused by corticosteroid use, in some cases they may exacerbate symptoms. Their use in patients who experience distinct depressive symptoms has been reported to be beneficial; their use in patients with any sign of mania, psychosis, or delirium as a component of the depressive syndrome may result in increased mania, psychosis, or confusion. Patients with worsening psychiatric symptoms on antidepressants may be treated with discontinuation of antidepressant therapy and the institution of neuroleptics at doses roughly equivalent to 15 mg of haloperidol daily.

E. Lithium carbonate. Lithium may be the most promising agent in the prevention and treatment of steroid-related psychiatric syndromes. Patients who are treated with lithium in conjunction with glucocorticoids may be less likely to develop psychiatric sequelae from the steroid use. Serum lithium levels must be monitored closely, however, as steroids can alter lithium levels by altering sodium balance. Lithium levels also may be affected by thiazide diuretics, which are commonly employed with steroid treatment.

F. Valproic acid. Although valproate may be effective in the prevention and treatment of steroid-induced psychiatric syndromes, particularly in patients who cannot tolerate or do not respond to lithium, case reports of its use are few.

Suggested Readings

Alcena, V., & Alexopoulos, G.S. (1985). Ulcerative colitis in association with chronic paranoid schizophrenia: A review of steroid-induced psychiatric disorders. *Journal of Clinical Gastroenterology, 7*, 400–404.

Boston Collaborative Drug Surveillance Program. (1972). Acute adverse reactions to prednisone in relation to dosage. *Clinical Psychopharmacology & Therapeutics, 13*, 694–698.

Brown, E.S., & Suppes, T. (1998). Mood symptoms during corticosteroid therapy: A review. *Harvard Review of Psychiatry, 5*(5), 239–246.

Falk, W.E., Mahnke, M.W., & Poskanzer, D.C. (1979). Lithium prophylaxis of corticotropin-induced psychosis. *Journal of the American Medical Association, 241,* 1011–1012.

Hall, R.C.W., Popkin, M.K., Stickney, S.K., et al. (1979). Presentation of the steroid psychosis. *Journal of Nervous and Mental Disease, 167,* 229–236.

Kahl, L. (1992). Arthritis and rheumatologic diseases. In M. Woodley, & A. Whelan (Eds.), *Manual of medical therapeutics* (27th ed.). Boston: Little, Brown, pp. 441–466.

Klein, J.F. (1992). Adverse psychiatric effects of systemic glucocorticoid therapy. *American Family Physician, 46,* 1469–1474.

Krauthammer, C., & Klerman, G.L. (1978). Secondary mania: Manic syndromes associated with antecedent physical illness or drugs. *Archives of General Psychiatry, 35*(11), 1333–1339.

Lagomasino, I.T., & Stern, T.A. (2001). Steroid psychosis: The neuropsychiatric complications of glucocorticoid use. *Medicine & Psychiatry, 4,* 35–43.

Lewis, D.A., & Smith, R.E. (1983). Steroid-induced psychiatric syndromes: A report of 14 cases and a review of the literature. *Journal of Affective Disorders, 5,* 319–332.

Ling, M.H.M., Perry, P.J., & Tsuang, M.T. (1981). Side effects of corticosteroid therapy: Psychiatric aspects. *Archives of General Psychiatry, 38,* 471–477.

Patten, S.B., & Neutel, C.I. (2000). Corticosteroid-induced adverse psychiatric effects: Incidence, diagnosis, and management. *Drug Safety, 22*(2), 111–122.

Physician's desk reference (49th ed.). (1995). Montvale, N.J.: Medical Economics Data Production Company.

Reus, V.I., & Wolkowitz, O.M. (1993). Behavioral side effects of corticosteroid therapy. *Psychiatric Annals, 23,* 703–708.

Stiefel, F.C., Breitbart, W.S., & Holland, J.C. (1989). Corticosteroids in cancer: Neuropsychiatric complications. *Cancer Investigation, 7,* 479–491.

Wada, K., Yamada, N., Sato, T., et al. (2001). Corticosteroid-induced psychiatric and mood disorders: Diagnosis defined by DSM-IV and clinical pictures. *Psychosomatics, 42*(6), 461–466.

Wada, K., Yamada, N., Suzuki, H., et al. (2000). Recurrent cases of corticosteroid-induced mood disorder: Clinical characteristics and treatment. *Journal of Clinical Psychiatry, 61*(4), 261–267.

CHAPTER 55

The Patient Receiving Psychotropics

Andrew A. Nierenberg and Andrea Kolsky

I. Introduction

Patients who take psychotropic medications need to be managed with tact and understanding. The patient's, and not just the physician's, perception of benefit must outweigh the experience of discomfort and perception of risks.

II. Explore the Meaning of Medications

The meaning of medications determines a patient's attitude toward taking the medication. A patient's attitude especially affects how psychotropic medication is taken, and it can ultimately affect outcome. It can be useful to ask "What is it like for you to take medication for your problem?" By elucidating dysfunctional attitudes about medication, the physician can correct misperceptions and help the patient feel understood.

A. Dysfunctional attitudes about medication

1. **Medication is a symbol and cause of defect.** Several beliefs along these lines can be elucidated.
   a. Taking medication means that something is fundamentally wrong with the patient as a person.
   b. Taking medication will create change so that they will no longer be the same person.
   c. Taking medication means that the individual is morally weak; instead, one should be able to take care of one's own problems.
   d. Taking medication is a crutch for "real problems" and should be stopped as soon as possible.
2. Medication is addictive. Along these lines several patients' **concerns about control may be manifest:**
   a. "If I need this medication, isn't that just like getting addicted?"
   b. "I don't want to have to take this medication."
   c. "The medication is going to control me."
   d. "I'm going to have to take this medication forever."
   These **negative meanings of medication-use lead to understandable non-compliance.** Rather than getting annoyed with patients, physicians can be helpful by educating patients and their family members about alternative meanings of medication.

B. Helpful alternative meanings of medication

1. Medication as a method to control a disorder
   a. Just as antihypertensive drugs control hypertension, so too can medication control psychiatric disorders and their symptoms, and reduce the likelihood of future adverse consequences.
   b. The medication can control symptoms and give patients more control over their lives.
   c. The medication can lift the burden of symptoms, make it easier to cope with stress, and improve functioning.

III. Explore the Meaning of the Diagnosis

No matter what the psychiatric diagnosis, people give meaning to their own diagnoses.

A. Even with limited time in a general medical practice, **simple and direct questions can lead to understanding and, ultimately, to better management.** Several questions can be asked to uncover the meaning of the illness to the patient.

    1. "What is it like for you to be told that you have [psychiatric diagnosis]?"

    2. "What does having [psychiatric diagnosis] mean to you?"

B. Alternatively, patients will have their own questions.

    1. "Why did I get [psychiatric disorder]?"

    2. "Did I do anything to cause this to happen to me?"

    3. "Will this be passed on to my children?"

    4. "What is my prognosis?"

    5. "How long will I need to take this medication?"

IV. Educate both Patient and Family

Useful information can be provided to the individual with the disorder.

A. We do not know the exact causes of [psychiatric disorder], but we do know that it has something to do with brain chemistry.

B. Medication and therapy can control the disorder, something like the use of antihypertensive medications for high blood pressure. Medication, exercise, and a healthy diet all contribute to help control high blood pressure. With [psychiatric disorder], medication, therapy, and stress reduction can all help.

C. Medication has to be taken as prescribed for it to be most effective. With some psychiatric disorders, side effects may appear before the benefit is achieved.

V. Track Target Symptoms

A. For each psychiatric disorder, one should track the course of the most important symptoms.

B. Consider using appropriate and validated self-report scales to quantify severity and measure improvement.

C. Systematically record the severity and the change in symptoms at each visit.

D. Ask patients if, since the last visit, they feel overall the same, better, or worse.

E. Document changes and the reasons for changes in the use of medications.

F. Meet as frequently as needed, usually more frequently at the beginning of a trial of medication, then decreasing the frequency as the patient improves and stabilizes. Make sure that the patient knows you are available by phone between visits. If the patient calls, record briefly the conversation and decide if the patient needs to be scheduled for an earlier than scheduled appointment.

VI. Track Side Effects

A. Ask simple and direct questions and briefly record the patient's responses.

    1. Do you feel [physically] differently in any way since our last visit?

    2. Do you have any new or troubling symptoms?

3. Have your side effects that were troublesome become better or worse?
   a. Antidepressants (see Chapter 66)
   b. Antianxiety agents
   Note: Be especially cautious with patients who drive and take benzodiazepines. Warn them that their driving could be impaired and that they should not drive if they feel that their coordination is not normal.
   c. Mood Stabilizers (see Chapter 21)
   d. Antipsychotics

VII. Track Compliance

A. Since at least half of all patients alter the way that they take their medications, it can be useful to **acknowledge the difficulty of taking medication every day.** Tell patients that if they are unable to take the medication regularly, you would like them to discuss that with you to explore alternative schedules that may make it less burdensome.
   1. Use q.d. or b.i.d. dosing when possible.
   2. If a patient is taking multiple drugs, have him or her take those drugs at the same time.

B. Track blood levels of selected medications. Limited data exist for only a few psychotropic medication blood levels.
   1. Antidepressants
   2. Antianxiety agents
   3. Mood stabilizers
   4. Antipsychotics

C. Inform patients about the need for long-term treatment to keep them well after they respond acutely (e.g., from depression, bipolar disorder, generalized anxiety disorder, or schizophrenia).

VIII. Track Stressors

A. Patients experience psychiatric disorders as a stress in and of itself. Alternatively, other stressors can exacerbate the psychiatric disorder. **Ongoing external stress will cause the psychiatric disorder to persist and may lead to non-response to medication.**
   1. Explore relationship, occupational, and financial sources of stress.
   2. Help the patient locate resources to solve these problems.

IX. Involve Family Members

Meet with both the family and the patient to discuss the diagnosis, benefits, and risks of psychotropic medication, and to track both improvement and side effects. Refer to support groups where available. Above all, listen to both the patient and the family members.

X. Negotiate Changes in Medication with Collaborative Empiricism

A. Negotiate with the patient over negotiable issues.
   1. Negotiate the speed of dose increases (e.g., how fast should the target dose be reached?)

2. Negotiate changes in the times the patient takes medication (e.g., morning, evening, and in-between; with or without meals).

3. Negotiate goals of treatment-improvement vs. back to pre-morbid self.

4. Negotiate an acceptable balance between benefits and side effects: does the patient feel that the benefit makes the side effects tolerable?

5. Negotiate prohibitions or restrictions of alcohol and drug use while taking psychotropic medications.

B. **Collaborative empiricism involves working together to see what works best.**

1. Inter-individual variation makes it difficult to predict exactly how well a patient will do with each psychotropic medication.

2. **Tell the patient that you have a reasonable idea what to expect from the medication but feedback from them and from their families is essential so that you and they can make the best decisions together.**

XI. Maintain a Non-judgmental Stance

Some physicians have a tendency to judge a patient who takes psychotropic medications. Because patients view physicians as authority figures, **physician attitudes and subtle communications of those attitudes can influence a patient profoundly.** A patient may fear judgment of non-compliance and, as a result, conceal problems that he or she has had with taking the medication as prescribed. A patient may want to please the physician by overstating improvement and understating side effects. It can be helpful when physicians explore their own feelings about prescribing psychotropic medications and clarify their understanding of the boundary between an individual patient's responsibility for his or her behavior and the influence of the psychiatric disorder. Inappropriate negative judgment can be minimized by using stress-diathesis and genetic-environmental models of psychiatric disorders.

XII. Track Relevant Medical Parameters

Like all medications, psychotropic drugs can have effects on physiological systems, such that certain tests should be obtained at baseline (to ensure safety) and then tracked (for those medications that can perturb those systems).

A. **Start doses low and gradually titrate as needed.**

B. **Monitor for withdrawal after discontinuation.**

C. **Monitor for drug–drug and drug–food interactions.**

D. **Prescribe limited numbers of pills and gradually increase when the patient become stable.**

1. Give 3 to 7 days' worth of samples, when available, along with a 1- to 2-week prescription initially.

2. Give 1- to 2-month supplies when starting long-term treatment when appropriate.

3. Give 3- to 6-month supplies for patients on maintenance treatments.

One word of caution: Some medications (e.g., tricyclic antidepressants) can be fatal if a 2-week supply is taken as an overdose. Always check for suicidal ideation; if present and the patient can be managed as an outpatient, prescribe very limited amounts of medication and meet with the patient more frequently.

E. **Use polypharmacy when necessary.**

Suggested Readings

Conrad, P. (1985). The meaning of medications: Another look at compliance. *Social Science & Medicine, 20,* 29–37.

Fisher, R., & Ury, W. (1991). *Getting to yes: Negotiating agreement without giving in* (2nd ed.). Boston: Houghton Mifflin.

Katz, J. (1984). *The silent world of doctor and patient.* New York: Free Press.

CHAPTER 56

The Patient Following a Traumatic Event

RAFAEL ORNSTEIN

I. Introduction

A. Definition

1. According to the *DSM-IV,* **a traumatic event involves "actual or threatened death or serious injury or a threat to the physical integrity of self or other."** Examples of trauma include the following:

    a. Exposure to military combat, violent assault (including rape and robbery), domestic violence, automobile accidents, childhood physical and sexual abuse or neglect, natural disasters, and sudden catastrophic medical illnesses

    b. Witnessing a traumatic event

    c. Being told about a trauma experienced by a loved one

2. Traumatic events are associated with experiences of overwhelming fear and helplessness. Because of the intensity of feelings associated with a traumatic event, perception of the event may be distorted; it may be experienced as fragments of sensations, time may be slowed or accelerated, feelings may be dissociated from the events as they are occurring, and there can be varying degrees of amnesia for all or part of the traumatic event.

II. Responses to Traumatic Stress

A. Acute and long-term responses to traumatic events are varied and multi-determined. Nearly every person can be expected to have some disruption in their mental functioning following a significantly traumatic event (i.e., a "normal" stress response). On average, most people are able to adapt following a traumatic event and return to their previous level of functioning, with or without some chronic symptoms. When the symptoms following a trauma impair functioning they often appear as syndromes, labeled in the *DSM-IV* as **acute stress disorder and post-traumatic stress disorder (PTSD).** Chronic exposure to trauma or trauma occurring in childhood can produce long-lasting personality disturbances. It is also common for traumatic events to cause psychiatric morbidity without meeting criteria for these syndromes; following a traumatic event individuals are at higher risk for depression, anxiety, somatoform disorders, and substance abuse.

1. The psychological disruption following a traumatic event takes the form of alternating states of mind; the person is overwhelmed with thoughts, feelings, or images of the trauma, along with states of numbness, denial, and avoidance.

    a. Trauma can present clinically as an extremely **labile mood,** tearfulness, and despair, alternating with a sense that the trauma "didn't really happen" or that "nothing feels real."

    b. A patient can appear "spacey" and **inattentive, or hypervigilant** and prone to startle. The individual can be oblivious to the consequences of the event or preoccupied with the trauma.

    c. **Traumatic memories have an intrusive quality;** they are unbidden and feel uncontrollable. They can intrude as **nightmares,** which are repetitive and disruptive to sleep. Memories can impair daily functioning and may be so vivid that patients feel as if they are re-occurring in the present, a so-called **flashback.** Traumatic memories are easily triggered by environmental cues that are associated with the traumatic event. Physiological arousal may occur with reminders of the trauma, involving intense feelings of fear, rapid palpitations, profuse sweating, and shortness of breath. Frequently a traumatized person will be concerned that he or she is "going crazy."

    d. Patients may attempt to avoid memories of the trauma. This can lead to an avoidance of talking and thinking about the trauma and avoidance of any environmental triggers. There may be a constriction of mood and affect as intense feelings of any kind can precipitate a traumatic recollection. Often patients feel detached and estranged from others and isolate themselves, even from close friends and family. There may be a feeling that "life has lost its meaning," and a feeling that the future is limited.

    e. Patients may complain of a set of symptoms related to an overall feeling of increased arousal; sleep is disrupted and there can be marked irritability and uncharacteristic outbursts of anger. Concentration and attention can be impaired.

    f. Under normal circumstances, intrusive preoccupations and avoidant behaviors resolve as individuals come to terms with the trauma and adapt to its consequences. Consistent themes emerge as patients confront the reality of the trauma, such as fear of re-traumatization, shame, humiliation, and helplessness. Frequently victims blame themselves as a way to maintain a feeling of control. Feelings of intense rage are common and can be overwhelming.

2. An **acute stress disorder** is diagnosed, according to *DSM-IV,* if the characteristic trauma response causes clinically significant impairment that lasts at least 2 days, persists up to 4 weeks, and occurs within 4 weeks of the traumatic experience. The features of an acute stress disorder include the following:

    a. Exposure to a traumatic event

    b. At least three of the following dissociative symptoms: (1) a sense of numbness and detachment, (2) being in a daze, (3) a feeling that one is unreal, (4) a feeling that one's environment is not real, and (5) an inability to remember important aspects of the trauma

    c. Intrusive re-experiencing of the trauma

    d. Avoidance of stimuli that lead to recollection of the trauma

    e. Symptoms of increased arousal and anxiety

3. The diagnosis of **PTSD** is made, according to *DSM-IV,* when the characteristic trauma response causes clinically significant impairment and lasts more than 1 month. The diagnosis is made on the basis of intrusive re-experiencing of the trauma, avoidance, numbing, and symptoms of hyperarousal. The disorder is considered **acute** if the symptoms have lasted less than 3 months and **chronic** if the symptoms last for more than 3 months. The onset of PTSD can be **delayed** if symptoms emerge after 6 months following a traumatic event.

4. **Disorders of Extreme Stress Not Otherwise Specified.** Children exposed to physical or sexual abuse or adults exposed to prolonged and repeated trauma may develop long-standing problems in psychological and interpersonal functioning. There can be difficulty tolerating feelings, especially the management of anger, leading to impulsive behavior. Dissociation, self-destructive behavior, and suicidal ideation are not uncommon. There may be attachments to powerful and abusive figures. New relationships may be difficult to form, as these persons can feel an intense need for

closeness but also fear being controlled or abandoned. There is a diminished sense of agency and a passive and helpless stance toward the world. Somatization is common. These patients are at risk to be repeatedly victimized.

B. Epidemiology

1. There is a 1–12% lifetime risk for developing PTSD in community samples.
2. Of those persons exposed to traumatic events, approximately 20% develop significant difficulties. For victims of rape and war veterans with combat experience, lifetime risk for developing PTSD begins around 30% and reaches 90% for brutalized prisoners of war.
3. An acute stress disorder puts a patient at risk for, but does not invariably lead to, PTSD. Those patients with PTSD may or may not have suffered from the acute disorder.

III. Evaluation Immediately Following a Traumatic Event

A. Immediately following a traumatic event the initial goal should be to help the patient regain a sense of mastery and control. Most people adapt to traumatic events without professional help. The intervention should focus on helping the patient face the reality of the traumatic event, identify useful coping skills, access social and community supports, and anticipate the characteristic symptoms that follow a traumatic event. Often a thorough and thoughtful evaluation can be the beginning of an effective intervention and provide an opportunity to assess the need for ongoing care. During the evaluation the physician should keep in mind that although the traumatic aspects of an event may appear self-evident, it is helpful to establish the personal meaning that the trauma has for the patient. It is important to identify what the patient hopes to gain from the encounter with the physician. An evaluation should include and be guided by the following principles:

1. **Rapport should be established with the patient.** Acknowledging the seriousness of the traumatic event, offering condolences if appropriate, and following usual social customs can set the patient at ease.
2. **Attention should be paid to the practical and immediate concerns** brought about by the traumatic event. The physical and medical status of the patient and any other victims should be evaluated. The availability of basic human necessities, such as food, shelter, and safety should also be established.
3. **Respect the patient's choice of whether or not to talk about the traumatic event**. Follow the patient's lead. Patients may "seal over" and appear detached from events; this should not be deliberately disrupted in a brief, one-time encounter. However the patient should be encouraged to talk about the events with the clinician and friends and family—when he or she is ready to do so.
4. A brief survey of the **patient's mental status** is important to determine if the patient can safely manage with currently available support. It is not uncommon for patients to either be overwhelmed with emotion or feel detached and numb. Patients can become markedly disorganized or surprisingly controlled. Suicidally-prone behavior should be monitored.
5. **The patient should be allowed to review the trauma and surrounding events.** The patient may share his or her feelings about the trauma, including feelings of helplessness, guilt, shame, and anger. Inquire about what specific actions were taken or not taken by the patient or others that could have affected the outcome of the traumatic event. **Identify the aspect of the trauma that was most distressing to the patient.**

Pay careful attention to the patient's ability to tolerate the telling of the story. The patient's characteristic coping style must be respected. It is important for patients to have a sense of control over the pace and intensity of the interview and at the same time for the physician to offer overwhelmed patients a sense of direction and structure.

6. **Risk factors** associated with the development of PTSD should be assessed. The stressor is the most important risk factor; sudden, severe, prolonged trauma, intentionally inflicted and intended to humiliate, puts the victim at risk for PTSD. Social support following an event is a critical variable in an individual's response. Previous trauma, low intelligence, and prior psychiatric history, especially conduct disorder, antisocial and narcissistic personality disorders, put patients at risk for PTSD.

7. **Know the patient's strengths** and customary manner of managing stress.

8. **Assess whether a patient is at risk for ongoing victimization.** For instance, the physician should be aware that spousal abuse is a common problem in all socioeconomic groups. A concerned but non-judgmental manner is crucial in allowing a victim of domestic violence to tell her story.

IV. Treatment Immediately Following a Traumatic Event

A. **The primary care provider should do the following things:**

1. **Maintain a calm, empathic, and hopeful attitude,** which can have a powerful effect on the patient immediately after a traumatic event. While acknowledging the profoundly disruptive effect of the trauma on the patient, the physician can also underline the fact that the patient is a survivor.

2. **Convey whatever information is known about the traumatic event to the patient.** Having the facts on hand can help the patient organize chaotic and confusing feelings.

3. **Tolerate the patient's feelings and help put them into context.** It can be greatly reassuring for a patient to know that feelings of fear, helplessness, guilt, shame, and anger are expectable responses to a traumatic event. The patient may need to be reassured that he or she is not "going crazy."

4. **Educate patients about the common responses to trauma,** which can help them feel more in control of their experiences. Patients should be told that they may experience insomnia, nightmares, intrusive memories, and irritability in the first few months or so after the trauma, but these symptoms should then begin to subside.

5. **Educate patients about possible maladaptive responses to trauma.** Alcohol abuse and other substance abuse are common as patients attempt to manage hyperarousal and intrusive symptoms.

6. **Review how the patient has managed crises in the past and help the patient recall and revitalize those strengths.** Following a trauma, patients frequently lose sight of previously attained coping mechanisms. Fatigue, terror, and loss may predispose patients to less adaptive ways of negotiating with the world. It can be helpful for the physician to focus on concrete tasks that may be facing the patient. For cases involving interpersonal traumatization, such as with a battered woman, the physician may need to help the patient consider and then access the legal system. Patients who face persistent threat should be encouraged to write out a "safety plan" that details concrete steps the patient will take to avoid future traumatization. These steps may include involving local law enforcement authorities. The physician can encourage the patient to take steps to protect himself or herself, but ultimately it is the patient who must make that decision.

7. **Encourage the patient to use existing supports.** Although the patient may feel ashamed and reluctant to call on friends or family, the physician may need to encourage those contacts. Frequently the patient's social network, family, friends, and wider community play an important role in recovery from trauma.

8. **Encourage the patient to return to his or her usual routine as soon as is reasonably possible.**

9. **Use medication sparingly.** There is no long-term benefit from heavily sedating patients following a trauma. Severe anxiety, agitation, and insomnia may be treated with benzodiazepines, such as lorazepam (Ativan) at doses of 1 mg b.i.d. and h.s. Supplies should be given for not more than several days and are contraindicated in patients with a history of alcohol or substance abuse.

10. **Schedule a follow-up office visit or phone call after a traumatic event.** It is helpful to orient the patient toward the future; it is reassuring to the patient not to feel alone in the process of recovery.

11. **Tell the patient that a referral to a psychiatrist or other mental health professional is available.** Patients with underlying psychiatric illness should be referred directly to a psychiatrist. Patients with a history of PTSD or a history of trauma should be monitored for difficulty in functioning. Patients who have suffered severe, intentional trauma, such as rape or domestic abuse, should have a follow-up appointment for psychological counseling. Patients whose symptoms persist or become debilitating will also require a referral. Be aware that recent research findings suggest that following a traumatic event, specific cognitive-behavioral therapies may help prevent the development of PTSD. Consult with a local mental health specialist to access such services, if available.

V. Evaluation and Treatment Weeks to Months Following a Traumatic Event

A. **It is very difficult to predict how an individual will respond to a traumatic event over time.** Some people have severe symptoms soon after the trauma, but go on to adapt very well. Some individuals do seemingly well after a trauma, but later develop PTSD months or even years after the event. An earlier trauma can leave a person vulnerable to the effects of a subsequent one. For example, a patient may do well following a car accident, despite suffering injuries, but then years later may develop a debilitating array of post-traumatic symptoms following a minor accident.

B. The time course of the patient's symptoms has important clinical implications. Symptoms may cause clinically significant impairment in the first month, as acute stress disorder, or in the following 2 months as PTSD. About half of patients will improve and return to an acceptable level of functioning, with some residual symptoms; the rest will go on to have chronic PTSD. After 3 to 4 months and definitely by 6 to 8 months PTSD is a chronic psychiatric illness.

C. Weeks to months following a traumatic event it is important to evaluate how the patient is adapting and to determine the extent of his or her post-traumatic symptoms.

1. Offer the patient an opportunity to recount the traumatic event, if not already done so, with the physician. It is important to allow the patient to modulate the telling of the story; it is not necessarily therapeutic for a patient to simply "get all of the feelings out." It is useful to note how much or how little the patient is able to talk about the

traumatic event. Ideally, the patient will find some relief in being able to talk about the event, and therefore, repeated tellings may have a therapeutic value. Some patients may be so overwhelmed they think or speak of nothing else; others may be so overwhelmed that they are not able to speak of the trauma at all.

2. Review the symptoms of PTSD with the patient and assess the severity and extent of the patient's symptoms. Are there intrusive symptoms, such as nightmares and flashbacks? How frequently? How does the patient manage thoughts and feelings about the trauma? Are there significant attempts to avoid these thoughts and feelings? Patients may not complain directly of feeling numb and detached, but these symptoms can be disabling. Does the patient have hyperarousal with hypervigilance, insomnia, and an exaggerated startle response?

3. Evaluate the patient's overall psychological, social, and occupational functioning. Has the patient been able to resume his or her usual activities? Is there inordinate difficulty in resuming routine activities that the patient associates with the trauma? How is the patient relating to family and friends? Is there an increase in social isolation or a feeling of alienation?

4. Formulate a differential diagnosis, as several psychiatric illnesses share characteristics of PTSD. Psychotic disorders, major depressive and bipolar affective disorders, other anxiety disorders, and factitious illnesses may present with symptoms that overlap or mimic PTSD.

5. Screen and treat the patient for co-morbid psychiatric illnesses that can complicate treatment and recovery.
   a. Alcohol abuse and other substance abuse
   b. Major depressive disorder
   c. Somatoform disorders
   d. Dissociative disorders
   e. Eating disorders associated with childhood sexual or physical abuse
   f. Other anxiety disorders

6. Anticipate that if a court case is pending, the patient's condition may remain static or deteriorate until the case is resolved. Increasingly, PTSD is being implicated in court cases involving personal injury claims. Even in cases where the diagnosis of PTSD is clear-cut, legal involvement complicates recovery.

7. Evaluate for ongoing traumatization. PTSD may leave patients less able to discriminate between threatening and non-threatening situations, leading to re-victimization.

C. **The treatment approach for patients, weeks to months following a traumatic event,** is similar to the one immediately following a trauma; establish rapport, review the traumatic event, educate the patient about the characteristic trauma response, and involve social and community supports. Critical treatment goals at this stage include helping the patient cope with post-traumatic symptoms, treating co-morbid conditions, and evaluating the need for referral to a mental health professional.

1. Monitor the intensity and frequency of the intrusive symptoms and take note of any stimuli that worsen or improve them. Avoidant symptoms need to be addressed directly; for instance, a patient who has been in a car accident may need ongoing, stepwise encouragement to return to driving. Outbursts of anger may need to be anticipated and actively controlled.

2. Medicate specific symptoms that interfere with functioning. Medication can help diminish the symptoms of PTSD and can play an important role in a comprehensive

treatment plan that includes social, psychological, and behavioral interventions. Treatment can be initiated with a selective serotonin reuptake inhibitor (SSRI), and other medications can be added as the patient's symptoms require. Depending on the treating physician's experience with psychopharmacology, he or she may want to refer to, or consult with, a psychiatrist if an initial SSRI trial is not adequate to relieve the patient's symptoms. A common combination of medication includes an SSRI, trazodone for sleep, and an anti-adrenergic for hyperarousal.

a. SSRIs are first-line treatment and have been found to be the most helpful in treating the intrusive, avoidant and hyperarousal symptoms of PTSD. Sertraline (Zoloft) 50-200 mg per day and paroxetine (Paxil) 20-60 mg, per day has been FDA-approved for PTSD, but fluoxetine, (Prozac) 20 mg per day and fluvoxamine (Luvox) 100-300 mg per day also appear helpful. Tricyclic antidepressants (TCAs) are somewhat helpful for intrusive symptoms and insomnia. Nefazodone (Serzone) 300-500 mg is frequently used although rigorous studies are pending. Venlafaxine (Effexor XR) 75-225 mg per day is also used though it has not been studied.

b. Anti-adrenergics, such as propranolol (Inderal) 20 to 60 mg per day, clonidine (Catapres) 0. 1 to 0.2 mg b.i.d. or h.s., or guanfacine (Tenex) 1 to 3 mg per day can be helpful with intrusive symptoms, especially nightmares.

c. Clonazepam (Klonopin), lorazepam (Ativan), or other benzodiazepines can be helpful for hyperarousal. Caution is advised in using these medications because tolerance and abuse are common complications. They are best used during episodes of acute distress. The use of benzodiazepines in patients with a history of alcohol or other substance abuse is contraindicated.

d. If insomnia is a persistent problem, trazodone (Desyrel) 50 to 100 mg or TCAs, such as doxepin (Sinequan) 25 to 50 mg or amitriptyline (Elavil) 25 to 50 mg h.s., can be helpful.

e. If mood lability or anger outbursts are particularly distressing, a trial of the anticonvulsants, valproic acid (Depakote) or carbamazepine (Tegretol), with therapeutic blood levels, may stabilize these symptoms.

f. Neuroleptics are not generally used in the treatment of PTSD. However, if the patient is prone to disorganized episodes of near psychotic levels, low-dose antipsychotic medication can be used and then discontinued as soon as possible. Risperidone (Risperdal) 0.5 to 2.0 mg per day is sufficient.

3. Co-morbid psychiatric conditions should be treated.

4. A referral to a mental health professional should be considered if the patient's symptoms become debilitating or persistent. Psychiatric treatment for PTSD involves social, psychological, behavioral, and pharmacological interventions. Cognitive-behavioral therapies, such as anxiety management, cognitive therapy, exposure therapy and psychoeducation, have been found to be the most effective psychotherapeutic tools and are often used in some combination. Psychotherapeutic approaches may include the following modalities:

a. Anxiety management (stress inoculation training) teaches patients techniques to cope with anxiety. These may include relaxation training, breathing exercises, assertiveness training, and thought-stopping.

b. Cognitive therapy focuses on identifying and changing underlying beliefs and automatic thoughts that may lead to overwhelming feelings. Common thoughts may include irrational guilt, a sense of personal failure, and a fear of losing control.

c. Exposure therapy helps the patient face the events, triggers, and memories that have become connected with the trauma and now bring up overwhelming fear. Patients are exposed to triggers either through mental exercises or real-life confrontations. Repeated exposures help patients learn to master their fear. It is a very effective treatment modality if patients can tolerate it.

    d. Psychoeducation involves teaching patients and families about the common responses to trauma.

    e. Psychodynamic psychotherapy may identify and address maladaptive patterns of adaptation. The patient's traumatic memory is modified by constructing a narrative of the event which allows for mastery of overwhelming feelings.

    f. Eye movement desentization and re-processing (EMDR) is a popular technique that involves patients silently recounting traumatic events while attending to rapidly alternating stimuli, such as a therapists hand moving back and forth. A controversial treatment, proponents claim a profound modification of traumatic memories; critics say the data is not yet conclusive.

    g. Group treatment can be helpful in providing social support and solutions to the problems that survivors face.

VI. Evaluation and Treatment Months to Years Following a Traumatic Event

A. Adaptation to trauma takes place over time. Individuals may be able to return to functioning and yet still bear invisible scars. For some there may be underlying depression or circumscribed phobias. Others, however, can successfully master and integrate the experience into their lives leading, at times, to personal growth. Even months or years later, new challenges or setbacks can trigger traumatic memories and feelings for survivors. Of particular relevance for primary care physicians PCPs, these patients may experience an emergence of trauma-related feelings in the context of their medical care. A patient with a childhood history of sexual abuse may become anxious at the time of a physical exam and fear being re-traumatized. Invasive procedures may be experienced by the patient as a replay of an abusive past. In these situations clinicians should gently inquire about a history of trauma and work with the patient so that he or she can feel more in control of the exam or procedure.

B. Chronic PTSD is a complex psychiatric illness. In almost all cases there are co-morbid psychiatric disorders. Ongoing re-traumatization is common and needs to be addressed before any improvement can be expected. Patients with debilitating, chronic PTSD should be referred to a mental health professional for comprehensive treatment. Treatment is helpful when it begins by addressing the patient's current life stressors and works to help the patient regain control of daily living.

C. Screening for PTSD. Patients often present without a complaint directly related to being traumatized and PTSD can be difficult to diagnose. Whenever an evaluation for anxiety or depression is indicated a brief trauma history should also be obtained; ask the patient if they have been assaulted, threatened, or otherwise exposed to traumatic events. Explore whether they have symptoms associated with PTSD. Inquiring about trauma should be done tactfully in a non-judgmental manner.

Suggested Readings

American Psychiatric Association. (1994). *Diagnostic and statistical manual of mental disorders* (4th ed.). Washington, DC: American Psychiatric Association, pp. 424–432.

Foa, E.B., Davidson, J.R.T., & Frances, A. (Eds.). (1999). The expert consensus guideline series: Treatment of posttraumatic stress disorder. *Journal of Clinical Psychiatry, 60*(suppl 16).

Foa, E.B., & Jaycox, L.H. (1999). Cognitive-behavioral treatments of posttraumatic stress disorder. In D. Speigal (Ed.), *Psychotherapeutic frontiers: New principles and practices.* Washington, D.C.: American Psychiatric Press, pp. 23–61.

Foa, E.B., Keane, T.C., & Friedman, M. (Eds.). (2000). *Effective treatments for PTSD: Practice guidelines from the International Society for Traumatic Stress Studies.* New York: Guilford Press.

Friedman, M.J. (1998). Current and future drug treatment for post-traumatic stress disorder patients. *Psychiatric Annals, 28,* 461–468.

Herman, J.L. (1993). Sequelae of prolonged and repeated trauma: Evidence for a complex post-traumatic syndrome (DESNOS). In J.R.T. Davidson, & E.B. Foa (Eds.), *Posttraumatic Stress Disorder. DSM-IV and beyond.* Washington, DC: American Psychiatric Press, pp. 213–228.

Horowitz, M.J. (1986). *Stress response syndromes.* Northvale, NJ: Jason Aronson.

Lange, J., Lange, C., & Cabatica, R. (2000). Primary care treatment of Post-Traumatic Stress Disorder. *American Family Physician, 62,* 1035–1040, 1046.

Mannar, C.R., Foy, D., Kagan, B., et al. (1993). An integrated approach for treating post-traumatic stress. In J.M. Oldham, M.B. Riba, & A. Tasman (Eds.), *Review of psychiatry, vol. 12.* Washington, DC: American Psychiatric Press, pp. 239–273.

Marshall, R.D., Beebe, K.L., Oldham, M., & Zaninelli, R. (2001). Efficacy and safety of paroxetine treatment for chronic PTSD: A fixed dose placebo-controlled study. *American Journal of Psychiatry, 158*(12), 1982–1988.

Meichenbaum, D. (1994). *A clinical handbook practical therapist manual for assessing and treating Post-Traumatic Stress Disorder.* Waterloo, Ontario: Institute Press.

Tomb, D.A., & Allen, S.N. (1994). Phenomenology of Posttraumatic Stress Disorder. *Psychiatric Clinics of North America, 17*(2), 237–250.

van der Kolk, B., McFarlane, A.C., & Weisaeth, L. (Eds.). (1996). *Traumatic stress.* New York: Guilford Press.

Wilson, J.P., Friedman, M.J., & Lindy, J. (Eds.). *Treating psychological trauma and PTSD.* New York: Guilford Press.

CHAPTER 57

The Patient Who Has Been Sexually Assaulted

ADELE C. VIGUERA AND PATRICIA MIAN

I. Introduction

A. Overview

1. **Rape is a legal term** rather than a medical diagnosis. Rape should be considered a **criminal act** with wide-ranging medical, psychological, legal, and social sequelae.
2. **The legal definition of rape varies by state,** but in general, the criteria for rape include lack of consent, use of threat of force, and any non-consensual contact involving the breasts, genitals, or anus with or without penetration.
3. **Any person, male or female, and any child of either gender can be considered a rape victim.**
4. **In general, hospital providers are not mandated reporters, and it is the patient's decision to report an assault to the police.** However, in certain situations, such as an assault involving an elder or a minor, providers are mandated to report the abuse.

II. Epidemiology

A. Incidence

1. **Rape is a violent crime with an increasing prevalence** and is part of a culture that is fraught with violence against women. The lifetime risk of rape or attempted rape among women in the United States varies from 2% to nearly 50% of all women. Most estimates fall between 13% and 25%. Only 50% of rapes are reported to legal authorities.
2. The incidence of male rape is not known. **Male sexual assault victims generally do not seek medical or legal help.** The care of men who have been sexually assaulted should follow the general guidelines for female victims except for the reference for gynecologic care. There are limited data that suggest that the psychological reactions of men to trauma are strikingly similar to those of women.
3. Research on violence against women shows a number of consistent patterns. **A woman is four times more likely to be assaulted by someone she knows than by a stranger.** The assailant is typically a male, most often a male intimate. This holds true for both sexual assault and physical assault and holds across ethnic groups and for both urban and rural populations.

III. Etiology

A. Evolutionary Theory

1. The causes of violence against women are multi-factorial and arise from interactions of biological, psychosocial, and social processes. Evolutionary theory posits that males who have difficulty obtaining partners are more likely to resort to sexual coercion or rape.

B. Neurophysiologic Theories

1. Physiologic and neurophysiologic correlates of violence include alterations in the functioning of neurotransmitters, such as serotonin, dopamine, norepinephrine, acetylcholine, and gamma-aminobutyric acid, which may interfere with cognition and or behavior.

C. Personality Theories

1. Studies have found a high incidence of psychopathology and personality disorders (most frequently antisocial personality disorder) among sexual offenders. In particular, distinctive personality profiles have been reported for rapists. These men typically are impulsive, self-centered, poorly educated and have low-status occupations. Rapists also tend to be hostile, resentful, and interpersonally alienated. Most investigators, however, have concluded that there is heterogenity among rapists and that sexual aggression is multi-determined.

2. **In most cases the motivation of the rapist appears to be related to issues of control, power, degradation and dominance of the victim** rather than the achievement of sexual relations that are not otherwise available.

IV. Evaluation of the Problem

A. The Clinician's Approach to the Sexual Assault Patient

1. The majority of sexual assault patients are evaluated in the emergency room setting, which is in general well equipped to manage such cases. Many emergency departments have a standardized kit for the collection of sexual assault evidence. Because of the complex implications of sexual assault, the patient requires medical care, collection of specimens for use as forensic evidence, and psychological support. Treatment of the victim should address physical injuries, pregnancy prophylaxis, sexually-transmitted diseases, and psychosocial sequelae.

   In general, the physical examination and the collection of evidence are performed by a gynecologist or an emergency department attending physician. Sexual Assault Nurse Examiner programs have been established in various areas of the country where certified nurses provide forensic evidence collection and expertise. Psychological support often is provided by a skilled nurse, clinical nurse specialist, or psychiatrist. The degree of psychological intervention is determined by the patient's needs.

2. **Sexual assault patients who come to the emergency department want emotional support, help in regaining a sense of control, and reassurance regarding their physical safety.** Clinicians must approach these patients in a manner that addresses these needs.

3. Since these patients often are frightened, it is important for them to know that they are safe and protected.

4. It is helpful for providers to begin to return a measure of autonomy and control to these patients. This can be done by explaining to the patient what to expect during the collection of evidence and during the physical exam.

5. It is helpful to have the patient identify his or her needs, mobilize support systems, and solve problems; each of these approaches reinforces self-esteem.

6. Since the patient will be faced with multiple decisions, such as who to tell about the incident, whether to press charges, and where to stay to feel safe, the clinician should provide the patient with as much information as possible to help the patient make the appropriate decisions.

V. Examination of the Patient

A. Documentation and Collection of Evidence

1. **Document briefly but accurately.**

   a. One clinician preferably, at the time of evidence collection, should document the circumstances of the assault, being sure to include the physical surroundings, the presence of threats (verbal or implied) and force, trauma, weapons, resistance, sexual acts, history of penetration and/or ejaculation, and penetration with objects or body parts. **One should use the patient's own words (quotations) when possible.** It is not generally recommended that one documents a description of the assailant or the time and length of the assault because inaccurate information could be used against the victim in court.

   b. **Do not include unnecessary social history or details** which are not relevant to the medical treatment or the legal documentation of the assault.

   c. **Make the chief complaint read "chief complaint of sexual assault,"** Don't use the word "*alleged*" which may be misconstrued in court. Alleged is a legal term, not a medical term **(Table 57-1)**.

2. **Collect the evidence. Data gathering should be accurate and thorough, since the medical record may be used as criminal evidence in court.** Most hospitals have protocols for evidence collection, and many states are developing standardized evidence collection kits. **Evidence collection** may include the following:

   a. Clothing and debris.

   b. Fingernail scrapings.

   c. Head hair sample and combing.

   d. Pubic hair sample and combing.

   e. Smears for sperm and/or acid phosphatase from any orifice involved (vaginal, oral, rectal). All specimens should be placed in a sealed paper container and given to the appropriate law enforcement agency, following the proper legal chain of evidence. With the patient's permission, photographs can be taken to further document physical trauma. When completed, the evidence must be secured according to the emergency department's protocol.

Table 57-1. Sexual Assault Documentation

1. Document the description of the event concisely
2. Document the physical and emotional trauma related to the assault
3. Use direct quotations from the patient
4. Write clearly
5. Do not provide a detailed description of the assailant
6. Do not provide irrelevant social details
7. Do not document perjorative information
8. Do not use judgmental language
   a. Instead of *alleged*, use *reported*
   b. Instead of *refused*, use *declined*
   c. Instead of *intercourse*, use *penetration*
   d. Instead of *in no acute distress*, use a description of the behavior

B. Medical History

1. The purpose of the history is to obtain information about potential injuries that require evaluation and treatment.

   a. **A wide range of injuries may have been sustained by the patient,** including gunshot or stab wounds, lacerations, bites, contusions of varying severity, and occult damage, such as venereal infection and pregnancy.

2. **A complete gynecologic history should be obtained,** including the following:

   a. Menstrual history and date of last menstrual period.

   b. Use of contraception.

   c. Elapsed time since the assault.

   d. Whether the patient has bathed, showered, defecated, or douched since the rape. These activities may interfere with the collection of specimens for evidence.

C. Physical Examination

1. The physical examination should be directed toward finding and documenting the following:

   a. Outward appearance of clothing, for example, any rips or stains.

   b. Signs of physical trauma. Diagrams drawn in the record and photographs are helpful.

   c. A pelvic examination should include a thorough search for signs of vaginal and cervical trauma and gonorrheal and chlamydial cultures; bimanual examination of the uterus and adnexa are no longer recommended.

D. Psychological Assessment

1. **The psychological reactions to a sexual assault or attempted sexual assault vary** and depend on many factors, such as where the woman is in the life cycle, a prior history of assault, the extent of family and other social supports, the presence of a psychiatric disorder, and substance abuse. Consider how the patient is coping with the trauma. Note the signs and symptoms of emotional distress and indicate behavior, such as crying, agitation, sadness, fearfulness, shaking, and preoccupation. The typical responses in the period immediately after a rape include the following:

   a. **Self-blame.** Seventy-five percent of women experience shame and humiliation about the assault ("If only I had not...").

   b. **Fear of being killed.**

   c. **Feelings of degradation and loss of self-esteem.**

   d. **Feelings of depersonalization or derealization.**

   e. **Recurrent intrusive thoughts.**

   f. **Anxiety and depression.**

2. In the aftermath of the assault, the patient may begin to manifest the more **chronic sequelae of the trauma,** such as the following:

   a. **Fear of walking or being alone**

   b. **Fear of people behind them and crowds**

   c. **Fear of the indoors or the outdoors, depending on where the rape occurred**

   d. **Sexual fears**

   e. **Intrusive nightmares** that recapitulate the assault

3. A patient's mental status exam should be an important part of this assessment.

4. In documenting the psychological assessment of the patient, **one should err on the side of writing too little rather than too much.** As the defense strategy is usually to discredit the victim, inconsistencies in the documentation or indications that the patient's character is questionable or unstable may be used against the patient. Unfavor-

able aspects of the patient's social history (divorce, use of recreational drugs) can be used to discredit the patient.

5. As in the general population, sexual assault patients can present with a spectrum of mental health and illness. Patients with a concurrent psychiatric disorder need appropriate intervention. Clinicians need to be aware that an acutely traumatized patient may exhibit symptoms that mimic a major psychiatric illness. **Unless a psychiatric disturbance is diagnosed by history or examination, inferences about psychiatric diagnosis should be avoided** because the emergency room record and medical record probably will be entered into evidence in a criminal trial and will be used against the patient.

VI. Psychiatric Differential Diagnosis

A. Anxiety Disorders

1. In the setting of trauma, one may see a new onset of anxiety disorders, such as panic attacks, agoraphobia (fear of public places), and generalized anxiety disorder, or an exacerbation of pre-existing illnesses. Among the anxiety disorders, **post-traumatic stress disorder (PTSD) is a common psychiatric sequela of trauma.** The criteria for this disorder include the following:

   a. The traumatic event is persistently re-experienced in a variety of ways, such as recurrent and intrusive distressing recollections of the event, including images and thoughts.

   b. Recurrent distressing dreams of the event.

   c. Acting or feeling as if the traumatic event were recurring (includes a sense of reliving the experience, hallucinations, illusions, and dissociative flashback episodes).

   d. Intense autonomic arousal after exposure to cues that resemble the traumatic event.

   e. Intense psychological distress after exposure to cues in the environment that elicit memories of the traumatic event.

   f. Persistent avoidance of stimuli and numbing of general responsiveness, including efforts to avoid thoughts, feelings, and conversations about the trauma; feelings of detachment or estrangement from others; and a restricted range of affect (e.g., unable to have loving feelings) or a sense of a foreshortened future (e.g., does not expect to have a career, marriage, children, or a normal life span).

   g. Persistent symptoms of increased arousal, such as an exaggerated startle response, difficulty concentrating, hypervigilance, irritability, and outbursts of anger.

   h. These symptoms must have persisted for at least a month and have caused significant impairment in overall functioning.

2. In one study, nearly 70% of rape victims developed PTSD. **Risk factors for developing PTSD** include: rape by a stranger, use of physical force, use of weapons, physical injury, and a history of depression and/or alcohol abuse. Assessment of these risk factors for PTSD can be readily indentified in an initial assessment of the patient.

B. Mood Disorders

1. Patients also may develop a major depressive disorder in response to trauma. Comorbidity of anxiety states and major depression is high. Patients should be evaluated for the symptoms of depression (see Chapter 14) and should be treated appropriately with pharmacotherapy and/or psychotherapy.

VII. Treatment Strategies

A. Medical

1. **Informed consent for treatment. Patients may decline to receive treatment,** but they should be given enough information to make an informed decision.

2. **Sexually-transmitted disease.** Baseline testing for sexually-transmitted diseases is no longer routinely recommended, unless clinically indicated. Instead, patients should be treated prophylactically with antibiotics for gonorrhea, chlamydia, and trichomoniasis. The clinician should test for hepatitis B (HbsAG and anti-HbsAG) as well.

   Before any prophylaxis with antibiotics is offered, a beta-human chorionic gonadotropin (HCG) should be obtained to determine pregnancy status.

   HIV prophylaxis is typically offered to the patient. Consultation with an infectious disease specialist is recommended to determine the most appropriate medication regimen, laboratory work-up, and follow-up (which is done on a case-by-case basis). HIV testing is not recommended in the acute setting. A patient who is overwhelmed and traumatized by sexual assault needs expert counseling and follow-up to make an informed decision about HIV testing. These referral resources should be provided.

3. **Pregnancy. Post-coital contraception is offered after a detailed menstrual history is taken and after the patient is advised about her options.** Medication is given if no birth control is being practiced, intercourse occurred within the past 72 hours, pregnancy is likely, and the victim would be at high risk if a pregnancy occurred. Currently, the recommended emergency contraception is known as Plan B which consists of 0.75 mg of levonorgesterel. One dose is given in the emergency department and one dose 12 hours later. Patients should be given a **follow-up gynecologic appointment** to review carefully the results of the various tests.

4. **After-care.** Written information about after-care resources and referrals should be given to the patient at the time of discharge from the emergency department.

B. Psychological

1. **A clinician evaluating a rape victim should have a low threshold for referring the patient to a psychiatrist or another mental health provider with expertise in trauma.** Facilitating a speedy and appropriate referral for both diagnostic and treatment purposes is perhaps the most crucial step in minimizing morbidity in patients who already feel alone and ashamed. Emergency rooms are identifying particular nurse specialists in this area to help other staff members with the proper management of these patients.

2. **Provide reassurance to the patient** that initial reactions, such as self-blame, are normal. **Prepare the patient for the possible sequelae of the trauma,** as was outlined previously, because the majority of rape victims will develop PTSD.

3. **Forewarn the patient that some people develop sexual problems,** such as aversion to sexual activity, vaginismus, and loss of orgasm. Emphasize to the patient that these are normal reactions to the trauma of sexual assault.

C. Legal

1. **Ultimately it is the victim's decision to pursue legal charges against the perpetrator.** This is a very personal decision. Physicians should be familiar with the state laws governing collection of evidence and should be prepared to provide information to the patient about reporting the crime.

2. In some areas, advocates from rape crisis centers are available to help the victim negotiate the legal process. Some states also have victim-witness advocacy programs through the court system.

D. Pharmacotherapy for the Psychological Sequelae of Sexual Assault

1. Benzodiazepines may help ameliorate the acute anxiety and agitation that follow a trauma and should be used liberally but are they not ideal for long-term treatment. Lorazepam 1 to 2 mg or diazepam 5 to 10 mg PO STAT and then twice daily and at bedtime may be helpful acutely.

2. Antidepressants, especially serotonin reuptake inhibitors (SSRIs), such as fluoxetine, paroxetine, and sertraline, should be considered a first-line pharmacologic intervention for the treatment of PTSD because of their efficacy, tolerability, and safety profile. Studies suggests that SSRIs have a broad spectrum of effect on PTSD symptoms, including hyperarousal symptoms, such as agitation, anxiety, and insomnia. SSRIs are also appropriate for the treatment of major depression and panic disorder.

VIII. Conclusions

Sexual assault is a complex event associated with significant morbidity. Immediate attention to the medical, legal, and psychological implications of this traumatic event will facilitate appropriate and timely management.

Suggested Readings

Breslau, N., Davis, G.C., Andreski, P., et al. (1997). Psychiatric sequelae of posttraumatic stress disorder in women. *Archives of General Psychiatry, 54,* 81–87.

Crowell, N.A., & Burgess, A.W. (1996). *Understanding violence against women.* Washington, DC: National Academy Press.

Herman, J.L. (1992). *Trauma and recovery.* New York: Basic Books.

Linden, J.A. (1999). Sexual assault. *Emergency Medicine Clinics of North America, 17,* 685–697.

van der Kolk, B.A. (1994). The body keeps score: Memory and the evolving psychobiology of posttraumatic stress. *Harvard Review of Psychiatry, 1*(5), 253–265.

Yehuda, R. (2002). Post-Traumatic Stress Disorder. *New England Journal of Medicine, 346,* 108–114.

Conducting Sexual Assault Evidence Collection Exams in Massachusetts. A Training Video, Sexual Assault Nurse Examiner Program. Massachusetts Department of Public Health 2002.

CHAPTER 58

Approach to Domestic Violence

JULIA M. READE

I. Introduction

Domestic violence is not a new or trivial problem in the United States. One-third to one-half of all marriages involve physical violence at some point, nearly one-fifth of homicides occur within the family, and half of those homicides involve a spouse killing a spouse. Although less well studied, homosexual partnerships appear to have similar rates of violence. The range and patterns of violent behavior are highly variable and may range from episodes of reciprocal hitting between the partners to lethal assaults.

A. **Women are injured or killed by domestic violence far more frequently than are men.** They are also more likely to be assaulted, raped, or killed by a current or former male partner than by a stranger.

B. **Domestic violence produces significant morbidity and accounts for huge numbers of physician and emergency room visits.** Abused women present with more physical symptoms, depression, anxiety, somatic complaints, and substance abuse than do non-abused women.

C. **Battered women enter the medical system at multiple points.**
   1. **Up to 20% of women making outpatient visits to an internist, 17% of pregnant women seeking routine obstetric care, and up to 64% of women on an inpatient psychiatric service are abused.**
   2. **Most of these women do not present with injuries but with various medical, behavioral, and psychiatric complaints.**
   3. A third of the women who present to an emergency room with any complaint are in an **abusive relationship.** Up to 40% of women who present with trauma have injuries secondary to battering.
   4. Among women who present with a first injury, **most go on to further abuse.** The violence is usually repetitive and escalates over time.

D. **Characteristics of Battered Women**
   1. Battered women constitute **a heterogeneous group** that encompasses all ages, income levels, ethnic backgrounds, educational backgrounds, and marital states.
   2. There are no victim-specific risk factors for being battered other than **involvement with a violent partner.**

E. **Characteristics of Battering Men**
   1. Batterers are **a demographically heterogeneous group.**
   2. They are **often needy, fragile men terrified by their dependency needs and enraged at their partners for any sign of autonomy.** They frequently have poor self-esteem, intense jealousy of their partners, and a need to dominate or control them.

3. A large percentage of **violent men abuse drugs or alcohol** and may **blame their behavior on disinhibition.** Their partners report, however, that they are also abusive when sober.

4. Although less well studied than their victims, battering men are **often excessively concerned with appearances.** They may take great pains to convince others of their congeniality and rectitude. Their violent behavior is often carefully concealed, and associates are disbelieving when presented with evidence of such an individual's brutality toward his partner.

5. **Clinically, abusive men often appear more intact and believable than their abused partners** and may accuse their partners of mental instability or a propensity to exaggeration.

6. **Most battering men minimize or deny their violent behavior when questioned** and frequently blame their partners for provoking them. Many have histories of behaving violently in other intimate relationships.

F. **Characteristics of Violent Relationships**

1. In most cases, **domestic violence does not begin right away.** It may emerge after the marriage, during a pregnancy, or after the birth of a child. It is frequently rationalized by both partners as being due to some external stressor and is thought to be unlikely to recur.

2. Most often the violence does recur and, in the view of some researchers, becomes **cyclical.** According to this model, a tension-building phase is followed by a violent outburst and then a period of reconciliation.

3. The **threats and violence are often terrifying and life-threatening** and may involve a variety of weapons, including fists, feet, clubs, knives, and guns. Some women are sexually assaulted, and any or all of the violence may take place in front of the couple's children.

4. The batterer is **often pathologically jealous** of his partner, accusing her of all manner of sexual infidelities, insisting that she account for all her actions, and frequently restricting her activities. She is often progressively restricted from outside relationships and contact with friends or family. She may be unable or not allowed to drive, work, make telephone calls, get medical care, and have access to money.

5. **The woman is often terrified to leave the relationship** or tell an outsider about the violence. She is frequently threatened by the batterer with death, the loss of her children, or his suicide if she tries to leave. When she does leave, a woman is often at highest risk for injury or death.

6. During periods of reconciliation **the batterer is often intensely remorseful** toward his partner, who may in turn feel sorry for him. At this juncture, feeling hopeful about the future, the woman may find it particularly difficult to leave the relationship.

G. **Why Women Stay in Violent Relationships**

1. A battered woman may be **trapped economically** and have no other source of housing, food, and child support.

2. **Many women blame themselves** for the violence and may stay in the relationship because they are convinced that they can remedy the problem by working harder to meet the male partner's needs.

3. For some women, the violence may be a commonplace, that is, something that is considered **the price of a relationship with a man.**

4. The woman may be **too frightened to leave.** Many women have tried to leave, only to find inadequate legal, medical, or social supports. Often leaving the relationship does not stop the violence but may instead escalate it.

H. **Consequences of Battering**

1. As a result of chronic verbal and physical abuse, **most women,** regardless of their pre-battering psychological make-up, **come to see themselves as worthless, incompetent, and unlovable.**

II. Evaluation of the Problem

A. **General Recommendations**

1. **The biggest problem in the evaluation of domestic violence lies with detection.** Despite ample evidence of the high rates of incidence and prevalence, **physicians have done a poor job of asking their patients routinely about abuse in current or former relationships.** Patients rarely volunteer information about abuse spontaneously but usually respond favorably to a physician who questions them in a tactful, empathic fashion.

2. **Clinicians' resistance to asking patients about domestic violence may stem from a variety of sources:** misconceptions about domestic violence (i.e., that a patient's high socioeconomic status precludes battering), fears that asking will offend the patient, fears that asking will "open up Pandora's box" and be too time-consuming, a stance that asking about violence is outside the purview of a medical professional. There may be unconscious responses to victims, which may include a sense of helplessness, fear of contamination or retaliation, and anxiety about the rage that violence often engenders. Many physicians have unresolved feelings about abuse that they may have endured or have perpetrated in their own relationships. Finally, many fear that "solving" the domestic violence will rest on the physician's shoulders.

3. **This resistance may result in harm to the patient. The diagnosis of battering may not be made so that the woman is left at serious risk of further harm,** her complaints may be belittled or taken out of context and misunderstood, she may be blamed and punished with inappropriate medication (anxiolytics, analgesics, or antipsychotics) which can produce iatrogenic abuse, and she may have inadequate follow-up, safety planning, and referral.

B. **Medical history.** A primary care physician (PCP) does not need to be an expert in domestic violence to make that diagnosis. Moreover, it is not up to the physician to "solve" the violence or rescue the victim from her batterer but to **screen** for abuse, document all findings, **assert that violence is not acceptable, and make appropriate referrals.**

1. As a matter of routine, **all patients should be asked about violence** in current and former relationships. These questions should be tactful and open-ended. Patients also should be asked about a history of sexual assault. Marital rape is not uncommon and often accompanies physical abuse.

2. **The index for suspicion should rise for women presenting with unusual injuries or repeated trauma and unlikely explanations for their injuries.** These patients may seem guarded or evasive when questioned about their partners.

3. **Multiple visits to the emergency room** for any reason should raise concern that a patient is being abused.

4. The sequelae of battering, and therefore a patient's presentation, may include **multiple somatic symptoms, chronic abdominal pain, chronic headache, pelvic pain, alcohol and substance abuse, musculoskeletal complaints, medical non-compliance, and a variety of psychiatric symptoms** (see below).

5. **Patients who disclose a history of abuse should be asked about the first episode, the most recent episode, and the most serious episode.** They should be asked about visits to the emergency room, any injuries they have sustained, and what weapons are in the house or are readily available. Patients with children should be asked if the children have been witness to, or targets of, the violence (in most states, physicians are mandated reporters for suspected child abuse). Patients also should be asked if they have been sexually assaulted.

C. **Interview. The physician needs time, willingness to listen, and tact.** The patient should be interviewed alone, and family members should be asked politely to wait elsewhere. **Under no circumstances should a woman be asked about suspected abuse in the presence of her partner.** This may put her at increased risk of harm, and she will not be free to answer fully or truthfully.

1. **Except when a physician is mandated to report abuse, patients should be assured of the confidentiality of the interview.** Many battered women fear that their attackers will gain access to their records.

2. Every effort should be made to **understand the patient's behavior in context.** She may be suspicious of the clinician, secretive or protective of her assailant, and, despite the clinician's recommendation, not ready to leave her partner. She may be reluctant to accept the physician's offer of help at the time, but if the encounter is a positive one in which she feels understood and is treated respectfully, she is more likely to return at a later date or avail herself of other resources.

3. **Physicians should think about their personal response to violence** and how it may affect their response to patients in violent relationships. Consultation with colleagues, continuing education courses, and an interdisciplinary treatment team all can be helpful and in many cases are necessary.

D. **Examination of the Patient**

1. There should be **a thorough physical examination** with careful documentation of the findings. This should include sketches in the chart of all injuries or photographs if possible, since the medical record may be needed in court. The physician should detail the patient's history without editorializing or ruling on its veracity.

2. **A mental status examination** should attend to symptoms of depression, anxiety, substance or alcohol abuse, post-traumatic stress disorder (PTSD), and psychosis. Many battered women live in a state of chronic stress and threat of harm akin to that experienced by soldiers in combat and show symptoms of hypervigilance and autonomic hyperarousal intermingled with episodes of psychic numbness, withdrawal, and apathy. Many abused women are suicidal or actively abuse substances.

3. The evaluation should include **a careful assessment of the woman's coping ability.** How did she deal with the violence in the past? Has she told anyone? What was the outcome? Has she made plans to leave? Is she able to function at home or at work? Have there been recent changes in her behavior or mental status?

4. What are the patient's **social supports?** Does she have friends, family, access to a car, use of a phone, mobility? Who can she trust and confide in?

5. What are the **current dangers?** Is the batterer pathologically jealous? Has there been an escalation in the violence or threats to kill the patient? Is there a weapon in the house?

III. Psychiatric Differential Diagnosis

There should be a low threshold for referral for psychiatric evaluation. As was noted above, battered women are at high risk for depression, suicide, anxiety disorders, PTSD, and alcohol and substance abuse.

IV. Diagnostic Criteria

The diagnosis is a clinical one but cannot be made unless the clinician routinely asks the right questions of his or her patients. Patients involved in violent relationships often elicit strong reactions from their caregivers, especially when they stay in violent relationships or engage in self-destructive behaviors. It is important to use consultation with colleagues who are knowledgeable about domestic violence and to remember that patients are not going to leave their batterers on the clinician's timetable.

V. Treatment Strategies

Treatment should be **tailored to the individual patient,** and appropriate referrals should be made. These patients are often best treated with an interdisciplinary team. The physician should make a clear statement that violence is unacceptable and that he or she is concerned about the safety and well-being of the patient. The physician should also make it clear that he or she understands that the patient is in a difficult situation and will provide care and referrals regardless of the decision the patient makes regarding her relationship.

A. **Primary psychiatric and medical disorders should be treated.** Some changes in approach may be necessary.
   1. **The physician may need to hospitalize a battered woman** earlier than he or she might do with a non-battered depressed or suicidal patient. The family may not be a good resource for monitoring symptoms, supervising medications, and containing self-destructive behavior.
   2. The physician must **exercise caution with prescriptions,** weighing the risks of abuse, overdose, and dulling of the patient's vigilance against the potential benefits.
   3. The physician and his or her office staff should **become familiar with hospital and community resources** for battered women and inform the patient of various options. These should include referrals to 24-hour hot lines, battered women's shelters or safe houses, battered women's advocates, legal advice, the police, and support groups. The National Domestic Violence Hotline (1-800-799-SAFE, or TDD: 1-800-787-3224) can provide useful information about different states' resources.
   4. Someone on the physician's staff should **review safety planning with the patient.** What will she do or where will she go in an emergency or when the violence erupts again? Does she want to press charges or obtain an order of protection against her assailant? If so, she should be referred to the police or a battered women's shelter that can provide an advocate to assist her. Has she thought about how to protect herself at

home (e.g., changing the lock on the door, obtaining an unlisted telephone number or caller ID) and at work?

5. The clinician also may need to **notify the appropriate state social services agency and the hospital's child protection team** if there is reason to suspect child abuse.

Selected Readings

Alpert, E.J. (1995). Violence in intimate relationships and the practicing internist: New "disease" or new agenda? *Annals of Internal Medicine, 123,* 774–781.

Campbell, J., Jones, A.S., Dienemann, J., et al. (2002). Intimate partner violence and physical health consequences. *Archives of Internal Medicine, 162,* 1157–1163.

Campbell, J.C. (2002). Health consequences of intimate partner violence. *Lancet, 359,* 1331–1336.

Carmen, E., & Rieker, P.P. (1989). A psychosocial model of the victim-to-patient process: Implications for treatment. *Psychiatric Clinics of North America, 12,* 431–443.

Council of Scientific Affairs, American Medical Association (1992). Violence against women: Relevance for medical practitioners. *Journal of the American Medical Association, 267,* 3184–3189.

Dickstein, I.J., & Nadelson, C.C. (1989). *Family violence: Emerging issues of a national crisis.* Washington, DC: American Psychiatric Association Press.

Flitcraft, A. (1995). From public health to personal health: Violence against women across the life span. *Annals of Internal Medicine, 123,* 800–801.

Hilberman, E. (1980). The "wife-beater's wife" reconsidered. *American Journal of Psychiatry, 137,* 1336–1347.

McLeer, S.V., & Anwar, R.A. (1987). The role of the emergency physician in the prevention of domestic violence. *Annals of Emergency Medicine, 16,* 1155–1161.

McLeer, S.V., Anwar, W.A., Herman, S., et al. (1989). Education is not enough: A system's failure in protecting battered women. *Annals of Emergency Medicine, 18,* 651–653.

CHAPTER 59
The Family in Crisis

ANNE K. FISHEL

I. Introduction

A family in crisis offers a unique opportunity for a clinician to intervene; such a family system is highly receptive to an outsider and to change, although the stakes can be high. The goals of family crisis intervention are to foster a healing process by promoting the family's resources (psychological and social), to prevent a deterioration in functioning, and to provide a realistic context for hopefulness about the future. In approaching a family in crisis, the clinician must first understand four fundamental concepts.

A. **The Definition of a Family**
1. **A family can be defined as a two- or three-generational system** in which the members are incorporated by birth, adoption, marriage, or its equivalent.
2. For the purposes of crisis intervention, **the relevant system must be taken into account.** The relevant system includes individuals within and outside the family who are actively involved in the presenting problem.

B. **The notion that crisis can be a dangerous opportunity.** According to Bingham Dai, a Chinese etymologist, the Chinese term for crisis is *we chai,* where *we* means "danger" and *chai* means "opportunity." **The opportunity in a crisis allows a family to move to a new level of flexibility and complexity and add something new to its repertoire of coping strategies.** The danger lies in the fact that despite the family's efforts to resolve the crisis, the family may deteriorate and its members may get hurt.

C. **The fact that an emergency and a crisis are different from each other.**
1. **An emergency is a subjective state. It is the feeling that an outside intervention is needed immediately.** A request for emergency help often takes the form of a family asking that a family member be hospitalized as soon as possible.
2. **A crisis is more subtle and can occur without an emergency state.** A crisis is the condition that arises when a change is impending and the system is too overwhelmed to respond. A crisis results when a stress impinges on a family that requires a change that is beyond its usual repertoire of coping strategies. The stress that precipitates a crisis is particular to a given family. Identifying and naming that stress constitute the clinician's first step toward helping a family in crisis.

D. **The notion that a crisis can be understood.** Identifying the stressor for a particular family in crisis gives the clinician a more neutral and direct entry into the family than does focusing on the pathology and symptoms. Frank Pittman, a psychiatrist and researcher of family crisis, suggests the following typology:
1. **Bolts from the blue.** The stressor is obvious and specific and arises from forces outside the family, such as an accidental death. The stress is a one-time occurrence that is as likely to strike a healthy family as one that is not healthy.

2. **Developmental crises.** The stressors in this case are normative and predictable, resulting in permanent changes in status and functioning, such as the birth of a child or the departure from home of the last child. Not every life-cycle transition results in a crisis. Instead, these normal passages become crises when there is a simultaneous accumulation of other major life events, as occurs when the birth of a child coincides with the death of the mother's father and the father's losing his job. A normal developmental transition may turn tumultuous if it occurs off schedule, as occurs when an adolescent has a baby or the mother of young children dies. Additionally, a developmental passage may be complicated by its similarity to difficulties in the previous generation.

3. **Structural crises.** These are recurrent crises in which problematic patterns within a family regularly become exacerbated. There may be no well-defined external stress to explain the current crisis. There are long-standing issues to contend with as well as pressing daily concerns. In this case, pervasive turmoil may make it difficult to establish a plan for change.

4. **Caretaker crises.** Caretaker crises occur when one family member is non-functional and dependent (e.g., has schizophrenia or Alzheimer's disease) and the illness has been diagnosed recently and is not fully accepted by the family members. Often the crisis is precipitated by a disagreement among family members or between the family and physician about what course of action to take regarding medication or hospitalization.

II. The Crisis Meeting

Throughout the meeting the clinician should look for opportunities to re-establish hope, indicate that the family has the resources and ability to solve the problem at hand, and show an appreciation for each family member's way of perceiving the world. This non-judgmental stance will go a long way toward lowering the stress engendered by a crisis.

A. **Setting the Stage**
   1. **Offer a rationale for the family meeting that is positive and non-blaming.** If an individual patient asks his or her family to attend a family meeting, he or she may invite them by saying, "I would appreciate your help." Or the clinician may telephone family members and say, "This problem of John's is affecting everyone, and we need everyone's ideas to help solve the problem."
   2. **Provide a context of safety and comfort by setting a time-frame for the meeting and offering certain rules of discourse.**
      a. The clinician may suggest that he or she will interrupt any **blaming comments** that are made.
      b. **The "I pass" tale can be introduced.** If anyone is asked a question that seems too intrusive, he or she is encouraged to "pass."
      c. The clinician may indicate in advance that he or she will be a **"traffic cop"** who will intervene to make sure that each person gets to speak without interruptions and that everyone has an equitable share of the time available.
   3. **Provide an introduction. One should introduce oneself, state briefly what one knows about the crisis, and make contact with each family member,** asking for names, ages, recent changes in daily routine, and how all the members occupy themselves during the day. However, if this phase is too long, the family may feel that the crisis is being minimized.

B. Getting the family's definition of the problem. It is imperative that early on in a family crisis meeting each family member be given the opportunity to explain, without interruptions and qualifications from others, his or her unique perspective on the problem at hand. An important task for the clinician in an emergency situation is to provide a safe haven where multiple and often opposing voices can be raised and heard. **The clinician may ask several questions to help family members speak about their current understanding of the problem.**

1. As an opening question, the clinician may say: "Often in families, everyone has a different view of the problem and different hopes for change. We need to hear from each of you how you see the difficulties."

2. It is important to discover why this is a problem and what aspect of the crisis is most difficult for each family member. For example, if you ask different family members about a girl's anorexia, the brother may worry about his sister's possible death, the father about the marital fights that focus on the daughter's food, and the mother about criticisms from her own mother about her mothering style.

3. The clinician can ask: "What have you already tried to do?" and "How have these attempted solutions helped or impeded matters?" Sometimes well-intentioned common-sense solutions make matters worse, as occurs when the parents of a school-phobic boy respond sympathetically to his anxiety by keeping him home from school.

4. "Who else has been concerned and has given advice or offered help?" This question is aimed at discovering the "relevant system," or the individuals inside and outside the family who will need to be included in the solution, by asking about their participation in the presenting problem.

5. "Have there been any other changes in the family in the last year, for example, illnesses, job loss, deaths, or moves?" Often a crisis occurs because there is an accumulation of stressors. It can be very helpful to put the current crisis into perspective by reminding the family of all the stressors that have recently coincided.

C. Expanding the family's definition of the problem. The crisis interview should provide not only an opportunity for family members to share their distress but also a place to build a new view of the problems and develop concomitant strategies for change and problem-solving. Several questions help create this shift from the family's current understanding of the problem to a new definition.

1. **Introduce a broader time perspective.** Each family member can be asked, "What would you like to see different in the family?" and "If things were to go really well in a few months and I were a fly on the wall, what might I observe?" These questions encourage family members to entertain a future perspective, which often gets discarded during a crisis, when the focus narrows to the present. In addition, the past may be brought in: "When were things different in this family? When did things start to change? What would have to change now to return the family to its previous state?"

2. **Ask "circular questions,"** that is, questions that focus not on the identified patient's problem but on the problem's impact on all the members of the relevant system. **Unlike linear questions (which isolate the problem in the identified patient), circular questions place a problem in a context.** In a patient with depression, for example, linear questions would include, "What is causing your depression?" and "Have there been any changes in your sleep, appetite, sexual interest, or concentration?" **Circular questions, by contrast, draw a web of inter-connectedness.** For example,

they include, "When you are depressed, who do you show your depression to, and how do you show it?" "When you scream at your wife, does she know that means that you are depressed?" "Meanwhile, what is your son doing while you are screaming at your wife?" "When he is very sympathetic to you and critical of his mother's response to you, how does your wife respond?" These questions attempt to reveal how everyone is participating in a father's depression and show that a change in anyone's behavior could affect the father.

3. As part of an effort to move the interview in a more positive direction, **exceptions to the problem should be asked about:** "When has the family come close to experiencing the problem but resisted its pull?" "What made it possible to resist the problem?" "What was everyone doing differently?" These questions may reveal a trajectory for change.

4. **Problem-solving questions** can be asked: "What is the smallest change you or another family member could make in the next week that would indicate that things were starting to move in a more positive direction?" The focus should be on establishing goals that are achievable. When a family is in a crisis, having something to do can start to relieve the feelings of hopelessness and being overwhelmed.

D. **Taking a break. A 10-minute recess provides an opportunity for both the clinician and the family to gain a perspective on the problem away from the charged emotional context of the crisis interview.** As the clinician leaves the room, the family is asked to review the session privately, discussing or contemplating which questions were left unasked and what might be a helpful next step. Meanwhile, the clinician can organize his or her thoughts and return to the room later with feedback. Such feedback should do the following:

1. **Comment on the family's strengths and coping abilities.** Conveying an appreciation of a family's positive qualities diminishes defensiveness, elicits cooperation, and promotes hopefulness. Also, **when one focuses on what is positive about the family as a whole, attention is shifted from the identified patient to the interconnectedness of the family members.** For example, a family that has talked a lot, even interrupting one another, may be praised for being lively and full of ideas. If nothing else, the fact that the family came together for a meeting can be commented on positively.

2. **Show an appreciation for the intensity of the family's concern or distress about its difficulties.**

3. **Identify the stressors and place the problem in a developmental perspective.** By identifying the stressors as the source of distress and acknowledging the distress as normal, one interrupts the cycle of blame, anger, and guilt which is usually counterproductive in problem-solving. A developmental perspective suggests that there are predictable transition points in the lives of all families (the birth of a child, a child entering adolescence, the death of a spouse) and that these transition points are times of increased stress.

4. **Use the family's own language and resources to suggest a plan of action.**
   a. **Point out the family's previous well-intentioned strategies** that have not been helpful.
   b. **Emphasize previous successful attempts to resist the problem** and prescribe more of the same.
   c. **Re-define the problem in a way that points to a new direction of action** that will be constructive.

E. **Ending the Interview**

1. **Offer the feedback outlined above.**
2. **Allow time for discussion** of the feedback, paying particular attention to the family's response to your re-definition of the problem and suggested actions for them to take.
3. **Negotiate decisions** regarding the plan for action which may include hospitalization, medication, individual or family therapy, or a problem-solving strategy you and the family have worked out together.
4. **Set up another meeting if appropriate,** suggesting the approximate number of meetings you want to schedule, raising the possibility of a subsequent referral for on-going individual or family therapy, and discussing who should attend the next meeting. **In general, it is useful for everyone who attended the first meeting and other individuals from the relevant system who were not present to attend a subsequent meeting.** The interval between the first crisis meeting and the second usually should be no more than a week.

III. Making a Referral for Family Therapy

A. **When to refer.** Obviously, there are times when it is not feasible for a primary care physician (PCP) to conduct a family crisis meeting. **Time constraints, lack of familiarity with a particular psychiatric disorder, and a patient's refusal to bring his or her family to the physician all make family meetings untenable.** In many instances, an immediate referral to a family therapist may be indicated. The following are guidelines for when to refer:

1. **When the identified patient is actively resistant to medical treatment** while the family is more agreeable. Alternatively, the family may be obstructing the identified patient's treatment.
2. **With certain individual psychiatric disorders** that are so entwined in family relationships that seeing only one member is like trying to conduct an orchestra when only the cellist shows up. Examples include eating disorders, substance abuse, a first psychotic break, and sexual difficulties, such as low sexual desire.
3. **When there is evidence that a serious trauma,** such as a divorce, the death of a parent, or a natural disaster that affects the whole family and has left one or more family members symptomatic a few months after the event.
4. **When someone makes a suicide attempt or gesture** it usually constitutes a powerful communication to the family. Family therapy can help decode the message and help the family make a decision about hospitalization. An individual meeting is also necessary to assess the patient's safety and ask about topics the patient may not be willing to discuss in front of other family members.
5. **When the family is having difficulty negotiating a life transition,** as occurs when a couple with young children are fighting fiercely and frequently over the equity of child care and work arrangements.
6. **When there is irreconcilable disagreement** in the family, such as a stalemate about whether to marry, divorce, have an abortion, or allow an adolescent to move out of the home.

B. **When Is Family Therapy Contraindicated?**

1. **With a violent patient.** While there is debate within the field about how to handle couples when abuse is part of the picture, the most conservative position is to refer each partner to individual therapy and refer the abuser to group therapy.

2. **When sexual abuse or incest is suspected.** In this case it is imperative to meet individually as long as the patient needs it. It is up to an abuse survivor to determine if and when he or she wants to confront the abuser.

C. **Information to Provide in Making a Referral**

1. **The family's resources** (individual capabilities, strengths as a family, and social supports). The availability of resources within and outside the family is the best predictor of a positive outcome in therapy.

   a. **The ability to use outside resources,** including the doctor: Has there been an approach that has been disastrous, such as excluding a grandparent, or saying something critical of a parent?

   b. **"Who is in the relevant system?"** "Is there anybody else you know of in the relevant system, that is, anyone else who has been involved in trying to solve the problem?"

   c. **Financial resources and insurance.**

2. **Your observations about the family's style**

   a. **Power hierarchy.** Do the parents have an egalitarian arrangement, or is one parent or grandparent clearly in charge?

   b. **Cultural matrix.** Since developmental changes, mental illness, and encounters with professionals all have different meanings according to a family's cultural background, it is important to be alert to this factor.

   c. **Expression of affect.** How does this family express emotion? Have its members cried readily in the doctor's office? A family therapist will try to make interventions fit the family's comfort level regarding affect expression.

3. **Your best assessment about "Why now?"** It is helpful to put the crisis in a context of what else is happening in the family currently.

D. **Family therapy is not a substitute for other therapies.** Even when it has been determined that a psychotic, depressed, anorectic, or chronically medically ill person's condition has been worsened by family interactions that can be addressed in family therapy, the patient's individual condition must be thoroughly evaluated medically and treated comprehensively. Medication, individual therapy, group therapy, Alcoholics Anonymous meetings, and hospitalization should not be ruled out because family therapy meetings have been scheduled.

Suggested Readings

Carter, E.A., McGoldrick, M., & Carter, B. (Eds.). (1998). *The expanded family life cycle: Individual, family and social perspectives.* Needham Heights, Mass.: Allyn and Bacon.

Fishel, A. (1999). How to start up the work. In A. Fishel (Ed.), *Treating the adolescent in family therapy: A developmental and narrative approach.* Northvale, N.J.: Jason Aronson.

Fishel, A., & Gordon, C. (1994). Treating the family in the emergency department. In S. Hyman, & G. Tesar (Eds.), *Manual of psychiatric emergencies.* Boston: Little, Brown, pp. 45–52.

Fraser, J.S. (1986). The crisis interview: Strategic rapid intervention. *Journal of Strategic Systemic Therapies, 5,* 71–87.

Gurman, A., & Kniskem, D. (Eds.). (1991). *Handbook of family therapy, vol.* 2. New York: Bruner Mazel.

Karpel, M. (1994). *Evaluating couples: A handbook for practitioners.* New York: W.W. Norton.

McDaniel, S., Hepworth, J., & Doherty, W. (1992). *Medical family therapy: A biopsychosocial approach to families with health problems.* New York: Basic Books.

McGoldrick, M., Giordano, J., & Peace, J.K. (Eds.). (1996). *Ethnicity and family therapy* (2nd ed.). New York, NY: Guilford Press.

Penn, P. (1982). Circular questioning. *Family Process, 21,* 267–279.

Pittman, F. (1986). *Turning points: Treating families in transition and crisis.* New York: Norton.

Rolland, J.S. (1987). Chronic illness and the life cycle: A conceptual framework. *Family Process, 26,* 203–221.

Walsh, F. (1998). *Strengthening family resilience.* New York: Guilford Press.

Weber, T., McKeever, J., & McDaniel, S. (1985). A beginner's guide to the problem-oriented first family interview. *Family Process, 25,* 257–264.

CHAPTER 60
The Violent Patient

KATHY M. SANDERS

I. Introduction

A. Violence is a complex issue with a variety of contributing factors (e.g., socioeconomic, medical, and psychiatric). While the majority of violent acts committed in the United States cannot be attributed to primary psychiatric pathology, temperament, poor impulse control, and episodic violence are associated with organic brain disorders, as are intoxication and/or withdrawal states, and psychiatric diagnoses. When violence is not managed by the legal authorities, emergency rooms, urgent care centers, and community medical health centers often become the sites in which violence is managed or contained. Increasingly, domestic violence and workplace violence are seen and managed by medical professionals in these settings.

II. Evaluation of the Problem

A. General recommendations. Safety, diagnosis, and management constitute a tripartite approach to violent patients and must occur rapidly and often simultaneously.
   1. **Safety** is the most important issue during the initial evaluation of a violent patient. Unless the patient is prevented from committing further episodes of violence or harm to himself or herself or to others, staff members will not be able to get close enough to adequately evaluate and manage the patient's aggression. **Control of the environment** for the safety of patient and staff is crucial.
   2. Making a quick but accurate **diagnosis** of the probable psychiatric, substance abuse, or medical causes that underlie violent behavior allows for specific interventions. Specificity allows prompt initiation of appropriate treatment and regaining of self-control. If violence is not due to medical or psychiatric disorders, it is best to have the legal authorities manage the situation.
   3. **Timely management** of aggressive and potentially violent patients is crucial. **Rapid tranquilization,** using neuroleptics and/or benzodiazepines, either with or without **restraint or seclusion,** allows the patient to regain behavioral control. Medical staff members are then able to pursue diagnostic work-ups and specific treatments.

B. Medical History
   1. Medical assessment during the acute management of violent, agitated, and threatening behavior starts by ruling out life-threatening causes.
      a. WWHHHHIMPS, a mnemonic adapted from Anderson (1980) and Wise and Rundell (1988), stands for **W**ithdrawal from barbiturates, **W**ernicke's encephalopathy, **H**ypoxia and **H**ypoperfusion of the brain, **H**ypertensive crisis, **H**ypoglycemia, **H**yper/hypothermia, **I**ntracranial bleed/mass, **M**eningitis/encephalitis, **P**oisoning, and **S**tatus epilepticus.

2. Numerous medical and neurologic causes of organic brain syndromes may result in agitated, aggressive, or violent behavior. A systematic review allows the clinician to rapidly rule out underlying organic causes that require specific treatment.

    a. **VINDICTIVE MAD** is a mnemonic cited by Cassem (1996) (Table 60-1).

C. Interview

1. Safe environment

   a. **Any potential weapon should be removed from the interview space.** If the patient has a knife or gun, it must be surrendered before the interview can proceed.

   b. **Attention must be paid to objects in the environment** (e.g., pens, envelope openers, heavy ashtrays, loose furniture, and books) that can be used as weapons.

Table 60-1. Differential Diagnosis of Medical and Neurologic Conditions Associated with Brain Dysfunction

General Etiology	Specific Etiologies
Vascular	Hypertensive encephalopathy, cerebral arteriosclerosis, intracranial hemorrhage or thromboses, circulatory collapse (shock), systemic lupus etythematosus, polyarteritis nodosa, thrombotic thrombocytopenic purpura
Infectious	Encephalitis, meningitis, general paresis, HIV
Neoplastic	Space-occupying lesions, such as gliomas, menigiomas, abscesses, metastases
Degenerative	Senile and presenile dementias (i.e., Alzheimer's and Pick's dementias, Huntington's chorea)
Intoxication	Chronic intoxication or withdrawal effects of sedative-hypnotic drugs, such as benzodiazepines, bromides, opiates, other classes of tranquilizers, anticholinergics, dissociative anesthetics, anticonvulsants
Congenital	Epilepsy, post-ictal states, aneurysm
Traumatic	Subdural and epidural hematomas, contusion, laceration, post-operative trauma, heat stroke
Intraventricular	Normal-pressure hydrocephalus, hemorrhage
Vitamin deficiency	Thiamine (Wernike-Korsakoff syndrome), niacin (pellagra), B_{12} (pernicious anemia)
Endocrine-metabolic	Diabetic coma and shock, uremia, myxedema, hyperthyroid and parathyroid dysfunctions, hypoglycemia, hepatic failure, porphyria, severe electrolyte or acid-base disturbances, remote side effect of carcinoma, Cushing's syndrome
Metals	Heavy metals (lead, manganese, mercury), carbon monoxide, toxins
Anoxia	Hypoxia and anoxia secondary to pulmonary or cardiac failure, anesthesia, anemia
Depression-other	Depressive pseudodementia, hysteria, catatonia

c. **Allow for adequate open spaces** for the patient and staff that ensure easy withdrawal from an escalating situation. The examination room should not be isolated. The door should remain ajar if necessary and should never be able to be locked from within. A "panic button" or alarm system should be readily available.

d. **Pay close attention to the patient's behavior for evidence of impending violence,** including the following:
   i. Loud, fast, threatening, and profane speech
   ii. Increased muscle tension, as evidenced by sitting on the edge of the chair, leaning forward or invading the personal space of the interviewer, fidgeting with the hands or feet, or clenching the jaw
   iii. Pacing, inability to stay seated, or talking to oneself
   iv. Slamming doors or knocking over furniture

e. When verbal interventions and re-direction do not help the patient remain calm, **the emergency use of restraints** (Table 60-2) often is needed while tranquilization is used to re-establish behavioral control.

Table 60-2. The Process of Secluding or Restraining a Patient

1. After verbal intervention or other means of controlling violent behavior have been considered or tried, a team of at least four staff members and one leader should be formed.

2. The staff should gather around the leader to project an image of confidence and control of the situation.

3. The leader should tell the patient that he or she must go to the seclusion room or be put into restraints, briefly state the reasons, and give directions.

4. The patient is given a few seconds to comply, and further negotiation or discussion is not allowed.

5. At a prearranged signal, each extremity is grabbed and controlled, and one staff member controls the patient's head.

6. The patient is brought to the floor in a backward motion without being injured.

7. Once the patient is on the floor, restraints are applied or the patient is carried to the seclusion room with uniform lifting of the body and control of extremities and the head.

8. The patient is searched, and street clothes and dangerous objects (such as rings, belts, shoes, and matches) are removed.

9. The patient is placed on his back with his head toward the door or facedown with the head away from the door.

10. Staff members exit one at a time in a coordinated manner.

11. After the seclusion or restraint procedure is completed, staff members should critique the process and discuss their feelings.

12. During visits by the staff, the patient should be assessed for the degree of control of his or her behavior and compliance with requests made by the staff.

13. The timing of gradual removal from seclusion or restraint is based on these assessments.

14. After the patient's removal from seclusion or restraint, the staff should discuss with the patient his or her feelings about the procedure, what led up to the behavior, and what could have prevented it.

2. **Examiner's behaviors**
   a. **Language**
      i. **Use calm, non-threatening language.** This is important in helping a potentially threatening, paranoid, and violent patient maintain self-control.
      ii. **Accept what the patient tells you.** Do not try to talk a paranoid patient out of delusional beliefs. Do not be confrontational.
      iii. **Express concern for the patient.** Make an alliance based on your interest in protecting the patient from further harm to himself or herself or to others.
      iv. **Attend to the physical comfort of the patient** by lowering the lights, offering food and water, or allowing a cigarette (if appropriate).
      v. **Do not make promises you cannot keep.**
   b. **Body language**
      i. **Avoid continuous unbroken eye contact with the patient.** Do not appear to stare. Eye contact may be experienced as a threatening and controlling activity by paranoid or angry patients.
      ii. **Pay attention to facial expressions and avoid extremes.** Control any winking or grimacing that may be misinterpreted.
      iii. **Do not crowd the patient,** keep your distance, and position yourself at a 45-degree angle to the patient.
      iv. **Respect interpersonal space.** Try to maintain equal altitudes during the interview by standing or sitting when the patient does.
      v. **Move slowly and deliberately.**
      vi. **Maintain a relaxed posture** (arms uncrossed in front of you with open palms). Do not put your hands in your pockets or clench your fists.
      vii. **Avoid touching the patient unnecessarily.** During the physical examination always tell the patient what you are going to do before touching the patient.
3. **A history of violence** should be obtained in a direct and honest manner once a rapport has been developed.
   a. **Routine screening questions**
      i. Have you ever thought of harming anyone?
      ii. Have you ever injured anyone?
      iii. What is the most violent thing you have ever done?
   b. **A prior history of violence or dangerous behavior is the best predictor of current behavior.** Taking a careful history to evaluate the nature, extent, and severity of the violence or aggression with attention to documentation allows the clinician to diagnose and make treatment recommendations. One should ask the following questions:
      i. When did the violent behavior begin? How often did it occur? What was the most recent episode?
      ii. Who are the targets?
      iii. Is there a recurring pattern or a recent escalation?
      iv. How serious have the injuries to the self or others been during violent episodes?
      v. Are there circumstances associated with the violence?
      vi. Have there been legal charges, jail time, or probation?
      vii. Is there a history of previous impulsivity, suicidality, destruction of property, or acting-out behavior (including criminal offenses and recklessness)?
      viii. Is there a history of violence in the family? Domestic violence? Child abuse? Gang-related involvement?
      ix. Is there a history of head injury, birth complications, serious childhood illnesses, or developmental delays or problems?

c. Were there previous evaluations or medical work-ups for violence in the past? Do you have access to those records? Gather medical, psychiatric, and criminal records.

d. Obtain corroborating evidence from as many sources as possible, including courts, probation officers, hospitals, health care professionals, family members, employers, and neighbors.

D. Examination of the Patient

1. Safe setting

a. **Safety cannot be over-emphasized.** When one is dealing with potentially violent, aggressive, or agitated patients, unpredictability should be anticipated. Trust your feelings when you do not feel safe with a patient and take the necessary precautions to manage the environment before you continue with the examination.

2. Mental status examination

a. **The mental status examination should focus on the sensorium, evidence of organicity or delirium, mood instability, agitated depression, impulsivity, agitation, paranoid states, the presence of thought disorders, command hallucinations, and intoxicated states.**

b. Violence is more likely to occur when a thought disorder is present. It is difficult to determine whether a patient with irrational, delusional, paranoid, or psychotic thinking will act on his or her thoughts and beliefs. When a thought disorder is part of the psychiatric pathology, careful attention to the possibility of violence and aggression is necessary.

c. Severe depression can result in impaired reality testing, fatalistic thinking, and psychosis that may increase the likelihood of acting-out in an aggressive or violent manner toward oneself or others.

d. If the patient admits to having violent thoughts, it is important to ascertain the severity of the intention, the presence of a plan, and the likelihood of action. Direct and honest discussion is a tool the clinician uses during the examination.

3. Pertinent laboratory and physical findings

a. During the emergent phase of the evaluation and management of violence, **the medical work-up follows from the clinical presentation, physical examination, and clinical history.** The following tests should be performed:

   i. Routine blood counts, chemistries, and toxicology

   ii. Organic brain work-up for dementia (see Chapter 22)

   iii. Other laboratory tests based on clinical suspicion

      (a) Electroencephalography (EEG) and brain imaging

      (b) Radiographic studies related to pertinent clinical findings or complaints, such as chest x-rays to look for pneumonia

      (c) Arterial blood gases

      (d) HIV testing (see Chapter 39)

      (e) Neuropsychological testing

      (f) Others as indicated by pertinent differentials

b. Once the acute phase of managing a patient with violent behavior is stabilized, clinical decisions about outpatient versus inpatient evaluation and treatment can be made.

   i. Initiate treatment of primary psychiatric disorders with psychotropic medication during an inpatient stay and then transition into outpatient care as the threat of violence or behavioral disturbance abates.

   ii. Close follow-up with adequate social supports may allow treatment to start on an outpatient basis.

III. Psychiatric Differential Diagnosis

A. Organic Mental Disorders (Table 60-1)

1. Primary central nervous system (CNS) disorders
2. Medical disorders affecting the CNS

B. Psychoactive Substance Use Disorders

1. Alcohol abuse is a common cause of violence in patients brought to the emergency room.

   a. When intoxicated, a patient may be disinhibited, aggressive, suicidal, and homicidal. When the patient sobers up, there may no longer be any ideas of harming, or intent to harm oneself or others. Because blackouts are associated with heavy alcohol use, containing an aggressive and intoxicated patient in a safe environment until the patient can be evaluated in a sober state is a public safety issue. Based on local community protocols and standards of practice, disruptive and intoxicated citizens are managed by the police or brought to the emergency room.

   b. In withdrawal states, patients may be irritable, agitated, delirious, or involved in aggressive or violent behavior.

   c. Dementia and hallucinosis may indicate permanent brain damage from chronic alcohol abuse and may persist whether the patient continues to drink or not.

2. Psychostimulants

   a. Cocaine intoxication and withdrawal states

   b. Amphetamine intoxication

3. Hallucinogens

   a. Phenyclidine (PCP) intoxication

   b. Inhalants, such as glue, volatile gases, and nitrous oxide

4. Sedative-hypnotics

   a. Disinhibition reactions with benzodiazepines

   b. Intoxication and withdrawal states

5. Opiates

   a. Opiate intoxication and withdrawal states

   b. Drug-procuring activities and risk of violence

   c. Scopolamine or other anticholinergic agents used to prepare heroin

6. Other prescription drugs

   a. Anticholinergics, such as benztropine (Cogentin) and trihexyphenidyl (Artane) may be abused by chronically mentally ill patients treated with neuroleptics.

   b. Steroids

C. Psychiatric Disorders

1. **Schizophrenia**

   a. Paranoid schizophrenia is characterized by paranoid delusions of persecution that may result in aggressive action by the patient toward the source of the patient's perceived persecution.

   b. Command auditory hallucinations induce actions on command.

   c. Impulsivity and disorganization are characteristic of the chronic deteriorating course of schizophrenia and may present as irritated, agitated, or aggressive behavior in an unpredictable manner.

2. **Mood disorders**

   a. Mania is an unstable and unpredictable mental state. These patients may display aggression based on feelings of omnipotence, paranoia, or other forms of psychotic and grandiose thinking.

    b. Psychotic depression or mixed bipolar states may result in unpredictable violence or aggression.

  3. **Disruptive behavioral disorders**

    a. Attention deficit hyperactivity disorder (ADHD) is thought of as an illness of childhood and adolescence. Some children who are diagnosed with this condition demonstrate inattentiveness and impulsivity, often resulting in aggressive and behavioral problems at home and in school.

      i. Adult residual ADHD is a recognized disorder that may underlie aggressive, impulsive, and harmful behaviors.

      ii. Any form of ADHD has a high incidence of co-morbid diagnoses involving substance abuse disorders and other psychiatric disorders.

    b. Conduct disorder is a behavioral problem of childhood and adolescence that may lead to an antisocial personality in adulthood.

  4. **Intermittent explosive disorder** is a general diagnosis for patients with a history of several episodes of aggressive behavior that were out of proportion to the precipitating stressors and were not due to other psychiatric disorders, substance abuse, or medical conditions.

  5. **Personality disorders**

    a. By definition, a personality disorder is a pattern of behavior and inner experience manifested by disordered cognitions, affects, impulse control, and interpersonal functioning, as well as significant distress or impairment in social, occupational, or other important areas of functioning.

    b. Any personality disorder can potentially lead to inappropriate behavior that may manifest as violence.

    c. The personality disorders that more commonly manifest as violence include the paranoid, antisocial, and borderline types.

IV. Treatment Strategies

A. Acute pharmacologic management

  1. In the initial management of violent or aggressive behavior, **the goal is to decrease further risk of harm to the patient, staff, or environment while performing the medical and psychiatric evaluation.**

  2. If the patient is mildly to moderately agitated, **oral benzodiazepines may be effective** in producing behavioral calm and may allow the clinical evaluation to proceed without further risk of violence.

    a. The use of benzodiazepines can be helpful in patients without known substance abuse problems or organic brain syndromes.

    b. The choice of which benzodiazepine to use is based on the pharmacologic profile.

      i. Alprazolam is fast-acting but it can be administered only orally.

      ii. Diazepam has a rapid onset but a long half-life, and this may cause problems for geriatric patients and for patients who need a clear sensorium for further evaluation. An advantage of using diazepam is a variable route of administration: oral, intramuscular (IM), and intravenous (IV).

      iii. Lorazepam is a highly reliable benzodiazepine because of its moderate half-life, lack of active metabolites, and ease of administration. It can be given by the sublingual, oral, IM, and IV routes.

      iv. The starting dose of the benzodiazepines depends on the age and underlying diagnosis of the patient. Generally, for mild to moderate agitation, the initial dose would be the lowest dose for that particular agent and would be further titrated on the basis of the response (e.g., alprazolam 0.5 mg, diazepam 5 mg, lorazepam 1 mg).

3. However, **if the agitation is moderate to severe or severe,** oral agents take too long and are not reliable in a non-compliant and resisting patient. In this situation, **parenteral preparations of benzodiazepines and/or neuroleptics** are indicated.

4. **The choice of which neuroleptic to use is based on the known diagnosis, the side effect profile of the neuroleptic, and the desired effect.**

   a. **Haloperidol is a high-potency neuroleptic** that has minimal side effects other than those related to dopamine blockade. It has a good safety profile in reference to cardiopulmonary side effects. It is flexibly administered using the oral, IM, or IV route.

      i. One or two doses of haloperidol 5 mg IM or IV will manage most incidents of aggression. The administration of the same dose every 30 to 60 minutes will calm most agitated patients.

      ii. When it is given intravenously, there are significantly fewer extrapyramidal reactions, such as dystonias and akathisia.

      iii. As in the use of other neuroleptics, attention should be paid to the possible occurrence of *torsades des pointes,* especially in alcoholics and patients with significant electrolyte imbalance, particularly hypomagnesemia.

   b. Other antipsychotics, such as droperidol, chlorpromazine, perphenazine, olanzapine, risperidone, and ziprasadone can be used in the acute setting.

      i. Droperidol is given only parenterally and has significant alpha-adrenergic activity, potentially lowering blood pressure and causing sedation. Dosage starts at 2.5 mg. It is highly effective and may be used in place of haloperidol if there has been a problem with the use of haloperidol in a particular patient. Electrocardographic monitoring must be used, as the FDA has warned about its association with QT_C prolongation.

      ii. Chlorpromazine has more anticholinergic side effects than do the other neuroleptics. Its sedative properties can be highly effective in patients who do not respond to the usual doses of the higher-potency neuroleptics.

      iii. Perphenazine, olanzapine, risperidone and/or ziprasadone has been limited by the requirement for an oral route of administration which meant using them in a cooperative patient. They are associated with fewer frequent extrapyramidal side effects, more sedation, and with the maintenance of behavioral calm after the acute phase. These drugs may be highly effective and are easily tolerated by patients in the early phases of decompensation. At present, the FDA has approved the use of IM preparations of both olanzapine and ziprasadone for the treatment of agitation.

   c. The combined use of haloperidol and lorazepam constitutes a safe, easy way to manage an agitated patient. These agents can be given in the same syringe and have synergistic effects. The potential of extrapyramidal side effects is lessened by their co-administration.

B. **Chronic management**

   1. **Diagnosis guides the more specific and lasting management** of an aggressive and violent patient.

   2. **Comprehensive neuropsychological testing** and cognitive-behavioral assessment help establish the appropriate treatment approach for each individual.

   3. The treatment approach includes **psychopharmacologic management; individual therapies** that may include cognitive re-training, behavioral management, and a supportive approach; **family interventions;** and **psychosocial supports**

that may include residential treatment, day treatment programs, and vocational rehabilitation.

4. **A variety of pharmacologic treatments are used in the chronic management of aggressive behavior.** The choice of agent depends on underlying diagnosis and the particular target symptoms.
   a. **Antipsychotics**
   b. **Anxiolytics**
      i. Benzodiazepines may be used.
      ii. Buspirone is a non-benzodiazepine, non-sedating anxiolytic that has unpredictable efficacy in a given patient. Usually trial and error will allow the clinician to determine whether this medication will be useful.
   c. **Anticonvulsants**
      i. Carbamazepine can be used safely in the therapeutic range. Attention should be paid to hematologic and hepatic function.
      ii. Valproic acid is well tolerated and has few side effects.
   d. **Lithium**
   e. **Beta-adrenergic blockers**
      i. Propranolol in high doses helps control chronic, recurrent aggressive and violent behaviors that often are refractory to other treatments.
      ii. Propranolol is used most successfully in patients with organic brain causes.
      iii. Propranolol requires several months of gradual dose increases up to 800 mg per day for a clinical trial to be completed.
   f. **Psychostimulants**
      i. Psychostimulants are effective in treating violence caused by impulsivity from adult residual ADHD.

5. **The combined use of patient-specific psychosocial therapies and medications provides the best approach to the long-term management of behavioral disorders.**

Selected References

Anderson, W.H. (1980). The physical examination in office practice. *American Journal of Psychiatry, 137,* 1188–1192.

Cummings, J.L., & Trimble, M.R. (2002). *Concise guide to neuropsychiatry and behavioral neurology* (2nd ed.). Washington DC: American Psychiatric Press.

Diagnostic and statistic manual of mental disorders IV-TR. (2000). Washington, DC: American Psychiatric Association.

Hyman, S.E. (1994). The violent patient. In S.E. Hyman, & G.E. Tesar (Eds), *Manual of psychiatric emergencies* (3rd ed.). Boston: Little, Brown, pp. 28–37.

Monahan, J., & Shah, S.A. (1989). Dangerousness and commitment of the mentally disordered in the United States. *Schizophrenia Bulletin, 15,* 541–553.

Feinstein, R., & Plutchik, R. (1990). Violence and suicide risk assessment in the psychiatric emergency room. *Comprehensive Psychiatry, 31,* 337–343.

Tardiff, K. (1996). *Concise guide to assessment and management of violent patient* (2nd ed.). Washington, DC: American Psychiatric Press.

Volavka, J. (1995). *Neurobiology of violence.* Washington, DC: American Psychiatric Press.

Rundell, J.R., & Wise, M.G. (2000). *Concise guide to consultation psychiatry* (3rd ed.). Washington, DC: American Psychiatric Press.

CHAPTER 61

Civil Commitment and the Patient Refusing Treatment

RONALD SCHOUTEN

I. Introduction

Individuals with serious mental illness may require hospitalization to protect themselves or others. One of the most difficult problems in this area is that symptoms of the illness may include a lack of insight into the need for hospitalization or treatment. The process of hospitalizing a person against his or her will is referred to as **involuntary civil commitment.** The law in this area can cause considerable confusion and frustration for the family and for the physician of a patient with serious mental illness. This frustration increases when caregivers realize that **involuntary commitment in most states does not automatically mean that the patient can be forced to accept treatment.**

A. **Legal Restrictions on Civil Commitment**
   1. Confinement of an individual against his or her will is considered to be a deprivation of fundamental rights guaranteed under the Constitution of the United States and state constitutions.
      a. Civil commitment is considered to be an act of the state government because it occurs under the authority of the state.
      b. Before a state can deprive someone of his or her fundamental rights, proper procedural protections (e.g., a court or administrative hearing before a neutral fact finder) must be granted. Such procedures collectively constitute due process, which is guaranteed by the Constitution.
   2. **In non-emergencies, the patient is entitled to a full hearing before he or she can be confined.**
   3. Lawsuits for deprivation of civil rights, false imprisonment, and negligence can arise from improper civil commitment.
   4. **An individual can only be involuntarily committed if he or she is a danger to self or others. The mere need for treatment, in the absence of risk of harm, is not sufficient.**

B. **The Right to Refuse Treatment**
   1. **All competent people have a right to make their own medical treatment decisions, and all adults are presumed to be competent.** Thus, a patient who requires involuntary commitment may still refuse treatment until such time as he or she is declared incompetent.
      a. This applies even to those individuals who are suffering from serious mental illness.
      b. The presumption of competency persists until a court has declared a person to be incompetent.

        i. **The clinical assessment that a person lacks the capacity to engage in certain activities (e.g., medical decision-making) does not mean that the person is incompetent in the eyes of the law; only a judge can make that declaration.**

        ii. Clinical assessments of capacity are generally relied upon by the courts.

        iii. **When a patient is believed to be incapacitated from making treatment decisions, the physician should seek an alternative decision-maker** rather than relying on the presumption of competence and allowing the patient to continue making treatment decisions.

2. Individuals who are incompetent still have a right to individual autonomy, which can be honored by following their preferences for treatment expressed when they were competent.

    a. Courts will appoint a **guardian** to make decisions on behalf of the incompetent individual. The incompetent individual is known as the **ward** once the guardianship is established.

    b. To better protect the autonomy of the patient, many states require that a substituted judgment analysis be used when treatment decisions are being made on behalf of the ward. This requires the decision-maker to determine what the incompetent patient would have chosen if competent under the circumstances.

II. The Civil Commitment Process

A. The details of the commitment process vary among the states. Physicians should become familiar with the applicable rules and procedures in their jurisdictions.

1. For example, in California an emergency commitment is valid for 72 hours, during which time the patient is evaluated to determine whether further commitment is necessary and justified. In Massachusetts, the emergency commitment is for 4 days.

2. States also differ in how mental illness is defined. Some states, for example, do not consider substance abuse and disorders like Alzheimer's disease as mental illnesses for the purpose of civil commitment, although confinement in substance abuse treatment facilities or public health facilities may be possible.

3. **Although the details differ, all states use the criteria of danger to self or others as the basis for involuntary commitment.** The danger must be the result of mental illness, rather than ordinary anger or antisocial behavior. As a result, a hired killer would not be an appropriate candidate for involuntary commitment to a psychiatric hospital should his murderous intentions become known, absent evidence that a mental illness other than a personality disorder contributed to his dangerousness.

B. The Dangerousness Criteria

1. **Danger to self** means attempts at serious self-harm or suicide, or credible threats to cause such self-harm.

    a. **Threats of self-injury** should be assessed for their seriousness. This includes a determination as to whether the patient has the means of carrying out the threat (e.g., access to a handgun) or has a history of serious suicide attempts. (See Chapter 15) A history of violence is the best predictor of future violence.

    b. A history of non-fatal wrist slashing or medication overdose should be taken seriously; successful suicide can occur as the result of a miscalculation of dosages, or the time when a rescuer may arrive.

    c. **The assessment of risk** should begin, but does not end, with questioning the patient about thoughts of self-injury. Individuals who are determined to kill themselves will avoid telling those who could put them in the hospital. The careful clinician relies upon the overall clinical picture, including life events, symptoms, substance abuse, and history of self-injury in making an assessment of dangerousness to self.

2. **Danger to others generally refers to threats or attempts to cause physical harm to others, or actual harm already inflicted.** In addition, it may include situations in which others are placed in reasonable fear that they will be harmed by the patient.

   a. **Explicit threats** to cause physical harm must be taken seriously. The dilemma is often whether such threats are the result of an illness or merely antisocial behavior. In the former case, the patient might be appropriate for civil commitment to a hospital. In the latter case, the threats are more properly within the realm of the criminal justice system.

   b. **Implied threats** ("If he knows what's good for him, he will stop following me") and conditional threats ("If I don't get the money they owe me, I'm going to blow somebody away") must be taken seriously, as well.

   c. **In many states, the law imposes a duty on clinicians to take steps to protect the safety of third parties against whom a patient issues threats.** Although these laws generally apply to mental health professionals, primary care physicians (PCPs) providing psychiatric care will likely find these same rules applying to them.

3. Individuals may also be involuntarily committed if they pose a substantial risk of harm because they are unable to provide for their own well-being in the community. In some states, this criterion is referred to as **the gravely disabled criterion.**

   a. Generally, mere difficulty caring for oneself is not enough to meet this criterion. The **risk of harm** (e.g., believing that one is invincible and therefore can walk into traffic) **must be substantial and imminent.** A likelihood of harm in the distant future is not sufficient.

   b. **Civil commitment under this criterion,** as well as the others, **is permissible only if no less restrictive alternative is available in the community.** Alternatives to civil commitment may include increased outpatient visits, voluntary hospitalization, day hospital programs, custodial care by relatives, or shelters.

III. Approach to Treatment Refusal

A. **The law concerning treatment refusal, like the law of civil commitment, varies among the states.**

1. **States generally draw a distinction between routine and ordinary medical care** (e.g., antibiotics and minor surgery), **and extraordinary or invasive care** (e.g., cancer chemotherapy and coronary artery bypass grafting). These distinctions will not always make clinical sense, but their origins can often be traced to specific cases that were brought before the court.

   a. Benzodiazepines and antidepressants are generally considered to be routine, ordinary, and non-invasive.

   b. Antipsychotic medication, electroconvulsive therapy, and psychosurgery are considered to constitute extraordinary, dangerous, and invasive treatments in many states.

2. States differ in what legal steps must be taken before a patient's refusal of treatment can be overridden.

   a. The basic rule in all stages is **that competent individuals have a right to make their own treatment decisions, including refusal of treatment that others believe is in the patient's best interest.** Exceptions to this rule exist in matters involving criminal law and the correctional system.

b. When a patient who appears to lack the capacity to make treatment decisions refuses routine and ordinary care, physicians can generally rely upon family members or significant others who know the patient to make a decision.

c. **When the care to be provided is extraordinary, invasive, or dangerous, many states require that a formal guardian be appointed to make the treatment decisions.**

   i. Guardianship is established after a hearing at which family members, treaters, and sometimes the patient will testify.

   ii. Not all states allow the guardian, once appointed, to make all decisions on behalf of the patient. In some states, extraordinary, invasive, or dangerous care can only be authorized by a judge after a full trial on the issue, with the guardian assigned to monitor the care.

   iii. Whereas some states require full adversarial proceedings and judicial involvement in these matters, others (including Federal courts) believe that professional judgment and administrative review satisfy the due process requirements without going to court.

B. **When a patient refuses psychiatric care,** it is helpful to ask certain questions.

1. **Does the patient's explanation for the refusal suggest a rational decision or incompetence?**

   a. Has the physician spent enough time with the patient to explain the treatment and reasons for it?

   b. Did the patient understand the information and explanations?

   c. Is the patient's decision the product of a logical thought process based upon his or her existing beliefs and experiences and the information provided?

2. If the answer to these questions is yes, then there is little basis to challenge the presumption that the patient is competent. In such cases, the physician should make every effort to persuade the patient to act in his or her best interests, as seen by the physician, without coercing the patient.

3. If there appears to be a basis for questioning the competency of the patient, an alternative decision-maker should be sought.

   a. Check with your hospital attorney or other legal advisor as to the law on these matters in your state.

   b. Check to see if the patient has a durable power of attorney or health care proxy, which gives someone else the power to make decisions on the patient's behalf in the event of incompetence.

   c. Determine if the proposed treatment is regarded under state law as invasive, extraordinary, or unduly burdensome. This will help decide what type of analysis will be undertaken (best interest vs. substituted judgment) and who the decision-maker will be (family member, guardian, or judge).

   d. The treating physician is generally asked to complete an affidavit concerning the issues of incompetency and the treatment recommendations that have been rejected by the patient. The affidavit is sometimes sufficient, but the physician may be called to testify about the contents of the affidavit.

4. Once the court has authorized treatment, it can proceed, even over the patient's objections.

5. If the guardian has been appointed to make decisions on behalf of the patient, the guardian's authority will be defined by the court. In those areas where the court has given the guardian authority, the guardian has the same authority to make decisions as the patient would have had if competent.

IV. Conclusion

A. Legal restrictions in these areas are designed to protect fundamental rights that are important to all of us, not to frustrate physicians or interfere with clinical care.

B. Although these restrictions can be frustrating, they are manageable under the following circumstances:
1. They are anticipated.
2. Physicians understand the legal requirements and how to meet them.
3. Physicians overcome their natural aversion to lawyers and take advantage of the legal representation available to them.

Suggested Readings

Appelbaum, P.S., & Gutheil, T.G. (2000). *Clinical handbook of psychiatry and the law* (3rd ed.). Baltimore: Williams & Wilkins.

Emanuel, E.J., & Emanuel, L.L. (1992). Proxy decision making for incompetent patients. An ethical and empirical analysis. *Journal of the American Medical Association, 267*(15), 2067–2071.

Fried, T.R., Bradley, E.H., Towle, V.R., & Allore, H. (2002). Understanding the treatment preferences of seriously ill patients. *New England Journal of Medicine, 346*(14), 1061–1066.

Greco, P.J., Schulman, K.A., Lavizzo-Mourey, R., et al. (1991). The Patient Self-determination Act and the future of advance directives. *Annals of Internal Medicine, 115,* 639–643.

Hundert, E.M. (1990). Competing medical and legal ethical values. In R. Rosner, & R. Weinstock (Eds.), *Ethical practice in psychiatry and the law.* New York: Plenum, pp. 53–72.

Spring, R.L., Lacoursiere, R.B., & Weissenberger, G. (1997). *Patients, psychiatrists, and lawyers: Law and the mental health system* (2nd ed.). Cincinnati: Anderson Publishing Co.

Werth, J.L., Jr. (2001). U.S. involuntary mental health commitment statutes: Requirements for persons perceived to be a potential harm to self. *Suicide & Life-Threatening Behavior, 31*(3), 348–357.

CHAPTER 62
The Management of Denial

BARBARA CANNON, JEFF C. HUFFMAN, AND THEODORE A. STERN

I. Introduction

In the medical setting, a patient's denial may have important clinical implications.

A. Patients manifest denial over a wide range of conditions.

1. The prevalence of denial has been poorly studied, but it appears to affect a significant proportion of medically ill patients.

2. A study of patients hospitalized for myocardial infarction (MI) found that 11% of the patients doubted that they actually had an MI and another 8% entirely denied having an MI.

3. Medical inpatients diagnosed with cancer deny their illness approximately 5–15% of the time. Such denial may be prolonged; one study found that 4% of patients denied having cancer six months after their diagnosis.

4. Denial of illness may also be manifest as treatment delay, which has been defined as waiting more than three months between the appearance of a specific symptom and seeking medical evaluation. Treatment delay is common (e.g., 35–50% of cancer patients delay evaluation of their symptoms for greater than three months), and, in breast cancer, delay in evaluation has been significantly associated with greater mortality rates.

5. Risk factors for denial may include older age, lower levels of education, history of risk-taking behavior, and inability to express negative emotions. However, fear or anxiety about the illness and its consequences may be the greatest risk factor for the development of denial.

B. Denial implies a disagreement between the patient and the physician about the presence, implications, or likely outcome of a disease.

C. A patient's denial should alert the physician that the patient may be having trouble coping with the stress of illness and death.

D. Physicians tend to criticize patients who deny. However, all adults, even highly functioning ones, use denial to cope with fear or anxiety.

E. Denial may be either adaptive or maladaptive.

1. In certain situations, denial may be linked with resiliency. Patients with initial denial after diagnoses of unstable angina and breast cancer have been found to have improved medical outcomes.

2. However, denial can also be maladaptive and lead to suboptimal treatment and poorer outcomes. **To judge whether denial is maladaptive, physicians should assess behavior rather than ideation.**

3. **Denial should be considered maladaptive when it interferes with: (a) treatment-seeking** (e.g., in treatment delay), **(b) treatment compliance** (e.g., with medications or dietary recommendations), **or (c) medical decision-making** (e.g., when diagnostic procedures are refused because the patient denies having an illness).

F. Denial is a complex process which must be understood in its clinical context. Patients may deny at some times but not at others, may deny some aspects of their condition but not others, and may deny to some people but not to others.

1. When an illness threatens critical relationships, patients may deny aspects of the illness to preserve those relationships.
2. A patient may deny to protect the physicians from feelings of impotence or grief. Physicians may collude in the denial.
3. Denial may be part of a patient's pattern of poor coping.
4. Denial and numbness, alternating with intrusive preoccupation, represent a normal response to an acute stress, such as the diagnosis of a life-threatening illness.

II. Differential Diagnosis of Denial

A. A patient who appears to deny may have poor communication with his or her physicians.

1. Physicians may give insufficient information to patients about their conditions. Patients often need to have bad news explained repeatedly as they try to master it.
2. A patient may not understand a physician's complex vocabulary, jargon, and syntax.
3. Physicians and patients may speak different languages.
4. A patient's hearing may be impaired.

B. A patient with cognitive impairment may be unable to assimilate information about his or her illnesses.

1. Delirium and intoxication impair a patient's attention.
2. Dementia and mental retardation impair a patient's ability to comprehend complex information.
3. Severe episodes of mental illness (e.g., depression, psychosis, or mania) may impair a patient's cognition.

C. Some patients hold alternative beliefs from their cultural or social groups or subgroups, a situation best understood as cross-cultural difference, not denial.

D. A patient may be non-compliant with a physician's recommendations without being in denial.

E. Anosognosia—denial or unawareness of a neurologic deficit—stems from specific cortical lesions.

1. Right parietal lesions and sometimes subcortical lesions can cause neglect of hemiplegic limbs, usually on the left side of the body.
2. Bilateral occipital lesions can produce denial of blindness (Anton's syndrome).

III. Assessing Denial

Physicians may guide their assessment of denial by asking the following questions:

A. How does the patient perceive his or her condition? Determine what the patient is doing about his or her conditions, not what is being avoided.

B. What is the context of denial?

1. What is the patient denying? The presence of disease? The likelihood of death or disability? The fear of death? The risk of a certain behavior?
2. To whom and in what setting is the patient denying?
3. What does the patient gain by denying?

C. What are a patient's social supports?

1. Are the patient's significant others able to cope with the stress of illness? Significant others who find the stress of a patient's illness overwhelming may need to have the patient deny that illness.
2. Does the patient have other community, religious, cultural, or professional supports?

D. Are the patient's denial behaviors likely to worsen the course of illness?

1. Is the patient seeking appropriate medical care?
2. How severe are the consequences of denial likely to be?

E. Is the patient able to care for him or herself?

1. Does the patient fail to perceive obvious physical problems with his or her body?
2. Does the patient's hygiene or physical condition suggest poor self-care?
3. Does the patient have a history of coping poorly with the stresses of daily life?

F. What aspect or consequence of illness does the patient fear most? Death? Disfigurement? Pain? Isolation? Loss of control? Loss of crucial relationships? Loss of self-regard?

G. How does the patient experience fear and anxiety about his or her illnesses?

1. A patient may deny fear and anxiety or experience others as being afraid. He or she may joke about their condition, minimize their distress, or engage in reckless behavior.
2. A patient may acknowledge a tolerable level of fear and anxiety.
3. A patient may worry or ruminate excessively about aspects of their illnesses. He or she may worry instead about their families and jobs.
4. A patient may suffer from panic or terror, often alternating with numbing or dissociation.
5. A patient may feel disorganized or confused or may feel unusual anger, bitterness, or another strong emotion.

H. How does the patient experience medical care? What are the patient's prior experiences with physicians and illness (in themselves and their loved ones)? A patient who has suffered trauma with illness may be fearful and apt to deny.

I. Is the patient psychiatrically ill? Most patients who deny do not have a psychiatric illness; however, in some patients psychiatric illness may contribute to denial.

IV. Strategies for Managing Denial

A. Physicians should strive to maintain a neutral stance toward patients who deny.

1. Approaching a patient with respect builds rapport.
2. Physicians should avoid power struggles and threats, which are harmful to patients.
3. Describing a patient's and a physician's clashing perspectives as differences of opinion tends to neutralize denial-related conflict.
4. Physicians should avoid taking denial personally. Denial most often reflects a patient's psychological state, not his or her opinion of a physician's competence.
5. Supporting a patient's wishes to get a second opinion shows respect for the patient's agency. For patients who choose to seek treatment elsewhere, welcoming them to return to treatment, if they choose, shows tolerance and acceptance.
6. With a patient who is beginning to acknowledge denial, physicians can normalize denial. Physicians can acknowledge to a patient that to some degree all individuals deny their vulnerability of illness and death.

B. Addressing denial requires effective communication.

1. Physicians should hear a patient's point of view and present their own. Active listening includes having each party repeat what the other has said (to clarify it and to reassure both parties that they have understood each other).
2. Physicians should assure that a patient has adequate information. Physicians should solicit questions and repeat information that a patient requires without intruding.

C. Support reduces a patient's need to deny. Physicians can do the following:

1. Assure the patient that they will be available throughout the course of illness and that they can effectively manage the illness or its symptoms.
2. Mobilize and support a patient's family and significant others. Families may need referral for additional support (to help manage stress and for other consequences of illness).
3. Encourage the patient's initiatives in coping with illness which are not harmful.
4. Encourage the patient's to engage in activities which build self-esteem.

D. Working with a patient's personal coping style is more likely to be effective than is working against it.

1. Identify a patient's strengths—courage, generosity, dedication to family or work, competence, intelligence—and encourage the patient to express them constructively.
2. Negotiate with the patient about participation in medical decision-making and control of medical treatment. Physicians should respect a patient's decision to take a less active role in medical management. In treating a patient who is used to being in control, physicians should allow the maximum control of treatment which does not compromise medical care.

E. Physicians should use psychiatric medications to target distress in a denying patient.

1. Benzodiazepines, such as clonazepam 0.5 mg b.i.d., can relieve anxiety. When a patient in an acute medical crisis is in denial, physicians should intervene early to relieve the anxiety with medication while proceeding with the evaluation and treatment.
2. Physicians can relieve a patient's extreme anxiety or terror with low-dose neuroleptics, such as haloperidol 0.5 to 2 mg every 4 hours p.r.n., not to exceed 6 mg/24 hours.
3. Physicians should assertively treat a patient with major depression with suitable antidepressant medication.
4. Psychiatric consultants can help manage severe psychiatric conditions, such as suicidality, psychosis, and mania.

F. Physicians should avoid confronting the patient in denial unless that denial leads to harmful behaviors.

1. Confronting the patient works best in the context of a good rapport. Even when physicians determine that a confrontation is necessary, they can consider deferring it until the patient and the physician have developed trust and a working alliance.
2. Confrontation consists of presenting to a patient in a neutral manner the difference between the patient's beliefs and actions and the beliefs and recommendations of the physician.

G. A small minority of denying patients who lack the capacity to make decisions about medical care may require guardianship.

1. Physicians should not restrict a patient's self-determination because of denial alone. Patients have the right to make judgments which seem foolish to others.
2. Physicians probably should pursue guardianship only when a patient does not acknowledge the simple facts of illness. If a patient merely does not comprehend the

significance or consequences of an illness, the physician probably should not pursue guardianship.

3. Physicians may need to take drastic interim measures, for example, combining sedation and restraints, for the patient whose incapacity to acknowledge the simple facts of illness puts him or her at risk for immediate, severe complications.

H. To assess whether they are colluding with a patient's denial, physicians may ask themselves the following questions:

1. Is the physician withdrawing either by physical absence or by avoiding discussion of a certain aspects of a patient's condition?

2. Does the physician find the patient's conditions personally threatening?

3. Does the physician respond to certain patients in unusual ways, such as with hostility or extreme concern?

I. Physicians should assess whether these interventions help the patient who denies.

1. Interventions probably work best if the patient more freely acknowledges his or her fears or changes their harmful behaviors.

2. Interventions probably are failing if the patient denies more or avoids medical contact more often.

Suggested Readings

Edelstein, E.L., Nathanson, D.L., & Stone, A.M. (Eds.). (1989). *Denial.* New York: Plenum Press.

Gavin, A.T., Fitzpatrick, D., Middleton, R.J., et al. (2002). Patients' denial of disease may pose difficulties for obtaining informed consent. *British Medical Journal, 324,* 974.

Goldbeck, R. (1997). Denial in physical illness. *Journal of Psychosomatic Research, 43,* 575–593.

Hackett, T.P., & Cassem, N.H. (1974). Development of a quantitative rating scale to assess denial. *Journal of Psychosomatic Research, 18*(93), 623–627.

Horowitz, M.J. (1985). Disasters and psychological responses to stress. *Psychiatric Annals, 15,* 161–167.

Kumkel, E.J., Woods, C.M., Rodgers, C., et al. (1997). Consultations for "maladaptive denial of illness" in patients with cancer: Psychiatric disorders that lead to noncompliance. *Psychooncology, 6,* 139–149.

Muskin, P.R., Feldhammer, T., Gelfand, J.L., et al. (1998). Maladaptive denial of physical illness: A useful new "diagnosis." *International Journal of Psychiatry in Medicine, 28,* 463–477.

Ness, D.E., & Ende, J. (1994). Denial in the medical interview: Recognition and management. *Journal of the American Medical Association, 272,* 1777–1781.

Weisman, A.D. (1972). *On dying and denying.* New York: Behavioral Publications.

CHAPTER 63

The Patient Seeking Disability Benefits

RONALD SCHOUTEN

I. Introduction

Physicians often are asked to certify that a patient has a psychiatric or physical disability. The reasons for this certification are varied and include the documentation of disability status in connection with a medical leave of absence, Social Security benefits, workers' compensation claims, short- and long-term disability insurance claims, and compliance with the Americans with Disabilities Act and the Family and Medical Leave Act. The subjective nature of psychiatric symptoms, such as complaints of stress, and the impact of those symptoms on the ability to work create special problems in the evaluation of a psychiatric disability. Numerous differences exist between the **standard clinical evaluation** and an **independent disability evaluation.** These differences are outlined below and summarized in Table 63-1.

A. The Clinical Evaluation

1. **Physicians generally assume that patients will report their symptoms accurately and without significant intentional exaggeration or understatement.** Trust in the accuracy of the patient's reporting is at the heart of the clinical assessment. As a

Table 63-1. Summary of Differences between Clinical Evaluations and Independent Disability Evaluations

Clinical Evaluations	Independent Disability Evaluations
Assumption of accuracy of the patient's self-report	Objective assessment of accuracy of the patient's self-report
Purpose of the evaluation is treatment	Purpose of the evaluation is assessment of the patient's claim
Patient is the primary source of information	Corroborating information is sought from other sources
Transference and countertransference are active	Transference and countertransference are active
Information obtained in the course of treatment is generally confidential	Information obtained in the course of evaluation is not confidential
Evaluation is conducted at the request of the patient seeking treatment	Evaluation is performed at the request of a third party
Payment for the evaluation comes from the patient, usually through a health insurer	Payment for the evaluation comes from the party requesting the evaluation

result, in most clinical evaluations physicians rely on the patient as the sole source of information. A request for corroborating information can offend the patient and harm the treatment relationship.

   a. Generally, a monetary issue is involved when a statement of disability is requested. This may involve either the payment of compensation during a period of disability or clearance to return to work. As a result, **some patients may be motivated to exaggerate, malinger, or minimize symptoms in accordance with their goals in pursuing a disability assessment.**

   b. While it is not the physician's job to guarantee the accuracy of patients' complaints in disability matters, other factors compel physicians to be objective and accurate in the assessment and documentation of disability.

      i. Certification of disability may remove a patient from the workforce permanently, often to the detriment of the patient's full recovery.

      ii. The physician may ultimately be called on to justify his or her assessment in court.

      iii. Inaccurate certification that a patient is no longer disabled and is fit to return to work can create a risk of harm to the patient and the patient's co-workers. Negligence in evaluation can provide the basis for a malpractice lawsuit against the physician.

2. **The focus of a clinical evaluation is the diagnosis and treatment of a disorder,** not the gathering of evidence for an administrative or legal proceeding.

3. **The physician has an obligation to serve as an advocate for the patient.** This can significantly limit the doctor's ability to be objective in situations in which the patient already has in mind the preferred outcome of the evaluation.

4. Patients may have certain expectations of their physicians and respond to them in ways which may not be readily understandable. Often these expectations and responses are products of the patient's experience with parents, caregivers, authority figures, and physicians. The unconscious patterns evident in a patient's relationship with a physician that reflect aspects of the patient's past are called **transference.** Similarly, a physician may unconsciously attribute feelings, experiences, and attitudes that reflect the physician's experiences with others to the patient. This is known as **countertransference.**

   a. Transference and countertransference occur in everyday life and in all types of medical practice, including primary care.

      i. If ignored, these phenomena can cause significant harm to the doctor-patient relationship and lead to an increased risk of malpractice in any type of medical practice. For example, a physician who has a low tolerance for complaining patients may become abrupt in the examination and treatment of an overly dependent patient. This may lead to poor judgment, errors in treatment, and rejection of the patient; each of these factors is associated with an increased risk of harm to the patient and with malpractice claims.

      ii. Transference and countertransference occur with all types of patients, not just those identified as psychiatric patients.

      iii. Transference and countertransference are particularly evident in, but are not limited to, the treatment of patients with psychiatric disorders. These phenomena can be most striking in patients who have certain personality traits or personality disorders, such as narcissistic, borderline, or dependent patients.

   b. **Transference and countertransference often have a major impact on the evaluation of disability.** This occurs in several ways.

      i. The patient may engender feelings of sympathy which cloud the physician's objectivity.

ii. Countertransference also can cloud the physician's judgment, leading to immediate rejection of the patient's complaints.

iii. The pressure to provide the patient with the answer he or she wants can be extreme and uncomfortable, especially in long-standing treatment relationships. The patient may expect the physician to respond to a request for assistance in a parental fashion, that is, by fulfilling the patient's needs and desires. For example, a patient may bring a request for disability certification or authorization to return to work to a physician with the attitude that "of course Dr. Smith will do this for me."

iv. Failure to provide a patient with the answer he or she wants can lead to disruption and perhaps destruction of the doctor-patient relationship.

v. Information discussed in the course of a clinical evaluation generally is held in confidence. Disability evaluation requires a breach of confidentiality in which personal information previously revealed to the physician with an expectation of confidentiality must be disclosed to third parties. This departure from previous practice in the relationship can have a negative impact on the treatment.

B. The Independent Disability Evaluation

1. **Objectivity is the key to credibility.**

   a. A fully objective evaluation requires collateral sources of information to corroborate or correct the information provided by the patient.

   b. The evaluator must have knowledge about the job and its essential functions as well as the psychological conditions common in that occupation. These data should be obtained from the patient and other sources.

   c. The treating clinician may not be able to provide an objective assessment because of the factors outlined in section I.A. above.

      i. The physician should be prepared to tell the patient that this is the case and provide a referral to someone who can perform an independent assessment.

      ii. The physician has an obligation to fill out attending physician statements and other forms even if he or she demurs from issuing an opinion about disability.

   d. Transference and countertransference issues arise in independent disability evaluations, just as they do in the clinical setting. An objective evaluator must be aware of these issues as factors in the patient's presentation and in his or her assessment of the patient.

2. **Unlike a clinical evaluation, an independent disability evaluation is conducted at the request of a third party** (e.g., employer, insurer, patient's attorney) rather than at the request of a patient seeking treatment. The patient should be informed that the content and conclusions of the evaluation will be reported to individuals and organizations that would not automatically be entitled to the information in the clinical setting.

3. Sources of information include the following:

   a. The patient

   b. Written and oral job descriptions from the employer

   c. Available medical records from treating clinicians, both present and past

   d. Information from managers, co-workers, and family members

II. The Psychiatric Disability Evaluation

A. Four things should be kept in mind as the evaluation proceeds.

1. The presence of a psychiatric diagnosis does not automatically confirm disability. An assessment of disability is an assessment of functional capacity, not merely a search for a diagnostic label.

2. The definition of disability differs, depending upon whether the evaluation is being done for Social Security Disability, private disability insurance, or workers' compensation. The physician performing disability evaluations should be aware of the definition applied by the program for which the evaluation is being conducted.

3. The level of disability may fluctuate over time. For example, individuals with bipolar mood disorder may be highly productive when symptom-free and totally disabled when symptomatic.

4. The physician should keep in mind that people become disabled by both mental illness and physical illness. Efforts at careful analysis and detection of malingering or exaggeration must not be allowed to obscure this fact.

B. One should start with a clear statement of the limitations on confidentiality.

1. This is both a legal and an ethical duty.

2. The release-of-information form documents that the patient has been warned about the limits on confidentiality. With or without these forms, a note that the limitations on confidentiality were discussed with the patient should be included in the record.

3. Even though confidentiality is limited, information should be shared only on a need-to-know basis. In other words, only information that is relevant to the matter in question should be included in the report or otherwise shared with the party requesting the evaluation. Details of childhood abuse and intimate sexual details, for example, are rarely necessary to provide a clear picture in a report of disability status.

C. More than one session may be required to complete the evaluation. This fact should be shared in advance with the evaluee and the party seeking the evaluation.

D. The assessment should proceed as follows:

1. Obtain a standard history and conduct standard physical and mental status examinations.

2. Document specific elements of the mental status examination relevant to performance at work, including the following:
   a. Concentration
   b. Interactions with others, including the examiner
   c. Mood and affect, including emotional lability
   d. Level of insight and judgment

3. Assess the likely impact of current medications and treatments.

4. Assess work-related abilities, including the following:
   a. Comprehension and ability to follow instructions
   b. Ability to perform repetitive tasks
   c. Capacity to maintain an adequate pace for a required workload
   d. Ability to perform complex and varied tasks
   e. Ability to relate to others beyond giving and receiving instructions
   f. Capacity to influence other people
   g. Ability to make generalizations, evaluations, and decisions without immediate supervision
   h. Ability to accept and carry out responsibility for direction, control, and planning

5. It may be necessary to employ ancillary assessment tools to perform a complete evaluation.
   a. Psychological and/or neuropsychological testing can be especially helpful in determining the level of function, the nature of an illness, and the presence of malingering.
   b. "Real-time" evaluations can be very useful in assessing functional capacity. These assessments can include occupational therapy evaluations of the ability to perform specific tasks or driving skills by qualified individuals, such as the state police.

E. The Report
1. The evaluating physician should determine whether the person requesting the evaluation wants an oral or a written report.
2. Key elements of the report include the following:
   a. Identifying information about the person being evaluated
   b. Documentation of the circumstances of the referral and the referral question
   c. Documentation of consent to the evaluation and the limitations on confidentiality
   d. Sources of information
   e. Provision of a job description and the nature of the job's essential functions
   f. Documentation of relevant history
   g. Documentation of the examination
   h. Observations relevant to disability versus fitness for duty
   i. Conclusions
   j. Recommendations

III. Disability Assessments in a Less Than Perfect World

A. There may be times when the treating physician feels compelled to perform the disability evaluation. In such cases, the following basic principles are helpful.
1. **Be honest with yourself, the patient, and the third party requesting the evaluation.** Ask the following questions:
   a. Do you have a full understanding of the nature of the evaluation question, the criteria, and the essential functions of the job?
   b. Do you have the information necessary to make an objective determination?
   c. Does your relationship with the patient allow you to conduct an objective evaluation?
   d. If the answer to any of these questions is no, the physician should feel free to decline to perform the evaluation.
2. Make a clear statement to the patient that this is not a standard clinical assessment and that you are required to seek additional information in order to form an objective and accurate opinion.
3. Make a clear statement in your report of the limitations on the basis for your opinion.

B. Keep in mind your varied obligations in performing evaluations of disability and fitness for duty.
1. Remember that your obligation to the patient is to certify disability only when it is appropriate and to return the patient to work only when it is safe to do so.
2. Remember that your obligation to the employer and the patient's co-workers is to return the patient to work only when it is safe and appropriate to do so.

Suggested Readings

Borgman Associates. (1995). *Managing disability, leave and absence issues.* Walnut Creek, CA: Council on Education in Management.

Carr, D.B. (1993). Assessing older drivers for physical and cognitive impairment. *Geriatrics, 48,* 46–51.

Crist, P.A.H., & Stoffel, V.C. (1992). The Americans with Disabilities Act of 1990 and employees with mental impairments: Personal efficacy and the environment. *American Journal of Occupational Therapy, 46,* 434–443.

Katz, R.T. (2001). Impairment and disability ratings in low back pain. *Physical Medicine and Rehabilitation Clinics of North America, 12,* 681–694.

Maffeo, P.A. (1990). Making non-discriminatory fitness for duty decisions about persons with disabilities under the Rehabilitation Act and the Americans with Disabilities Act. *American Journal of Law & Medicine, 16,* 279–326.

Melhorn, J., & Mark, M.D. (2001). Impairment and disability evaluations: Understanding the process. *Journal of Bone & Joint Surgery, 83-A*(12), 1905–1911.

Mintz, J., Mintz, L.I., Arruda, M.J., & Hwang, S.S. (1992). Treatments of depression and the functional capacity to work. *Archives of General Psychiatry, 49,* 761–768.

Pederson, M.T., Muldoon, S., & Curtiss, E.C. (1993). Request for medical evaluation: An approach for on-site occupational health professionals. *American Academy of Occupational Health Nursing Journal, 41,* 241–244.

Ravid, R., Menon, S. (1993). Guidelines for disclosure of patient information under the Americans With Disabilities Act. *Hospital & Community Psychiatry, 44,* 280–281.

Rigaud, M.C., & Flynn, C.F. (1995). Fitness for duty (FFD) evaluation in industrial and military workers. *Psychiatric Annals, 25,* 246–250.

Schouten, R. (1993). Pitfalls of clinical practice: The treating clinician as expert witness. *Harvard Review of Psychiatry, 1,* 64–65.

Strasburger, L., Gutheil, T.G., & Brodsky, A. (1997). On wearing two hats: Role conflict in serving as both psychotherapist and expert witness. *American Journal of Psychiatry, 154,* 448–456.

Zuckerman, D. (1993). Reasonable accommodations for people with mental illness under the ADA. *Mental & Physical Disability Law Reports, 17,* 311–320.

CHAPTER 64
The Homeless Patient

MICHAEL F. BIERER AND JENNIFER M. LAFAYETTE

I. Introduction

A. Definitions

1. **Homelessness is not synonymous with mental illness** and does not imply severe distress or dysfunction. Instead, homelessness refers to a person's housing status, and there are many contrasting situations which fit this broad definition. Despite the non-specific nature of the term, consideration of a patient's homeless condition is critical to the ability to provide effective care. An understanding of the relative frequency of clinical disorders within the population is helpful. Homelessness complicates both the diagnostic and the therapeutic process.

2. **Homelessness occurs along a continuum; each homeless individual's circumstances must be ascertained on a case-by-case basis.** Someone sleeping in a doorway on the street meets a stringent definition of homelessness (literal homelessness), while someone sleeping transiently in a series of friends' apartments meets another definition (Table 64-1). Shelters or missions that provide beds also run the gamut from violent, chaotic, crowded shelters with hundreds of mattresses (where people may stay for no more than a few nights) to more stable, individualized accommodations.

3. **Shelters vary in regard to the types of services offered,** which in turn affect the experience of being homeless. Some may provide minimal services, such as sandwiches and showers, while others may provide social and nursing services, a clinic, job training, computer classes, and/or housing search services. These support services play a crucial role in the primary provider's care of patients.

Table 64-1. Definitions of Homelessness

1. An individual who lacks a fixed, regular, and adequate nighttime residence; or

2. An individual who has a primary nighttime residence that is

    A. A supervised or publicly operated shelter designed to provide temporary living accommodations (including welfare hotels, congregate shelters, and transitional housing for the mentally ill);

    B. An institution that provides a temporary residence for individuals intended to be institutionalized; or

    C. A public or private place not designed for, or ordinarily used as, a regular sleeping accommodation.

SOURCE: From U.S. Congress, House. 1987. PL 100-77, the Stewart B. McKinney Homeless Assistance Act. Conference report to accompany H.R. 558, 100th Cong., 1st Sess.

B. Prevalence of homelessness

1. Many studies have investigated the point and lifetime prevalences of homelessness. The number of people counted as homeless depends on the definition used and the methods employed. A survey by Link and colleagues (1994) found that 7.4% of adult Americans have experienced literal homelessness (sleeping in the street, abandoned buildings, or shelters) in their lifetimes. This is one of the highest estimates of prevalence published to date. Other studies suggest that several hundred thousand to over a million people are homeless at any moment in the United States, and the number experiencing homelessness during a 1-year period may be three times as high.

2. The high prevalence, combined with emerging policies that may broaden health insurance coverage for the economically disadvantaged, means that homelessness will increasingly become a concern of every primary care provider (PCP).

C. Demographics of the Homeless

1. **Single adults make up the majority of the homeless,** although families have accounted for a growing proportion of the homeless over the last several decades.

2. **Ethnic minorities are overrepresented.**

3. **Veterans,** whether combat-exposed or not, **make up 30–40% of homeless men.**

4. **Composition varies locally.** Who becomes homeless depends on local housing markets and the specifics of the social "safety net," which may vary state by state or even neighborhood by neighborhood. The numbers of people who move in and out of homelessness will thus reach different equilibria, depending on local factors.

5. **The common characteristic of the homeless is poverty.** All studies demonstrate that homeless people are the most economically disadvantaged group in the United States.

6. Although the homeless often eat and sleep in crowded conditions, **social isolation is common** among these persons. The majority of homeless adult individuals report having one or no confidant, friend, or family member with whom they are in contact. This isolation may reflect primary character traits or may be a learned response to an environment marked by assault and intrusion.

7. **Up to 55% of homeless patients do not have health insurance. Those without health insurance are less likely to receive ambulatory medical care or to comply with prescribed medications.**

II. Prevalence of Psychiatric Diagnoses among the Homeless

Knowledge of likely psychiatric diagnoses may assist in the management of a homeless patient. Any generalization from the published literature should be made with caution, however, because the characteristics of a homeless group are specific to time and place. Many surveys and studies have been performed to assess psychiatric morbidity. In general, the following statements can be made:

A. About a quarter of homeless adults report a history of psychiatric hospitalizations.

B. The duration of homelessness is correlated with the likelihood of major psychiatric disease.

C. Homeless adults have a high prevalence of personality disorders, with antisocial personality disorder present in 17% of homeless individuals.

D. The lifetime prevalences of schizophrenia, major depression, bipolar disorder, and organic brain syndromes range from 10–40%. Schizophrenia and mania are the least prevalent among these disorders but are the most strongly associated with homelessness. Compared with matched housed samples, homeless adults have about 30 times the prevalence of schizophrenia or mania and 5 times the prevalence of major depression.

E. Alcohol abuse typically is present in a third to two-thirds of homeless adults but can be as high as 90% in some samples.

F. Abuse of drugs other than alcohol is less common, with the prevalence ranging up to 25%.

G. The concurrence of psychiatric disease with substance use disorders is common. Among homeless men with a mental illness, the majority has a concurrent alcohol disorder; about one-fourth have a substance abuse problem other than alcoholism. Among homeless substance abusers, about a third have a psychiatric disorder.

H. Sexual assault is 20 times more common among homeless women than it is among the non-homeless. Among homeless women, the lifetime prevalence of physical and/or sexual assault is at least 10% and it may be as high as 95%. Whether predating the onset of homelessness or resulting from the vulnerability caused by living on the street, the problem is extensive.

I. Greater than 90% of homeless families are headed by women. Many have a history of abuse, major family disruptions, and limited support systems. They have high rates of depression, post-traumatic stress disorder (PTSD), and substance abuse and dependence. About one-third have made a suicide attempt at some time in their lives.

J. Up to 50% of children in homeless families have delayed development, anxiety, depression, or learning difficulties. They rarely receive psychiatric care.

III. Medical Overview

Compared with appropriate samples of housed controls, homeless adults have more chronic and acute illnesses.

A. Tuberculosis rates rival those found in developing countries, ranging from 25 to 100 times those of the non-homeless. One-third of homeless adults have a positive Mantoux test or purified protein derivative (PPD) test. The likelihood of a positive PPD rises with the duration of time spent in shelters.

B. Skin diseases associated with venous stasis and poor hygiene, such as chronic ulcers and cellulitis, are 15 times more common among the homeless.

C. Chronic lung disease associated with smoking is 15 times more prevalent among the homeless.

D. Trauma is common. Over a three-year period, 10% of homeless people suffer concussions, 10% have fractures, and a third are threatened with weapons. As was mentioned above, sexual assault is common.

E. Among people attending outpatient clinics, the homeless are approximately twice as likely to have **serious chronic medical diseases** (e.g., AIDS, diabetes, cancer, stroke) than are the non-homeless.

F. Homeless adults with psychiatric disease have **more physical diseases** and make more use of medical facilities than do those without psychiatric disease.

G. The homeless face a **mortality rate nearly four times higher** than that of the general population.

H. Homeless patients with HIV infection, renal disease, liver disease, and arrhythmias have the highest mortality rates.

IV. Implications of Homelessness for Primary Care Practice

A. Compliance with basic recommendations may be difficult. Medications, if affordable, may be difficult to store safely. Many medications are stolen irrespective of their intrinsic "street value." Access to refrigeration for storage of drugs may be limited. There may be no place to carry out therapeutic recommendations, such as leg elevation, dressing changes for wound care, and bed rest. Finally, a visible sign of vulnerability, such as an arm sling, may mark a patient as an easy victim who may be carrying medications.

B. Compliance with appointments may represent a challenge. Homeless people often spend days waiting for food, shelter, clothing, hygiene facilities, and transportation. Attending a doctor's appointment may mean giving up a basic necessity, such as a meal or a bed; patients may rationally choose not to forgo sustenance. Appointment slips are often lost, and phone calls or postal card reminders are frequently an impossibility. Moreover, many aspects of medical offices may discourage the homeless from keeping appointments. Tolerance for bureaucratic paperwork may be exhausted by the time a homeless patient gets to the office. Patients may be made uncomfortable by their sense that their appearance or hygiene is disturbing to others in a waiting room; and others, including the clinic staff, may corroborate this by revealing uneasiness in the presence of the homeless.

C. The patient's priorities may be conditioned by homelessness. A homeless patient's assessment of the importance of medical issues may not coincide with that of the provider. For instance, the work-up of any asymptomatic problem, such as a lung nodule or hypertension, may rank far lower in priority than obtaining shoes, a dry pair of socks, or a safe sleeping arrangement for the night.

D. A sense of hopelessness and inevitability, especially among the chronically homeless, may seem justified to a patient who sees little reason to hope for a better situation in the future. This sense of resignation can be generalized to medical symptoms and problems. While this hopelessness may be part of a treatable disease, such as major depression, it is often a stubborn reality which presents an important challenge to the practice of primary care. A corollary of the effect of chronicity is that the more recent the occurrence of homelessness, the more likely it is that it may be reversed; if it is caused by a medical or psychiatric problem, the problem itself may well be reversible.

E. A higher mortality rate among the homeless in general and the day-to-day uncertainties may alter the impact of basic health promotion and disease prevention involved in primary care practice. As difficult as it may be for non-homeless patients to change their behavior for a seemingly nebulous health or mortality benefit in the indefinite future, that benefit may be overshadowed completely by the other forces that mediate high mortality rates among the homeless.

V. Assessment of the Homeless Patient

A. Interview
   1. The interview should attend to the major considerations listed above in order to negotiate a realistic role for primary care and an effective care plan.
      a. How may the daily routine of homelessness contribute to the problem being evaluated?
         i. **Medical illnesses may be exacerbated by homelessness.** For instance, does standing in food lines exacerbate lower extremity pain? Is disturbed sleep part of

the etiology of headache? Are skin lesions on the hands a result of reaching into trash bins for recyclables?

    ii. **Psychiatric diagnosis may be complex.** The interaction of the environment with symptoms is specially problematic. Many diagnostic criteria for psychiatric diseases may be unreliable among the homeless unless their symptoms are interpreted in a wider context. Though unemployment and transience are characteristic of antisocial personality disorder, they are nearly universal traits among the homeless and may lack specificity for this disorder unless they are present before homelessness. Similarly, impaired sleep may be inevitable, and the poor concentration, lack of energy, and decreased libido and interest that result may appear to be part of major depression. Vigilance may be more a necessity than a manifestation of anxiety or paranoia.

    iii. It may be impossible to distinguish whether a psychiatric entity is primary or secondary to the environment. The threat and occurrence of repeated assault, for example, may produce a condition indistinguishable from refractory depression. Until the patient's circumstances change, diagnosis and resolution may be unattainable.

  b. How does the problem interact with the homeless environment or routine? **The impact of a symptom may be magnified by homelessness.** Diarrhea, for instance, may be an overwhelming problem when toilets are blocks away. The loud snoring characteristic of sleep apnea may cause ejection of the patient from a shelter if enough people complain.

  c. **What facilities or resources are available where the patient sleeps?** Is there a shower, a clinic, or a refrigerator (for medication storage)? Can a shelter counselor or someone else hold medicines, remind the patient of appointments, arrange transportation, or act as a communications link? Can visiting nursing services be arranged?

  d. **What matters most to the patient?** Does the patient share the provider's assessment that a condition is problematic? If the PCP fails to address a patient's foot pain which immediately affects nearly all aspects of that patient's daily life, other problems, even if life-threatening, may not get onto the patient's agenda. Similarly, a physician may assess a behavior, such as drinking alcohol to fall asleep, as a problem while the patient does not perceive that behavior to have negative consequences.

  e. **What are realistic goals?** What effort or intervention makes sense to the patient? What can the patient and doctor realistically hope to accomplish?

  f. It is wise to enter into a "contract" incrementally, as it is difficult to predict the degree of compliance a patient will be able to achieve. For example, it may sometimes be appropriate to wait to make referrals to specialists until the patient and provider have arrived at a reliable mechanism for follow-up.

2. **The patient's comfort should be attended to during the interview.**

  a. Should the door be open?

  b. Is the patient hungry or thirsty?

  c. What are the consequences of running late and of missing meals, shelter, or transportation?

3. **The meaning of confidentiality should be emphasized.** Homeless people in general lead lives exposed to public view and may be reassured by an explicit promise that their privacy is being protected.

4. **There are concrete strategies for communicating with the patient.**

  a. **Collect important data,** including the following:

    i. Places where the patient takes meals (churches, soup kitchens, restaurants, bars)

    ii. Places where the patient sleeps

    iii. Phone numbers

iv. Aliases

v. Contacts (people willing to transmit messages)

- Specific names of counselors or others whom the patient sees regularly and where they can be reached
- "Representative payee," if one exists, who receives a check for the patient and whom the patient is highly likely to see

b. **Obtain written releases permitting communication with others.** It may be helpful to have patients sign a statement identifying the care provider and asserting that they would like the provider to communicate with them. Acquaintances or shelter staff members may otherwise try to shield patients from inquiries. Without such a release, some shelters will not acknowledge that an individual is sleeping there even when told that communicating with the patient is a medical necessity.

B. **Medical history.** Difficulties with access to care and infrequent attention to preventive health measures raise several concerns. In addition to the usual historical information, special note should be made of the following:

1. PPD test
2. Vaccines (flu, pneumonia vaccine, tetanus)
3. Sexually transmitted diseases and current risk behaviors
4. Addiction treatment history
5. Trauma
6. Insurance and benefits or entitlements and income sources

C. **Examination of the Patient**

1. Touching may be jarring for the patient because of previous trauma, paranoia, or the habit of guarding privacy.
2. Because medical contact may be novel, an explanation of what is occurring and why, especially during the physical examination, may be welcome.
3. Many conditions are particularly common or important in the homeless. In addition to a routine or focused examination, consider inspecting the following:
   a. The feet, for early tinea, fissures, or infections
   b. The skin and hair, for infestations
   c. The mouth, for dental neglect, periodontal disease, and cancer
   d. Multiple organ systems, for signs of drug or alcohol abuse

VI. Treatment Strategies

A. **When possible, provide the essentials for further compliance.**

1. Make follow-up or referral appointments before the patient leaves the office and give the patient an appointment slip.
2. Provide the patient with needed items: medications, devices (slings, canes), transportation vouchers, essential clothing (e.g., clean socks).

B. In treating psychiatric symptoms, **be conscious of the patient's probable need to remain alert.** Non-sedating drugs should be used when possible.

C. **Use simple dosing schedules when possible.** The relative scarcity of wristwatches and the inconvenience of multiple dosage schedules make once-daily dosing preferable.

D. **Use networks and community supports that are integrated into the fabric of the patient's life.** If you do not make use of supports and services beyond your office practice, homelessness may become an insurmountable problem for the delivery of medical or psychiatric care. Specifically, schedule a follow-up evaluation after the institution of psychiatric medication. Even when the right medication is prescribed, its use may be doomed to failure by under- or over-medication or by the appearance of unwanted side effects. These negative clinical experiences may lead not only to non-compliance with the specific medication but also to frustration about, and bias against, future medical or psychiatric care. **Arranging for follow-up that the patient feels will work may be the key to psychiatric care.**

1. Communicate with the facility where the patient stays to find out who can help. Dial the number with the patient in your office to see if it works. Communicate your plans for follow-up or monitoring.

2. Some patients will receive the most successful treatment in a specialized homeless clinic. Over 120 **Health Care for the Homeless (HCH) programs** nationwide receive federal support. These programs vary by city but should be explored with individual patients. Interdisciplinary teams within these programs can provide information, physical and mental health care, substance abuse treatment, and support to facilitate care for the homeless patient. Information about the nearest HCH can be obtained from Health Care for the Homeless Information Resource Center (888) 439-3300, ext. 247 or through their website at http://www.hchirc.com.

3. **Shelters** and soup kitchens may provide other services. There may be shelters for pregnant or parenting women, couples with children, women who need to escape an abusive situation, runaway or "throw-away" youth, and people with psychiatric diseases. These shelters often have enriched services to care for particular needs.

4. **Specialty psychiatric services** may be available. Some areas have mental health workers and psychiatric clinics that focus on the homeless. They may work with the local HCH or have expertise in outreach-oriented assertive case management and patient advocacy. These organizations may have services to help not only with psychiatric issues but also with many of the daily challenges that face homeless people and their families.

E. **By attending to the considerations outlined above, it is possible to arrive at a treatment plan that involves and satisfies the patient and will not be derailed by the rigid constraints of homelessness.**

Suggested Readings

Bassuk, E.L., Rubin, L., & Lauriat, A.S. (1986). Characteristics of sheltered homeless families. *American Journal of Public Health, 76*(9), 1097–1101.

Bassuk, E.L., Weinreb, L.F., Buckner, J.C., et al. (1996). The characteristics and needs of sheltered homeless and low-income housed mothers. *Journal of the American Medical Association, 276,* 640–646.

Breakey, W.R., Fischer, P.J., Kramer, M., et al. (1989). Health and mental health problems of homeless men and women in Baltimore. *Journal of the American Medical Association, 262,* 1352–1357.

Dickey, B. (2000). Review of programs for persons who are homeless and mentally ill. *Harvard Review of Psychiatry, 8*(5), 242–250.

Hibbs, J.R., Benner, L., Klugman, L., et al. (1994). Mortality in a cohort of homeless adults in Philadelphia. *New England Journal of Medicine, 331,* 304–309.

Hwang, S.W., Lebow, J.M., Bierer, M.F., et al. (1998). Risk factors for death in homeless adults in Boston. *Archives of Internal Medicine, 158,* 1454–1460.

Institute of Medicine. (1988). *Homelessness, health and human needs.* Washington, DC: National Academy Press.

Koegel, P., Burnam, A., & Farr, R.K. (1988). The prevalence of specific psychiatric disorders among homeless individuals in the inner city of Los Angeles. *Archives of General Psychiatry, 45,* 1085–1092.

Kushel, M.B., Vittinghoff, E., & Haas, J.S. (2001). Factors associated with the health care utilization of homeless persons. *Journal of the American Medical Association, 285*(2), 200–206.

Link, B.G., Susser, E., Stueve, A., et al. (1994). Lifetime and five-year prevalence of homelessness in the United States. *American Journal of Public Health, 84,* 1907–1912.

Winkelby, M.A., & Fleshin, D. (1993). Physical, addictive and psychiatric disorders among homeless veterans and nonveterans. *Public Health Report, 1,* 30–35.

Wright, J.D. (1989). *Address unknown: The homeless in America.* New York: Aldine de Gruyter.

CHAPTER 65
The Celebrity Patient

BARBARA A. DUNDERDALE, JAMES E. GROVES, AND THEODORE A. STERN

I. Introduction

Celebrities come in standard sizes—small, medium, and large—but the problems they create in the medical setting depend less on their size than on the worldliness and sense of humor of the caregiver. Even with a head of state, the difficulties posed for a seasoned clinician may be easier to deal with than the stress placed on a new house officer emergently admitting the mayor's father-in-law. **The key concept in treating any "special" patient is maintaining the usual standard of care and not letting the patient's "specialness" interfere with normal medical procedure.**

II. The Impact of Publicity

A. **Difficulty in treating celebrities usually occurs not because they are entitled, demanding, or seductive, which they may be, but because of the publicity that surrounds them.** Whether the patient is an all-star quarterback or a famous actress, the clinician who inherits the ultimate responsibility for the care of a celebrity suddenly realizes that when very important persons (VIPs) get worse or die, they do so in full view of a curious and critical public.

B. The way caregivers deal with the stresses of a career in medicine depends in part on their mastery of the distressing feelings that difficult patients stir up: fear, rage, depression, and hatred. While treating a celebrity carries certain perks, such as hobnobbing with the rich and famous, knowing their secrets, and vicariously tasting power, such experiences can be as vexing as taking care of a "hateful patient." The skills and wisdom a clinician needs to cope with a hostile patient differ from those needed to manage a seductive patient (see Chapters 12 and 13), but both sets of skills may be needed to cope with a VIP.

C. **The issue of publicity magnifies any worries the caregiver may have about his or her competence.** With "ordinary" patients minor errors in diagnosis and treatment may go unnoticed, but with a celebrity there is a public or "jury" looking over the caregiver's shoulder and second-guessing every diagnosis and treatment. These issues are particularly troublesome when the individual is a political leader, because leadership depends on a person's mental and physical health. When legitimacy to govern is called into question by an injury or illness, caregivers necessarily become a part of the legitimating structure of the government.

D. Publicity affects the clinician even if the patient is only a local VIP, such as a colleague in the same hospital. The good opinion of friends and co-workers may be even more important than that of the faceless crowd.

III. The Impact of Celebrity

The typology of celebrities referred to here is independent of size. In other words, a VIP may be very important in the outside world yet reasonable, grateful, and gracious with the health care team. (Conversely, the care of a physician's distant relative can be maddening if family politics clouds the medical encounter.) Celebrity often is a matter of money, sex, and power, and some celebrities are experts at manipulating the world around them. If the patient is of this type—and egotistical—the clinician may have to set firm limits on manipulation to protect the patient's health.

A. Narcissism and the Celebrity

1. Although psychiatric diagnosis is designed for the clinical situation, one type of personality disorder can serve as a useful model for a clinician who takes care of a celebrity: the narcissistic personality. Celebrities are not necessarily diagnosed as having a narcissistic personality disorder, but **the situation surrounding a celebrity brings out narcissistic traits both in the staff caring for the patient and in the family and staff the celebrity brings into the medical environment.** Some celebrities arrive in the center of a crowd, and inevitably there are going to be narcissistic people in that coterie. This phenomenon is seen especially with patients who are film stars at the zenith, politicians active on the national level, and individuals with suddenly acquired or fabulous wealth.

2. **DSM-IV defines narcissistic personality disorder in terms of the grandiosity and lack of empathy** demonstrated in at least five of the following traits:
   a. Arrogance
   b. Lust for power through beauty, love, brilliance, or money
   c. Conviction of "specialness"
   d. Hunger for admiration
   e. Entitlement
   f. Exploitation and manipulativeness
   g. Stunted empathy, or the inability to "feel into" the other person
   h. Enviousness
   i. Displays of contempt

3. Especially under the stress of publicity, these traits are brought out in some of the individuals in a celebrity's coterie. Such individuals—in their own argot *energy creatures* or *drama queens*—create discord and anxiety in the system. The clinician cannot prevent this, but being aware of the phenomenon keeps the situation from compromising patient care.

4. While physicians are used to hearing about the medical staff's empathy or lack of it, the converse phenomenon is salient here. It can be a bruising experience when someone important treats a caregiver unempathetically. In dealing with individuals with a narcissistic personality disorder, **the only thing the staff can count on is that at some point the narcissistic individual will treat a caregiver as a thing, an object, a tool, or a slave.**

B. The coterie surrounding the celebrity. A celebrity may arrive on the medical scene accompanied by an entourage including any and all of the following:

1. The celebrity's **personal medical staff,** including physicians, nurses, and others who may be jealous of their prerogatives

2. **Public relations specialists,** who try to put the best possible "spin" on anything that occurs in the celebrity's life

3. **The press,** whose duty it is to discover things, especially things public relations specialists wish to conceal

4. **Security experts,** whose job it is to be jumpy and suspicious

5. **Family members,** who may expect to be regarded as demi-celebrities

6. **Personal staff,** including the adviser, the chief of staff, the executive secretary, the in-house attorney, the translator, the cook, the valet, and even the personal trainer, who, although "outside the walls" of the medical situation, play supporting roles and are beholden to the celebrity.

C. **Managing the Coterie**

1. The person who will take care of a celebrity must ask the patient explicitly who is to be privy to information, who is "in the loop." In a non-celebrity situation, the next of kin is clearly the only person other than the patient who is privy to information. **With a celebrity, there often is a second individual on whom the celebrity depends almost as much as a next of kin: a senior aide, press agent, or chief of staff.** If the patient agrees, conferences that convey clinical information should be held with both the next of kin and the chief power person in the presence of the patient. There are two domains in the celebrity's life—personal and public—and there is no getting around the difficulties posed by the addition of the public domain to the private situation of medical care.

2. From the outset, the physician needs to have immediate access to the next of kin and, if the patient wishes it, the chief of staff on an around-the-clock basis. This issue of access must be spelled out; with the patient's approval, the physician must be assured of clear and unbroken communication with the patient's "power people" and the next of kin.

IV. The Timing and the Place

A. Two kinds of encounters occur in the treatment of a VIP: emergencies and elective events.

1. **In a way, emergencies are easier to manage because the "celebrity" surrounding the celebrity gets shooed out of the medical arena.** Then, after emergency treatment, there can ensue an accelerated version of the non-emergency scenario set forth below.

2. **The typical situation is an encounter that is planned.** Here two pre-existing, relatively autonomous power structures—the celebrity's coterie and the medical treatment system—come together around a single task. The basic script is, "Let's have my people talk to your people." The two heads of the power structures designate various individuals to collaborate with one another at lower levels. Large medical centers usually have an expert in celebrity care, and this person knows which questions to ask, such as, "Will you bring your own translator, or do we provide one?"

B. Large urban tertiary care settings typically have ready-made resources to cope with a celebrity patient. These hospitals often have a public relations team in place with standard protocols for dealing with such situations. An effective working relationship with this team is vital, and the physician can delegate most of the non-medical details of management to the individual who heads this team. The team must be sensitive to other services and departments in the hospital who want to contribute and interact directly with the VIP patient. Multiple interactions and interruptions may not be in the best interest of the ill patient. But this must be delicately managed to preserve good working relationships between departments, because when things are back to normal, people must continue to work cooperatively with one another.

V. A Checklist of Non-medical Concerns

A. Anticipation of, and planning for, the arrival of a "special" patient is the key, and so the following checklist of non-medical concerns can help the treating physician.

1. **Level of security.** Is this encounter necessarily public? Does even the fact of hospitalization need to be protected? The answers determine much of the planning detailed below.

2. **Transport.** Depending on the level of security, getting the patient anonymously in and out of the medical setting requires thought. This is actually one of the easiest tasks. Oxygen masks, eye patches, bulky facial bandages, and back door routes are effective and close at hand. In the hospital, transportation is a bit more difficult but can be managed along the same lines. (Whenever possible, however, it is best to have tests and procedures "come to" the patient rather than *vice versa.*)

3. **Data sequestration.** Information about any patient flows through the medical setting in an enormous and unrealized volume on paper, in computers, and by word of mouth. Even if information is protected on a need-to-know basis, the hospital staff can be especially problematic. Thus, the use of an alias is often wise, along with special computer passwords, locked charts, and other measures that limit access to data. The pseudonym is a tool with some risk to the patient's safety and should be unique and keyed to only one patient identification number.

4. **Language and culture.** If the VIP is from a foreign culture (even if the celebrity is fluent in English), translators will have to be made available to members of the coterie who are not fluent. These translators must be fluent not only in the two languages but also in the two cultures. Generally, the hospital's translators are best, since they have some familiarity with medical issues and can prevent meaningful information from getting lost in the translation.

5. **Diet.** Like language, diet and other amenities may need special handling and even "translation" if the patient is from a distant culture. During the planning phase of the hospitalization, the role of relevant outside vendors, such as restaurants, may have to be explored.

6. **Accommodations.** The hospital may have its own suites for VIPs, but the celebrity's staff should be asked about its expectations for the arrangements, which may be very elaborate in terms of space, decor, supplies, communications, and media hook-ups. The coterie are often expecting more than the celebrity. One can graciously remind the celebrity staff that this is a hospital first, and this is why they are here. If family or staff will be staying in the suite with the celebrity patient overnight, an explanation of normative hospital practices may be needed as a frame of reference. The staff should anticipate unusual events, such as sudden demand for international phone lines and a massive flood of flowers and gifts for the patient.

7. **Visitors.** If possible, issues of visitation should be negotiated with the patient in advance. Otherwise, the VIP's chief of staff and next of kin should be prepared to decide who gets to visit and ideally prepare a list of visitors. (The physician and the patient decide when visitors will come and for how long, and it is wise to schedule plenty of "visitor-free" time so that the patient is not overwhelmed.) If the patient is a caregiver hospitalized in his or her own institution, a plan needs to be instituted to prevent colleagues and friends on the staff from dropping in at any time: a no visitors sign, for instance.

8. **Leadership of the medical staff.** The physician's staff and other medical personnel will have complex reactions to the celebrity that have to be anticipated and addressed on an ongoing basis. The patient's right to privacy will require tactful emphasis and re-emphasis. Also, some caregivers may see the caregiving institution's accommodating reactions to a celebrity as unegalitarian or even immoral and feel resentful of it.

9. **Billing.** Billing issues surface frequently here, especially in the care of foreign patients. There are cultural expectations about payment, and those of the patient and his or her coterie may have to be anticipated and dealt with. (Sometimes the physician is asked to take care of other members of the entourage as well, rather like a "package deal.")

B. This checklist is only a beginning guide to issues that may arise, **and the more planning that is done, the better. Just as important, however, is the caregiver's management of his or her personal feelings about the encounter with the VIP.** This is true for all caregivers dealing with a celebrity patient, and the physician's "countertransference" will serve as a paradigm for other caregivers.

VI. Inside the Celebrity's Physician

A. Becoming a treating physician requires both healthy aggression and romantic vision. Idealized images of doctoring support caregivers through the rigors of training and practice. From childhood on individuals carry inside themselves a romantic narrative of being a hero that is so deep in the unconscious that it sounds corny to an adult. These ideals or archaic images lie dormant in most situations because they are childish and therefore embarrassing to the adult consciousness. However, **the sudden glare of publicity or abrupt access to power can unearth less mature aspects of the physician's personality which for lack of a better word can be termed narcissistic.**

B. This is not to say that caregivers are forbidden excitement, fantasies, and wishes while treating celebrity patients, but there is a need to know what those wishes are and to keep them actively in mind so that they do not influence clinical behavior. An inevitable example of this occurs when the physician is called on to set forth medical restrictions, something that is so much a part of doctoring that it is taken for granted. In the case of a celebrity patient, the physician may pull back from laying down medical restrictions because of an unconscious fear of disapproval from a powerful patient.

C. The King Midas Phenomenon

1. In one version of the fable, the feckless Midas, presumably after his adventures with the golden touch, is again cursed by the gods and made to grow the ears of an ass. Every morning before dawn the king's barber trims the ears so that they can be hidden under the royal coif. This is done, of course, with the barber sworn to secrecy under pain of death. One day the barber can no longer contain this great secret and goes down to the river. There he digs a hole in the riverbank and whispers into it many times, "The king has ass's ears! The king has ass's ears!" Then he fills the hole and, greatly relieved, goes away. But out of the mound of earth he has just tamped down grows a beautiful narcissus in full flower, and to all passersby it whispers, "The king has ass's ears! The king has ass's ears!"

a. The point of this fable is not to warn a celebrity's physician against gossiping; it is to show that **even under pain of death a normal person needs to confide in others, especially about stressful experiences.**

b. Generally, **the best and safest confidants are colleagues, preferably those familiar with the issue of celebrity patients.**

D. Consultation and Other Data Gathering

1. Requesting consultations on the patient by physicians and other professionals is a major responsibility of a VIP's physician. As with laboratory tests and other studies, there are two competing tendencies generated by a VIP patient: too much and too little.

2. **Anxiety about overlooking something may lead to a greater than ordinary utilization of studies, and the desire to spare a "special" patient trouble or social overexposure may lead to stinting on evaluations.** The issue becomes one of balancing these two forces to come up with the right studies and consultations; this is a judgment call by the treating physician.

VII. Variant VIPs

Although it is impossible to anticipate all varieties of celebrities, three are worth noting here because they raise special issues.

A. The Medical Celebrity

1. This individual, often another caregiver in the physician's medical setting, is probably the most challenging VIP to deal with because caregivers tend to identify closely with other caregivers. Overidentification with the caregiver-patient may lead to unwise deviations from routine care. Sometimes the caregiver will take a distant stance as a defense against identifying with somebody "who could be me."

2. A major problem cited in most of the literature on the care of medical personnel is the assumption by caregivers that less needs to be explained about the illness, injury, treatment, and caregiving routine than is the case with other patients. Actually, the converse is true, and colleagues may hesitate to ask questions for fear of being thought ignorant. The best policy is to explain everything in detail, preceded if necessary with "You're probably aware of this, but . . ."

B. The Family Member

1. Although physicians know not to take care of their own family members because of overidentification and lack of objectivity, in a surprisingly large number of instances a doctor will end up involved in the care of a relative.

2. The issues are almost identical to those in the discussion of medical VIPs above, because the medical VIP is part of the physician's "medical family" and is the focus of much of the same social pressure. Except in a medical emergency, however, this practice is unwise and should be avoided.

C. The Negative Celebrity

1. This involves a medical encounter with an accused or convicted individual whose celebrity revolves around a crime. Here the notorious individual, while in custody, is brought as a patient to the medical setting.

2. There can be media coverage, a "coterie"—in this instance law enforcement officers and members of the patient's (sometimes quite dysfunctional) family—and conflicting demands on the treating physician that pit the individual's role as a public figure against the patient's right to privacy and appropriate care.

3. Additional complications with negative VIPs may arise around "malingering," because symptoms and complaints may have not just a medical cause but a role in "buying time" out of the penal system.

4. There may be conflict between the medical routine (patient transport, procedures) and security needs (guards, restraints).

5. Similarly, there is sometimes a conflict in gathering and recording data that may be used not only for medical purposes but also as legal evidence.

6. The individual's presence may cause anxiety about the personal safety of other patients, their families, and the staff generally. Although rarely "rational," these feelings have to be dealt with.

7. Realizing that a negative celebrity is a variant of the VIP prepares the physician to monitor the patient's rights in the ways described above and to use the standard algorithm for celebrity care.

VIII. Ten Commandments for a VIP's Doctor

A. Anticipation of potential problems by caregivers and careful planning in advance of the encounter are crucial.

B. Also imperative are teamwork and a conscious commitment by the staff to deliver a consistent standard of care to the patient that is equal to that of any other patient in the institution.

C. These are generalizations, but to be more specific, the following rules are offered.

1. **First and foremost, follow standard procedure.** In clinical decisions pretend that the celebrity issue does not exist. In other words, ask yourself how you would handle any given clinical decision if you and your patient were in perfect obscurity and only you and the patient would know the result. Any deviation from routine, even a seemingly trivial one, such as crossing off serial stool guaiacs from standard orders, should serve as a red flag that the patient's specialness is becoming a problem.

2. **Downplay specialness.** Be honest, brief, and understated; use your communication skills and bedside manner to damp down the ambient hysteria a VIP stirs up in the medical setting. Stay calm, speak slowly, use pastel nouns and gentle verbs, and understate any issue that you can without damaging the truth. Utilize thoughtful pauses to collect yourself before speaking. Keep a low profile and model for your staff and the celebrity's coterie a respectful and collaborative attitude.

3. **Ask yourself what flavor of celebrity this is.** Is this a normal personality who through luck and skill has made it big? Is this an arrogant, driven individual who succeeded in order to defeat feelings of vulnerability and smallness? Is this someone who succeeded in order to get revenge or destroy others? The answer places the patient on a continuum ranging in psychiatric jargon from normal to pathologic "narcissism." This is like any other diagnosis that one needs to know for effective patient management.

4. **Ask yourself what your particular vulnerabilities are regarding the celebrity phenomenon.** Do you most want the VIP's praise, or are you most hoping to impress your colleagues? Are you trying to show your parents that you are wonderful after all? Of course all these factors are going to be present, but what is your besetting flaw? Once you know, you can lower your expectations accordingly.

5. **Get mentoring.** Search out your oldest, wisest teacher, preferably someone conversant with the medical problems of the celebrity. Run all issues great and small by this

trusted individual not only for the advice you will get back but also for the relief you will feel from telling the ongoing story of the celebrity's care.

6. **Manage information flow and delegate publicity.** All information goes through the patient first and then the next of kin. If the patient is a celebrity, let the hospital's public relations people handle the public part of the information flow after clearance from the patient or the patient's next of kin. If part of your duty to the patient involves speaking with the media, clear the content with the patient first, rehearse the delivery, downplay your individual role, and be brief.

7. **Know what you want from the VIP.** A conscious grasp of the wish for power or money will prepare you to respond appropriately (usually declining with thanks) to blandishments offered by the celebrity's coterie. There is of course the inevitable Rolex that seems to surface during the care of a potentate, but the more subtle temptations are hard to foresee. Still, try to know what *you* want; this helps keep your motives pure.

8. **Do not overlook the issue of substance abuse simply because the patient is a big shot.** Similarly, other health-related risk factors may need to be explored.

9. **Do not avoid sexual issues.** This VIP is your patient, not your parent, and if you would ordinarily raise sexual issues as part of the care, you must also do so in this case.

10. **Do not forget to listen.** Because of the stress the patient's celebrity places on the clinician, there may be a tendency to skimp on the most important part of any caregiver's job: providing comfort. Just because the patient is important or special does not protect that individual from the terror that illness or injury can bring, or change the need for privacy. In this crisis a caregiver may become one of the few individuals with whom the VIP can talk intimately.

IX. Conclusion

VIPs embody a paradox for caregivers. **These patients are special because of power or position and at the same time ordinary because disease and death are universal levelers.** It is best for the treating physician to keep these contradictory ideas in mind, simultaneously acknowledging the nature of social status and, when being the doctor, ignoring it. While treating VIPs is taxing, it has rich, intangible rewards, not the least of which is the bittersweet experience of rediscovering one's own foibles and humanity. In these situations, it is not just the celebrity's cardiologist who is reminded that "The king's heart is in the hands of the Lord" (Proverbs 21:1).

Suggested Readings

American Psychiatric Association. (1994). *Diagnostic and statistical manual of mental disorders* (4th ed.). Washington, DC: American Psychiatric Association.

Groves, J.E., Dunderdale, B.A., & Stern, T.A. (2002). Celebrity patients, VIPs, and potentates. *Primary Care Companion, Journal of Clinical Psychiatry, 4,* 215–223.

Groves, J.E. (1986–1987). Physician, sketch thyself. *Harvard Medical Alumni Bulletin, 60,* 36–38.

Kucharski, A. (1984). On being sick and famous. *Political Psychology, 5,* 69–81.

La Puma, J., Stocking, C.B., La Voie, D., & Darling, C.A. (1991). When physicians treat members of their own families. *New England Journal of Medicine, 325,* 1290–1294.

Marzuk, P. (1987). When the patient is a physician. *New England Journal of Medicine, 317,* 1409–1411.

Rundle, R.L., & Binkley, C. (1999). America's most luxurious hospitals. *Wall Street Journal,* pp. W1, W14.

Therapeutic Complications and Considerations

CHAPTER 66

Management of Antidepressant-Induced Side Effects

JORDAN W. SMOLLER, MARK H. POLLACK, AND DARA K. LEE

I. Importance of Management of Side Effects

A. **Enhanced compliance.** Treatment-emergent side effects may limit a patient's compliance with psychotropic medication, resulting in suboptimal treatment.

B. **Adequacy of dosing.** Without management of side effects, patients may not tolerate therapeutic doses of medication. The result may be a prolongation of acute symptoms and illness relapse from the precipitous discontinuation of therapy.

C. Effective relief of unpleasant side effects can enhance the doctor-patient relationship and **prevent the premature abandonment of treatment.**

II. General Principles of Management of Side Effects

A. **Anticipate the probable side effects.** Straightforward reassuring explanations of probable side effects and their management can increase a patient's confidence in the physician and reduce feelings of anxiety and discouragement when side effects develop.
   1. Review the most common side effects (e.g., increased anxiety, gastrointestinal [GI] distress, sleep disturbance with selective serotonin reuptake inhibitors [SSRIs]) and any serious side effects that are associated with a given medication or class of medication (e.g., risk of seizure with bupropion and of priapism with trazodone). This also serves to provide informed consent for the use of psychotropic medication.
   2. Reassure the patient that management strategies are available to minimize the adverse effects that occur.

B. **Select the appropriate drugs.** This can prevent undesirable side effects. For example, the newer antidepressants (SSRIs, bupropion, venlafaxine, nefazodone) generally have a more favorable side effect profile than do the agents, such as the tricyclic antidepressants (TCAs) and monoamine oxidase inhibitors (MAOIs), which became available more than 30 years ago (Table 66-1). The newer agents are often more suitable for patients with a co-morbid medical disease which may be exacerbated by the adverse effects (including cardiotoxicity and anticholinergic effects) associated with the older antidepressants. Among the TCAs, the secondary amines (e.g., desipramine and nortriptyline) are better tolerated than are the tertiary amines (e.g., amitriptyline, doxepin, and imipramine).

C. **Use the lowest effective dose during the initial phase of treatment and gradually titrate the dose.** Since adverse effects usually are dose-dependent, this strategy may minimize side effects. However, inadequate dosing or dose reduction during maintenance therapy below the levels needed to achieve remission can result in undertreatment and an increased risk of relapse.

Table 66-1. Adverse Effects of Antidepressants

	Orthostatic Hypotension	Cardiac Conduction	Anticholinergic	Sedation	Weight Gain	Nervousness/ Insomnia	GI Distress	Sexual Dysfunction
Older agents								
TCAs								
Amitriptyline	++++	++++	++++	++++	++++	++	++	++
Imipramine	++++	++++	+++	+++	+++	++	++	++
Doxepin	+++	++	+++	++++	++++	++	++	++
Clomipramine	+++	+++	++++	++++	+++	+++	+++	+++
Desipramine	++	++	++	++	++	++	+	+++
Nortriptyline	++	++	+++	+++	++	+++	+	++
Protriptyline	+++	+++	+++	++	++	+++	+	++
MAOI								
Phenelzine	++++	+	++	+++	++++	++	++	++
Tranylcypromine	+++	+	+	++	++	+++	++	++
Newer agents								
SSRIs								
Fluoxetine	+	+	+	++	+	++	+++	+++
Sertraline	+	+	+	++	+	++	+++	+++
Paroxetine	+	+	++	++	+	++	+++	+++
Fluvoxamine	+	+	+	++	+	++	+++	+++
Citalopram	+	+	+	++	+	++	+++	+++
Escitalopram	+	+	+	+	++	++	+++	+++
Others								
Bupropion	+	+	+	+	+	+++	++	+
Trazodone	+++	++	+	++++	+	+	++	+
Nefazodone	++	+	+	++	+	+	++	+
Venlafaxine	+	+	+	++	+	++	+++	+++
Mirtazapine	++	+	+	+++	+++	+	+	+

NOTE: Relative likelihood of adverse effects: +, none to minimal; ++, low; +++, moderate; ++++, high.

D. Follow the maxim "start low, go slow," especially among special patient populations (e.g., children, the elderly, the neurologically-impaired, and the medically ill). These patients may not be able to tolerate the usual dose of psychotropics.

E. Use adjunctive agents to manage side effects rather than switching antidepressants, which may delay the therapeutic response. Switching can be appropriate when persistent side effects preclude treatment with therapeutic doses of an antidepressant.

F. Reassure the patient and employ temporary treatments of side effects that may "buy time" until the adverse effects diminish spontaneously, since side effects often abate with time.

G. Be aware that the symptoms of underlying mood and anxiety disorders (e.g., insomnia, GI distress, fatigue) **may be difficult to distinguish from medication side effects.** Symptoms that begin after medication is initiated and worsen in a dose-dependent fashion are more likely to be medication-related.

III. Cardiovascular Effects

A. Orthostatic hypotension is more common with the use of MAOIs, TCAs, and trazodone than it is with the use of SSRIs. Patients who complain of light-headedness, dizziness, or near syncope should have their orthostatic vital signs measured. Hypotension is of greatest concern in the elderly, in those on antihypertensive medications that may prevent compensatory hemodynamic reflexes, and in patients with cardiac and cerebrovascular disease. The hypotension may or may not be dose-dependent, and tolerance to this effect may not develop. For TCAs and trazodone, alpha-adrenergic blockade is the primary mechanism underlying hypotension. Management strategies include the following:

1. **Select agents with a lower propensity for alpha-adrenergic blockade**: the newer antidepressants (e.g., SSRIs, venlafaxine, bupropion). Among the TCAs, nortriptyline may have the lowest propensity to induce hypotension.

2. **Consider other potential causes of orthostasis,** such as dehydration, hypoadrenalism, hypothyroidism, and the concomitant use of antihypertensives.

3. **Gradually escalate the dose.**

4. Apply the following non-pharmacologic measures:

   a. **Educate patients about the possibility of orthostasis.** During periods of dosage adjustment, patients should be advised to rise slowly from a prone or sitting position and to sit or lie down if they experience light-headedness.

   b. **Consider the use of support hose** and calf muscle-strengthening exercises to prevent venous pooling.

   c. **Maintain adequate hydration.**

5. When these measures fail, pharmacologic measures may be effective. Although controlled data are lacking, the following may be helpful for some patients:

   a. **Use agents which increase intravascular volume.** Administration of these agents requires caution in patients with cardiac or renal dysfunction.

      i. **Fludrocortisone acetate** (0.05 to 0.2 mg q.d.), a mineralocorticoid, increases fluid volume and may reverse hypotension in 1 to 2 weeks. Patients should be monitored for the development of hypertension, edema, and electrolyte abnormalities.

      ii. Increase **dietary salt** intake.

   b. **Use thyroid hormones** (triiodothyronine 25 to 50 mcg/day or thyroxine 0.1 to 0.2 mg/day).

   c. **Use stimulants** (methylphenidate 10 to 40 mg/day or dextroamphetamine 2.5 to 20 mg/day). These agents should in general not be combined with MAOIs.

   d. **Ingest caffeine.** Caffeine may elevate blood pressure in patients on MAOIs.

   e. **Use metoclopramide** (10 mg t.i.d.). This drug carries a risk of tardive dyskinesia and should be reserved for refractory cases.

   f. **Use yohimbine** (2.7 to 10.8 mg q.d. to t.i.d.), an alpha-2 antagonist. This agent should not be used in patients on MAOIs.

B. Hypertension

1. **Venlafaxine** has been reported to produce blood pressure elevation in a dose-dependent fashion. Sustained increases in diastolic blood pressure (> 90 mmHg and ≥ 10 mmHg above baseline for three consecutive visits) occur in 3% of patients at doses of < 100 mg/day but in up to 13% of patients at doses of > 300 mg/day. Elevations are typically in the range of 2 to 7 mmHg and usually do not exceed 10 to 15 mmHg. Baseline blood pressure generally does not predict treatment-related hypertension, although patients with pre-existing hypertension should be monitored closely. Patients receiving higher doses of venlafaxine should have periodic blood pressure monitoring (every 1 to 2 weeks for the first month and then at regular follow-up visits). Management of hypertension consists of dose reduction, switching to an alternative agent, or the adjunctive use of an antihypertensive.

2. **Hypertensive crisis may occur in patients on MAOIs (e.g., phenelzine, tranyl-cypromine) who ingest sympathomimetic drugs or consume sufficient amounts of dietary tyramine** (Tables 66-2 and 66-3). Prescription of these medications is best undertaken by a psychiatrist or a physician familiar with their use. Spontaneous hypertensive reactions occur rarely in patients on MAOIs. The signs of hypertensive reaction include severe occipital headache, stiff neck, flushing, palpitations, retro-orbital pain, nausea, and sweating. Extreme elevations of blood pressure can lead to intracerebral bleeding. **The use of serotonergic medications (e.g., SSRIs) or narcotics (especially meperidine and dextromethorphan) in combination with an**

Table 66-2. Relative Restrictions of Foods and Beverages with MAOI Use

Restriction	Foods
Absolute	Aged cheeses; aged and cured meats; banana peel; broad bean pods; improperly stored or spoiled meats, poultry, and fish; Marmite; sauerkraut; soy sauce and other soybean condiments; tap beer
Moderate	Red or white wine (no more than 8 ounces per day), bottled or canned beer, including non-alcoholic varieties (no more than two per day)
Unnecessary	Avocados; bananas; beef or chicken bouillon; chocolate; fresh and mild cheeses, e.g., ricotta, cottage, cream cheese, processed slices; fresh meat, poultry, or fish; gravy (fresh); monosodium glutamate; peanuts; properly stored pickled or smoked fish, e.g., herring; raspberries; soy milk; yeast extracts (except Marmite)

SOURCE: Adapted from Gardner, D.M., et al. (1996). The making of a user-friendly diet. *Journal of Clinical Psychiatry, 57,* 99–104.

Table 66-3. Some Important MAOI-Drug Interactions	
Drug	*Interaction May Cause*
Sympathomimetic amines (indirect are most dangerous)	
Indirect (e.g., amphetamines, ephedrine, pseudoephedrine, dopamine, alpha-methyldopa, L-dopa, metaraminol, methylphenidate, phentermine, phenylpropanolamine)	Hypertensive crisis
Direct (e.g., epinephrine, norepinephrine, phenylephrine, isoproteronol)	Hypertensive crisis
Antidepressants	
Tricyclics	Hypertensive crisis/serotonin syndrome
Venlafaxine	Hypertensive crisis/serotonin syndrome
Bupropion	Hypertensive crisis
SSRIs	Serotonin syndrome
Nefazodone	Potential serotonin syndrome
Mirtazapine	Potential hypertensive crisis/serotonin syndrome
Opiolds/Analgesics	
Meperidine	Serotonin syndrome
Dextromethorphan	Serotonin syndrome
Tramadol	Hypertensive crisis/serotonin syndrome
Anorexigens	
Sibutramine	Hypertensive crises/serotonin syndrome
Barbiturates	Prolonged sedative-hypnotic effects
Oral hypoglycemics	Enhanced hypoglycemic effect
Sumatriptan	Enhanced effect of sumatriptan

MAOI is contraindicated and may produce a serotonin syndrome with hyperthermia, agitation and/or delirium, hyperreflexia, neuromuscular irritability, seizures, hypotension, coma, and even death. For prevention and management, the following steps should be taken:

a. **Patients should be provided with lists of contraindicated foods and medications for reference purposes.**

b. **Patients should be instructed to go immediately to a medical office or emergency room if the symptoms of a hypertensive reaction occur.**

c. **Patients should be instructed not to lie down if a hypertensive reaction is suspected,** as this can increase intracranial pressure.

C. **Disturbances of Rate and Rhythm**

1. **Sinus tachycardia** may occur in patients on TCAs, MAOIs, venlafaxine, or bupropion; however, it is rarely clinically significant. **Decreases in heart rate** occasionally are observed in patients on nefazodone and SSRIs but rarely require medical

attention except in patients with underlying sinoatrial (SA) or atrioventricular (AV) node dysfunction.

2. **Conduction defects and arrhythmias** may be exacerbated in some patients on TCAs or trazodone. Toxic levels of TCAs, underlying conduction disease (especially multifascicular block), and the period after a myocardial infarction (MI) are risk factors for TCA-related arrhythmias. Patients over age 40 and those with a history of cardiac disease should have a baseline electrocardiogram (ECG) to rule out QTc prolongation and other manifestations of conduction system disease. In general, the newer antidepressants (SSRIs, nefazodone, venlafaxine, bupropion) have relatively little risk of cardiotoxicity and are preferred for patients with a history of heart disease. Trazodone has been associated with ventricular arrhythmias in patients with pre-existing cardiac disease.

IV. Gastrointestinal Adverse Effects

These effects may occur with all antidepressants but usually abate within a few days or weeks. Specific ameliorative strategies are summarized in Table 66-4.

A. **Nausea and dyspepsia** are common adverse effects of the newer antidepressants and can be relieved in some cases by the use of divided dosing or dosing with meals.

Table 66-4. Strategies for the Treatment of Gastrointestinal Distress

Nausea and dyspepsia

  Dose with meals or use divided doses

    Over-the-counter antacids (e.g., Maalox, Mylanta)

    H_2 blockers

      Famotidine (Pepcid) 20–40 mg q.d.

      Rantidine (Zantac) 150 mg q.d.–b.i.d.

      Metoclopramide (Reglan) 5–10 mg q.d.–b.i.d.

Diarrhea

  Diphenoxylate hydrochloride (Lomotil) 5 mg b.i.d.–q.i.d.

  Loperamide (Imodium A-D) 2–4 mg b.i.d.–q.i.d.

  Cypropheptadine (Periactin) 2–4 mg q.d.–b.i.d.

  Lactobacillus acidophilus (1 capsule/meal)

Constipation

  Increased fluid intake and fiber

  Over-the-counter laxatives:

    Metamucil 1–2 tbsp every morning

    Docussate sodium (Colace) 100 mg b.i.d.–q.i.d.

    Milk of Magnesia 30 mL PO q.d.

Bethanechol (Urecholine) 10–30 mg q.d.–t.i.d.

Abbreviations: q.d., every day; b.i.d., twice a day; t.i.d., three times a day; q.i.d., four times a day.

SOURCE: Adapted from Pollack, M.H., & Smoller, J.W. (1996). Management of antidepressant-induced side effects. In M.K. Pollack, M.W. Otto, & J.F. Rosenbaum (Eds.), *Challenges in clinical practice: Pharmacologic and psychosocial strategies*. New York: Guilford Press, pp. 451–480.

Mirtazapine appears to be less likely to cause nausea. Adjunctive agents that are sometimes helpful include **antacids, bismuth salicylate, and H₂ blockers** (e.g., famotidine 20 to 40 mg/day or ranitidine 150 mg q.d.–b.i.d.). Metoclopramide (5 to 10 mg q.d.–b.i.d.) has been used for antidepressant-induced dyspepsia and nausea but should be limited to short-term use because of the risk of extrapyramidal symptoms and even tardive dyskinesia caused by its dopamine-blocking effects.

B. Diarrhea is more commonly seen with newer serotonergic antidepressants, such as the SSRIs, that lack anticholinergic effects. Management strategies include the use of antidiarrheal agents, such as diphenoxylate hydrochloride (5 mg b.i.d.–q.i.d.) and loperamide (2 to 4 mg b.i.d.–q.i.d.). For SSRI-induced diarrhea, the serotonin and histamine antagonist cyproheptadine (2 to 4 mg q.d.–b.i.d.) and *Lactobacillus acidophilus* culture (one capsule with meals) have been helpful for some patients.

C. Constipation most commonly occurs as an anticholinergic side effect of TCAs but can be seen with all antidepressants. In elderly patients, severe constipation and paralytic ileus may develop and pose serious risks. Maintaining adequate hydration and intake of dietary bulk, as well as physical activity, can prevent or relieve constipation. If necessary, over-the-counter bulk laxatives (e.g., Metamucil 1 to 2 tablespoons every morning) or stool softeners (e.g., docussate sodium 100 mg b.i.d.–t.i.d.) may be useful. Bethanechol (10 to 30 mg q.d.–t.i.d.) relieves constipation caused by anticholinergic antidepressants in some patients. Intermittent and short-term use of cathartic laxatives (e.g., milk of magnesia 30 mL PO q.d.) can be effective, but chronic use may reduce intestinal motility and worsen constipation.

V. Weight Gain

Weight gain may be a common cause of medication non-compliance and is most commonly associated with TCAs (especially the tertiary amines, such as amitriptyline, imipramine, and doxepin) and MAOIs (especially phenelzine). Weight gain may be related to the antihistaminic effects of these agents and has been reported with the newer antidepressant mirtazapine, which also has antihistaminic properties. The SSRIs, bupropion, venlafaxine, and nefazodone are less likely to cause weight gain, and some patients experience minor weight loss on these agents. If weight gain occurs during antidepressant administration, dietary modification and increased exercise should be recommended. Patients should avoid the use of high-calorie beverages to treat a dry mouth. Low doses of agents that have both antidepressant and anorectic effects (e.g., methylphenidate, bupropion) can be added to a non-MAOI antidepressant to limit weight gain. In addition some patients experience weight loss with addition of the anticonvulsant topiramate, initiated at 25 mg q.d. and titrated up slowly against side effects, such as sedation and mental cloudiness, to doses of 50–200 mg/day. Patients whose weight gain is attributable to edema can be treated with leg elevation or the judicious use of a diuretic, such as hydrochlorothiazide (12.5 to 25 mg q.d.) or amiloride (5 to 10 mg q.d.).

VI. Central Nervous System Effects

A. High-frequency **tremor** can occur as a side effect of TCAs, SSRIs, and MAOIs and may be exacerbated by anxiety or caffeine. Anxiolytic interventions and limitation of caffeine intake can be helpful. Pharmacologic strategies include the use of beta-blockers (e.g., propranolol 10 to 20 mg b.i.d.–t.i.d. or atenolol 25 to 100 mg q.d.) or low doses of benzodiazepines (e.g., lorazepam 1 to 2 mg b.i.d.–q.i.d. or clonazepam 0.5 to 2.0 mg q.d.–b.i.d.).

B. **Jitteriness and increased anxiety** are commonly seen with the initiation or dose escalation of TCAs, SSRIs, venlafaxine, and bupropion, particularly in patients with preexisting anxiety. Anticipation of this possibility and provision of reassurance are important factors in the prevention of medication non-compliance. Jitteriness usually remits within a few days to weeks and can be minimized by initiating treatment at low doses (e.g., 10 to 25 mg of imipramine or 5 to 10 mg of fluoxetine) with a gradual upward titration to allow for acclimation. The concomitant use of benzodiazepines (e.g., clonazepam 0.5 mg q.d.–b.i.d.) or gabapentin 300 mg q.d.–b.i.d. at the start of treatment may prevent initial jitteriness. Some patients on SSRIs or venlafaxine may experience an akathisia-like motor restlessness which may respond to the addition of propranolol (20 to 40 mg b.i.d.–q.i.d.), gabapentin 300–600 mg q.d.–b.i.d, or clonazepam (0.5 to 2.0 mg q.d.–b.i.d.). Limiting caffeine intake may be helpful.

C. **Fatigue and sedation** can represent medication side effects or the symptoms of an underlying mood or anxiety disorder; this distinction may be difficult to make. TCAs (especially those with greater antihistaminic or antiadrenergic properties), MAOIs (phenelzine more than tranylcypromine), trazodone, nefazodone, and mirtazapine are the most likely to produce sedation, but all antidepressants have this potential. Sedation can be exploited as a means of improving sleep in anxious and depressed patients, but daytime fatigue may be troublesome and oversedation may predispose the elderly to dangerous falls. Management strategies include (Table 66-5) the following:

1. Consideration of the role of underlying psychiatric or medical illness or of drug interactions.

2. Moving most or all doses of a sedating agent to bedtime. However, MAOIs, bupropion, venlafaxine, fluvoxamine, and nefazodone generally should still be given in divided doses.

3. When nighttime insomnia causes daytime sedation, adding a hypnotic (e.g., lorazepam 1 to 2 mg q.h.s., zolpidem 5 to 10 mg q.h.s., or trazodone 50 to 100 mg q.h.s.) can be helpful.

4. Caffeine intake can be increased early in the day or at times when sedation is most problematic.

5. For patients not on MAOIs, the addition of modafinil, a non-stimulant wake-promoting agent (at 100–200 mg b.i.d), low doses of stimulating antidepressants (e.g., desipramine 25 to 50 mg q.d., or bupropion 75 to 100 mg q.d.–b.i.d.) or psychostimulants (e.g., methylphenidate 10 to 20 mg b.i.d.) may target both refractory depression and fatigue. TCA plasma levels may be markedly elevated when TCAs are combined with SSRIs; combined use should be initiated with low doses of the TCA and with the plasma levels monitored.

6. The use of other agents, including dopaminergic agonists (e.g., amantadine 100 mg t.i.d.–q.i.d., pergolide 0.5 to 2.0 mg q.d.) or triiodothyronine (25 to 50 μg/day), can be helpful. The latter is contraindicated in patients with known or suspected coronary artery disease.

D. **Sleep disturbance and nightmares** as well as hypnopompic or hypnagogic phenomena may be related to antidepressant treatment and may improve if dosing is moved to earlier in the day. Insomnia occurs most commonly with SSRIs, bupropion, venlafaxine, and MAOIs and less often with TCAs, nefazodone, trazodone, and mirtazapine. Sleep

---

Table 66-5. Strategies for the Treatment of Antidepressant-Induced Fatigue and Sedation

Consider the role of underlying illness or drug interactions

Bedtime dosing

Adding a hypnotic

    Lorazepam (Ativan) 1–2 mg q.h.s

    Zolpidem (Ambien) 5–10 mg q.h.s.

    Trazodone (Desyrel) 50–100 mg q.h.s.

Increasing caffeine intake

Adding modafanil (Provigil) 100–200 mg b.i.d

Adding a stimulant antidepressant to an SSRI

    Desipramine (Norpramin) 25–50 mg q.d.

    Bupropion (Wellbutrin) 75–100 mg q.d.–b.i.d.

Adding a psychostimulant to an SSRI

    Methylphenidate (Ritalin) 10–20 mg b.i.d.

Thyroid supplementation of an SSRI or MAOI

    Triiodothyronine 25–50 µg/day

Adding dopaminergic agonists to an SSRI or MAOI

    Amantadine (Symmetrel) 100 mg t.i.d.–q.i.d.

    Pergolide (Permax) 0.5–2.0 mg q.d.–b.i.d.

Abbreviations: q.d., every day; b.i.d., twice a day; t.i.d., three times a day; q.i.d., four times a day.

SOURCE: Adapted from Pollack, M.H., & Smoller, J.W. (1996). Management of antidepressant-induced side effects. In M.K. Pollack, M.W. Otto, & J.F. Rosenbaum (Eds.), *Challenges in clinical practice: Pharmacologic and psychosocial strategies.* New York: Guilford Press, pp. 451–480.

---

hygiene and stimulus control measures, including reducing caffeine intake, avoiding daytime naps, limiting fluid intake before bedtime to minimize nocturia, and restricting bedroom activities to sleep and sexual relations, may be effective for insomnia. The adjunctive use of a benzodiazepine or zolpidem (5 to 10 mg q.h.s.) as a hypnotic, gabapentin (300–600 mg q.h.s), or trazodone (50 to 200 mg q.h.s.) can reduce insomnia.

E. Myoclonus (sudden jerking or twitching movements of limbs) may be relieved by dosage reduction or, for nocturnal myoclonus, by moving dosing away from bedtime. Clonazepam (0.5 to 2.0 mg q.h.s.) may relieve nocturnal myoclonus; anecdotally, trazodone (50 to 300 mg q.d.), cyproheptadine (4 to 16 mg q.d.), gabapentin, valproate, and carbamazepine (at therapeutic levels) have been used successfully to treat myoclonus.

F. Paresthesias (numbness or tingling) may occur with antidepressant use and have been associated most frequently with MAOIs. Pyridoxine deficiency may be causative in some cases, and supplemental pyridoxine (50 to 150 mg q.h.s.) may be helpful. Low doses of a benzodiazepine (e.g., clonazepam 0.5 to 2.0 mg q.d.–b.i.d.) are a useful alternative.

G. **Hypomania or mania** may occur during treatment with antidepressants in approximately 1% or less of patients without a history of bipolar disorder. Patients with a history of bipolar disorder who are not on mood-stabilizing medication (e.g., lithium or valproate) are at much higher risk. Treatment of depression in such patients is best managed by a psychiatrist. Limited data suggest that TCAs may be most likely to cause "switching" into mania among bipolar patients, with lower rates observed for bupropion, MAOIs, and perhaps SSRIs. The signs and symptoms of hypomania or mania include an elevated or irritable mood, racing thoughts, a decreased need for sleep, impulsive behavior, and rapid, pressured speech. Mild hypomania may remit with dose reduction or discontinuation of antidepressants, but more severe presentations may require treatment with mood stabilizers, benzodiazepines, and even antipsychotic medications. Psychiatric consultation for these patients is indicated.

H. **Suicidal ideation** has been reported as a rare adverse effect of antidepressant treatment but it does not appear to be associated with a specific antidepressant. Suicidal ideation in patients on antidepressants may be attributable primarily to an underlying psychiatric disorder, such as depression, panic disorder, and borderline personality disorder. If suicidality worsens after the initiation of antidepressant treatment, clinicians should be alert to the possible contribution of antidepressant-related akathisia or agitation, which may develop with rapid dose escalation. In such cases, starting at lower doses, slowly titrating upwards, and using adjunctive benzodiazepines or beta-blockers may be effective. Antidepressant-induced mania can increase the risk of self-harm. Psychiatric consultation usually is indicated for these patients.

VII. Anticholinergic Effects

A. Anticholinergic activity varies greatly among antidepressants and is **greatest for the tertiary amine TCAs** (e.g., amitriptyline, imipramine, doxepin) and minimal for most newer antidepressants (SSRIs, venlafaxine, bupropion, trazodone, nefazodone, and mirtazapine). Among the TCAs, nortriptyline and desipramine are the least anticholinergic. Tolerance often develops to many of the anticholinergic side effects over time.

B. **Dry mouth** (xerostomia) may result in the development of bad breath, stomatitis, and dental caries. **Sugarless gum and sugarless hard candy may stimulate salivation without producing weight gain or dental caries.** Artificial saliva preparations can be used. Cholinergic agonists, such as bethanecol (10 to 30 mg q.d.–t.i.d.) and pilocarpine (oral tablets or a 1% pilocarpine rinse prepared by mixing 4% pilocarpine solution and water in a 1:3 mixture) may be useful, but patients with uncontrolled asthma should not be treated with cholinergic agonists. The adverse effects of cholinergic agonists may include abdominal cramping, diarrhea, rhinitis, flushing, and tearing. Bethanecol (10 mg q.d.–t.i.d.) has been used safely to treat anticholinergic side effects in elderly patients. Dry eyes can be treated with artificial tear solutions.

C. **Blurred vision** usually abates with time, but when it is persistent, it can be managed with pilocarpine 1% drops (one drop three times daily) or bethanecol (10 to 25 mg q.d.–t.i.d.). Patients with narrow-angle glaucoma may experience dangerous elevations of intraocular pressure on anticholinergic medications, and so newer antidepressants that lack anticholinergic activity generally should be utilized in affected patients.

D. **Urinary hesitancy and retention,** sometimes complicated by urinary tract infections and even renal damage, can occur in patients on anticholinergic agents, including the

TCAs. The elderly and patients with prostatic hypertrophy or other reasons for compromise of urinary outflow are at particular risk. Although less likely to cause difficulties because of their minimal anticholinergic activity, newer antidepressants and MAOIs have occasionally been associated with urinary hesitancy or retention. Bethanecol (10 to 30 mg t.i.d.) can be used for urinary hesitancy in the absence of outflow obstruction but should be avoided in patients with prostatic hypertrophy because the bladder may be damaged by forceful contractions against a fixed obstruction. Severe urinary retention mandates the discontinuation of the antidepressant.

E. **Central nervous system (CNS) anticholinergic toxicity** can present with confusion, memory loss, delirium, and even psychosis, variably accompanied by other signs of anticholinergic excess (e.g., increased temperature, dry skin, flushing, and urinary retention). High-risk patients include the elderly, in whom anticholinergic medications should always be minimized if possible. Children and brain-injured patients are also at increased risk for difficulties. Management includes decreasing or discontinuing anticholinergic medication and, in emergencies, administering physostigmine (1 to 2 mg slow IV push over 2 minutes) every 30 minutes or 1 to 2 mg IM every hour. Physostigmine administration requires close monitoring of vital signs and mental status; life support and cardiac monitoring equipment should be available in case bronchoconstriction, hemodynamic instability, or seizures develop. Agitation may respond to a benzodiazepine (e.g., lorazepam 0.5 to 2.0 mg PO or IM every 30 to 60 minutes as needed).

VIII. Sexual Side Effects

A. **Sexual dysfunction is increasingly recognized as a common side effect of many antidepressants** and may occur in one-third or more of these patients. Sexual dysfunction may be underreported unless it is specifically asked about and can be an occult cause of medical non-compliance. Patients should be encouraged to report such side effects and should be reassured that if it occurs, **sexual dysfunction is often treatable and certainly is reversible with drug discontinuation.** Antidepressants with a lower propensity for causing sexual dysfunction include bupropion, nefazodone, and mirtazapine.

B. **Decreased libido** may occur as a symptom of a mood or anxiety disorder as well as secondary to antidepressant administration. When it persists or worsens after other depressive symptoms have been relieved, an adverse medication effect should be suspected.

C. **Erectile dysfunction** may result from the anticholinergic and/or anti-alpha-adrenergic effects of antidepressants. **Priapism** can occur with a number of antidepressants or antipsychotics but has been **reported to occur mostly frequently with trazodone** (approximately 1 in 1000 to 10,000 men). Trazodone-related priapism usually occurs within the first 4 weeks of therapy but has been reported as late as 18 months into treatment and appears to be independent of dose. Men who are prescribed trazodone should be warned about this potential side effect and instructed to discontinue the medication immediately if unusual erectile or urinary symptoms occur. Priapism is a medical emergency that requires evaluation by a urologist. Surgical intervention may be necessary, although priapism may respond to intracavernosal injection of alpha-adrenergic agonists, such as metaraminol, that promote venoconstriction and detumescence.

D. **Ejaculatory dysfunction** associated with antidepressants includes delayed, retrograde, or painful ejaculation as well as anhedonic ejaculation (without orgasm).

E. **Delayed orgasm and anorgasmia** have been associated with TCAs, MAOIs, SSRIs, and atypical antidepressants and may be serotoninergically mediated. Occasionally, **spontaneous orgasms** during yawning have been reported with the SSRIs, trazodone, and clomipramine.

F. Several strategies have been used successfully to treat the sexual side effects of antidepressants although controlled trials supporting their use are lacking for most of these (Table 66-6).

1. The use of **sildefanil**, an agent indicated for male erectile dysfunction, has been demonstrated effective for the treatment of antidepressant-induced sexual dysfunction, including libido, erectile, ejaculatory, and orgasm disturbance in men and preliminarily in women. It is typically dosed at 50–100 mg p.r.n. 1–2 hours prior to sexual relations. It is contraindicated in patients with unstable coronary ischemia and in those receiving nitrates.

2. The use of **adjunctive bupropion** has been effective in relieving SSRI-induced sexual dysfunction, but this agent should not be combined with MAOIs. Although SSRIs may decrease the metabolism of bupropion and thus lower the seizure threshold, this has not represented a clinically significant problem. However, adjunctive bupropion should be initiated at low doses to minimize adverse interactions.

3. The use of **yohimbine**, an alpha$_2$-adrenergic antagonist, can improve erectile and orgasmic dysfunction. Treatment is initiated at 2.7 mg q.d. and increased by 2.7 mg

---

Table 66-6. Agents Used in the Treatment of Antidepressant-Induced Sexual Dysfunction

Agent (Proprietary Name)	Dose
Sildenafil (Viagra)	50–100 mg p.r.n.
Yohimbine (Yocon)	5.4 mg q.d.–t.i.d.
Bupropion (Wellbutrin-SR)	100–200 mg q.d.–b.i.d.
Modafanil (Provigil)	100–200 mg q.d.–b.i.d.
Buspirone (BuSpar)	5–20 mg t.i.d.
Cyproheptadine (Periactin)	4–16 mg q.d.
Dopaminergic agonists	
Amantadine (Symmetrel)	100 mg b.i.d.–t.i.d.
Pergolide (Permax)	0.05–2.0 mg q.d.–b.i.d.
Methylphenidate (Ritalin)	5–10 mg q.d.–q.i.d.
Cholinergic agonists	
Bethanechol (Urecholine)	10–80 mg b.i.d.
Nefazodone (Serzone)	50–100 mg p.r.n.
Mirtazapine (Remeron)	15–30 mg p.r.n.

Abbreviations: p.r.n., as needed; q.d., every day; b.i.d., twice a day; t.i.d.. three times a day; q.i.d., four times a day.

SOURCE: Adapted from Pollack, M.H., & Smoller, J.W. (1996). Management of antidepressant-induced side effects. In M.K. Pollack, M.W. Otto, & J.F. Rosenbaum (Eds.), *Challenges in clinical practice: Pharmacologic and psychosocial strategies.* New York: Guilford Press, pp. 451–480.

q.d. every 2 to 3 days up to 5.4 mg t.i.d. if necessary. A full response may take several weeks to develop, and the side effects include anxiety and even panic attacks, nausea, light-headedness, and sweating. Yohimbine also can be used on an as-needed basis 1 to 2 hours before intercourse. It is contraindicated in patients on MAOIs.

4. The use of dopamine agonists may improve libido, as well as erectile, ejaculatory, and orgasmic dysfunction. Examples include **amantadine** (100 mg b.i.d.–t.i.d.), **pergolide** (0.05 mg titrated up by 0.1 mg every 2 to 3 days up to 2 to 5 mg per day in divided dosing), and ropinirole (0.25 mg titrated up to 2–4 mg over 4 weeks as tolerated), methylphenidate (Ritalin) (5 to 10 mg q.d.–q.i.d.).

5. The non-stimulant wakefulness-promoting agent modafanil (Provigil) may be helpful in treating antidepressant induced sexual dysfunction; it is administered at doses of 100–200 mg q.d.–b.i.d.

6. The use of adjunctive **buspirone** (5 to 20 mg t.i.d.) may improve sexual dysfunction in some patients.

7. The use of **cyproheptadine,** an antihistamine with serotonin antagonist properties, may relieve anorgasmia, improve libido, and reverse ejaculatory and erectile dysfunction induced by SSRIs, TCAs, and MAOIs. Side effects include sedation and weight gain. Serotonin antagonism occasionally may interfere with the antidepressant efficacy of SSRIs. Dosing begins at 2 mg q.h.s. and may be increased up to 4 to 16 mg/day in once- or twice-daily dosing.

8. The use of **cholinergic agonists, such as bethanechol** (10 to 30 mg/day in b.i.d. dosing) or neostigmine (7.5 to 15 mg 30 minutes before sexual intercourse) may enhance libido and improve erectile and ejaculatory function in men.

9. The use of "drug holidays" has been reported to relieve sexual dysfunction in patients treated with the shorter-acting SSRIs, paroxetine and sertraline. Patients may temporarily discontinue the antidepressant on Thursday to allow a washout and a return of sexual function for the weekend and resume the medication on Sunday. The half-life of fluoxetine is considerably longer than that of paroxetine, sertraline, and fluvoxamine, so that brief drug holidays do not appear to reverse sexual dysfunction in fluoxetine-treated patients. Caution should be exercised in recommending drug holidays, as patients may experience withdrawal symptoms or relapse after abrupt drug discontinuation.

10. Switching to an antidepressant such as bupropion, nefazodone, or mirtazapine with a low risk of sexual side effects can be helpful.

IX. Dermatologic Side Effects

A. Up to 5–10% of patients experience cutaneous reactions to antidepressants, usually in the form of **erythematous maculopapular rashes,** which tend to occur early in treatment and usually are self-limited even when the antidepressant is continued. The decision about whether to continue the medication depends on the level of patient discomfort, evidence of systemic involvement, and history of therapeutic response to other agents. Pruritis associated with localized maculopapular rashes may respond to an antihistamine (e.g., diphenhydramine 25 to 50 mg q.d.–t.i.d.) or the occasional administration of a topical steroid cream containing 1% hydrocortisone.

B. Reactions that progress beyond a localized maculopapular rash or are associated with signs of systemic involvement (e.g., fever, leukocytosis, and elevated liver function tests) may indicate a generalized immune response and generally necessitate discontinuation of the medication. When another antidepressant is substituted, it is prudent to select an agent from a different class to minimize the risk of cross-reactivity.

C. Less commonly, severe reactions, including generalized urticaria, erythema multiforme, and toxic epidermal necrolysis, may occur. Cutaneous erythematous plaques with atypical lymphoid infiltrates and pseuodolymphomas have been reported in some patients on SSRIs and benzodiazepines. The development of severe or atypical dermatologic reactions should prompt discontinuation of the offending agent and dermatologic consultation.

X. Hair Loss

Hair loss may occur with a variety of psychotropic agents. While the mechanism is unknown in most cases, multivitamins containing supplemental selenium and zinc (e.g., Centrum Silver) have been reported to be helpful for some patients. Use of topical agents (e.g., minoxidil [Rogaine]) may be helpful as well.

XI. Excessive Sweating

Excessive sweating may occur with the use of any antidepressant. Daily showering or the use of talcum power may provide some relief. The alpha-adrenergic antagonists, terazosin (1 to 2 mg q.h.s.) and doxazosin (1 to 2 mg q.h.s.), have been used successfully to reduce antidepressant-induced sweating, and clonidine (0.1 to 0.25 mg q.d.–q.i.d.) may be helpful for some patients. These medications should be initiated at low doses to minimize the risk of hypotension. A solution of aluminum chloride hexahydrate (20% weight per volume) in anhydrous alcohol (Drysol), a potent antiperspirant, can be used to control excessive sweating localized to the axilla or palms.

XII. Headache

Headache is a relatively common side effect of newer antidepressants and may respond to acetaminophen or non-steroidal anti-inflammatory drugs. New-onset severe headache in a patient on an MAOI may signal the onset of a hypertensive crisis which requires immediate attention.

XIII. Discontinuation Effects

Discontinuation effects, though generally mild and short-lived, may occur with any antidepressant and can be distressing for some patients. Abrupt discontinuation of TCAs, MAOIs, SSRIs, and venlafaxine has been associated with symptoms that include a "flu-like" syndrome with malaise, dizziness, headache, nausea, fatigue, and weakness as well as confusion, sleep disturbance, "electric shock-like" paresthesias, and rapid re-crudescence of mood and anxiety symptoms. Because of its longer half-life, discontinuation symptoms may be less common with the SSRI fluoxetine. Discontinuation symptoms can be avoided by gradually tapering antidepressants (e.g., by 25% of the dose every 3 to 7 days). In some cases resumption of medication followed by more gradual tapering may be necessary.

Suggested Readings

Dording, C.M., Mischoulon, D., Petersen, T.J., et al. (2002). The pharmacologic management of SSRI-induced side effects: A survey of psychiatrists. *Annals of Clinical Psychiatry, 14,* 143–147.

Fava, M., & Rosenbaum, J.F. (1996). Treatment-emergent side effects of the newer antidepressants. *Psychiatric Clinics of North America, 3,* 13–29.

McElroy, S.L., Keck, P.E., Jr., & Friedman, L.M. (1996). Practical management of antidepressant side effects: An update. In R.E. Hales, & S.C. Yudofsky (Eds.), *Practical clinical strategies in treating depression and anxiety disorders in a managed care environment.* Washington, DC: American Psychiatric Association, pp. 39–48.

Nurnberg, H.G., & Hensley, P.L. (2003). Selective phosphodiesterase type-5 inhibitor treatment of serotonergic reuptake inhibitor antidepressant-associated sexual dysfunction: A review of diagnosis, treatment, and relevance. *CNS Spectrums, 3,* 194–202.

Pollack, M.H., & Smoller, J.W. (1996). Management of antidepressant-induced side effects. In M.K. Pollack, M.W. Otto, & J.F. Rosenbaum (Eds.), *Challenges in clinical practice: Pharmacologic and psychosocial strategies.* New York: Guilford Press, pp. 451–480.

CHAPTER 67

Cardiovascular Side Effects of Psychotropic Agents

JEFF C. HUFFMAN, GEORGE E. TESAR, AND THEODORE A. STERN

I. Introduction

A. Historically, psychotropic agents have been recognized for their potentially adverse effects on the heart and the cardiovascular (CV) system. Some antidepressants (e.g., tricyclic antidepressants [TCAs]), antipsychotics (e.g., low-potency neuroleptics), and mood-stabilizing agents (e.g., lithium and carbamazepine) can compromise CV performance at toxic or even therapeutic doses in patients with pre-existing CV disease.

B. Drugs with a safer CV profile have supplanted many of the older psychotropic agents. When the use of a potentially toxic psychotropic agent is necessary, knowledge of its specific CV activity and careful monitoring of CV performance help promote its safe use.

C. This chapter reviews the following areas:
   1. The potential **adverse effects of psychotropic agents** on the heart and the CV system
   2. The known **mechanisms of psychotropic action** on the heart and the CV system
   3. **Risk factors for psychotropic-associated CV toxicity**
   4. **Recommendations for the treatment of a patient with CV disease who requires psychotropic medication**

D. The discussion is organized around the classification of psychotropic agents into the following major treatment categories:
   1. Antidepressants
   2. Antipsychotics
   3. Mood stabilizers
   4. Anxiolytics
   5. Psychostimulants
   6. Agents used to treat substance abuse

II. Antidepressants (Table 67-1)

A. The antidepressants of choice are selective serotonin reuptake inhibitors (SSRIs).
   1. **Classification.** The SSRIs currently available in the United States for the treatment of depression are listed in Table 67-2 and include fluoxetine (Prozac), sertraline (Zoloft), citalopram (Celexa), escitalopram (Lexapro), and paroxetine (Paxil). Fluvoxamine (Luvox), an SSRI that is available elsewhere in the world for the treatment of depression, has been approved in the United States only for the treatment of obsessive-compulsive disorder (OCD).
   2. **Indications. SSRIs have been approved for the treatment of depression. They are also effective for a variety of anxiety disorders,** such as panic and OCD.

(text continues on page 638)

Table 67-1. The Use of Antidepressants in Patients with Cardiovascular Disease

Cardiac Status	Psychiatric Condition	Drug of Choice on Basis of Available Data	Alternatives	Comments
Bundle branch block	Depression	Citalopram Bupropion Sertraline	Fluoxetine Mirtazapine Paroxetine Escitalopram	All TCAs prolong H-V interval and increase risk of OH in the presence of bundle branch block
	Psychosis/delirium	Risperidone Olanzapine Quetiapine	High-potency neuroleptics	Low-potency neuroleptics produce same risk as do TCAs
	Bipolar disorder	Divalproex	Lithium	Carbamazepine probably produces same risk as do TCAs
Ventricular arrhythmias same as bundle branch block	Depression	Bupropion Fluoxetine Paroxetine Sertraline	Mirtazapine Nefazodone Venlafaxine	Trazodone may increase PVC frequency TCAs can have antiarrhythmic effect SSRIs may raise levels of beta-blockers, ecainide, flecainide, and propafenone
	Psychosis/delirium	High-potency neuroleptics	Risperidone	Low-potency neuroleptics could theoretically have an antiarrhythmic effect
	Bipolar disorder	Divalproex	Lithium	Carbamazepine probably produces same risk as do TCAs
Orthostatic hypotension	Depression	Bupropion Citalopram Sertraline	Mirtazapine Fluoxetine Paroxetine Escitalopram	Use nortriptyline if TCA necessary
	Psychosis/delirium	Olanzapine	High-potency neuroleptics	Risperidone and quetiapine associated with moderate rates of OH All typical neuroleptics (low-potency more than high-potency) and clozapine can aggravate pre-existent OH
	Bipolar disorder	Divalproex	Lithium	Carbamazepine probably produces same risk as do TCAs

Condition	Disorder			Comments
Coronary artery disease	Depression	Bupropion Citalopram Sertraline Quetiapine Olazapine Risperidone	Mirtazapine Escitalopram	TCAs increase risk of angina or MI because of anticholinergic effects and potential OH SSRIs (especially fluoxetine and paroxetine) may raise levels of beta-blockers, ecainide, flecainide, and propafenone
	Psychosis/delirium		High-potency neuroleptics	Low-potency neuroleptics produce same risk as do TCAs Olanzapine may be better for short-term use (less OH, potentially less QTc prolongation) Risperidone may be better for long-term use (potentially less weight gain and diabetes risk)
	Bipolar disorder	Divalproex	Lithium	Carbamazepine produces same risk as do TCAs
Left ventricular dysfunction	Depression	Citalopram Bupropion Sertraline	Fluoxetine Mirtazapine Paroxetine Escitalopram	No antidepressant absolutely contraindicated
	Psychosis/delirium	Typical neuroleptics	Risperidone Clozapine	No contraindications
	Bipolar disorder	Divalproex	Carbamazepine Clozapine	No contraindications
Congestive heart failure	Depression	Citalopram Bupropion Sertraline	Fluoxetine Mirtazapine Paroxetine Escitalopram	Use nortriptyline if TCA necessary
	Psychosis/delirium	High-potency neuroleptics	Risperidone	Avoid low-potency neuroleptics Avoid clozapine
	Bipolar disorder	Divalproex	Carbamazepine Lithium	Lithium levels may be difficult to control in presence of renal failure and diuretic therapy

(continued)

Table 67-1. The Use of Antidepressants in Patients with Cardiovascular Disease (Continued)

Cardiac Status	Psychiatric Condition	Drug of Choice on Basis of Available Data	Alternatives	Comments
Essential hypertension	Depression	Bupropion Sertraline Citalopram	Mirtazapine Escitalopram Fluoxetine Paroxetine	Venlafaxine could aggravate hypertension SSRIs can raise levels of beta-blockers
	Psychosis/ delirium	High-potency neuroleptics Low-potency neuroleptics	Risperidone Clozapine	Low-potency neuroleptics may help lower blood pressure
	Bipolar disorder	Divalproex	Carbamazepine Lithium	
Recent acute myocardial infarction	Depression	Citalopram Bupropion Sertraline	Mirtazapine Nefazodone Fluoxetine Escitalopram	Paroxetine has mild anticholinergic effects TCAs should be avoided for 4 to 6 weeks post-MI if possible (if used at all) Sertraline best studied in this population
	Psychosis/ depression	High-potency neuroleptics	Risperidone Clozapine Lithium	
	Bipolar disorder	Divalproex		
Sick sinus syndrome	Depression	Bupropion Mirtazapine Quetiapine Olanzapine	Citalopram Escitalopram Fluoxetine Paroxetine	SSRIs may be relatively contraindicated because of their rare association with bradycardia
	Psychosis/ delirium	Risperidone	Typical neuroleptics	

Condition	Indication			
Atrioventricular block (second- or third-degree)	Bipolar disorder	Divalproex	Carbamazepine	Lithium should be avoided because of sinus node effect
	Depression	Bupropion Citalopram Sertraline	Mirtazapine Paroxetine Escitalopram Venlafaxine Fluoxetine	TCAs absolutely contraindicated
	Psychosis/delirium	Risperidone Olanzapine Quetiapine		Low-potency neuroleptics *absolutely* contraindicated High-potency neuroleptics *relatively* contraindicated
Atrial fibrillation	Bipolar disorder	Divalproex	Lithium	Carbamazepine absolutely contraindicated
	Depression	Citalopram Bupropion Sertraline	Fluoxetine Mirtazapine Paroxetine Escitalopram	
	Psychosis/delirium	High-potency neuroleptics	Risperidone	
	Bipolar disorder	Divalproex Lithium		Lithium effect on sinus node may be beneficial
Prolonged QTc interval	Depression	Bupropion Citalopram Sertraline	Escitalopram Mirtazapine Fluoxetine Paroxetine	Avoid TCAs
	Psychosis/delirium	Olanzapine	Risperidone	Avoid typical neuroleptics or use high-potency if necessary
	Bipolar disorder	Divalproex	Lithium	Avoid carbamazepine

NOTE: HV, His-ventricular; OH, orthostatic hypotension; MI, myocardial infarction; TCA, tricyclic antidepressant.

Table 67-2. Psychotropic Agents and Their Effects on the Heart and Cardiovascular System

Generic Name	Trade Name	Treatment Class	Effects on Heart and Cardio-vascular System[a]	Comments
Amitriptyline	Elavil	Antidepressant (TCA)	1c, 3c, 5	Highly anticholinergic TCA
Aripiprazole	Abilify	Atypical neuroleptic	1a	Not yet systematically tested in patients with cardiovascular disease
Bupropion	Wellbutrin; Zyban	Antidepressant		Also effective for smoking cessation
Buspirone	Buspar	Anxiolytic		Reported to cause increased BP when used in combination with MAOI and hypertension and anxiety when used with clomipramine
Carbamazepine	Tegretol	Mood stabilizer	1a, 5	Serum levels may be raised by the following drugs: calcium channel-blockers, cimetidine, erythromycin, isoniazid, propoxyphene, SSRIs
Chlorpromazine	Thorazine	Low-potency neuroleptic	1c, 3c, 5	
Citalopram	Celexa	Antidepressant (SSRI)		Least drug-drug interactions of the SSRIs
Clomipramine	Anafranil	Antidepressant (TCA)	1c, 3c, 5	
Clozapine	Clozaril	Atypical neuroleptic	1c, 3c	Parkinson's disease patients may need to start at as little as 6.5 mg q.d. Associated with myocarditis, pericarditis, and pericardial effusion
Desipramine	Norpramin	Antidepressant (TCA)	1c, 3a, 5	
Dextroamphetamine	Dexedrine	Psychostimulant	2c, 3b	CV effects are dose-related
Disulfiram	Antabuse	Anti-alcohol agent		Alcohol-disulfiram interaction may have profound effects on heart and CV system

Divalproex sodium	Depakote	Mood stabilizer		
Donepezil	Aricept	Acetylcholinesterase inhibitor	4b	Case report of heat block associated with overdose May slow the cause of mild-moderate dementia Should be administered with caution to patients with bradycardiac arrhythmias (e.g., sick sinus syndrome)
Doxepin	Adapin; Sinequan	Antidepressant	1c, 3c, 5	
Droperidol	Inapsine	High-potency neuroleptic	1b	More OH and sedation than with haloperidol; black-box warning for potential QTc prolongation
Duoxetine	Cymbalta	Antidepressant		Currently an investigational agent; not yet systematically tested in patients with cardiovascular disease
Fluoxetine	Prozac	Antidepressant (SSRI)		Reports of bradycardia and syncope; may increase levels of ecainide, flecainide, metoprolol, propafenone, propranolol, thioridazine, timolol, and TCAs; also effective for OCD
Fluphenazine	Prolixin	High-potency neuroleptic		
Fluvoxamine	Luvox	Antidepressant (SSRI)		May increase levels of clozapine, warfarin
Haloperidol	Haldol	High-potency neuroleptic		Prolonged QTc and torsades des pointes arrhythmia reported with high-dose IV use
Imipramine	Tofanil	Antidepressant (TCA)	1c, 3b, 5	Has been shown to have antiarrhythmic effect
Lamotrigine	Lamictal	Mood stabilizer		
Lithium	Eskalith; Lithobid	Mood stabilizer	4a	Trivial effects on repolarization; reports of sinus arrest in elderly; rare reports of myocarditis
Loxapine	Loxitane	Mid-potency neuroleptic	1b, 3b	
Methylphenidate	Ritalin	Psychostimulant	2b, 3b	Hypertension and tachycardia are dose-related

(continued)

Table 67-2. Psychotropic Agents and Their Effects on the Heart and Cardiovascular System (Continued)

Generic Name	Trade Name	Treatment Class	Effects on Heart and Cardio-vascular System[a]	Comments
Mirtazapine	Remeron	Hypnotic and antidepressant agent		Not yet systematically tested on patients with cardiovascular disease
Molindone	Moban	Mid-potency neuroleptic	1a, 3b	May increase levels of propanolol May be associated with less weight gain than other neuroleptics
Naltrexone	ReVia	Anti-alcohol agent		
Nefazodone	Serzone	Antidepressant		May increase blood levels of following agents: calcium channel-blockers, carbamazepine, lidocaine, quinidine, and TCAs Absolutely contraindicated with astemizole, cisapride, and terfenadine
Nortriptyline	Pamelor	Antidepressant (TCA)	1a, 3a, 5	Less likely to cause OH than other TCAs
Olanzapine	Zyprexa	Atypical neuroleptic	1a, 3b	
Paroxetine	Paxil	Antidepressant (SSRI)	3b	See fluoxetine, has mild anticholinergic effects
Pemoline	Cylert	Psychostimulant		Fewer CV effects than methylphenidate or dextroamphetamine
Perphenazine	Trilafon	Mid-potency neuroleptic	1a, 3a, 5	
Phenelzine	Nardil	Antidepressant (MAOI)	1c	Hypertensive crisis possible
Pimozide	Orap	High-potency neuroleptic		Calcium channel-blocking properties
Protriptyline	Vivactil	Antidepressant (TCA)	1b, 3c, 5	
Quetiapine	Seroquel	Atypical neuroleptic	1b	Effective in sleep apnea
Risperidone	Risperdal	Atypical neuroleptic	1b	

Drug	Brand	Class	Codes	Comments
S-adenosyl methionine (SAM-e)		Antidepressant		Natural substance used for the treatment of depression; has not been FDA-evaluated or approved
Escitalopram	Lexapro	Antidepressant (SSRI)		Like citalopram, has fewest drug-drug interactions of the SSRIs
St. John's wort		Antidepressant		Natural substance used for the treatment of depression; not FDA-evaluated or approved. Combination with SSRIs or MAOIs should be avoided
Sertraline	Zoloft	Antidepressant (SSRI)		Has less inhibition of cytochrome P450 isoenzymes than fluoxetine. Has the most data of any antidepressant for safe and effective use post-MI
Thioridazine	Mellaril	Low-potency neuroleptic	1c, 3c, 5	Associated with prolonged QT interval and torsade des pointes arrhythmia
Thiothixene	Navane	High-potency neuroleptic		
Topiramate	Topamax	Mood stabilizer		Co-administration with diuretic acetatolomide may increase risk of renal stone formation
Tranylcypromine	Parnate	Antidepressant (MAOI)	1b, 2	Hypertensive crisis possible
Trazodone	Desyrel	Antidepressant	1b	Also good as a hypnotic
Venlafaxine	Effexor	Antidepressant	2b	Untreated hypertension is a relative contraindication
Ziprasidone	Geodon	Atypical neuroleptic	1a	Associated with greater QT interval prolongation than other neuroleptics

[a]1, hypotensive effect; 2, hypertensive effect; 3, tachycardia; 4, bradycardia; 5, quinidine-like slowing of conduction through bundle of His; a, weak, b, intermediate; c, strong.

Because of their favorable side-effects profile, they are considered by most experts to be the drugs of choice for the treatment of uncomplicated major depression, especially in patients with underlying CV disease and other medical illnesses.

3. **Mechanism of action. The SSRIs inhibit the reuptake of serotonin** after it has been released by the presynaptic nerve terminal into the synaptic cleft. These agents affect other central neurotransmitter systems, but their principal activity is on the serotoninergic system. Citalopram and escitalopram are the most highly selective SSRIs.

4. **CV effects. SSRIs are remarkably free of significant CV effects.** SSRIs do not cause orthostatic hypotension (OH), tachycardia, or widening of cardiac intervals. **There have been isolated case reports of bradycardia associated with syncope** in patients treated with SSRIs. Such rhythm disturbances have largely occurred in elderly patients or those taking significant overdoses of SSRIs. However, systematic studies of SSRI administration in the elderly have found these agents to be well tolerated, with low rates of CV events. Furthermore, reviews of SSRI overdoses have found low rates of bradycardia and other CV effects. Based on this data, it appears that SSRIs have a relatively safe CV profile. However, elderly patients, especially those with sinus node disease, should be monitored carefully when treated with an SSRI.

   SSRIs appear to be safe in the period after myocardial infarction (MI). Three recent studies of SSRIs in post-MI patients have found these agents to be safe in this population. Specifically, these agents did not adversely affect left ventricular (LV) function, blood pressure (BP), heart rate, or QTc intervals. When compared to placebo, SSRIs were not associated with elevated rages of reinfarction or other CV events in these studies.

   SSRIs generally have few anticholinergic side effects. However, paroxetine has mild anticholinergic effects, which can include tachycardia. Therefore, in patients with significant cardiac disease, an SSRI other than paroxetine may be preferable to avoid these effects.

5. **Drug Interactions**
   a. SSRIs may affect levels of other agents through interactions at the cytochrome P450 hepatic isoenzyme system. The cytochrome P450 system is made up of numerous isoenzymes that help to metabolize medications. The **three most relevant isoenzymes are the 2D6, the 3A4, and the 1A2 isoenzymes.**
   b. **2D6 metabolism:** Fluoxetine is the greatest inhibitor of the cytochrome 2D6 isoenzyme, followed by paroxetine. Sertraline, and especially citalopram and escitalopram, cause minimal inhibition of the 2D6 isoenzyme.
   c. **2D6 inhibition by SSRIs can lead to elevated levels of** the following cardioactive agents: **ecanide, flecanide, metoprolol, profafenone, propranolol, thioridazine, timolol, and TCAs.** Therefore, an SSRI with little inhibition of the 2D6 isoenzyme system (e.g., citalopram) should be prescribed for patients concurrently taking these cardioactive medications.
   d. **3A4 metabolism:** Fluvoxamine is the greatest inhibitor of 3A4 metabolism; fluoxetine causes moderate inhibition. The other SSRIs have minimal actions at this isoenzyme.
   e. **3A4 inhibition by SSRIs can cause elevated levels of** the following cardioactive agents: **amiodarone, calcium channel-blockers, cyclosporine, lidocaine, quinidine, and some TCAs.**
   f. **1A2 metabolism:** Fluvoxamine is the only SSRI causing clinically significant inhibition of this isoenzyme.

g. **1A2 inhibition by SSRIs can lead to elevated levels of aminophylline, clozapine, theophylline, and warfarin.** Therefore, a different SSRI should be used in patients taking these agents.

h. **In addition, the combined use of SSRIs and monoamine oxidase inhibitors (MAOIs) is absolutely contraindicated because it can produce a serotonin syndrome** (manifest by agitation, hyperreflexia, hypertension, tachycardia, and delirium). Case reports suggest that the combined use of an SSRI and **the selective MAOI L-deprenyl (selegiline; El-depryl)** is safe as long as the dose of the MAOI remains below 10 mg daily.

B. **Second-choice antidepressants. Bupropion (Wellbutrin), mirtazapine (Remeron), and venlafaxine (Effexor)** (Table 67-1) have few clinically significant effects on the heart or CV system but are designated as second-choice antidepressants because they are newer than the SSRIs or are less widely used.

1. **Bupropion (Wellbutrin).** Bupropion, an antidepressant agent that has effects on nor-epinephrine and dopamine, has no serious CV toxicity. More recently, bupropion has also been found to be effective for smoking cessation. Bupropion has no significant drug-drug interactions, and is not associated with anticholinergic effects, orthostatic hypotension (OH), or cardiac conduction abnormalities. It is associated with a slightly increased risk of seizures, and therefore its use in patients with known seizure disorder, head trauma, or bulimia should be avoided. To further reduce this risk of seizure, single doses greater than 150 mg or total daily doses greater than 450 mg should be avoided.

2. **Mirtazapine (Remeron).** Mirtazapine, a newer antidepressant, also appears to have little CV toxicity. This agent has effects on serotonin and norepinephrine through $5\text{-}HT_2$, $5\text{-}HT_3$ and alpha$_1$ receptor blockade. It has negligible anticholinergic effects, and only rarely reported OH as a result of its alpha$_1$-blocking properties. Recent meta-analysis found that mirtazapine was associated with significantly fewer anticholinergic and cardiac adverse effects than the TCA amitriptyline.

3. **Venlafaxine (Effexor).** Chemically unrelated to other antidepressants, venlafaxine potentiates central neurotransmitters through its potent inhibition of both serotonin and norepiniphrine reuptake. It produces a dose-related sustained elevation of supine diastolic BP in up to 7% of individuals treated within the recommended therapeutic dose range (200 to 300 mg). BP should be measured before and during treatment in all patients who receive venlafaxine, especially those with hypertension. Venlafaxine has not been tested in patients with coronary artery and other CV diseases.

C. **Tricyclic Antidepressants**

1. **Classification.** Available for the treatment of depression since the 1960s, the TCAs are often subdivided into the tertiary and secondary forms on the basis of the number of methyl groups on the terminal amino side chain; the tertiary amine TCAs have two methyl groups, and the secondary amines have one methyl group (Table 67-3). **The tertiary amine TCAs (e.g., amitriptyline [Elavil], doxepin [Sinequan], imipramine [Tofranil], trimipramine [Surmontil])** typically cause more sedation and anticholinergic side effects (e.g., dry mouth, constipation, blurred vision, tachycardia, and confusion) than do the **secondary amine TCAs (e.g., desipramine [Nor-pramin], nortriptyline [Pamelor],** and **protriptyline [Vivactil]).** The exception to this generalization is **protriptyline,** which is second only to **amitriptyline** in anticholinergic potency (Table 67-4).

Table 67-3. Tricyclic Antidepressants

Tertiary amines
    Amitriptyline
    Doxepin
    Imipramine
    Trimipramine
Secondary amines
    Desipramine
    Nortriptyline
    Protriptyline

Table 67-4. Relative Affinities for Muscarinic Anticholinergic Receptors

Drug	*Affinity*[a]
Atropine (reference)	42.0
Amitriptyline	5.6
Protriptyline	4.0
Clomipramine	2.7
Trimipramine	1.7
Doxepin	1.2
Imipramine	1.1
Paroxetine	0.93
Nortriptyline	0.67
Desipramine	0.50
Maprotiline	0.18
Sertraline	0.16
Amoxapine	0.10
Fluoxetine	0.05
Nefazodone	0.0091
Fluvoxamine	0.0042
Bupropion	0.0021
Trazodone	0.00031
Venlafaxine	0.0

[a]Affinity = $10^7 \times 1/K_d$ (K_d is the equilibrium-dissociation constant in molarity).
SOURCE: From Richelson (1996).

2. **CV effects.** All TCAs affect the heart and CV system. At therapeutic doses, TCAs produce a statistically significant increase in heart rate, a drop in postural BP, and a slowing of cardiac conduction. The extent to which these changes assume clinical significance is based largely upon the presence of pre-existent CV disease, not solely on the intrinsic properties of the drugs.

    a. **Nortriptyline** has a reputation as being the least "cardiotoxic" TCA on the basis of a demonstrated, although incompletely understood tendency to cause less OH than other TCAs; nortriptyline also is less anticholinergic than all TCAs other than desipramine (Table 67-4).

3. **Risk factors.** The following factors increase the risk of clinically significant CV disturbance during TCA treatment:

    a. **Tachycardia** (heart rate > 90 beats per minute)

    b. **Postural BP drop** > 10 mmHg

    c. **Prolonged cardiac conduction,** as evidenced by any of the following:

        i. **PR interval ≥ 200 milliseconds**

        ii. **QRS > 100 milliseconds** (i.e., an intraventricular conduction delay or a bundle branch block, including a right bundle)

        iii. **QTc > 440 milliseconds**

    d. **Ejection fraction (EF) < 60%.** In patients with congestive heart failure (CHF), all TCAs increase the risk of OH without further compromising the EF.

    e. **The 4- to 6-week interval after a MI.** In the absence of conduction abnormalities and reduced LV performance, a history of MI is not by itself a contraindication to the use of TCAs.

4. **Recommendations for Clinical Use**

    a. **Treatment selection.** TCAs are a treatment alternative for depressed patients who do not respond to first- or second-line antidepressants (i.e., SSRIs, bupropion, venlafaxine, and mirtazapine). When a TCA must be selected, nortriptyline is the TCA of choice.

    b. **Work-up.** Screen for the risk factors listed in section II.C.3 above. Check baseline heart rate, postural BP measurements, and an electrocardiogram (ECG) on all patients before starting a TCA.

    c. **Treatment guidelines.** TCAs are relatively contraindicated if risk factors are present. Treatment may be conducted safely, however, with appropriate monitoring. The following measures are recommended if risk factors are present and a TCA is to be prescribed.

        i. Use nortriptyline.

        ii. Start at 10 mg daily and increase the dose gradually. For example, add 10 mg h.s. every 5 to 7 days up to the therapeutic dose (usually 50 to 100 mg daily).

        iii. Monitor heart rate, postural BP, and conduction intervals before each dose increase.

        iv. Monitor serum nortriptyline blood levels (therapeutic range, 70 to 150 ng/mL).

        v. Discontinue the TCA if conduction times (PR, QRS, or QT intervals) increase by more than 25% of their baseline values.

D. Monoamine Oxidase Inhibitors

1. **Classification.** The MAOIs currently available in the United States for the treatment of depression are **phenelzine (Nardil) and tranylcypromine (Parnate)** (Table 67-1).

2. **Indications.** Approved for the treatment of depression. MAOIs are also very effective for the treatment of panic and phobic disorders. If one MAOI is ineffective, it is worth trying another.

3. **Mechanism of action.** MAOIs augment the concentration of central catecholamines available to post-synaptic receptors by inhibiting MAO activity and thus slowing catecholamine metabolism.

4. **CV Effects**

   a. **Cardiac conduction.** No direct effect on cardiac conduction and no chronotropic effects have been found. MAOIs may inhibit the heart rate response to postural challenge.

   b. **Blood Pressure**

      i. **Orthostatic hypotension.** Significant postural, as well as supine hypotension, can occur during treament with MAOIs.

      ii. **Hypertension and hypertensive crisis.** Significant hypertension can occur in response to the concurrent use of MAOIs and tyramine-containing foods or certain drugs (Table 67-5). The concomitant use of an MAOI and the agents listed in Table 67-5 is contraindicated. Hypertensive episodes associated with tranylcypromine have been reported. It has been postulated that tranylcypromine autoinduces hypertension because of its amphetamine-like structure.

5. **Overdose. A serotonin-like syndrome** has been reported to occur up to 12 to 24 hours after an MAOI overdose.

E. **Other antidepressants**

   1. **Trazodone (Desyrel).** Trazodone acts through serotonin reuptake inhibition and $5-HT_2$ receptor blockade. At doses used for an antidepressant effect (300–600 mg), most patients find this agent too sedating; trazodone is more commonly used as a non-habit-forming sedative at 50 to 100 mg h.s. than as an antidepressant. Trazodone has neither anticholinergic properties nor adverse effects on cardiac conduction. There have been reports of an association, however, between trazodone use and the aggravation of pre-existent premature ventricular contractions (PVCs). Trazodone also can cause OH by virtue of its comparatively high affinity for post-synaptic $alpha_1$ receptors.

   2. **Nefazodone (Serzone).** Nefazodone is structurally related to trazadone and chemically unrelated to other antidepressants. Nefazodone blocks serotonin type 2 ($5-HT_2$) receptors post-synaptically and inhibits the neuronal reuptake of serotonin and norepinephrine pre-synaptically. No serious adverse CV effects at therapeutic or toxic doses have been reported following its use. However, its clinical use has waned due to potential hepatotoxicity, an effect that prompted the FDA to issue a black box warning. Nefazodone may inhibit the metabolism and increase the blood levels of the following agents that can affect the heart and CV system: calcium channel-blockers, carbamazepine, lidocaine, quinidine, and TCAs. The concurrent use of nefazodone and the following drugs is absolutely contraindicated because of possible precipitation of *torsades des pointes* (TDP) arrhythmia: **astemizole, cisapride, and terfenadine.**

F. **Agents under Investigation**

   1. **Duloxetine.** Duloxetine, like venlafaxine, is a dual serotonin and norepinephrine-reuptake inhibitor. Pharmacologic studies of duloxetine suggest that it is a more potent reuptake inhibitor of both serotonin and norepinephrine than venlafaxine. Preliminary studies have also found that treatment with duloxetine may have beneficial effects on pain and on urinary incontinence. These preliminary studies have found that duloxetine is not associated with adverse CV side effects; however, duloxetine has not yet been tested in patients with significant CV disease.

> **Table 67-5. Drugs and Foods Contraindicated during Therapeutic Use of Monoamine Oxidase Inhibitor Drugs**
>
> **Foods**
>
> Absolutely restricted
>> Aged cheeses
>> Aged and cured meats
>> Improperly stored or spoiled meats, fish, or poultry
>> Banana peel; broad bean pods
>> Marmite
>> Sauerkraut
>> Soy sauce and other soy condiments
>> Draft beer
>
> Consume in moderation
>> Red or white wine (no more than two 4-ounce glasses per day)
>> Bottled or canned beer, including non-alcoholic
>>> (no more than two 12-ounce servings per day)
>
> **Medications**
>
> Alpha antagonists
>
> Alpha-methyldopa
>
> Beta-blockers
>
> Dextromethorphan
>
> Direct-acting sympathomimetics
>> Epinephrine
>> Norepinephrine
>> Phenylephrine
>> Isoproterenol
>> Methoxamine
>> Guanethidine
>> Macrodantin
>> Meperidine
>> Reserpine
>> SSRI (fluoxetine, fluvoxamine, paroxetine, sertraline)
>> Sulfisoxazole
>
> SOURCE: Adapted from Gardner et al. (1996) and Lipson & Stern (1991).

2. **Natural remedies used for depression. St. John's wort** (*Hypericum perforatum*) is a natural substance that has been used in the treatment of depression. St. John's wort's antidepressant mechanism appears to include weak serotonin reuptake inhibition. Recent meta-analyses and double-blind studies have suggested that St. John's wort may have limited efficacy in depression, especially moderate to severe depression. St. John's wort is generally well tolerated, but does have some significant drug-drug interactions. **St. Johns's wort may lower blood concentrations of the**

following agents: **warfarin, digoxin, protease inhibitors (especially indinavir), theophylline, and the TCA, amitriptyline.** It has also been **associated with serotonin syndrome** in patients concurrently taking serotonergic agents (e.g., SSRIs).

3. **S-adenosyl methionine (SAM-e)** is an amino acid that has also been used in the treatment of depression. Its mechanism of action is unclear; SAM-e appears to be involved in methylation reactions in the body and may affect levels of melatonin, serotonin, and dopamine. Limited studies have found SAM-e to have similar efficacy as TCAs in the treatment of depression. There have been reports of **serotonin syndrome** with this agent in combination with TCAs. No other drug-drug interactions have been discovered.

G. **Electroconvulsive therapy (ECT).** When practiced appropriately, ECT is a safe and effective treatment for patients who are refractory to antidepressant medication or who require emergent life-saving antidepressant treatment. This form of treatment is not without risks, especially in individuals with pre-existent CV or cerebrovascular disease. A variety of CV disturbances have been reported to occur as a result of ECT. **Exaggerated hypertensive responses, circulatory collapse, acute MI, and a variety of arrhythmias have been reported.** However, CV disease is not an absolute contraindication to ECT, as long as careful attention is paid to the pre-treatment evaluation and post-treatment management of potential CV complications.

III. Antipsychotics

Antipsychotic agents are classified into the typical neuroleptic agents (high-potency and low-potency) and the atypical agents. The typical neuroleptics are characterized by their principal neurotransmitter effect: blockade of post-synaptic central dopamine D_2 receptors. The atypical neuroleptics effect a variety of neurotransmitter systems and have comparatively little effect on D_2 receptor subtypes. Atypical agents have become the treatments of choice for most psychotic disorders because of their favorable side effect profiles. The **cardiac side effects most often associated with antipsychotics are OH, anticholinergic side effects (including tachycardia), and QTc-interval prolongation** (increasing the risk of TDP and other arrhythmias).

A. **Atypical neuroleptics.** There are currently six atypical antipsychotics approved for use in the United States: **aripiprazole (Abilify), clozapine (Clozaril), olanzapine (Zyprexa), risperidone (Risperdal), ziprasidone (Geodon), and quetiapine (Seroquel).** Atypical antipsychotics differ from typical neuroleptics by their greater blockade of serotonin at $5-HT_2$ receptors and by less efficacy in blocking dopamine at D_2 receptors. Clinically, atypicals appear to be as effective as typical antipsychotics in the treatment of psychotic symptoms and delirium. In addition, they maybe more effective than typical agents in alleviating the negative symptoms (e.g., flattened affect, apathy, and withdrawal) of schizophrenia, and they are less likely to produce the movement disorders caused by traditional neuroleptics (e.g., acute dystonia and tardive dyskinesia). Despite some similarities, each of the atypical antipsychotics have distinctive receptor-binding capacities, side effect profiles, and potential for CV toxicity (Table 67-6).

1. **Aripiprazole (Abilify).** The newest antipsychotic, approved in late 2002, aripiprazole not only blocks $5-HT_2$ receptors, but it also functions as a $5-HT_{1a}$ partial agonist, a property it shares with ziprasidone. Aripiprazole has been safe, effective and well

Table 67-6. Cardiac Effects of Atypical Antipsychotics.[a]			
Medication	Anticholinergic Effects	Orthostasis	QTc Prolongation
Clozapine[b]	+++	+++	–
Olanzapine	+	+	–
Quetiapine	–	++	+
Risperidone	–	++	+
Ziprasidone	–	+/–	++

+++ = severe   ++ = moderate   + = mild   – = little to none

[a]Aripiprazole not included because of limited clinical experience with this agent at the time of this writing.
[b]Clozapine also has multiple other potential cardiovascular effects, including myocarditis, tachycardia, and pericardial effusion.

tolerated in clinical trials, but thus far there has been no study of its safety specifically in patients with cardiac disease. Preliminary studies thus far have found that aripiprazole does not cause significant OH, anticholinergic effects, or QTc prolongation. It does not appear to have significant effects on drug levels of other agents. However, given that aripiprazole is metabolized by the cytochrome 2D6 and 3A4 isoenzymes, the cardioactive agent **quinidine may elevate blood levels of aripiprazole.** Both further study of this agent and clinical experience will serve to reveal more about its cardiac safety profile.

2. **Clozapine (Clozaril).** In addition to acting principally at $5-HT_2$ rather than D_2 receptors, clozapine has a comparatively high affinity for central histaminic and muscarinic cholinergic receptors. A major drawback of clozapine treatment is the occurrence of **agranulocytosis in 1–2% of these patients.** This necessitates weekly monitoring of blood counts for the duration of therapy. **An increased risk of seizure** is another significant adverse effect. A variety of adverse CV events have been associated with clozapine.

a. **Tachycardia.** Up to 25% of clozapine-treated patients exhibit sustained tachycardia, with an average increase of 10 to 15 beats per minute.

b. **ECG changes.** Some patients develop reversible ECG repolarization changes, including flattening or inversion of T waves and ST segment depression. The clinical significance of these changes is unknown.

c. **Orthostatic hypotension.** Clinically significant OH has been reported to occur unexpectedly at a single daily dose of 25 mg. The elderly, those with Parkinson's disease, and patients with compromised autonomic function caused by medications or disease are at greater risk of developing OH. It is therefore recommended that all patients start at 12.5 mg daily and undergo a slow and gradual dosage titration. Some patients with Parkinson's disease may not be able to tolerate more than 6.25 mg daily.

d. **Myocarditis.** Clozapine has been associated with an elevated risk of the development of myocarditis, prompting addition of a black-box warning about this association to its package literature. The risk of myocarditis is relatively small (approximately one case per 10,000 patients) but it represents a significantly greater risk than would be expected in the general population. Myocarditis most commonly occurs in the first month of therapy, but approximately one-third of patients develop myocarditis after the first month.

e. **Pericarditis/Pericardial Effusion.** Clozapine, uncommonly, has also been associated with these CV effects; causality has yet to be determined.

f. **Drug Interactions.** Clozapine does not have specific drug-drug interactions with cardioactive agents, but clozapine may potentiate the hypotensive effects of antihypertensive agents. Concurrent administration of clozapine with other agents that may cause bone marrow suppression should be avoided.

3. **Olanzapine (Zyprexa).** Olanzapine has a similar chemical structure to clozapine; it primarily causes 5-HT$_2$ receptor blockade. Unlike clozapine, olanzapine is not associated with agranulocytosis or seizures. However, it has been associated with significant weight gain in some patients (associated with its H$_1$ receptor blockade) and the development of new-onset diabetes. Olanzapine is associated with **mild to moderate anticholinergic effects,** but it is not associated with OH. Furthermore, olanzapine was found to cause minimal QTc prolongation when administered to healthy volunteers (see Table 67-3). In this study, olanzapine caused the least QTc prolongation of the four atypical antipsychotics studied. However, it is difficult to extrapolate this data to those with cardiac disease or conduction abnormalities. Olanzapine does not appear to have significant drug-drug interactions with cardioactive agents.

4. **Risperidone (Risperdal).** Risperidone blocks 5-HT$_2$ receptors more than it does D$_2$ receptors. It is associated with a lower incidence of extrapyramidal symptoms (EPS) than typical antipsychotics, especially at low dose, but it generates more EPS than other atypicals. Because of blocking activity at alpha$_1$ receptors, **risperidone is commonly associated with OH.** However, it does not have significant anticholinergic effects. Its use has also been associated with QT prolongation, but only in selected cases and only at doses well above the recommended therapeutic range of 4 to 6 mg daily. Risperidone does not have significant drug-drug interactions with cardioactive agents; as with clozapine, hypotensive effects of antihypertensives may be potentiated with concurrent use of risperidone.

5. **Quetiapine (Seroquel).** Quetiapine has a novel receptor-binding profile, that includes mild antagonism of both 5-HT$_2$ and D$_2$ receptors. In addition, quetiapine blocks H$_1$ and alpha$_1$ receptors. **Quetiapine is associated with mild-moderate OH** as a result of its alpha$_1$ blockade. It is not associated with anticholinergic effects, and does not have other associated CV toxicity. Quetiapine does not have significant drug-drug interactions with cardioactive agents.

6. **Ziprasidone (Geodon).** A relatively new atypical antipsychotic (introduced in 2001), ziprasidone has a receptor-binding profile similar to that of aripiprazole. Ziprasidone blocks 5-HT$_2$ receptors, and also serves as a 5-HT$_{1a}$ partial agonist. Ziprasidone has minimal anticholinergic effects, and is not associated with OH. However, ziprasidone appears to have greater propensity to prolong the QTc interval than other atypical antipsychotics (see Table 67-7) and should generally be avoided in patients with prolonged QTc intervals, conduction disease, history of ventricular arrhythmia, hypokalemia, hypomagnesemia, or other risk factors for TDP. At this writing, there have been no reports of TDP with ziprasidone.

B. **Typical Neuroleptic Agents**

1. **Classification.** The typical antipsychotic agents are organized in Table 67-8 according to dosage equivalence (i.e., potency). Neuroleptic potency (Table 67-8) is a function of binding affinity for D$_2$ receptors in the central nervous system (CNS). Clinically, the low-potency neuroleptics produce less EPS and more anticholinergic, CV, and

Table 67-7. QTc Prolongation with Antipsychotics		
Drug	Mean QTc Increase (msec)	% with > 60 msec Increase
Thioridazine (Mellaril)	35.8	30
Ziprasidone (Geodon)	20.6	21
Quetiapine (Seroquel)	14.5	11
Risperidone (Risperdal)	10.0	4
Olanzapine (Zyprexa)	6.4	4
Haloperidol (Haldol)	4.7	4

sedating effects than do the high-potency neuroleptics. Because of a comparatively low index of cardiac toxicity, high-potency neuroleptics have been used widely to treat a variety of psychotic disorders, as well as delirium and agitation in medical and surgical settings. Other neuroleptic and neuroleptic-like agents not used as antipsychotics, but capable of producing neuroleptic side effects, are listed in Table 67-9.

2. **Indications.** The indications for these agents include acute psychosis, schizophrenia, mania, and delirium.

3. **Mechanism of action.** Traditionally, antipsychotic agents have been presumed to exert their clinical effects via dopamine blockade at CNS D_2 receptors. The efficacy of the atypical antipsychotic agents (whose principal neurotransmitter effects occur at serotonin but not dopamine receptors) suggests alternative mechanisms of action.

Table 67-8. Typical Antipsychotic Agents			
Potency	Generic Name	Trade Name	Dosage Equivalence, mg
Low	Chlorpromazine	Thorazine	100
	Thioridazine	Mellaril	100
	Chlorprothixene	Taractan	75
	Mesoridazine	Serentil	50
Intermediate	Loxapine	Loxitane	10
	Molindone	Moban	10
	Perphenazine	Trilafon	8
High	Trifluoperazine	Stelazine	5
	Thiothixene	Navane	5
	Fluphenazine	Prolixin	2
	Haloperidol	Haldol	2
	Pimozide	Orap	1

SOURCE: Adapted from Hyman, S.E., & Tesar, G.E. (1994). *Manual of psychiatric emergencies* (3rd ed.). Boston: Little, Brown.

Table 67-9. Agents with Neuroleptic Properties Not Typically Used for Antipsychotic Purposes

Droperidol (Inapsine)

Metoclopramide (Reglan)

Prochlorperazine (Compazine)

Promethazine (Phenergan)

Trimethobenzamide (Tigan)

---

4. **CV Effects**
   a. **Cardiac conduction.** All typical neuroleptic agents can affect cardiac conduction through their anticholinergic or quinidine-like properties. **Low-potency neuroleptics are highly anticholinergic** and cause slowing of electrical conduction across the bundle of His to roughly the same degree as do TCAs. High-potency neuroleptic agents have comparatively little anticholinergic effect and rarely produce conduction defects except at very high doses. Therefore, **high-potency neuroleptics are preferred for patients with cardiac conduction disturbances.**
   b. **Blood pressure.** Low-potency neuroleptics can cause clinically significant OH, particularly in patients who are dehydrated or who are taking other BP-lowering agents. High-potency neuroleptics are much less likely to lower blood pressure, although the presence of other risk factors (e.g., dehydration) increases the risk of OH.
   c. **Drug interactions. The combined use of a low-potency neuroleptic** (e.g., chlorpromazine, thioridazine) **and a tertiary amine TCA** (e.g., amitriptyline, imipramine) **should be avoided because of the high potential for additive anticholinergic and quinidine-like toxicities. Similarly, the concurrent use of a low-potency neuroleptic and a type Ia antiarrhythmic agent** (e.g., quinidine, disopyramide, procainamide) **should be avoided.** If combined use is necessary, consideration should be given to the reduction of the type Ia antiarrhythmic dose so that the neuroleptic dose can be pushed to a therapeutic level.
   d. **Intravenous (IV) Administration.** Some typical antipsychotics can be administered intravenously; this is most frequently done for the symptomatic treatment of delirium. Haloperidol is the most frequently used antipsychotic for this indication; because it is a high-potency neuroleptic, the risk of OH, anticholinergic effects, or quinidine-life effects is low. However, **IV haloperidol, especially in high doses, has been associated with the development of TDP.** Given this risk, patients who receive IV haloperidol should have their potassium maintained at a level of 4 mmol/L or greater and their magnesium at 2 mmol/L or greater to reduce the risk of TDP. Furthermore, ECGs should be obtained at baseline and during treatment; prolongation of the QTc by 25%, or intervals greater than 500 milliseconds may prompt use of alternative agents (e.g., sublingual olanzapine).

IV. Mood Stabilizers

Mood stabilizers are agents that are used to control mania and the cyclic mood changes of manic-depressive (bipolar) disorder. The best known and longest used of these agents is **lithium (Eskalith, Lithobid).** More recently, anticonvulsants, such as **carbamazepine (Tegretol)** and **divalproex sodium (Depakote),** have been found to be useful, particularly in the approximately 40% of individuals who do not respond favorably to lithium. **Lamotrigine (Lamictal),** a glutamate antagonist anti-convulsant, and **topiramate (Topamax),** an anticonvulsant with effects on both GABA and glutamate, may also have mood-stabilizing properties.

A. Lithium

1. **CV effects.** Lithium has trivial effects on the normal heart and CV system. In 20% of treated patients, lithium produces benign, reversible flattening or inversion of T-waves, possibly as a result of displacement of intracellular potassium. Perhaps the most common clinically significant adverse effect is **sinus node dysfunction,** a potential manifestation of lithium toxicity. Reports of bradycardia and sinus arrest in elderly patients who previously were well controlled with stable doses and blood levels of lithium suggest progression of underlying sinus node disease aggravated by lithium. There are also a few reports of lithium-associated **myocarditis.**

2. **Toxicity.** Lithium toxicity may be problematic for lithium-treated patients who have hypertension, CHF, and/or renal failure. Several factors can contribute to the elevation of serum lithium levels: reduced glomerular filtration; sodium restriction; and the use of thiazide diuretics, ACE inhibitors, and NSAIDs. In the event of lithium toxicity, lithium should be withheld until the symptoms of toxicity (e.g., nausea, tremor, diarrhea, confusion) remit and should be resumed at a level 25% lower than the previous dose. Depending on the serum level and the clinical condition (i.e., neurotoxicity), dialysis may be required.

B. Carbamazepine and Oxcarbazepine (Trileptal). Carbamazepine's TCA-like structure is believed to account for some of its potentially adverse effects on the heart and CV system. Like TCAs it has quinidine-like properties that can produce **conduction abnormalities** at toxic doses and even at therapeutic doses in individuals with pre-existent conduction abnormalities. Carbamazepine use should be monitored carefully in patients with pre-existent conduction disease and during concurrent use with **drugs that can raise carbamazepine serum levels (e.g., calcium channel-blockers, cimetidine, erythromycin, isoniazid, propoxyphene,** and **SSRIs). Carbamazepine may also lower plasma levels of a number of drugs,** such as phenytoin, valproic acid, and cyclosporine. **Oxcarbazepine** is a newer anticonvulsant that is a metabolite of carbamazepine. Oxcarbazepine does not appear to be associated with conduction abnormalities or other CV toxicity. It also has fewer drug-drug interactions than carbamazepine; **however, oxcarbazepine can lower blood levels of dihydropyridine calcium channel-blockers.**

C. Divalproex sodium (Depakote). In a recent controlled, multi-center trial, divalproex sodium compared favorably with lithium for patients with acute mania. It is currently the alternative of choice for bipolar patients who are resistant to, or cannot tolerate, lithium therapy. Its therapeutic activity is believed to be related to increased brain levels of gamma-aminobutyric acid (GABA). In therapeutic doses it has no adverse effects on the heart and CV system, although with overdose it has been associated with heart block.

D. Lamotrigine (Lamictal). Lamotrigine is a central glutamate antagonist with no reported adverse effects on the heart or CV system. It may have particular efficacy in patients with bipolar depression. Levels of lamotrigine are increased when valproic acid is co-administered and decreased with concurrent administration of phenytoin or carbamazepine.

E. Topiramate (Topamax). Topiramate is an anticonvulsant that appears to increase GABA levels, inhibit glutamate receptor binding, and block sodium channels. It also has no reported adverse effects on the CV system. It appears to be effective as an adjunctive mood-stabilizer. Topiramate should be used with caution in combination with the diuretic **acetazolamide,** as both increase the propensity for the formation of **kidney stones.** As with lamotrigine, levels of topiramate are increased by valproic acid and decreased by carbamazepine and phenytoin.

V. Anxiolytics and Sedative-Hypnotic Agents

A variety of agents, including the barbiturates and benzodiazepines, have been used to control anxiety and tension. Many of these agents can be used to initiate and to maintain sleep. **Antihistamines,** which frequently are used to induce sleep, generally are effective only during short-term use; with long-term use or **in high doses their anticholinergic properties can cause confusion and tachycardia.** The principal adverse CV effects of anxiolytics and sedative-hypnotics occur during their sudden or precipitate withdrawal; seizures and/or dangerous autonomic hyperactivity may develop.

A. **Barbiturates.** The barbiturates, which have been largely replaced by the benzodiazepines, have comparatively high abuse potential and a dangerously low toxic-to-therapeutic ratio. They have no direct CV toxicity but in overdose can cause CV collapse.

B. **Benzodiazepines.** The benzodiazepines (e.g., diazepam, lorazepam) have no adverse effects on the heart or CV system. In fact, they are used therapeutically to dampen noradrenergic activity in patients with tachyarrhythmias or acute MI. In addition, benzodiazepines have been found to inhibit platelet-activating factor-induced aggregation of human platelets.

C. **Buspirone (Buspar).** Buspirone is a non-benzodiazepine anxiolytic that is indicated for the treatment of generalized anxiety. It is exceptionally safe and has no direct CV effects; however, it has been reported to cause **increased BP when used in combination with an MAOI, and hypertension and anxiety when used with clomipramine and other serotoninergic agents.**

VI. Psychostimulants and Related Compounds

A. **Classifications and indications. Dextroamphetamine (Dexedrine), methylphenidate (Ritalin), pemoline (Cylert), and mixed amphetamine and dextroamphetamine salts (Adderall)** are most commonly used for attention deficit disorder (ADD) in both children and adults, narcolepsy, and certain types of depression (e.g., treatment-resistant depression and depression secondary to prolonged illness in hospitalized medical and surgical patients).

B. **Pharmacology and mechanism of action.** Dextroamphetamine (DAMP) and methylphenidate (MPD) are rapidly absorbed from the gastrointestinal (GI) tract and undergo rapid hepatic metabolism. Their half-lives are short: $t_{1/2} = 12$ hours for DAMP and 4 hours for MPD. Similarly, the mixed salts found in **Adderall** have a $t_{1/2}$ of approximately 7 to 8 hours. These agents stimulate pre-synaptic release of dopamine and to a lesser extent norepinephrine. **Pemoline** is believed to have similar pharmacologic activity, although it has minimal sympathomimetic effects.

C. **CV effects. DAMP, MPD, and Adderall produce dose-related effects on heart rate and BP.** MPD and Adderall may produce **sustained tachycardia and mild elevation of mean BP,** whereas DAMP tends to cause **BP elevation** while simultaneously **slowing heart rate.** The risk of CV stimulation is low at the doses usually prescribed for the depressed medically ill, typically 20 mg per day or less of DAMP or MPD. Pre-existing tachycardia, ventricular arrhythmia, and poorly controlled hypertension are relative contraindications to the use of Adderall, DAMP, and MPD. If a psychostimulant is indicated in the presence of these contraindications, pemoline is a good alternative, since it causes little if any CV activation.

D. Modafanil (Provigil). Modafanil is a wakefulness-promoting agent that was recently approved for the treatment of narcolepsy. Its mechanism of action is poorly understood; it has little structural similarity to psychostimulants and does not affect dopamine, norepinephrine, or serotonin receptors. Modafanil does not appear to have the sympathomimetic properties of psychostimulants, but it has been associated with **rare CV adverse effects (chest pain and palpitations),** especially in those with mitral valve prolapse. Modafanil has not yet been evaluated in patients with hypertension, unstable angina, or recent MI; therefore, it should be used with great caution in such patients. **Modafanil may lower cyclosporine levels** (from cytochrome 3A4 induction) **and may raise propranolol levels** (from 3C19 inhibition).

VII. Agents Used to Treat Substance Abuse

A. Disulfiram (Antabuse). Used in the treatment of alcoholism, disulfiram blocks the metabolism of alcohol, resulting in a rapid accumulation of acetaldehyde. This accounts for the unpleasant experience a disulfiram-treated patient has when ingesting even a small amount of alcohol. The typical symptoms of an alcohol-disulfiram interaction include flushing, throbbing headache, vomiting, sweating, chest pain, palpitations, dyspnea, tachycardia, hypotension, syncope, weakness, vertigo, blurred vision, and confusion. **Given the potential for significant hypotension, tachycardia, and syncope when alcohol is ingested, disulfiram is contraindicated in an alcoholic who has significant CAD or cardiac arrhythmia.**

B. Naltrexone (ReVia). Naltrexone is an opioid antagonist used for alcohol and opioid dependence. When alcohol is used concurrently with naltrexone, there is no toxic reaction, but instead diminished release of endogenous opioids, results in reduced craving and euphoria. Naltrexone does not have significant CV toxicity or interactions with cardioactive agents.

C. Narcotic and benzodiazepine antagonists. Buprenorphine (Buprenex), naloxone hydrochloride (Narcan), and flumazenil (Romazicon) do not directly affect CV function. Abrupt reversal of narcotic or benzodiazepine toxicity, however, can precipitate drug withdrawal and its attendant autonomic hyperactivity. Therefore, these agents should be used cautiously in patients with pre-existing cardiac disease.

Suggested Readings

Alpert, J.E., Bernstein, J.G., & Rosenbaum, J.F. (1997). Psychopharmacologic issues in the medical setting. In N.H. Cassem, T.A. Stern, J.F. Rosembaum, & M.S. Jellinek (Eds.), *Massachusetts General Hospital handbook of general hospital psychiatry* (4th ed.). St. Louis, MO: Mosby.

Anton, J. (2001). Pharmacologic approaches to the management of alcoholism. *Journal of Clinical Psychiatry, 62*(suppl 20), 11–17.

Dec, G.W., & Stern, T.A. (1990). Tricyclic antidepressants in the intensive care unit. *Journal of Intensive Care Medicine, 5,* 69–81.

Ereshefsky, L., Riesenman, C., & Lam, Y.W.F. (1996). Serotonin selective reuptake inhibitor drug interactions and the cytochrome P450 system. *Journal of Clinical Psychiatry, 57*(suppl 8), 17–25.

Gardner, D.M., Shulman, K.I., Walker, S.E., et al. (1996). The making of a user-friendly MAOI diet. *Journal of Clinical Psychiatry, 57,* 99–104.

Glassman, A.H. (1998). Cardiovascular effects of antidepressant drugs: Updated. *Journal of Clinical Psychiatry, 59*(suppl 15), 13–18.

Goodnick, P.J., & Jerry, J.M. (2002). Aripiprazole: Profile on efficacy and safety. *Expert Opinions in Pharmacotherapy, 3,* 1773–1781.

Hyman, S.E., & Tesar, G.E. (1994). *Manual of psychiatric emergencies* (3rd ed.). Boston: Little, Brown.

Lipson, R.E., & Stern, T.A. (1991). Management of monoamine oxidase inhibitor-treated patients in the emergency and critical care setting. *Journal of Intensive Care Medicine, 6,* 117–125.

Meltzer, H.Y., Davidson, M., Glassman, A.H., et al. (2002). Assessing cardiovascular risks versus clinical benefits of atypical antipsychotic drug treatment. *Journal of Clinical Psychiatry, 63*(suppl 9), 25–29.

Mitchell, P.B., & Malhi, G.S. (2002). The expanding pharmacopoeia for bipolar disorder. *Annual Review of Medicine, 53,* 173–188.

CHAPTER 68

Drug-Drug Interactions: The Interface between Psychotropics and Other Agents

JONATHAN E. ALPERT

I. Introduction

Drug-drug interactions, which are characterized by alterations in drug plasma levels and/or drug effects, can occur whenever two or more prescribed, illicit, or over-the-counter agents are used concurrently. While many drug-drug interactions involve drugs administered within minutes to hours of each other, some drugs are implicated in interactions days to weeks after their discontinuation by virtue of their long half-lives or long-term impact on the activity of metabolic enzymes. Evaluation for potential drug-drug interactions therefore should include a thorough history of recent as well as current drug use.

II. Relevance to Clinical Decisions

A. **Drug-drug interactions involving psychotropic medications are ubiquitous.** Nevertheless, the treatment of patients with co-morbid psychiatric and medical disorders frequently requires multiple medications.

B. Fortunately, **most drug-drug interactions** involving psychotropic and other medications **do not contraindicate the combined use of those drugs.** Awareness of such interactions should, however, prompt close attention to dosing and monitoring.

C. **The anticipated clinical significance of drug-drug interactions must be judged in comparison to the influence of other factors that may alter drug responses,** including age, gender, nutritional status, disease states, smoking and alcohol use, and genetic polymorphism in the activity of drug metabolic enzymes. These factors often account for considerable inter-individual variability in the response to medications; in this context, the additional impact of drug-drug interactions may be small.

D. In the approach to a patient on multiple medications, **consideration of potential drug-drug interactions is crucial when the following situations occur:**

1. **Medications with a low therapeutic index are used,** that is, drugs for which the margin between a toxic dose and a therapeutic dose is small. These drugs include digoxin (Lanoxin), warfarin (Coumadin), theophylline (Slo-bid, Theodur), carbamazepine (Tegretol), and lithium (Eskalith, Lithobid, Lithonate).

2. **Medications with a narrow therapeutic window are used,** that is, drugs that are thought to be relatively ineffective at doses below and above a specified therapeutic range. These drugs include nortriptyline (Pamelor).

3. **Drugs associated with rare but catastrophic drug-drug interactions,** for example, hypertensive crises (monoamine oxidase inhibitors [MAOIs]) and torsades des pointes (pimozide [Orap]) , cisapride [Propulsid]), **are administered.**

4. **A perplexing clinical picture,** including mental status changes and unexplained clinical deterioration, **develops.**

5. **Unexpectedly extreme or variable drug plasma levels are detected.**

6. **Refractoriness of a condition** to standard pharmacologic management **occurs.**

7. **Elderly or medically unstable patients are placed at risk** for adverse effects, such as hypotension and urinary retention, which are especially hazardous.

8. **Clinical states** (e.g., congestive heart failure [CHF]) **are present in which hepatic or renal elimination of drugs may be markedly altered.**

9. **Concurrent or recent abuse of drugs, alcohol, or tobacco is a complicating factor.**

10. **A polydrug overdose is suspected.**

E. **Becoming well acquainted with the potentially catastrophic as well as the most common interactions is appropriate;** resources that may be consulted for the more esoteric interactions include:

1. Commercially available software packages

2. Websites (e.g., www.drug-interactions.com)

3. Publications (e.g., *Physician's Desk Reference; Medical Letter*)

F. **Drug-drug interactions are not intrinsically undesirable and some may be used to advantage:**

1. Management of overdose (e.g., naloxone reversal of opiate overdose)

2. Treatment of side effects (e.g., reduction of nausea on a serotonergic agent with a 5-HT$_3$ receptor antagonist)

3. Enhancement of drug levels/duration of action (e.g., ketoconazole or grapefruit juice taken with cyclosporine)

III. Classification

Drug-drug interactions may be described as idiosyncratic, pharmacodynamic, or pharmacokinetic on the basis of the presumed mechanism of interaction.

A. **Idiosyncratic interactions** are interactions which occur unpredictably in a small number of patients and **are unexpected** from the known pharmacokinetic and pharmacologic properties of the drugs involved.

1. Evidence for such interactions is often inconclusive and is based on a small number of case reports of complex patients on complicated medical regimens.

2. Examples include reported cases of neurotoxicity when **lithium** and **verapamil** (Calan, Isoptin) were co-administered.

B. **Pharmacodynamic interactions** are interactions which **involve a known pharmacologic effect.** These interactions are mediated by a direct effect on tissue receptor sites and may be additive, synergistic, or antagonistic.

1. Knowledge about pharmacodynamic interactions often is based on predictions from basic and pre-clinical studies and subsequent confirmation in clinical case reports.

2. Examples of pharmacodynamic drug-drug interactions include the following:

a. Depression of cardiac conduction when drugs with quinidine-like effects are co-administered (e.g., low-potency antipsychotics such as chlorpromazine [Thorazine] and class I antiarrhythmics, such as disopyramide [Norpace])

b. Respiratory depression when alcohol and benzodiazepines are used concurrently

c. Interference with the treatment of Parkinson's disease or hyperprolactinemia when dopamine agonists are co-administered with dopamine-blocking antipsychotic drugs

d. Anticholinergic toxicity when drugs that share antimuscarinic properties, including tricyclic antidepressants (TCAs), low-potency antipsychotics, and diphenhydramine (Benadryl), are combined

C. **Pharmacokinetic interactions** are interactions that **involve a change in the plasma level and/or tissue distribution of drugs** rather than in their pharmacologic activity. Pharmacokinetic interactions are mediated by effects on drug **absorption, distribution, metabolism, or excretion.**

1. **Absorption.** Drug-drug interactions that affect drug absorption may reduce or enhance the bioavailability of orally administered drugs. Examples include the effects of drugs that do the following:

    a. **Accelerate gastric emptying** (**metoclopramide** [Reglan], **cisapride** [Propulsid]) or diminish intestinal motility (**TCAs, morphine, cannabis**), potentially promoting greater contact with and absorption from the mucosal surface of the small intestine

    b. **Bind to other drugs** (cholestyramine [Questran], orlistat, charcoal, kaolin-pectin), forming complexes that pass unabsorbed through the intestinal lumen

    c. **Alter gastric pH** (aluminum hydroxide, magnesium hydroxide, sodium bicarbonate), potentially altering the non-polar, un-ionized fraction of drug available for absorption

    d. **Inhibit metabolic enzymes** present in the stomach or intestine (e.g., MAO), potentially retarding local degradation of other drugs or exogenous substances (e.g., pressor amines in aged, cured, spoiled or fermented foods) and thus enhancing their absorption

2. **Distribution.** Drug distribution from the systemic circulation to tissue is determined by a variety of factors that influence the concentration of free (unbound) drug in plasma, regional blood flow, the physiochemical properties of a drug (e.g., lipophilicity), and drug transport proteins that regulate entry into target tissues. Examples of drug-drug interactions that may influence distribution include the following:

    a. **Competition for protein-binding sites** by two or more drugs may result in displacement of a previously bound drug which in the unbound state becomes available for pharmacologic activity. Most psychotropic drugs are more than 80% protein-bound, and many are more than 90% protein-bound ("highly protein-bound") to albumin, alpha-1-acid glycoproteins, or lipoproteins. Exceptions include **lithium, gabapentin** (Neurotonin), **topiramate** (Topamax) and **venlafaxine** (Effexor), which **are minimally protein-bound**, and citalopram (Celexa), fluvoxamine (Luvox), bupropion (Wellbutrin, Zyban), lamotrigine (Lamictal), molindone (Moban), and carbamazepine, which are only moderately (60–85%) protein-bound. While potentially vital in the dosing and monitoring of drugs with a low therapeutic index, the practical significance of protein-binding interactions for clinical management is often small, since the transient rise in plasma concentrations resulting from the displacement of a previously bound drug is offset by the rapid redistribution of active drug to tissue, where it is metabolized and excreted.

    b. **Alterations in regional blood flow** produced by one drug may impede or enhance the delivery of other drugs to relevant receptors in tissue.

    c. **Competition for or other interference with active transport to tissue** (e.g., across the blood-brain barrier) may hinder the access of some agents to relevant receptor sites.

    d. **Effects on drug transport proteins** (e.g., P-glycoprotein) that appear to regulate permeability of intestinal epithelia, lymphocytes, and the blood-brain barrier. Agents such as St. John's wort may alter the pharmacokinetics of other agents via an effect on P-glycoprotein.

3. **Metabolism.** Most drugs undergo several types of biotransformation, usually enzyme-mediated, resulting in metabolites that may or may not be pharmacologically active. Many clinically important pharmacokinetic drug-drug interactions involving psychotropic drugs are based on interference with this process.

a. **Phase I metabolic reactions, including oxidation, reduction, and hydrolysis reactions, produce intermediate metabolites,** which then undergo **phase II metabolic reactions, including conjugation and acetylation,** that result in highly polar water-soluble metabolites suitable for renal excretion. Most psychotropic drugs undergo both phase I and phase II reactions. Exceptions include **lithium** and gabapentin, which are not subject to hepatic metabolism, and the **3-hydroxy substituted benzodiazepines (lorazepam** [Ativan], **oxazepam** [Serax], and **temazepam** [Restoril]), which undergo only phase II metabolism.

b. A growing understanding of drug metabolic enzymes, particularly the **cytochrome P450 isoenzymes,** has contributed to more rational prediction of drug-drug interactions (see **section IV** below).

c. Some drugs are closely associated with metabolic inhibition or the induction of other medications and therefore are frequently involved in drug-drug interactions. Common **inhibitors of hepatic metabolic enzymes include** the following:

    i. **Macrolide antibiotics** (e.g., erythromycin, clarithromycin [Biaxin], troleandomycin [Tao]) and fluoroquinolones (e.g., ciprofloxacin [Cipro])

    ii. **Antifungals** (e.g., ketaconazole [Nizoral], miconazole [Monistat, Fungoid], and itraconazole [Sporanox])

    iii. **Antimalarials**

    iv. **Antiretrovirals** (e.g., ritonavir)

    v. **Selective serotonin reuptake inhibitors (SSRIs)** (except venlafaxine [Effexor], citalopram [Celexa], and escitalopram [Lexapro])

    vi. **Lipophilic, hepatically metabolized beta-blockers** (propranolol [Inderal], metoprolol [Lopressor, Toprol], pindolol [Visken], timolol [Blocadren, Timolide, Timoptic], labetalol [Normodyne, Trandate]) but not those excreted unchanged by the kidney (atenolol [Tenormin], sotalol [Betapace], nadolol [Corgard])

    vii. **Calcium channel blockers** (diltiazem [Cardizem], verapamil [Calan, Isoptin])

    viiii. **Cimetidine** (Tagamet)

    ix. **Isoniazid** (Nydrazid)

    x. **Psychostimulants** (methylphenidate [Ritalin], dextroamphetamine [Dexedrine])

    xi. **Valproic acid** (Depakene) and divalproex sodium (Depakote)

    xii. **Disulfiram** (Antabuse)

    xiii. **Acute alcohol ingestion**

    xiv. **Grapefruit juice**

The introduction of these agents produces a typically abrupt elevation in the blood levels of the co-administered drugs whose metabolism they inhibit. Their discontinuation is associated with a rapid fall in those blood levels.

d. **Common inducers of hepatic metabolic enzymes** include the following:

    i. Chronic ethanol or tobacco

    ii. Barbiturates (phenobarbital, secobarbital)

    iii. Anticonvulsants (carbamazepine, phenytoin [Dilantin], primidone [Mysoline])

    iv. Rifampin

    v. St. John's wort

    vi. Cruciferous vegatables (e.g., brussels sprouts) and charbroiled meats

The introduction of these agents produces a characteristically slow decline over days to weeks in the blood levels of the co-administered drugs whose metabolism they induce. Their discontinuation is associated with a gradual increase in those levels.

4. **Excretion. Drug-drug interactions based on interference with renal excretion have little relevance in regard to most psychotropic drugs,** since the majority of

these agents present for excretion in the form of inactive metabolites with only a small fraction of the parent compound.

    a. **The principal exception is lithium,** in which drug-drug interactions involving renal excretion may alter lithium levels substantially (see section V.A. 1 below).

    b. Drug-drug interactions involving renal excretion are sometimes utilized in the emergency management of drug overdose. Acidification of urine with agents such as ammonium chloride enhances the excretion of weak bases, such as phencyclidine (PCP) and amphetamines, while alkalization with agents such as acetazolamide (Diamox) promotes the excretion of weak acids, such as phenobarbital.

IV. Interactions Involving Cytochrome P450 Isoenzymes

A subset of important pharmacokinetic drug-drug interactions involve the cytochrome P450 isoenzymes, which are located largely on microsomal membranes and are responsible for the oxidative metabolism of over 80% of all psychotropic and non-psychotropic drugs and toxins as well as the metabolism of endogenous substances, such as prostaglandins, fatty acids, and steroids. Much remains to be learned about companion metabolic enzyme systems, such as the uridine diphosphate-glucurnosyltransferases (UGTs) and flavin-containing monoxygenases (FMOs). The substrates, inhibitors, and inducers of P450 isoenzymes 1A2 and 2D6 and the 3A and the 2C subclasses have been particularly well characterized (Table 68-1). Drug-drug interactions involving P450 mechanisms, together with other relevant drug-drug interactions, are outlined in section V below.

V. Drug-Drug Interactions According to Psychotropic Drug Class

A. Mood stabilizers. The principal mood stabilizers—**lithium, valproate, and carbamazepine**—are involved in a number of significant drug-drug interactions (Table 68-2) by virtue of their pharmacokinetic properties

    1. **Pharmacokinetics**

        a. **Elimination. Lithium is more than 95% eliminated by the kidney** with reabsorption in the proximal tubules and to a lesser extent in the loop of Henle, while both valproate and carbamazepine are metabolized hepatically.

        b. **Metabolic induction. Carbamazepine is a potent inducer of oxidative metabolism,** while to a lesser extent valproate inhibits these microsomal enzymes.

        c. **Active metabolite.** Carbamazepine is associated with an active metabolite, carbamazepine-10,11-epoxide, with anticonvulsant and possibly other central nervous system (CNS) effects.

        d. **Protein binding.** Lithium and gabapentin are not protein-bound, carbamazepine and lamotrigine are only moderately protein-bound, and valproate is moderately to highly protein-bound.

B. Antidepressants

    1. **Serotonin reuptake inhibitors and TCAs.** The SSRIs, with the exception of venlafaxine (Effexor), citalopram (Celexa) and escitalopram (Lexapro), are inhibitors of cytochrome P450 isoenzymes and therefore play a role in a wide variety of pharmacokinetic drug-drug interactions. In addition the "serotonin syndrome" is a rare but potentially fatal complication associated with the combined use of highly serotoninergic agents and the contraindicated overlapping use of MAOIs and SSRIs. The

Table 68-1. Selected Substrates, Inhibitors, and Inducers of Cytochrome P450 Isoenzyme Metabolisms

		Substrates	
1A2	*2C*	*2D6*	*3A3/4*
Acetaminophen	Angiotensin II	Calcium channel	Alprazolam
Aminophylline	blockers	blockers	Buspirone
Caffeine	Celecoxib	Alfentanil	Calcium channel
Clozapine	Diazepam	Codeine	blockers
Haloperidol	Diclofenac	Dextromethorphan	Carbamazepine
Olanzapine	Glyburide	Encainide	Cisapride
Phenacetin	Glipizide	Flecainide	Cyclosporine
Phenothiazines	Mephenytoin	Hydrocodone	Diazepam
Tacrine	Naproxen	Metoprolol	Disopyramide
Tertiary TCAs	NSAIDs	MCPP	Lidocaine
Theophylline	Omeprazole	Phenothiazines	Loratadine
	Phenytoin	Propafenone	Lovastatin
	Piraxicam	Propranolol	Macrolide antibiotics
	Propranolol	Risperidone	Methadone
	Rosiglitazone	Secondary TCAs	Midazolam
	S-Warfarin	Tertiary TCAs	Nefazodone
	Tertiary TCAs	Timolol	Oral contraceptive
	Tolbutamide	Tramadol	pills
			Propafenone
			Quinidine
			Sildenafil
			Steroids
			Tacrolimus
			Tamoxifen
			Tertiary TCAs
			Triazolam
			Vinblastine
			Zaleplon
			Zolpidem

Table 68-1. *(Continued)*

Inhibitors			
1A2	*2C*	*2D6*	*3A3/4*
Cimetidine	Cimetidine	Antimalarials	Cimetidine
Fluvoxamine	Fluoxetine	Bupropion	Clarithromycin
Fluoroquinolones	Fluvoxamine	Fluoxetine	Erythromycin
Omeprazole	Ketaconazole	Haloperidol	Fluvoxamine
	Paroxetine	Moclobemide	Itraconazole
	Ritonavir	Methadone	Ketaconazole
	Sertraline	Perphenazine	Lovastatin
		Protease inhibitors	Grapefruit juice
		Quinidine	Nefazodone
		Secondary TCAs	Troleandomycin
		Sertraline	
		Thioridazine	

Inducers			
Omeprazole	Rifampin		Carbamazepine
Tobacco			Oxcarbazepine
			Phenobarbital
			Phenytoin
			Rifampin
			Ritonavir (chronic)
			St. John's wort

Selected drug brand names in order of appearance: olanzapine (Zyprexa), tacrine (Cognex), fluvoxamine (Luvox), diclofenac (Voltaren), mephenytoin (Mesantoin), omeprazole (Prilosec), ketaconazole (Nizoral), flecainide (Tambocor), hydrocodone (Vicodin), maprotiline (Ludiomil), propafenone (Rythmol), risperidone (Risperdal), timolol (Timoptic), trazodone (Desyrel), venlafaxine (Effexor), perphenazine (Trilafon), thioridazine (Mellaril), alprazolam (Xanax), amiodarone (Cordarone), carbamazepine (Tegretol), cisapride (Propulsid), disopyramide (Norpace), ethosuximide (Zarontin), loratadine (Clarion), lovastatin (Mevacor), midazolam (Versed), sildenafil (Viagra), nefazodone (Serzone), triazolam (Halcion), zolpidem (Ambien), zaleplon (Sonata), clarithromycin (Biaxin), itraconazole (Sporanox), troleandomycin (Tao), oxcarbazepine (Trileptal).

SOURCE: Devane, C.L., & Nemeroff, C.B. (2000). 2000 guide to psychotropic drug interactions. *Primary Psychiatry, 7,* 10; Ereshefsky, L. (1996). Drug interactions of antidepressants. *Psychiatric Annals, 26,* 342; Ketter, T.A., Flockhart, D.A., Post, R.M., et al. (1996). The emerging role of cytochrome P450 3A in psychopharmacology. *Journal of Clinical Psychopharmacology, 15,* 387; Markowitz, J.S., & DeVane, C.L. (2001). The emerging recognition of herb-drug interactions with a focus on St. John's wort (Hypericum perforatum). *Psychopharmacology Bulletin, 35,* 53; Riesemnan, C.L. (1995). Antidepressant drug interactions and the cytochrome P450 system: A critical appraisal. *Pharmacotherapy, 15,* 845; Nemeroff, C.B., DeVane, C.L., & Pollock, B.G. (1996). Newer antidepressants and the cytochrome P450 system. *American Journal of Psychiatry, 153,* 311; Preskorn, S.H., & Magnus, R.D. (1994). Inhibition of hepatic P450 isoenzymes by serotonin selective reuptake inhibitors: *In vitro* and *in vivo* findings and their implications for patient care. *Psychopharmacology Bulletin, 30,* 251.

Table 68-2. Drug-Drug Interactions Involving the Mood Stabilizers[a]

Mood Stabilizers	Potential Interactions
Lithium	
ACE inhibitors	Increased lithium levels
Angiotensin II receptor antagonists	
Cox 2 inhibitors	
Ethacrynic acid	
Metronidazole	
NSAID[b]	
Spectinomycin	
Spironolactone	
Tetracycline	
Thiazide diuretics[c]	
Triamterene	
Aminophylline	Decreased lithium levels
Acetazolamide	
Osmotic diuretics	
Sodium bicarbonate	
Theophylline	
Antidepressants (TCAs, SSRIs, MAOIs)	Augmented antidepressant effect
Neuromuscular blockers (succinylcholine, pancuronium, decamethonium)	Prolonged muscle paralysis
Antithyroid drugs (propylthiouracil, methimazole)	Increased antithyroid effect
Serotoninergic agents (e.g., clomipramine)	Rare emergence of "serotonin syndrome"
Myelosuppressive drugs (e.g., AZT, carbamazepine)	Masked myleosuppression while on lithium
Antipsychotics	Rare neurotoxicity[d]
Calcium channel blockers	
Methyldopa	
Valproate	
Aspirin	Increased valproate levels or unbound fraction of valproate (aspirin)
Cimetidine	
SSRIs (fluoxetine)	
Carbamazepine	Decreased valproate levels; increased levels of 10-, 11-epoxide carbamazepine metabolite, phenobarbital, and lamotrigine (rash) due to valproate
Lamotrigine	
Phenobarbital	
Phenytoin	
Rifampin	

Table 68-2. *(Continued)*

Mood Stabilizers	Potential Interactions
Carbamazepine	
Antifungal agents	Increased carbamazepine levels
Fluvoxamine	
Isoniazid	
Macrolide antibiotics	
Nefazodone	
Propoxyphene	
SSRIs	
Verapamil	
Valproate	Increased levels of 10-, 11-epoxide metabolite of carbamazepine
	Decreased carbamazepine levels
Phenobarbital	
Phenytoin	
Primidone	
Antidepressants	Induction of metabolism by carbamazepine
Antipsychotics	
Benzodiazepines	
Carbamazepine	
Corticosteroids	
Cyclosporine	
Doxycycline	
Ethosuximide	
Methadone	
Oral contraceptives	
Phenytoin	
Tetracycline	
Theophylline	
Thyroid hormones	
Valproate	
Warfarin	
Furosemide	Increased risk of hyponatremia
Thiazide diuretics	

[a]Selected drug brand names in order of appearance: metronidazole (Flagyl), methimazole (Tapazole), lamotrigine (Lamictal), astemizole (Hismanal), diltiazem (Cardizem), verapamil (Calan, Isoptin), isotretinoin (Accutane), primidone (Mysoline), ethosuximide (Zarontin), doxycycline (Vibramycin), furosemide (Lasix).
[b]Sulindac may be less likely than other NSAIDs to interfere with lithium excretion.
[c]Thiazide-like diuretics, such as indapamide, also raise lithium levels.
[d]Possible increased risk of neuroleptic malignant syndrome (NMS) with lithium-haloperidol co-administration.

TCAs are substrates of the cytochrome P450 enzymes, and therefore TCA plasma levels may be altered by inhibition and induction of this system by other drugs. The potential for pharmacodynamic drug-drug interactions is higher for the TCAs than it is for other antidepressants by virtue of their broad spectrum of activity on muscarinic, histaminergic, and alpha-$_1$-adrenergic receptors and on monoamine reuptake mechanisms and cardiac conduction. Significant drug-drug interactions involving TCA and SSRI antidepressants are presented in Table 68-3.

Table 68-3. Drug-Drug Interactions with Tricyclic Antidepressants (TCAs) and Selective Serotonin Reuptake Inhibitors (SSRIs) and Related Agents[a]

Drug Class	Potential Interactions
Tricyclic antidepressants	
Acetazolamide	Increased TCA levels
Antifungals	
Antipsychotics	
Cimetidine	
Diltiazem	
Disulfiram	
Glucocorticoids	
Macrolide antibiotics	
Propafenone	
Psychostimulants	
Quinidine	
Salicylates	
SSRIs (see below)	
Thiazides	
Thyroid hormone	
Verapamil	
Carbamazepine	Decreased TCA levels
Phenobarbital	
Phenytoin	
Primidone	
Rifampin	
Tobacco	
Antiarrhythmics (type I)	Prolonged cardiac conduction, ventricular arrhythmias
Antipsychotics (low-potency)	
Sympathomimetic amines (epinephrine, isoproterenol)	Arrhythmias, hypertension

Table 68-3. *(Continued)*

Drug Class	Potential Interactions
Tricyclic antidepressants *(continued)*	
Clonidine	Attenuated antihypertensive effects
Guanethidine	
Antihypertensives	Hypotension
Vasodilators	
Antipsychotics (low-potency)	
Anticholinergic drugs (low-potency antipsychotics, benztropine, diphenhydramine)	Anticholinergic toxicity
Sulfonylurea hypoglycemics	Hypoglycemia
MAOIs	Delirium, fever, convulsions
Alcohol	Increased CNS depression
Anxiolytics	
Sedative/hypnotics	
SSRIs and related newer agents	
Secondary amine TCAs Amoxapine	Increased TCA levels with fluoxetine, paroxetine, bupropion, sertraline (2D6)
Desipramine Nortriptyline Protriptyline	
Tertiary amine TCAs Amitriptyline Clomipramine Doxepin Imipramine	Increased TCA levels with fluvoxamine, nefazodone, sertraline, fluoxetine, paroxetine, bupropion (1A2, 2C, 2D6, 3A)
Antipsychotics Phenothiazines	Increased levels with fluoxetine, paroxetine, bupropion and sertraline (2D6)
Quetiapine Ziprasidone	Increased levels with nefazodone fluvoxamine (3A4)
Olanzapine Clozapine Haloperidol	Increased antipsychotic levels with fluvoxamine (1A2)
Benzodiazepines and other sedative/hypnotics	
Alprazolam Diazepam Midazolam	Increased benzodiazepine and zolpidem and zaleplon levels with fluvoxamine, nefazodone, sertraline, fluoxetine (3A, 2C)

(continued)

Table 68-3. Drug-Drug Interactions with Tricyclic Antidepressants (TCAs) and Selective Serotonin Reuptake Inhibitors (SSRIs) and Related Agents[a] (Cont.)

Drug Class	Potential Interactions
Triazolam	
Zaleplon	
Zolpidem	
Methylxanthines	Increased methylxanthine levels with
Aminophylline	fluvoxamine (1A2)
Theophylline	
Antiarrhythmics (Type IC):	Increased antiarrhythmic levels with
Ecainide	fluoxetine, paroxetine, sertraline,
Flecainide	bupropion (2D6)
Propafenone	
Beta-blockers (lipophilic):	Increased beta-blocker levels with fluoxetine,
Metoprolol	paroxetine, sertraline, bupropion (2D6)
Propranolol	
Timolol	
Calcium channel blockers:	Increased calcium channel blocker levels
Diltiazem	with fluvoxamine, nefazodone, sertraline,
Nifedepine	fluoxetine (3A3/4)
Verapamil	
Carbamazepine	Increased carbamazepine levels with
	fluvoxamine, nefazodone, sertraline,
	fluoxetine (3A3/4)
Phenytoin	Increased phenytoin levels with
	fluoxetine, sertraline, fluvoxamine (2C)
Warfarin	Variable, potential effects; likely to be
	multifactorial including P450 effects

[a]Selected drug brand names in order of appearance: diltiazem (Cardizem), disulfiram (Antabuse), propafenone (Rythmol), verapamil (Calan, Isoptin), primidone (Mysoline), clonidine (Catapres), amoxapine (Asendin), protriptyline (Vivactil), clomipramine (Anafranil), doxepin (Sinequan), risperidone (Risperidal), midazolam (Versed), triazolam (Halcion), zolpidem (Ambien), astemizole (Hismanal), cisapride (Propulsid), flecainide (Tambocor), nifedipine (Procardia).

2. **Monoamine oxidase inhibitors.** Among the psychotropics, the MAOIs are most closely associated with potentially fatal drug-drug interactions.

   a. **Hypertensive (hyperadrenergic) crisis.** Abrupt elevation of blood pressure, severe headache, nausea, vomiting, diaphoresis, cardiac arrhythmias, intracranial hemorrhage, and myocardial infarction can occur when a variety of prescribed over-the-counter sympathomimetics, particularly indirect sympathomimetics, are used concurrently with MAOIs. Sympathomimetic drugs include L-dopa, dopamine, cocaine, amphetamines, phenylpropanolamine, oxymetazoline (Afrin), phentermine, mephentermine, metaraminol (Aramine), ephedrine, pseudoephedrine, phenylephrine (Neo-

Synephrine), norepinephrine, isoproterenol, and epinephrine. Generally safe over-the-counter allergy, cold, and cough medications include plain chlorpheniramine (Chlor-Trimeton), brompheniramine (Dimetane), and guaifenesin (Robitussin). The widely available combined preparations that include decongestants or dextromethorphan (DM) must be avoided scrupulously. Although dextromethorphan is not associated with hypertensive crises, its use with MAOIs has been linked to acute confusional states.

b. **Serotonin syndrome.** Myoclonus, rigidity, confusion, nausea, hyperthermia, autonomic instability, coma, and death may occur when highly serotonergic agents including the SSRIs, venlafaxine (Effexor), clomipramine (Anafranil), or tryptophan are combined with the MAOIs. A minimum wash-out interval of 2 weeks is necessary following discontinuation of MAOIs before the initiation of one of these drugs. Reciprocally, a minimum of 2 weeks must elapse after discontinuing most serotonergic drugs before starting an MAOI. In the case of fluoxetine, a minimum delay of 5 weeks is necessary because of its long half-life. Although not associated with a "serotonin syndrome" the combination of buspirone (Buspar) with MAOIs has been associated with episodes of blood pressure elevation. Although the serotonin syndrome may occur when two potent serotonergic agents are used simultaneously in the absence of an MAOI, this fortunately appears to be a rare occurrence.

c. **Meperidine (Demerol).** Agitation, convulsions, blood pressure instability, hyperpyrexia, respiratory depression, peripheral vascular collapse, coma, and death may occur when meperidine is administered concurrently with the MAOIs. Other narcotic analgesics (e.g., codeine, morphine) appear to be safer, although their analgesic and CNS-depressant effects may be potentiated and dose adjustments may be necessary.

d. **TCAs.** Cases of adverse but reversible events, including fever, delirium, convulsions, hypotension, and dyspnea, have been reported when MAOIs and TCAs have been combined. The concurrent use of these two classes of antidepressants generally is contraindicated. However, the very cautious addition of an MAOI to an established treatment with a TCA has been carried out successfully in treating exceptionally treatment-resistant depressed patients.

e. **Other drugs.** The effects of CNS depressants, insulin, sulfonylurea hypoglycemic drugs, and antihypertensive or vasodilator medications may be potentiated, with the exception of guanethidine (Esimil, Ismelin), whose antihypertensive effects may be blocked. There have been reported cases of hypertension and bradycardia in patients on beta-blockers and of hypertension and mental status changes in patients on reserpine and methyldopa. The beta-agonistic effects, including tachycardia, palpitations, and anxiety, of methylxanthines and inhaled bronchodilators may be enhanced.

Phenelzine (Nardil) may potentiate neuromuscular blockage in patients on succinylcholine.

3. **Atypical antidepressants.** While nefazodone (Serzone) inhibits cytochrome P450 3A4 and bupropion inhibits P450 2D6, the atypical antidepressants, including mirtazapine (Remeron) and trazodone (Desyrel), are not known to be inhibitors of specific cytochrome P450 isoenzymes. Hypotension can occur on a pharmacodynamic basis when trazodone is administered with antihypertensive agents. Although bupropion and trazodone have been cautiously administered with MAOIs, the safety of these combinations is not well established.

C. **Antipsychotics.** Antipsychotics (neuroleptics) are extensively metabolized by the liver, and most, with the exception of molindone (Moban) are highly protein-bound.

Lower-potency agents are more likely than are high-potency agents to participate in pharmacodynamic interactions with drugs such as TCAs, causing hypotension, anticholinergic effects, sedation, and prolonged cardiac conduction. With respect to pharmacokinetic mechanisms, the atypical antipsychotics clozapine (Clozaril) and olanzapine (Zyprexa) appear to be subject mainly to drug-drug interactions that interfere with cytochrome P450 1A2 activity, while the atypical agent risperidone (Risperdal) is subject to interactions that affect P450 2D6 and both quetiapine (Seroquel) and ziprasidone (Geodon) may participate in interactions that affect P450 3A4. In addition, the lower potency agents, intravenous (IV) haloperidol or droperidol, and some of the newer atypicals, including ziprasadone, may prolong the QT interval, particularly when combined with other agents that have similar properties (e.g., TCAs). Plasma levels of the butyrophenone haloperidol and the phenothiazines may also be altered by interactions involving P450 isoenzymes. Because of great inter-individual variability in antipsychotic blood levels and their high therapeutic index, pharmacokinetic interactions of this kind are relevant mainly to the treatment of patients maintained on neuroleptic doses in the low therapeutic range and patients who are very sensitive to side effects in whom fluctuations in antipsychotic blood levels could significantly alter the clinical status. Drug-drug interactions involving the antipsychotics are presented in Table 68-4.

D. Anxiolytics

1. **Pharmacodynamic interactions**

   a. The most common and potentially serious drug-drug interactions involving the benzodiazepine anxiolytics are the additive (CNS) depressant effects that occur when these agents are co-administered with barbiturates, ethanol, narcotics, antihistamines, TCAs, and zolpidem (Ambien) or zaleplon (Sonata). These effects commonly include sedation and psychomotor impairment. At high doses and in severely compromised patients, however, fatal respiratory depression may occur.

   b. Flumazenil (Romazicon) is a competitive inhibitor of the benzodiazepine receptor and therefore antagonizes benzodiazepine effects. The anticholinesterase physostigmine also blocks benzodiazepine binding in the brain and therefore can reverse the CNS depression caused by benzodiazepines.

2. **Pharmacokinetic interactions.** While rarely life-threatening, alterations in blood levels of the benzodiazepines may account for the emergence of side effects, such as unsteadiness and slurred speech, and for the loss of anti-anxiety or hypnotic efficacy when a new drug is co-administered.

   a. **Absorption.** Antacid suspensions (aluminum and magnesium hydroxide) may delay the rate, but less likely the extent, of the absorption of orally administered benzodiazepines.

   b. **Metabolic induction.** Inducers of phase I metabolic processes, including carbamazepine, phenobarbital, and rifampin, may reduce the levels of the majority of benzodiazepines, which are subject to oxidative metabolism, while leaving levels of lorazepam, oxazepam, and temazepam unchanged.

   c. **Metabolic inhibition**

      i. Inhibitors of phase I oxidative processes, including cimetidine (Tagamet), isoniazid, disulfiram (Antabuse), estrogens, and hepatically-metabolized beta-blockers (e.g., propranolol, metoprolol), may increase the levels of those benzodiazepines, whose clearance relies on oxidative metabolism.

Table 68-4. Drug-Drug Interactions with Antipsychotic Medications[a]

	Potential Pharmacokinetic Interactions
Antidepressants (TCAs, SSRIs)	Mutually increased levels of antipsychotic and antidepressant or beta-blocking agents (see Table 68-1)
Beta-blockers (lipophilic)	
Cimetidine	Variable effects on antipsychotic levels
Carbamazepine	Decreased antipsychotic drug levels
Phenobarbital	
Phenytoin	
Rifampin	
Tobacco	
Antacids (gel type)	Reduced or delayed absorption of antipsychotics (Al^{3+}, Mg^{2+})
	Other Potential Drug-drug Interactions
Antiarrhythmics (type I)	Prolonged cardiac conduction and ventricular arrhythmias (low-potency antipsychotics)
TCAs	
Calcium channel blockers	Prolonged cardiac conduction and ventricular arrhythmias (pimozide [Orap], thioridazine [Mellaril], mesoridazine [Serentil])
Antihypertensives	Increased risk of hypotension (low-potency antipsychotics, risperidone)
Epinephrine	
MAOIs	
TCAs	
Trazodone	
Vasodilators	
Clonidine	Blockade of antihypertensive effect
Guanethidine	
Bromocriptine	Mutual interference with dopamine receptor-mediated effects
L-Dopa	
Anticholinergics	Anticholinergic toxicity (low-potency antipsychotics)
Myelosuppressive agents	Additive risk of leukopenia/agranulocytosis (clozapine)
Lithium	Rare neurotoxicity, possible elevated NMS risk (haloperidol)
Antidepressants	Enhanced effectiveness in treatment of psychotic depression

[a]Selected drug brand names in order of appearance: trazodone (Desyrel), clonidine (Catapres), bromocriptine (Parlodel).

ii. Specific inhibitors of the cytochrome P450 3A3/4 subclass (Table 68-1), including the macrolide antibiotics, antifungals, nefazodone (Serzone), and fluvoxamine (Luvox), may increase plasma levels of the triazalobenzodiazepines (alprazolam [Xanax], triazolam [Halcion], midazolam [Versed]), whose clearance depends on hydroxylation catalyzed by the P450 3A3/4 isoenzymes. Levels of diazepam (Valium) may be affected, although diazepam also is metabolized through the P450 2C subclass.

iii. Specific inhibitors of the cytochrome P450 2C class (Table 68-1), including omeprazole (Prilosec), as well as ketaconazole (Nizoral) and certain SSRIs, including fluoxetine, fluvoxamine, and sertraline, may increase plasma levels of diazepam by interfering with N-demethylation.

iv. Inhibitors of glucuronide conjugation (phase II metabolism), including valproate and probenecid, may increase plasma levels of the 3-hydroxy substituted benzodiazepines (lorazepam [Ativan], oxazepam [Serax], and temazepam [Restoril]), which are not altered by inhibitors of phase I metabolism.

v. Increased levels of digoxin have been reported when co-administered with benzodiazepines (diazepam, alprazolam)

3. **Idiosyncratic interactions.** Absence seizures have been described in some patients on valproate and clonazepam (Klonopin), although this drug combination is widely and safely used in patients with bipolar disorder or seizure disorders.

E. **Miscellaneous**

1. **Zolpidem (Ambien).** Additive CNS depressant effects are likely to occur when other sedating agents, including alcohol, barbiturates, and benzodiazepines, are co-administered with zolpidem, which interacts with the gamma-aminobutyric acid–benzodiazepine complex. The sedative and hypnotic effects of zolpidem are reversed by the benzodiazepine receptor antagonist flumazenil (Romazicon). As with the triazolo-benzodiazepines, zolpidem levels are potentially affected by drug-drug interactions involving cytochrome P450 3A4.

2. **Tacrine (Cognex)** is a substrate for cytochrome P450 1A2 (Table 68-1) and may compete with other drugs for this hepatic microsomal isoenzyme. Elevated levels of theophylline have been reported in this context.

3. **Disulfiram (Antabuse).** In addition to inhibiting aldehyde dehydrogenase and its resultant accumulation of acetaldehyde after ethanol ingestion, disulfiram inhibits other hepatic microsomal enzymes, interfering with the metabolism of a variety of drugs, including warfarin, phenytoin, benzodiazepines (except those bypassing phase I metabolism), antipsychotics, and antidepressants. The severity of the disulfiram-alcohol reaction is increased by a variety of agents, including MAOIs, vasodilators, alpha- or beta-adrenergic antagonists, and paraldehyde. Severe confusional states may occur when metronidazole (Flagyl) is administered within 2 weeks of disulfiram, and therefore concurrent use is contraindicated.

Suggested Readings

Alderman, C.P. (2000). Patient-oriented strategies for the prevention of drug interactions. *Drug Safety, 22,* 103–109.

Alpert, J.E., Bernstein, J.O., & Rosenbaum, J.F. (1997). Psychopharmacological issues in the medical setting. In N.H. Cassem, T.A. Stern, J.F. Rosenbaum, & M.S. Jellinek (Eds.),

Massachusetts General Hospital handbook of general hospital psychiatry (4th ed.). St. Louis: Mosby, pp. 249–303.

Bernard, S.A., & Bruera, E. (2000). Drug interactions in palliative care. *Journal of Clinical Oncology, 18,* 1780–1799.

Blackwell, B. (1991). Monoamine oxidase inhibitor interactions with other drugs. *Journal of Clinical Psychopharmacology, 11,* 55–59.

Callahan, A.M., Fava, M., & Rosenbaum, J.F. (1993). Drug interactions in psychopharmacology. *Psychiatric Clinics of North America, 16,* 647–671.

Ciraulo, D.A., Shader, R.I., Greenblatt, D.J., et al. (Eds.). (1995). *Drug interactions in psychiatry* (2nd ed.). Baltimore: Williams & Wilkins.

Cozza, K.L., & Armstrong, S.C. (2001). *The cytochrome P450 system: Drug interaction principles for medical practice.* Washington, DC: American Psychiatric Press.

DeVane, C.L., & Nemeroff, C.B. (2000). 2000 guide to psychotropic drug interactions. *Primary Psychiatry, 7,* 10.

Ereshefsky, L. (1996). Drug interactions of antidepressants. *Psychiatric Annals, 26,* 342–350.

Fugh-Berman, A. (2000). Herb-drug interactions. *Lancet, 355,* 134–138.

Greenblatt, D.J., von Moltke, L.L., Harmatz, J.S., & Shader, R.I. (1999). Human cytochromes and some newer antidepressants: Kinetics, metabolism and drug interactions. *Journal of Clinical Psychopharmacology, 19*(5 suppl 1), 23S–35S.

Hyman, S.E., Arana, G.W., & Rosenbaum, J.F. (1995). *Handbook of psychiatric drug therapy* (3rd ed.). Boston: Little, Brown.

Keck, P.E., & Arnold, L.M. (2000). The serotonin syndrome. *Psychiatric Annals, 30,* 333–343.

Livingston, M.G., & Livingston, H.M. (1997). Monoamine oxidase inhibitors. An update on drug interactions. *Drug Safety, 14,* 219–227.

Markowitz, J.S., & DeVane, C.L. (2001). The emerging recognition of herb-drug interactions with a focus on St. John's wort *(Hypericum perforatum). Psychopharmacology Bulletin, 35,* 53–64.

Stoudemire, A. (1996). New antidepressant drugs and the treatment of depression in the medically ill patient. *Psychiatric Clinics of North America, 19,* 495–514.

Tseng, A.L., & Foisy, M.M. (1999). Significant interactions with new antiretrovirals and psychotropic drugs. *Annals of Pharmacotherapy, 33,* 461–473.

Von Moltke, L.L., & Greenblatt, D.J. (2000). Drug transporters in psychopharmacology—are they important? *Journal of Clinical Psychopharmacology, 20,* 291–294.

CHAPTER 69

Natural Medications in Psychiatry

DAVID MISCHOULON AND ANDREW A. NIERENBERG

I. Introduction

A. Definition
So-called "natural," "complementary," or "alternative" medications are derived from natural products, but are not approved by the U.S. Food and Drug Administration (FDA) for their purported indications. These medications may include plants, herbs, hormones, vitamins, fatty acids, and homeopathic preparations, as well as other products.

B. Indications
Natural medications are available for almost any medical problem. However, **there are relatively fewer medications for psychiatric disorders** (though this is one of the most popular indications for alternative therapies). **Psychiatric treatments are available primarily for mood disorders, anxiety and sleep disorders, dementia, and some psychotic disorders.**

C. The History of Natural Remedies
Natural medications have been in use all over the world for thousands of years, and are especially popular in Europe, Asia, and South America. **Recently, their popularity has grown dramatically in the United States,** and they are widely featured on television, newspapers, books, and Internet sites. **The National Institutes of Health (NIH) recently recognized that one-fourth of the people in the United States use non-traditional treatments (medications as well as other treatments, such as acupuncture),** and more than 70% of the population worldwide uses such treatments. In 1990, more visits were made to alternative practitioners nationwide than to primary care physicians (PCPs). Unfortunately, traditional medical education has largely neglected the topic of natural remedies in didactic curricula, though increasing numbers of medical schools, **residency training programs, and continuing medical education programs are beginning to incorporate alternative medicine into their didactics.** As physicians, we need to inform ourselves about the topic from medical, scientific, and cultural standpoints.

D. Reasons for the Growing Popularity of Natural Medicines
1. **Increasing numbers of patients are becoming dissatisfied with the medical profession** and with orthodox medicine, largely due to a perceived emphasis on managed care and profits rather than with healing.
2. **There has been a cultural shift in how patients view their role vis-à-vis the medical establishment,** with growing emphasis on taking a more active role, rather than on assuming the traditional "passive" stance when working with a physician.

3. **Natural remedies are readily available without a prescription,** and this provides a heightened sense of independence. Patients may now "prescribe" for themselves if they wish, and bypass the medical establishment.

4. **There are growing numbers of non-physician practitioners who recommend these medications** without having the need to consult with a medical doctor.

5. **The remedies are generally easy to obtain,** and are often cheaper than obtaining prescription treatments.

E. **The Importance of Learning About Natural Medicines**

Because **natural remedies are so widely used,** particularly for psychiatric conditions, physicians need to understand the therapeutic potential and the safety profiles of these medications. In addition, **physicians need to consider the meaning of natural remedies to their patients.** A working knowledge of these agents will facilitate communication between patient and physician when the use of these agents is considered. Understanding the actions and hazards of natural medicines will also help guide their prescription or discontinuation.

II. Problems Associated with Use of Natural Medications

A. **Effectiveness Issues**

1. **The actual benefits of natural remedies are not clear,** largely because most of the available data are in the form of small (often uncontrolled) clinical studies, case reports, and practitioner anecdotes. Few systematic studies have addressed the question of effectiveness, or the question of superiority to placebo.

2. **Manufacturers, suppliers, and the United States government have traditionally avoided sponsoring clinical research,** though in recent years there has been an increase in government and industry sponsorship of such trials in the United States.

B. **Safety Issues**

1. Many people mistakenly believe that a natural medication is automatically safe to use. **While there are relatively few reports of serious adverse effects from these medications, there are increasing reports of toxicity** in people who take these medications—even when the medications were used at recommended doses.

2. **There are limited data regarding the safety and efficacy of combining natural medications with conventional medications or with other natural medications.** However, there have been reports of serious—even tragic—interactions that have resulted with such combinations.

3. **Natural medications are generally not regulated by the FDA,** except for homeopathy. However, what little regulation exists tends to focus on safety, rather than efficacy. Therefore, many manufacturers are free to make misleading claims.

4. **There is no guidance from systematic study for optimal doses, contraindications, interactions, and potential toxicities.**

5. **There is much variability among different preparations** made by different manufacturers. Different preparations vary in potency, quality, and purity—and hence in effectiveness.

C. **Cost Issues**

Some treatments can be very costly, and may even cost more than conventional medications, particularly if there is a need for higher doses. **Insurance companies**

generally do not cover natural treatments, so patients usually have to pay out-of-pocket. These treatments can therefore be more costly in the long run, and less cost-effective, especially in cases where they prove ineffective.

III. The Different Medications

A. Natural Antidepressants

1. **St. John's Wort (SJW) (*Hypericum perforatum L.*)**
   a. **Efficacy**
      i. **SJW has been shown to be effective for mild-to-moderate depression,** and to have greater efficacy than placebo, based on over 20 placebo-controlled trials that showed an approximate 55% response rate. A recent large-scale controlled study, however, suggested that SJW was no more effective than placebo for major depression, in a population of varying depressive severity.
      ii. **SJW has been shown to have equal efficacy to low-dose tricyclic antidepressants (TCAs),** in several active control studies (vs. imipramine 75 mg or equivalent). Responses were about 80% vs. 63% (SJW was not as effective as amitriptyline).
      iii. There have been at least three published studies comparing SJW to SSRIs. In two studies, SJW yielded a comparable response rate to fluoxetine and sertraline. However, a recent study comparing SJW to sertraline and placebo suggested no advantage for either medication when compared to placebo in moderately severe major depressive disorder (MDD).
   b. **Active components**
      Polycyclic phenols, hypericin, pseudohypericin, and hyperforin are presumed to be among the psychotropically-active components of SJW. Hypericin and hyperforin are generally believed to be the principal active components. Most SJW preparations are standardized to one or the other.
   c. **Mechanism of action**
      Mechanisms of action are believed to include regulation of cytokine production (change levels of IL-6, IL-1ß, decreased cortisol); decreased 5-HT receptor density; decrease reuptake of neurotransmitters; there is also some minimal MAOI activity, and for this reason, **SJW should not be combined with SSRIs, as serotonin syndrome may result.** The metabolism of SJW is not well understood, but it is presumed to be hepatic.
   d. **Dosing**
      Recommended doses range from 900 to 1,800 mg/day, usually divided on a b.i.d. or t.i.d. basis. However, different preparations may vary in the amount of active product.
   e. **Adverse effects**
      Adverse effects from SJW may include dry mouth, dizziness, constipation, and phototoxicity. There are limited data regarding safety in overdose. There are several case reports of a switch to mania in bipolar patients who took SJW without a concomitant mood stabilizer. Serotonin syndrome has occurred when SJW was combined with SSRIs.
   f. **Drug-drug interactions**
      A number of cases of adverse drug-drug interactions with SJW have emerged in the past few years. **Hyperforin induces CYP-3A4 expression, and may reduce the therapeutic activity of a number of medications, including warfarin, cyclosporine, oral contraceptives, theophylline, fenprocoumon, digoxin, indinavir, and Camptosar.** There are cases of transplant rejection resulting from SJW-cyclosporine interactions.

Transplant recipients and HIV-positive individuals receiving protease inhibitors should not use SJW.

g. **Summary**

   Overall, SJW appears to be better than placebo, and comparable to low-dose TCAs, and perhaps to SSRIs. However, recent studies suggest that its effectiveness may be limited to milder forms of depression. **Its safety profile is generally favorable, though dangerous interactions need to be considered.**

2. **S-Adenosyl Methionine (SAMe)**

   a. **Efficacy**

   SAMe has a mood-elevating effect in depressed patients. A small number of clinical studies suggest that **doses up to 1,600 mg/day** of parenteral (intravenous [IV] and intramuscular [IM]) and oral SAMe preparations **are superior to placebo and as effective as TCAs.** However, some early studies are problematic, due to instability of oral SAMe preparations. SAMe may have a relatively faster onset of action than conventional agents; some patients have shown improvement in as little as one to two weeks. The combination of SAMe and low-dose TCAs may result in earlier onset of action than TCA alone.

   Other indications for SAMe may include: treatment of cognitive deficits in dementia; relief of distress during the purpuerium; reduction of psychological distress during opioid detoxification; reduction of depression in alcoholics; use in medically ill depressed patients for whom conventional antidepressants may be contraindicated; and use for arthritis or other disease of the joints.

   b. **Active components**

   SAMe is a major methyl donor in the brain. It functions by donating methyl groups to hormones, neurotransmitters, nucleic acids, proteins, and phospholipids. **SAMe levels depend on levels of the vitamins folate and B_{12}.** Deficiencies in folate and B_{12} are also associated with development of depression and/or refractoriness to treatment (see next section).

   c. **Mechanism of action**

   SAMe is thought to exert its antidepressant effect by donating methyl groups in the reactions that result in the synthesis of norepinephrine, serotonin, and dopamine, deficiencies of which have been associated with mood disorders.

   d. **Dosing**

   Recommended doses of SAMe, based on clinical studies, range from **400–1,600 mg/day.** Real-world experience, however, suggests that some patients may need even higher doses. **SAMe is relatively expensive** ($0.75–1.25 for a 200 mg tablet) and the cost may be prohibitive to many patients, particularly those requiring higher doses.

   e. **Adverse effects**

   SAMe is well tolerated, relatively free of adverse effects, and it has no apparent hepatotoxicity. **Side effects include mild insomnia, lack of appetite, constipation, nausea, dry mouth, sweating, dizziness, and nervousness.** There are some reports of increased anxiety, mania or hypomania in patients with bipolar depression.

   f. **Drug-drug interactions**

   So far, there are **no reports of adverse drug-drug interactions** with SAMe.

   g. **Summary**

   SAMe appears to be safe and effective for depression, but larger studies are needed to establish this with certainty.

3. **Folic Acid and Vitamin B_{12}**

   a. **Efficacy**

   Between 10% and 30% of depressed patients may have low serum folate, and this may result in a decreased response rate to antidepressants. B_{12} deficiency may re-

sult in an earlier age of onset of depression. Replenishment of these vitamins in depressed patients with vitamin B-deficiencies has resulted in improved response rates with antidepressant treatment. Folate supplementation in normofolatemic patients has been shown to augment the antidepressant effect of SSRIs.

b. **Active components**

The vitamins folate and B$_{12}$ are obtained in the diet, and play important roles in the synthesis of CNS neurotransmitters, such as serotonin, norepinephrine, and dopamine.

c. **Mechanism of action**

Folic acid is required for synthesis of SAMe (and hence for synthesis of norepinephrine [NE], dopamine [DA], and serotonin [5-HT]). Vitamin B$_{12}$ is converted to methylcobalamin, which is a co-factor in the synthesis of CNS neurotransmitters. Replenishment of these vitamins results in optimal synthesis of the different neurotrasmitters, and may thus help to reverse depression.

d. **Dose**

The recommended dose of folate is 400 μg daily. The recommended dose of B$_{12}$ is 6 μg daily. Excess doses are eliminated in the urine.

e. **Adverse effects**

There appear to be **no adverse effects** associated with replenishment of these vitamins.

f. **Drug-drug interactions**

There are no known adverse interactions between these vitamins and other medications.

g. **Summary**

Physicians should check serum levels of B$_{12}$ and folate in depressed patients who have not responded to treatment, particularly if they have concurrent medical illness or alcoholism, and/or appear to be at risk of deficiencies. Correction of folate and B$_{12}$ deficiency may help alleviate depressive symptoms and/or improve response to antidepressant therapy .

4. **Essential Fatty Acids (EFAs)**

a. **Efficacy**

Initial evidence in support of the omega fatty acids was based on the finding of lower rates of depression in countries where large amounts of fish are consumed. **Omega-3 fatty acids are thought to have a protective role against unipolar depression and bipolar disorder.** One small double-blind placebo-controlled trial with 30 patients with bipolar disorder has been performed. Of those who received a 9 g/day of an omega-3 fatty acid mix, only one had a recurrence, and this group had a longer period of remission. **Omega-3 and omega-6 fatty acid mixtures may help alleviate psychotic symptoms,** as suggested by case reports and small studies showing variable results when omega fatty acids are used alone or as an adjunct to neuroleptics.

b. **Active components**

Omega-3 and omega-6 fatty acids are the two essential fatty acid types thought to possess psychotropic effects. **Among the omega-3 fatty acids, eicosapentanoic acid (EPA) and docosahexanoic acid (DHA) are thought to be the most psychotropically active,** with most recent evidence favoring EPA.

c. **Mechanism of action**

Several mechanisms of action have been proposed for the omega-3 fatty acids. **They may function similarly to mood stabilizers such as lithium, by inhibiting G-protein signal transduction and thus regulating the phosphatidylinositol cascade inside the cell.**

d. **Dose**

Commercially available preparations of omega-3 may have **up to 1,000 mg of different omega-3 fatty acids per capsule.** The ratio of EPA and DHA vary greatly among different preparations. Earlier studies have used high doses (as much as 9–10 grams/day) of omega-3, but recent studies suggest that doses of 1 gram or less may be satisfactory for treatment of mood disorders.

e. **Adverse effects**

Mild dose-related GI distress has been the only side effect reported from omega-fatty acids thus far.

f. **Drug-drug interactions**

No adverse interactions have been reported with omega-3 fatty acids.

g. **Summary**

Overall, this is a promising treatment, particularly in view of the wide variety of illness potentially treatable, and the tolerable side-effect profile. Larger studies are needed in order to better assess the effectiveness and safety of the different omega-fatty acids.

5. **Inositol**

a. **Efficacy**

Inositol has been studied for various indications, and has been found, in small, double-blind placebo-controlled trials, to be **effective for depression, panic disorder, bulimia, and OCD, at doses ranging from 12 to 18 grams/day.** It appears to have no effect in schizophrenia, attention deficit hyperactivity disorder (ADHD), Alzheimer's disease, autism, or ECT-induced cognitive impairment.

b. **Active components**

Inositol is a **polyol precursor in brain second messenger systems.**

c. **Mechanism of action**

Administration of inositol may reverse desensitization of serotonin receptors. Effects on the inositol cascade, similar to those induced by mood stabilizers, may also be involved in its therapeutic action.

d. **Dose**

High doses (12–18 grams/day) have been recommended, based on clinical trials.

e. **Adverse effects**

Inositol has **no apparent toxicity,** and a mild side-effect profile (GI upset, headache, insomnia, dizziness, sedation).

f. **Drug-drug interactions**

No adverse interactions have been reported with inositol.

g. **Summary**

Overall, inositol is a promising treatment with multiple possible indications, but trials so far are small. Trials with larger patient samples are required for better understanding of this drug's effectiveness.

B. **Natural Anxiolytic-Hypnotics**

1. **Valerian (*Valeriana officinalis*)**

a. **Efficacy**

Valerian has been shown in a few small controlled clinical trials to be **an effective sedative and mild hypnotic.** It is not considered ideal for acute treatment of insomnia, but promotes natural sleep after several weeks of use. Valerian is very popular among Hispanics.

b. **Active components**

The active components of valerian are thought to be **valepotriates and sesquiterpenes.**

c. **Mechanism of action**

Valerian is **thought to function similarly to benzodiazepines.** It may decrease GABA breakdown, and cause changes in sleep EEG. The net clinical effect appears to be a decrease in sleep latency, and improved sleep quality. The metabolism of valerian is not well understood.

d. Dose

Recommended doses are from **450 to 600 mg, about 2 hours before bedtime.**

e. Adverse effects

There appears to be no dependence or daytime drowsiness associated with valerian. Valerian was compared with flunitrazepam in one study, and found to have the same efficacy, but fewer side effects. The relatively uncommon side effects reported with valerian include **blurry vision, dystonias, and hepatotoxicity.** It is important to remember that Mexican or Indian valerian should not be used, as some components may present a carcinogenic risk.

f. Drug-drug interactions

No adverse drug-drug interactions have been reported with valerian.

g. Summary

Overall, data are promising, but we need more double-blind trials, and trials comparing valerian to more conventional anxiolytic/hypnotics. Limitations to double-blinding have included valerian's **distinctive and powerful smell** (due to isovaleric acid). Placebos with similar smells have been developed.

2. Kava (*Piper methysticum*)

a. Efficacy

Kava originated in the Polynesian Islands, and is a staple of tribal rituals. It is said by tribal members that "with Kava in you, you can't hate." Evidence suggests that **kava has a calming and relaxing effect without altering consciousness.** A few controlled double-blind studies have shown **effectiveness for mild anxiety states including agoraphobia, specific phobia, generalized anxiety disorder (GAD), and adjustment disorder.** It does not appear to be as effective for more severe anxiety or panic disorder.

b. Active components

The active components are thought to be **kavapyrones.** Their half-life varies from 90 minutes to several hours. Bioavailability can vary up to ten-fold, depending on the preparation.

c. Mechanism of action

Kava's active components are believed to act as **central muscle relaxants and anticonvulsants. They bind GABA receptors, and inhibit uptake of norepinephrine.**

Their net effect is to reduce the excitability of limbic system, perhaps as well as benzodiazepines, but without dependence or withdrawal.

d. Dose

Recommended doses range **from 60 to 300 mg/day.**

e. Adverse effects

Mild side effects associated with kava include **GI upset, headaches, and dizziness.** Toxic reactions with high doses or prolonged use may include **ataxia, hair loss, visual and respiratory problems, and kava dermopathy** (a transient yellowing of the skin, perhaps related to cholesterol metabolism). Most of these toxic effects are reversible if use is discontinued.

Recently, there have emerged at least two dozen cases of **hepatotoxicity** related to kava, including, in some extreme cases, the need for liver transplant. In some cases, a direct relationship between kava and liver disease was not clear, and some individuals were reported to have been taking excessive doses of the medication. Consequently, several countries have mandated removal of kava from the market. The FDA is currently investigating the safety of kava so as to determine need for stricter regulation.

The sudden emergence of kava-related liver toxicity may reflect increasing use of kava, particularly in the absence of physician supervision. Until more information is available, physicians and consumers should proceed with caution regarding use and prescription of kava. It is recommended that **duration of use of kava not exceed 3 months. Individuals with a history of liver disease, alcohol use, or who are taking concurrent medications with potential liver toxicity should avoid kava.**

f. **Drug-drug interactions**

No adverse interactions have been reported with kava.

g. **Summary**

Kava appears more effective than placebo for mild anxiety states, but we need more studies to compare it to other anxiolytics. Serious questions of safety have emerged in the past year, and those using kava should do so only under the supervision of a physician, and preferably for short periods.

3. **Melatonin**

a. **Efficacy**

Melatonin is believed to be **an effective hypnotic, which works within one hour** of administration, regardless of the time. It is commonly used by travelers to reset their biological clock when traveling across time zones (this is its main source of popularity).

b. **Active components**

Melatonin is **a hormone derived from serotonin,** and made in the pineal gland.

c. **Mechanism of action**

Melatonin is thought to be involved in **organization of circadian rhythms**. This may involve interaction with the suprachiasmatic nucleus. Its net effect is to reset the circadian pacemaker, and attenuate the alerting process. It may also have a direct soporific effect.

d. **Dose**

The optimal dose of melatonin is unclear. Some studies suggest that **0.25 to 0.30 mg/day** can decrease sleep latency. However, many preparations have as much as 5 mg of melatonin.

e. **Adverse effects**

Although generally benign, **daytime sleepiness or confusion** may result with high doses. Other more serious adverse effects reported include **inhibition of fertility, decreased sex drive, hypothermia, and retinal damage.** It is contraindicated in pregnant women and those with immunocompromised status (e.g., HIV-positive individuals and people who take steroids or other immunosuppressant drugs).

f. **Drug-drug interactions**

None reported.

g. **Summary**

Melatonin is a promising treatment, generally accepted as safe and effective, but we need more trials to say with certainty. It is one of the few alternative treatments studied in children, and may have a potential use in children with sleep disorders.

C. **Medications for Premenstrual Syndrome (PMS)/Menopausal Symptoms**

1. **Black Cohosh (*Cimicifuga racemosa*)**

a. **Efficacy**

Black cohosh is a herbaceous plant **used for alleviation of physical and psychological menopausal symptoms.** Five placebo-controlled studies show efficacy of doses of 40 mg/day, as measured by changes in various psychometric scales.

b. **Active components**

The active components are thought to be **triterpenoids, isoflavones, and aglycones.**

c. **Mechanism of action**

The mechanism of action may involve **suppression of luteinizing hormone** (in the pituitary gland). There is also some evidence of an anti-breast cancer effect.

d. **Dose**

Recommended dose is **between 40 to 200 mg/day.**

e. **Adverse effects**

Reported adverse effects include **GI upset, headache, dizziness, and weight gain.** No specific toxicity is associated, but data are limited. Duration of use is **not recommended to exceed 3 months.** Contraindications include pregnancy, heart disease, and hypertension.

f. **Drug-drug interactions**

No adverse interactions have been reported with black cohosh.

g. **Summary**

This is a promising treatment, but is relatively understudied and requires further investigation.

2. **Chaste Tree Berry (CTB) (*Vitex agnus castus*)**

a. **Efficacy**

CTB is the dried fruit of the chaste tree. It helped medieval monks keep their vow of chastity, by **decreasing their sex drive.** It is **used for premenstrual syndrome (PMS) alleviation.** In one controlled double-blind study of 175 mg/day chasteberry vs. pyridoxine (vitamin B_6), both groups reported decreased PMS symptoms, based on a psychometric scale for assessing PMS.

b. **Active components**

The clinically active ingredient of CTB is **not known.**

c. **Mechanism of action**

The effect of chaste tree berry **may be due to prolactin inhibition** (based on one study of women). There may also be a role for D_2 dopaminergic receptor interactions.

d. **Dose**

Recommended doses range is **from 20 to 400 mg/day.**

e. **Adverse effects**

No adverse effects have been reported with CTB.

f. **Drug-drug interactions**

No adverse interactions have been reported with CTB.

g. **Summary**

We need more systematic trials to better assess the usefulness of CTB.

D. **Cognition-Enhancing Remedies**

1. **Ginkgo Biloba**

a. **Efficacy**

Ginkgo is derived from the seed of the ginkgo biloba tree. It has been used in traditional Chinese medicine for over 2000 years. It is **used for treatment of cognitive deficits and affective symptoms in organic brain diseases,** such as Alzheimer's disease and vascular dementias. Target symptoms include memory, abstract thinking, and affective symptoms. **Ginkgo may also improve learning capacity.**

Many double-blind trials (more than 30) suggest that dementia symptoms improve with ginkgo. However, standards for testing response have changed over time. The German Federal Health Agency Mandates of 1991 decreed that improvement in dementia symptoms (e.g., memory and abstraction) was not enough. Improvement in activities of daily living (ADL) and reduced need for care are necessary for the medication to be considered effective. Hence, many older studies became uninformative, as they did not meet the new criteria for improvement.

A recent year-long randomized, double-blind study with 309 patients suggested that **ginkgo may stabilize and improve cognitive performance and social functioning in demented patients.** Changes were modest but significant, and were noticeable by caretakers. Some studies have compared ginkgo with other nootropics, and found comparable efficacy, but ginkgo seems to have fewer side effects. For these reasons, **24–28% of physicians recommend ginkgo.** Family physicians in particular tend to favor ginkgo over other nootropics.

Ginkgo may also have a potential role in treatment of antidepressant-induced sexual dysfunction. In males and females on several antidepressants, low-dose ginkgo resulted in improvement in all aspects of the sexual cycle (desire, arousal, orgasm, and resolution).

b. **Active components**

The active ingredients of ginkgo include **flavonoids and terpene lactones.**

c. **Mechanism of action**

The mechanism of action of ginkgo is thought to be **multi-fold.** Beneficial effects include:

   i. **Stimulation of still functional nerve cells.**
   ii. **Protection from pathologic effects,** such as hypoxia, ischemia, seizures, and peripheral damage.
   iii. **Membrane/receptor stabilization.**
   iv. **Free radical scavenging.**
   v. **Inhibition of platelet activating factor** (by Ginkgolide B). For this reason, ginkgo should be avoided in individuals with bleeding disorders, or those who are taking anticoagulants.

d. **Dose**

Recommended doses are **from 120 to 240 mg/day, divided in a b.i.d. to t.i.d. regimen.** A minimal 8-week course is recommended, and the patient should be re-evaluated every three months during use. Full assessment of the therapeutic effect may require up to one year of use.

e. **Adverse effects**

Adverse effects are mild and **may include GI upset, headache, irritability, and dizziness.**

f. **Drug-drug interactions**

Ginkgo may potentiate the effect of anticoagulants, and may thus result in hemorrhage.

g. **Summary**

Overall, ginkgo **appears effective, with very low toxicity,** and limited interactions with other drugs. **It may have a potential role in amelioration of antidepressant-induced sexual dysfunction.** Its full role remains to be clarified.

E. Homeopathy

1. Efficacy

Homeopathy was developed in Germany 200 years ago, by Samuel Hahnemann. It is the second most utilized health care system worldwide. **Homeopathic remedies are derived from plants and minerals. They are regulated by the FDA** (for safety), and sold over-the-counter. Homeopathic remedies are administered orally, and allowed to dissolve on or under the tongue. Improvement tends to be gradual, on the order of weeks to months. Transient aggravation of symptoms may occur early in treatment. Most research has focussed on physical rather than mental health.

One study examined 12 patients with various psychiatric disorders, including social phobia, panic, major depressive disorder (MDD), attention deficit disorder (ADD), and chronic fatigue. There is also a meta-analysis of 107 trials. These data suggest that **homeopathy may be useful,** but most studies are not rigorously designed.

2. **Active components**
   Varies with preparation.

3. **Mechanism of action**
   Homeopathy is believed to function under some unusual paradoxes. For instance, **potency is believed to be proportional to the degree of dilution.** Preparation therefore involves dilution to minute quantities. The Principle of Similars suggests that symptoms represent the body's attempt to heal itself. Therefore, **the medication must paradoxically cause the symptoms it intends to alleviate.** The homeopath obtains a careful history, with the goal of finding the one medication or combination of medications which will help the body heal its symptoms. Personality, diet (particularly the use of milk products), sleep pattern, reaction to temperature and weather are considered in the assessment and formulation.

   The homeopathic mechanism is controversial and not well understood. Homeopathy has drawn on various disciplines (including quantum theory!) to explain it, but none has proven entirely convincing. The general belief is that since small amounts of crystals can cause lattice changes in water, by the same reasoning, small amounts of medication may cause major changes in disease states.

4. **Dose**
   Varies depending on preparation.

5. **Adverse effects**
   Apparently, side effects are benign, except for the initial worsening of symptoms, which can often result in discontinuation of treatment.

6. **Drug-drug interactions**
   There are no known drug interactions or overdose risk, probably due to the minute quantities of medication used.

7. **Summary**
   Homeopathy has shown promising results in some cases, but further studies are needed. For long-term use of these remedies, many choose to seek assistance from a homeopathic practitioner, in view of the frequent need for combination treatments.

IV. Conclusions and Recommendations for Practitioners

Natural medications are a rapidly growing field in psychopharmacology. Over time, they may prove a valuable addition to the pharmacological armamentarium. **Early research data and anecdotal reports have been promising.** But to recommend them as effective and safe, we need more systematic, controlled studies on adequate patient samples. **Recent studies suggest effectiveness for mild-moderate illness.** In the past few years, the NIH and NIMH have been supporting large-scale studies, and these will hopefully yield more useful guidelines and recommendations for clinicians.

At this time, the best candidates for alternative treatments may include mildly symptomatic patients with a strong interest in natural remedies, and patients who have failed multiple trials of conventional remedies, or who are highly intolerant of side effects. But it is worth noting that this latter group is often the most difficult to treat, and alternative agents seem best suited to the mildly ill.

Physicians should routinely inquire about patients' use of natural medications, as many patients will not volunteer information about their use of these remedies. It is important to emphasize to patients the relatively unproven status of these drugs, and that it is unclear whether natural medications are appropriate or preferable to conventional psychotropics. Special care should be taken with patients on multiple medications, in view of the emerging reports of interactions and toxicity.

Suggested Readings

Alpert, J.E., & Fava, M. (1997). Nutrition and depression: The role of folate. *Nutrition Reviews, 55,* 145–149.

Alpert, J.E., Mischoulon, D., Rubenstein, G.E.F., et al. (2002). Folinic acid (Leucovorin) as an adjunctive treatment for SSRI-refractory depression. *Annals of Clinical Psychiatry, 14*(1), 33–38.

Baldessarini, R.J. (1987). The neuropharmacology of S-adenosyl-L-methionine. *American Journal of Medicine, 83,* 95–103.

Benjamin, J., Agam, G., Levine, J., et al. (1995). Inositol treatment in psychiatry. *Psychopharmacology Bulletin, 31,* 167–175.

Brenner, R., Azbel, V., Madhusoodanan, S., & Pawlowska, M. (2000). Comparison of an extract of hypericum (LI 160) and sertraline in the treatment of depression: A double-blind, randomized pilot study. *Clinical Therapeutics, 22*(4), 411–419.

Chatterjee, S.S., Bhattacharya, S.K., Wonnermann, M., et al. (1998). Hyperforin as a possible antidepressant component of hypericum extracts. *Life Science, 63,* 499–510.

Cohen, A. (1996). Treatment of antidepressant-induced sexual dysfunction: A new scientific study shows benefits of ginkgo biloba. *Healthwatch, 5*(1).

Comas-Diza, L. (1989). Culturally relevant issues and treatment implications for Hispanics. In D.R. Koslow, & E.P. Salett (Eds.), *Crossing cultures in mental health.* Washington, DC: SIETAR International, pp. 31–48.

Coppen, A., & Bailey, J. (2000). Enhancement of the antidepressant action of fluoxetine by folic acid: A randomised, placebo controlled trial. *Journal of Affective Disorders, 60,* 121–130.

Davidson, J.R., Morrison, R.M., Shore, J., et al. (1997). Homeopathic treatment of depression and anxiety. *Alternative Therapies in Health and Medicine, 3,* 46–49.

Eisenberg, D.M., Kessler, R.C., Foster, C., et al. (1993). Unconventional medicine in the United States: Prevalence, costs, and patterns of use. *New England Journal of Medicine, 328,* 246–252.

Eisenberg, D.M. (1997). Advising patients who seek alternative medical therapies. *Annals of Internal Medicine, 127,* 61–69.

Ernst, E. (1998). Harmless herbs? A review of the recent literature. *American Journal of Medicine, 104,* 170–178.

Ernst, E. (2002). St John's Wort supplements endanger the success of organ transplantation. *Archives of Surgery, 137*(3), 316–319.

Farrel, R.J., & Lamb, J. (1990). Herbal remedies. *British Medical Journal, 300,* 47–48.

Fava, M., Borus, J.S., Alpert, J.E., et al. (1997). Folate, B12, and homocysteine in major depressive disorder. *American Journal of Psychiatry, 154,* 426–428.

Furnham, A., & Bhagrath, R. (1993). A comparison of health beliefs and behaviours of clients of orthodox and complementary medicine. *British Journal of Clinical Psychology, 32,* 237–246.

Furnham, A., & Smith, C. (1988). Choosing alternative medicine: A comparison of the beliefs of patients visiting a general practitioner and a homeopath. *Social Science & Medicine, 26,* 685–689.

Hypericum Depression Trial Study Group. (2002). Effect of hypericum perforatum (St. John's Wort) in major depressive disorder. A randomized controlled trial. *Journal of the American Medical Association, 287,* 1807–1814.

Itil, T., & Martorano, D. (1995). Natural substances in psychiatry (Ginkgo biloba in dementia). *Psychopharmacologh Bulletin, 31*(1), 147–158.

Jenike, M.A. (1994). Hypericum: A novel antidepressant. *Journal of Geriatric Psychiatry and Neurology, 7,* S1–S68.

Jonas, W., & Jacobs, J. (1996). *Healing with homeopathy.* New York: Warner.

Kaufeler, R., Meier, B., & Brattstrom, A. (2001). Efficacy and tolerability of Ze 117 St. John's wort extract in comparison with placebo, imipramine and fluoxetine for the treatment of mild to moderate depression according to ICD-10. An overview. *Pharmacopsychiatry, 34*(suppl 1), S49–50.

Kleijnen, J., Knipschild, P., & ter Riet, G. (1991). Clinical trials of homeopathy. *British Medical Journal, 302,* 316–323.

Krippner, S. (1995). A cross cultural comparison of four healing models. *Alternative Therapies in Health and Medicine, 1,* 21–29.

Laakmann, G., Schule, C., Baghai, T., et al. (1998). St. John's Wort in mild to moderate depression: The relevance of hyperforin for the clinical efficacy. *Pharmacopsychiatry, 31*(suppl 1), 54–59.

Leathwood, P.D., & Chauffard, F. (1985). Aqueous extract of valerian reduces latency to fall asleep in man. *Planta Medica, 2,* 144–148.

LeBars, P.L., Katz, M.M., Berman, N., et al. (1997). A placebo-controlled, double-blind, randomized trial of an extract of Ginkgo biloba for dementia. North American EGb Study Group. *Journal of the American Medical Association, 278,* 1327–1332.

Linde, K., Ramirez, G., Mulrow, C.D., et al. (1996). St. John's wort for depression—an overview and meta-analysis of randomized clinical trials. *British Medical Journal, 313,* 253–258.

MacGregor, F.B., Abernethy, V.E., Dahabra, S., et al. (1989). Hepatotoxicity of herbal medicines. *British Medical Journal, 299,* 1156–1157.

Mathews, J.D., Riley, M.D., Fejo, L., et al. (1988). Effects of the heavy usage of kava on physical health: Summary of a pilot survey in an aboriginal community. *Medical Journal of Australia, 148,* 548–555.

Matsumoto, J. (1995). Molecular mechanism of biological responses to homeopathic medicines. *Medical Hypotheses, 45,* 292–296.

Maurer, K., Ihl, R., Dierks, T., & Frolich, L. (1997). Clinical efficacy of Ginkgo biloba special extract EGb 761 in dementia of the Alzheimer type. *Journal of Psychiatric Research, 31,* 645–655.

Mischoulon, D., & Fava, M. (2002). The role of S-adenosyl methionine (SAMe) in the treatment of depression: A review of the evidence. *American Journal of Clinical Nutrition, 76*(5), 1158s–1161s.

Mischoulon, D., & Nierenberg, A.A. (2000). Natural medications in psychiatry. In T.A. Stern, & J.B. Herman (Eds.), *Psychiatry update and board preparation.* New York: McGraw-Hill, pp. 399–408.

Mischoulon, D., & Rosenbaum, J. (Eds.). (2002). *Natural medications for psychiatric disorders: Considering the alternatives.* Philadelphia: Lippincott Williams & Wilkins.

National Institutes of Health Office of Alternative Medicine. (1997). Clinical Practice Guidelines in complementary and alternative medicine. An analysis of opportunities and obstacles. Practice and Policy Guidelines panel. *Archives of Family Medicine, 6,* 149–154.

Nierenberg, A.A. (1998). St. John's Wort: A putative over-the-counter herbal antidepressant. *Journal of Depressive Disorders, Index & Reviews III, 3,* 16–17.

Norton, S.A., & Ruze, P. (1994). Kava dermopathy. *Journal of the American Academy of Dermatology, 31,* 89–97.

Peet, M., Laugharne, J.D., Mellor, J., & Ramchand, C.N. (1996). Essential fatty acid deficiency in erythrocyte membranes from chronic schizophrenic patients, and the clinical effects of dietary supplementation. *Prostaglandins Leukotrienes & Essential Fatty Acids, 55,* 71–75.

Sack, R.L., Hughes, R.J., Edgar, D.M., & Lewy, A.J. (1997). Sleep-promoting effects of melatonin: At what dose, in whom, under what conditions, and by what mechanisms? *Sleep, 20,* 908–915.

Schrader, E. (2000). Equivalence of St John's wort extract (Ze 117) and fluoxetine: A randomized, controlled study in mild-moderate depression. *International Clinics of Psychopharmacology, 15*(2), 61–68.

Schulz, V., Hänsel, R., & Tyler, V.E. (1998). *Rational phytotherapy: A physicians' guide to herbal medicine* (3rd ed.). Berlin: Springer.

Schwartz, G.E., & Russek, L.G. (1997). Dynamical energy systems and modern physics: Fostering the science and spirit of complementary and alternative medicine. *Alternative Therapies in Health and Medicine, 3,* 46–56.

Shelton, R.C., Keller, M.B., Gelenberg, A., et al. (2001). Effectiveness of St John's wort in major depression: A randomized controlled trial. *Journal of the American Medical Association, 285*(15), 1978–1986.

Singh, Y.N. (1992). Kava: An overview. *Journal of Ethnopharmacology, 37,* 13–45.

Spillman, M., & Fava, M. (1996). S-adenosyl-methionine (ademethionine) in psychiatric disorders. *CNS Drugs, 6,* 416–425.

Stoppe, G., Sandholzer, H., Staedt, J., et al. (1996). Prescribing practice with cognition enhancers in outpatient care: Are there differences regarding type of dementia?—Results of a representative survey in lower Saxony, Germany. *Pharmacopsychiatry, 29,* 150–155.

Volz, H.P. (1997). Controlled clinical trials of hypericum extracts in depressed patients—An overview. *Pharmacopsychiatry, 30*(suppl 2), 72–76.

Volz, H.P., & Laux, P. (2000). Potential treatment for subthreshold and mild depression: A comparison of St. John's wort extracts and fluoxetine. *Comprehensive Psychiatry, 41*(2 suppl 1), 133–137.

Wetzel, M.S., Eisenberg, D.M., & Kaptchuk, T.J. (1998). Courses involving complementary and alternative medicine at US medical schools. *Journal of the American Medical Association, 280,* 784–787.

Whitmore, S.M., & Leake, N.B. (1996). Complementary therapies: An adjunct to traditional therapies [letter]. *Nurse Practitioner, 21,* 12–13.

Williams, L.L., Kiecolt-Glaser, J.K., Horrocks, L.A., et al. (1992). Quantitative association between altered plasma esterified omega-6 fatty acid proportions and psychological stress. *Prostaglandins Leukotrienes & Essential Fatty Acids, 47,* 165–170.

CHAPTER 70

Treatment Decisions at the End of Life

SCOTT Y. H. KIM AND ALEXANDRA F. M. CIST

I. Introduction

Modern medicine prolongs the dying process, and this may increase rather than decrease the suffering of a dying patient. Fearing such a fate, a patient may even ask the doctor to actively hasten death.

A. With long-term knowledge of the patient and the patient's family, the primary care physician (PCP) plays an important role in helping the patient make necessary, but difficult, treatment decisions at the end of life.

B. The primary responsibilities of the physician to a terminally ill patient are to optimize palliative care and to assist the patient and the patient's family with the dying process (see Chapter 51).

C. Treatment decisions at the end of life often involve perplexing questions of medical ethics.

II. Definitions

A. **Withholding and withdrawing life-sustaining treatment** are both morally and legally permissible, although withdrawal of interventions is psychologically more difficult. Both practices, when properly done, are widely recognized ways to prevent unnecessary, avoidable suffering in a dying patient.

B. **In physician-assisted suicide,** the physician provides the sufficient means of death (e.g., a large amount of barbiturates) to the patient, who performs the final act (e.g., ingestion). In **voluntary active euthanasia,** a competent, informed, and consenting patient is killed by the direct action of another person. Giving large doses of narcotics to decrease pain or ease dyspnea, even if it shortens life, is not considered euthanasia.

III. Autonomy at the Bedside

The autonomous choice of the patient has become a central concept in medical ethics. For clinical purposes, **an autonomous choice is made when a competent, informed choice expresses the patient's considered preferences.** Because the concept of autonomy has legal origins, it can misleadingly frame the clinical situation as an adversarial one. This mind-set must be resisted. It is crucial to remember that while the choice is made by an individual, **an autonomous choice does not take place in a vacuum; it must be nurtured through a continued thoughtful dialogue involving the patient, the patient's relatives and/or surrogates (when available), and the physician.**

A. Is the patient competent? Does the patient have the cognitive and evaluative capacity to make momentous decisions that may affect him or her irreversibly?

1. **Competency is a legal concept.** The physician in effect assesses whether a patient will be found competent by a court of law. Patients are presumed to be competent. However, if a question of competence arises, especially if a serious medical or ethical question is at stake, the "competency evaluation" should be done by someone with experience in this area.

2. **Loss of competence (i.e., the capacity to make medical decisions) is common in patients with a terminal illness.** While coma and persistent vegetative states obviously render a person incompetent, other organic mental syndromes occur in patients with a severe illness (e.g., dementia in AIDS patients or delirium secondary to medication side effects).

3. **Depression** merits special mention because it is common (though not normal), treatable, and known to cause cognitive deficits and/or distortions that interfere with the capacity to make rational choices.

   a. Among HIV-positive patients, psychological distress (including depression, hopelessness, and suicidal ideation) is a better predictor of a patient's interest in physician-assisted suicide than is physical disability. **A terminally ill patient who desires death is likely to be clinically depressed.**

   b. Diagnosis can be difficult because the neurovegetative signs and symptoms of depression overlap with symptoms of serious medical illness (e.g., problems of sleep and appetite, and fatigue). **Attention should be paid to the symptoms most likely to interfere with a patient's ability to accurately appreciate his or her medical situation:** anhedonia, hopelessness, helplessness, suicidal ideation, worthlessness, and a general lack of mood reactivity to situations or events that should evoke at least a transient alteration in mood. A history of depression or suicidality and a family history of mood disorders aid in the diagnosis.

B. Is the patient adequately informed? While this question usually is included in the competency evaluation, the issue of **whether a patient is adequately informed is only part of the larger issue of the overall quality of communication between the patient and the doctor.** Human communication is a complex affair, especially when it involves asymmetry in power and knowledge between parties in emotionally loaded situations. Less than one-half of terminally ill patients have discussions about prognosis or cardiopulmonary resuscitation (CPR) with their physicians, and most physicians are ignorant of their terminally ill patients' wishes regarding CPR (SUPPORT study, 1995).

1. **All decisions involving medical ethics begin with the best facts available.** The physician initially determines the diagnosis, prognosis, and treatment options. Then the physician must determine the following: **Is the patient's condition reversible? Are the treatment options beneficial or useless and/or harmful?** The goal is to arrive at a judgment based on the best available information; consultation is important.

2. **The most important stage of delivering clinical information is the process of exploration that follows the delivery.** The physician must carefully explore the patient's concerns and questions. **This is best accomplished in a quiet room, while sitting down, at a time specially set aside for this purpose.** Simple, respectful, non-judgmental follow-up questions such as "What do you mean?" and "Can you talk more about what you mean by…?" may be the keys to ensuring that the patient has an adequate understanding of the situation.

3. **The physician should be aware that his or her own feelings about death and dying may influence his or her interpretation of the medical situation** to the patient or the patient's surrogate.
   a. Physicians tend to underestimate their patients' perceptions of quality of life and are poor at predicting preferences regarding resuscitation.
   b. The death of a patient may be felt as a personal failure by the physician.
   c. The common thought "If I were the patient, I'd probably feel that way too" usually is not helpful and, in combination with superficial "respect" for the patient's rights, can lead to premature decisions, in effect abandoning patients to their rights.
4. Initially, denial can be useful for a patient; the physician should wait for the patient's defenses to adapt before taking a more direct approach. Repeated interviews may be necessary.
5. An "informed" patient is not someone to whom "value-neutral" facts have been delivered at a single point in time, but someone who has an ongoing supportive relationship with the doctor. This is important to remember, since clinical situations are fluid and changing.

C. **What is the patient's considered preference?** The patient's stated preference may not represent his or her real and final preference. Arriving at a considered preference may entail clarifying a vague wish, uncovering a hidden preference, aligning with one desire over another in working through an ambivalence, or even forming a new preference. **The focus should be on the meaning of the patient's request.** Two-thirds of Dutch patients who explicitly ask for voluntary euthanasia or physician-assisted suicide eventually change their minds (Table 70-1). Be sensitive to expressions such as "I have no options, no choice . . . I feel trapped. . ." and "I'm at the end of my rope." These are expressions of powerlessness and desperation that may indicate a need to address one or more of the following areas:

1. **Are the patient's symptoms** (e.g., pain, nausea, dyspnea, fatigue, insomnia, constipation) **being aggressively treated?** The SUPPORT study (1995) found that half of the terminally ill patients who died in the hospital were in moderate to severe pain in their last days. The assurance of aggressive palliative care may itself be therapeutic.
2. **Are psychiatric issues being addressed?**
   a. **Depression** must be sought and treated. Even if it does not render a person incompetent, it can color a person's preferences.

Table 70-1. Assessment of Factors Influencing a Patient's Stated Preference

1. Are all symptoms being treated aggressively?
2. Are psychiatric issues being addressed, especially depression, personality styles, and disorders?
3. How is the patient perceiving his or her social supports?
4. What is the patient's world view?
5. Have the patient's stated reasons for wanting to die been explored?
6. Have the dynamics of the patient-doctor relationship been explored?

b. **Anxiety** is common in the terminally ill. The physician must explore a patient's fears of abandonment, anticipated suffering (especially pain), and separation from loved ones.

c. The presence of a **personality disorder** makes the assessment of a patient's considered preferences extraordinarily difficult. A self-destructive person who mistrusts the world may view himself or herself as worthless and see no option but a hastened death; an abused person may re-enact past abuse; a histrionic patient's request to die may be a desperate request for love and care, and a narcissitic patient's fear of dependency may show itself as a need for an unrealistic level of control. When the treatment team is divided or when the patient evokes intense negative emotions in the clinician, the diagnosis of a personality disorder should be considered. Rather than feeling frustrated, angry, resentful, and guilty, the physician can turn those feelings into useful data. Psychiatric consultation is warranted in such cases.

d. Terminal illness often takes away essential features of the patient (e.g., via bodily loss, loss of social roles); the painful working through of this **grieving process** is a sensitive and vulnerable process for the patient.

e. **Substance abuse,** often complicated by concomitant personality disorders, predisposes a patient to being undertreated for pain.

3. **What are the perceived social supports?**

a. Since a terminally ill patient often fears that a prolonged process of dying will place a financial burden on the family, the patient's social network should be evaluated.

b. Determine whether the family dynamics affect the patient's stated preference. Is the patient feeling abandoned and angry? Is the patient concerned about being a burden on the family? Are the family members feeling guilty and therefore requesting overly aggressive treatment?

c. Is there a local disease-specific support group that could provide advice, support, or equipment?

4. **Is the patient's stated preference consistent with a life pattern or a stated world view?** Be respectful of, but do not presume to know without thorough exploration, the patient's cultural values that may be affecting his or her choices.

5. **Is it clear what the patient means by "loss of dignity** . . . intolerable suffering," "being a burden," and other terms which may have a variety of meanings? After a respectful exploration, the physician not only will come to know the patient's value system better, but may discover misconceptions and frustrations which can be addressed.

6. **Attempt to understand the perspective of the patient** and family before addressing their seemingly "unrealistic" concerns, as a way of optimizing realistic hopes and planning for realistic fears.

7. **Are the dynamics of the patient-doctor relationship interfering with decision-making?** Might the patient's seemingly irrational insistence on over-aggressive treatment be based on a lack of trust in the health care system? By contrast, a patient's request for death may represent a request for more attention and caring from the doctor.

IV. Advance Directives

When a terminally ill patient is incompetent, the approach is still one of attempting to preserve the patient's self-determination.

A. An advance directive is a mechanism designed to extend patient autonomy. It documents what should be done when a person becomes incompetent or appoints a surrogate or health care proxy who will judge what the patient would want if the patient were competent **(substituted judgment),** or it may do both.

1. Hospitals are required by federal law (Patient Self-Determination Act of 1991) to ask and inform patients about advance directives.

2. While widely promoted, the use of, and research into, advance directives is still relatively new. Some limitations may exist: An advance directive may not cover enough specific situations, and so translating the directive into specific orders may be difficult. There is poor compliance in both filling out the directive and adhering to it on the part of surrogates and doctors. Finally, it is not clear how well surrogates represent a patient's wishes.

3. Advance directives serve the valuable function of initiating the important dialogue between the patient, the patient's surrogates, and the physician regarding treatment decisions at the end of life. The process of thinking through an advance directive is probably as important as the content of the directive. The discussion regarding advance directives ideally should take place before a life-threatening illness occurs.

4. When advising patients about end-of-life treatment options, physicians unfamiliar with the capabilities and limitations of life-sustaining treatments should consider consultation with a critical care specialist (e.g., consult a specialist for a patient with early amyotropic lateral sclerosis well before respiratory compromise develops).

5. The option of a time-limited therapeutic trial of life-sustaining therapy might be offered, with the understanding that the therapy can be withdrawn if the desired benefits are not achieved.

B. In the absence of a formal advance directive, close relatives and the patient's doctor must combine their best substituted judgment with the patient's best interests. When a patient is alert but incompetent (e.g., in psychotic depression), strong consideration should be given to obtaining **formal guardianship.** This provides stability in decision-making as the patient's clinical condition fluctuates.

V. Premature Requests for Limiting Life-Sustaining Treatment

Sometimes a patient and/or family may request the withdrawal or withholding of life-sustaining or life-saving treatment when in the opinion of the physician the condition of the patient is reversible. **A competent adult has the legal right to refuse treatment even if that decision will lead to harm.** The goal is to ensure a truly autonomous choice, remembering that autonomy is not simply a superficial assessment of "whatever the patient says," but a careful evaluation that occurs in the context of a stable and meaningful doctor-patient relationship (Figs. 70-1 and 70-2).

VI. Physician-Assisted Suicide and Euthanasia

When a patient requests physician-assisted suicide or voluntary active euthanasia, the physician faces one of the most difficult questions in medical ethics.

A. Policy Considerations

1. **Legal issues.** At the time of this writing, only the state of Oregon permits assisted suicide for terminally ill patients. The U.S. Supreme Court has ruled that there is no constitutional right to assisted suicide.

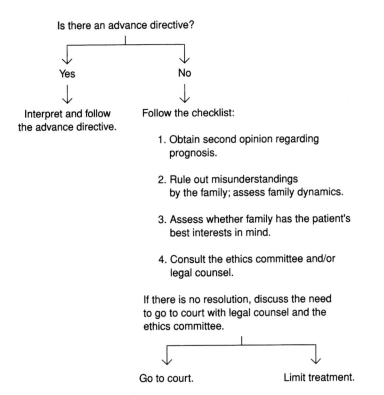

Figure 70-1. When there is a question of premature limitation of life-sustaining treatment in an unconscious patient.

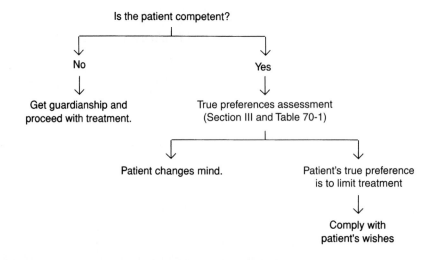

Figure 70-2. When there is a question of premature limitation of life-sustaining treatment in a conscious patient.

> **Table 70-2. Assessment of Requests for Physician-Assisted Suicide and Voluntary Active Euthanasia**
>
> 1. Is there a meaningful doctor-patient relationship?
> 2. Has the wish to die been fully and repeatedly explored over several sessions?
> 3. Have there been adequate consultations to:
>   a. Maximize palliative care
>   b. Address psychiatric issues
> 4. Is the family in agreement with the patient?
>
> SOURCE: Derived from Block, S.D., & Billings, J.A. (1994). Patient requests to hasten death: Evaluation and management in terminal care. *Archives of Internal Medicine, 154,* 2039–2047.

2. **Professional standards.** Most professional physician organizations have issued statements against physician-assisted suicide and voluntary active euthanasia, including the American Medical Association and the American Geriatric Society.

3. It is notable that ethnic minorities, the poor, and the elderly tend to be skeptical about the legalization of these practices.

B. **Palliative Care.** Improving the delivery of comprehensive palliative care should make requests for voluntary euthanasia and physician-assisted suicide extremely rare. **A request for physician-assisted suicide or voluntary active euthanasia should prompt a thorough assessment to discern the patient's truly autonomous wishes** (Table 70-2). Refusing to hasten a patient's death does not constitute abandonment of the patient, but the refusal must be accompanied by redoubled efforts to provide appropriate palliative care, including adequate pain relief. Knowing that a patient desires a hastened death does not justify withholding pain medications for fear of suicide. (See Chapter 51)

VII. Resolving Conflicts about Forgoing Life-Sustaining Treatment

A physician is under no obligation to provide a useless or harmful treatment. However, the meaning of futility is still under debate, and a strictly "medical" definition is difficult to formulate. The law is evolving on this issue. In the Wanglie case in Minnesota, the court sided with a man who stated that it would have been his wife's wish (she was in a persistent vegetative state) to have life-sustaining treatment continued. In the Gilgunn case in Massachusetts, the trial court decided that if a patient were going to die in a short period of time with or without treatment, physicians were not negligent in not offering that treatment.

A. When the patient or family wants "everything done" and the effort will cause more suffering without changing the trajectory of the course of dying, the physician has the obligation to make the situation as clear as possible to the patient and/or surrogates. The apparent impasse usually can be resolved (Table 70-3). The physician should do the following:

1. **Use jargon-free language** and explore any misconceptions the patient and family may have. The physician also should review in specific and concrete terms the patient's course up to that point to reinforce the reality of the situation. Listen carefully

---

Table 70-3. When a Patient or Family Seeks a Futile Intervention: A Checklist

1. Is there true futility?
   a. Obtain consultations from specialists to confirm or revise the prognosis.
   b. Assess the physician's countertransference feelings toward the patient.
2. Honestly assess the working alliance with the patient and/or family.
3. Review the clinical situation with the patient and/or family in jargon-free, concrete terms with appropriate exploratory follow-up questions.
4. Listen carefully to the patient and/or family's telling of "the story" and their values.
5. Assess family dynamics.
6. Obtain an ethics committee consultation with or without legal counsel.

---

to the patient's and/or family's perception of the patient's course and their expectations. A working alliance among the patient, family, and the physician is crucial.

2. **Explore the family dynamics.** The loss of a loved one is paradoxically more difficult for the members of the family who have had a strained (by guilt, suspicion, distance) relationship with the patient.

3. **Deal with countertransference** (i.e., the doctor's feelings toward the patient) issues which may lead the treatment team to conclude prematurely that a treatment is futile. For instance, an active IV drug abuser with endocarditis who has failed to keep a "contract" with doctors to "stay clean" and now needs a valve replacement may erroneously seem to be a "hopeless case" to the treatment team.

4. **Consult with other physicians and the hospital ethics committee when the question of futility arises.**

B. **Rarely, there may be a genuine impasse.** At times, an intervention is deemed futile by the treating team, the consultants, and the hospital ethics committee but the patient or family may desire that treatment.

1. At this point, legal counsel should be sought (if not involved already).

2. A compromise, such as a transfer to another facility, may be considered.

3. An effort should still be made to understand what the impasse is based on (e.g., unusual religious convictions, or unresolvable family dynamics). The way the decision gets made will have a lasting impact on the surviving family members. Thus, every effort should be made to maintain a therapeutic connection and avoid abandonment of the family.

VIII. Final Remarks

A. **A good time to discuss end-of-life treatment decisions with a patient is before the crisis occurs.**

B. Even after big decisions have been made, it is useful to remember the following:

1. It is normal to feel ambivalent; after all, these are often tragic situations.

2. Clinical situations evolve; one must remain open and flexible.

C. It is never inappropriate to seek help from the hospital ethics committee or legal counsel.

D. Good documentation is important.

Suggested Readings

Appelbaum, P.S., & Grisso, T. (1988). Assessing patients' capacities to consent to treatment. *New England Journal of Medicine, 319,* 1635–1638.

Block, S.D., & Billings, J.A. (1994). Patient requests to hasten death: Evaluation and management in terminal care. *Archives of Internal Medicine, 154,* 2039–2047.

Breitbart, W., Rosenfeld, B.D., & Passik, S.D. (1996). Interest in physician-assisted suicide among ambulatory HIV-infected patients. *American Journal of Psychiatry, 153,* 238–242.

Cassem, E.H. (1985). Appropriate treatment limits in advanced cancer. In J.A. Billings (Ed.), *Outpatient management of advanced cancer.* Philadelphia: Lippincott, pp. 139–151.

Chochinov, H.M., Wilson, K.G., Erms, M.E., et al. (1995). Desire for death in the terminally ill. *American Journal of Psychiatry, 152,* 1185–1191.

Council on Scientific Affairs, American Medical Association. (1996). Good care of the dying patient. *Journal of the American Medical Association, 275,* 474–478.

Emanuel, E.J., Fairclough, D., & Emanuel, L.L. (2000). Attitudes and desires related to euthanasia and physician-assisted suicide among terminally ill patients and their caregivers. *Journal of the American Medical Association, 284,* 2460–2468.

Emanuel, L.L., Barry, M.J., Stoelde, J.D., et al. (1991). Advance directive for medical care—a case for greater use. *New England Journal of Medicine, 324,* 889–895.

Groves, J.E. (1978). Taking care of the hateful patient. *New England Journal of Medicine, 298,* 883–887.

King, D., Conwell, Y., & Kim, S. (2000). Family matters: A social systems perspective on physician-assisted suicide and the older adult. *Psychology, Public Policy, and Law, 6,* 434–451.

Lynn, J., & Teno, J.M. (1993). After the Patient Self-Determination Act, the need for empirical research on formal advance directives. *Hastings Center Reports, 23,* 20–24.

Muskin, P.R. (1998). The request to die: Role for a psychodynamic perspective on physician-assisted suicide. *Journal of the American Medical Association, 279,* 323–328.

Paris, J.J., Cassem, E.H., Dec, G.W., & Reardon, F.E. (1999). Use of a DNR order over family objections: The case of *Gilgunn v. MGH. Journal of Intensive Care Medicine, 14,* 41–45.

Rothchild, E. (1998). Family dynamics in decisions to withhold or withdraw treatment. In M.D. Steinberg, & S. Youngner (Eds.), *End-of-life decisions: A psychosocial perspective.* Washington, DC: American Psychiatric Press.

Sullivan, M.D., & Youngner, S.J. (1994). Depression, competence, and the right to refuse lifesaving medical treatment. *American Journal of Psychiatry, 151,* 971–978.

SUPPORT Principal Investigators. (1995). A controlled trial to improve care for seriously ill hospitalized patients: The study to understand prognoses and preferences for outcomes and risks of treatments (SUPPORT). *Journal of the American Medical Association, 274,* 1591–1598.

Truog, R.D., Brett, A.S., & Frader, J. (1992). The problem with futility. *New England Journal of Medicine, 326,* 1560–1564.

Truog, R.D., Cist, A.F.M., Brackett, S.E., et al. (2001). Recommendations for end-of-life care in the intensive care unit: The Ethics Committee of the Society of Critical Care Medicine. *Critical Care Medicine, 29,* 2332–2348.

Van der Maas, P.J., Van Delden, J.J., Pijnenborg, L., et al. (1991). Euthanasia and other medical decisions concerning the end of life. *Lancet, 338,* 669–674.

Quality-of-Life Enhancing Strategies

CHAPTER 71

Encouraging Your Patients to Live Healthier Lives

ANDREW B. LITTMAN

I. Introduction

Enormous advances have been made in technological and pharmacological interventions for chronic diseases. Despite these innovations, **much of the decrease in mortality from these diseases over the past few decades has been due to population-based reductions of major risk factors for chronic disease** (e.g., smoking, hypertension, and elevated serum lipid levels).

A. **Reduction of risk factors** (e.g., by stopping cigarette smoking, lowering cholesterol, treating hypertension, tightening glycemic control in diabetics, increasing physical activity levels, and treating co-morbid psychiatric disorders) improves quality of life and decreases mortality rates.

1. Reduction of serum lipids with pharmacologic trials in both asymptomatic individuals and those with coronary artery disease (CAD) has led to reductions in CAD and overall mortality.

B. **Diagnosis and treatment of co-morbid psychiatric symptoms or disorders** in patients seen in the general medical sector has proven valuable. Treatment of those conditions boosts the capacity of affected individuals to modify their lifestyle and dramatically improve their quality of life.

C. Besides recognition of the benefit of treatment of traditional risk factors and psychiatric co-morbidity, there is abundant data regarding the possible **benefits of various dietary, vitamin, and non-traditional treatments.** A large percentage of our patients seek or currently practice a host of non-traditional treatments.

D. Assessment of patient-created, physician-created, and systemic barriers in assisting patients to **lifestyle change is advised.**

II. What Factors Are Associated with Lifestyle Change?

With clear and explicit recommendations for the need to make a behavior change (e.g., stopping smoking, eating less saturated fat, and increasing physical activity), many patients change. However, over time many individuals are unable to maintain the new and more healthful behavior, and some appear incapable of change.

A. **Clear and understandable information about the health risks of various health behaviors needs to be provided to patients** by their physician. It should be personally, relevantly, and empathetically communicated.

B. **When patients feel vulnerable to the behavioral risk causing illness and are able to change that risk, and when the benefits of the behavioral change are greater than**

its costs, then the motivation to change becomes great enough to induce and to sustain change.

　　1. **Secondary prevention of illness** (i.e., after the disease is already present) with behavior modification is invariably easier to effect than is primary prevention (asymptomatic individuals).

C. **Social support of change** in various settings (e.g., home, work, or other social networks) can either greatly facilitate or hamper behavioral change.

　　1. When changing behaviors, the threat of loss of social support can make the interpersonal costs of behavioral change too great to effect a change.

　　2. Evaluation of co-existing marital, family, or work site conflict needs to be considered when these conflicts appear to stand in the way of lifestyle change.

　　3. Organized programs of behavioral change in medical settings or at work can act as important bridges to provide social support for patients during critical and vulnerable periods of change.

D. Since patients are at different stages in the process of readiness for undertaking behavior change, **strategies for assessing the patient's stage in the process of behavioral change** (Prochaska) are helpful.

　　1. **Precontemplation**—no interest in behavior change, denies impact of behavior on self or health

　　2. **Contemplation**—thinks about changing health behavior, low confidence in ability to change, has fears and concerns about changing

　　3. **Preparation**—preparing to change, is ready for lifestyle intervention with little help

　　4. **Action** has just recently changed health behavior but can return to old behaviors fairly easily (relapse)

　　5. **Maintenance**—has changed health behaviors quite some time ago and is not at major risk for relapse

E. **Assistance should be based on a patient's current stage in the process of change.** Specific examples of the skills required to address the patient's current stage of change and to help them progress to smoking cessation are discussed in Chapter 72.

　　1. **Precontemplators have little or no motivation or desire to change** and deny the impact of the health behavior on their health. Many clinicians have the mistaken belief that those patients should be "passed over" in order to work with more "motivated" patients. In contrast, we have found that these patients can usually be engaged non-judgmentally to discuss the base for their decision. This calm, evenhanded, but firm discussion can move some patients to become contemplators. Those who persist in this mode, especially if it is pervasive in other areas of health behavior and life overall, warrant psychiatric consultation to look for frequently found and treatable underlying causes. Denial of illness, its differential diagnosis, and its treatment are discussed in Chapter 62.

　　2. **Contemplators usually have specific concerns or fears about changing their health behavior that interfere with change.** Detailed discussion of past attempts at change and the alternatives for dealing with difficulties often prepares patients for change. Specific health behavior barriers to successful change are noted in the next paragraph.

　　3. **Preparation to change is health-behavior specific,** although certain features are common. Understanding the principles of behavioral therapy is critical in promoting

lifestyle change for any health behavior. The principles of behavior therapy are discussed in Chapter 9.

    a. Those ready to change should be encouraged to set a specific date for introduction of that change.

    b. Those ready to change with a history of relapse on prior attempts early in the attempt should receive specific skills training in how to deal with the roadblock that interfered with past attempts at change. Treatment recommendations for improving patient compliance are discussed in Chapter 74.

    c. **Those attempting to change should receive a follow-up appointment or phone call at whatever time they have relapsed historically when changing or within the first 2 weeks after changing, whichever is first.**

    d. Those patients with low confidence in their abilities to change, who request specialized treatment or make repeated unsuccessful attempts at change, will benefit from specialized programs to assist in health behavior change. Direct referral to a program with which the physician has regular contact has a greater likelihood of success in making the referral stick (see Chapter 4).

F. Since patients who have taken action and attempted to change their lifestyle are at high risk for relapse in the weeks and months following their behavioral change, **relapse prevention,** the term for an intervention that attempts to block the return to the unhealthy behavior pattern, is crucial.

    1. Debriefing of situations that preceded the return to the unhealthy behavior is discussed and multiple and varied strategies are devised to block the relapse.

        a. Celebration of joyous events can cause individuals to feel that they deserve to relapse.

        b. Acute stressors (e.g., family illnesses or personal emergencies) may also lead to relapse.

    2. **Mindfulness, self-observation, and self-monitoring** can be developed to recognize the emotional, cognitive, and behavioral antecedents (triggers) of unhealthy behaviors and relapse.

    3. **The skills of assertiveness, avoidance, meditation, and role rehearsal are critical** in managing the tendency toward relapse.

    4. Acceptance of the inevitability of situations leading toward relapse is critical so as to be able to contain slips in behavior, instead of a downwards spiral to complete and chronic return of old behaviors. Punitive reactions to the slips from the patient, family, or physician will only lead to further slips. One can learn from the slips about an individual's specific vulnerabilities and attain earlier recognition of the triggers so as to prevent future slips.

G. Those patients who have failed all of the preceding interventions, or who have current psychiatric symptomatology, will benefit from **psychiatric referral** to evaluate psychiatric co-morbidity or other emotional or behavioral causes of inability to change lifestyle. Most of the time, the patient's psychiatric symptomatology will be misunderstood by both the patient, the patient's family, and the primary care physician (PCP) as the patient being stuck, overly negative, indecisive, angry, defensive, or difficult to engage. Characteristically, the presenting features of co-morbid psychiatric conditions involve difficulties in management of a patient's medical conditions for the following reasons.

    1. **Psychiatric conditions are directly detrimental to behavioral change;** one of the symptoms of the untreated or partially treated psychiatric condition is oftentimes the treatment target of the lifestyle change desired. For example, overeating or inactivity

resulting from untreated depressive syndromes requires treatment of the depressive disorder for lasting behavioral change to occur.

2. The sadness, worry, negativism, or impulsivity in patients with various psychiatric co-morbidities can have a negative impact on attempts at behavioral change.

   a. The hopelessness, pessimism, and lack of confidence commonly seen in those with depressive conditions, both major depressive disorder and chronic depressions (e.g., dysthymia), can inhibit motivation to the degree that makes it impossible for patients to expose themselves to and to adopt a new behavioral routine. If an attempt at change can be mustered, any slip or deviation from the plan of change can lead to a crisis of confidence for those with depression and lead to relapse.

   b. The exaggerated worry, indecision, and hypervigilance of patients with the anxiety disorders (e.g., generalized anxiety, panic, obsessive-compulsive, or post-traumatic stress disorder) makes it difficult for patients to commit to a lifestyle modification plan without undue internal and interpersonal struggle.

   c. Impulsivity, irritability, hyperreactivity to stressors, distrust, and post-traumatic stress make it difficult for some patients to commit to and organize lifestyle change.

   d. The relative equanimity and confidence necessary to deal with the inherent slips and relapses in behavioral change are nearly impossible without treatment of impulse control difficulties and anger outbursts.

III. What Are Strategies for Lifestyle Change?

A. Strategies for helping patients quit cigarette smoking are discussed in Chapter 72.

B. Strategies for treating eating disorders, including obesity, and strategies to lose weight are discussed in Chapters 20 and 48.

C. Strategies for helping your patient begin an exercise program are discussed in Chapter 73.

D. Strategies for the treatment of systemic arterial hypertension consist primarily of compliance to the medical regimen, discussed in Chapter 74.

1. The non-pharmacological therapies of weight loss and sodium restriction are strategies effective in significantly lowering blood pressure. Relaxation, stress management, and nutritional supplementation have virtually no impact on hypertension.

E. Strategies for helping your patient to manage mental stress are discussed in Chapter 11.

IV. The Physician's Role in Risk-Factor Reduction

Studies show that physicians perform suboptimally with risk-factor reduction in their patients. Even in areas of risk-factor reduction where there are established national consensus guidelines, many physicians have difficulty adhering to these guidelines. What are the causes for this?

A. Many physicians have never received training and have little experience in behavioral intervention counseling skills. They also believe that they are ineffective in producing behavioral change in their patients.

1. These skills can be taught and their use markedly improves outcomes in behavioral change.

B. Some physicians are more comfortable when vigorously treating patients with acute exacerbations of chronic illnesses than when they are treating patients in a preventive mode.

C. Physicians increasingly wish to integrate risk factor modification into their practices. However, **physicians are increasingly busy and more pressured to be productive, leaving precious little or no time to help patients modify their lifestyle.**

D. Some physicians believe that patients do not wish to be helped to modify their behavior. They believe delving into this arena will drive patients away or induce patient dissatisfaction with their practice.

1. Patients look to their physicians for advice and help about modifying their lifestyles. **Patients view discussion about prevention as evidence of a caring and concerned physician.**

E. Physicians commonly are disheartened and frustrated by attempts to address risk factor reduction in patients because of difficulties dealing with patient's negativism, pessimism, or hopelessness. Understanding those reactions as possible manifestations of frequent psychiatric co-morbidity can help physicians to engage in treating these difficult patients.

F. Physicians are reimbursed for procedures and management of acute illnesses of complex severity at higher levels than they are for cognitive services of a preventive nature. The lack of reimbursement of preventive measures, especially of a non-pharmacological nature, only exacerbates this imbalance.

V. Conclusions

Major systemic barriers are present that block the implementation of lifestyle modification programs to large numbers of patients.

A. It is rare for medical practices to be organized with disease management systems that provide an infrastructure for the integrated management of risk factors for specific medical diagnoses and associated conditions. These systems of care require multidisciplinary teams with collaborative styles of interaction.

1. Recent studies, such as MULTIFIT, demonstrate that an integrated system treatment program for those with established cardiovascular disease can reduce cardiovascular risk factors and slow the progression of atherosclerosis when compared with routine medical care. In addition, the costs for the preventive care were relatively inexpensive when compared with the expensive interventions employed by these patients.

B. Current medical practices are not organized to facilitate behavioral change programs. Training for staff to facilitate behavioral change has not generally occurred. In addition, the environment of the general medical practice is not organized to track these behaviors or deliver this type of care.

C. There is a theoretical and practical opportunity for farsighted managed care organizations to recognize financial savings and improve patient satisfaction associated with integrated systems of treatment of these disorders.

Suggested Readings

DeBusk, R.F., Miller, N.H., Superko, H.R., et al. (1994). A case management system for coronary risk factor modification following acute myocardial infarction. *Annals of Internal Medicine, 120,* 721–729.

Expert panel on detection, evaluation, and treatment of high blood cholesterol in adults. (1993). Summary of the second report of the National Cholesterol Education Program (NCEP) Expert

Panel on detection, evaluation, and treatment of high blood cholesterol in adults (adult treatment panel II). *Journal of the American Medical Association, 268,* 3015–3023.

Littman, A.B. (1993). Prevention of disability due to cardiovascular diseases. *Heart Disease and Stroke, 2,* 274–277.

Milani, R., Littman, A.B., & Lavie, C.J. (1993). Depressive symptoms predict functional improvement following cardiac rehabilitation and exercise program. *Journal of Cardiopulmonary Rehabilitation, 13,* 406–411.

Ockene, I.S., & Ockene, J.K. (1996). Barriers to lifestyle change, and the need to develop an integrated approach to prevention. *Cardiology Clinics, 14*(1), 159–169.

CHAPTER 72
Smoking Cessation Strategies

ANDREW B. LITTMAN

I. Introduction

Cigarette smoking remains the single most preventable cause of death in the United States.

A. Cigarette smoking is responsible for an **increased risk of numerous medical conditions**, including cancers, pulmonary disease, and cardiovascular disorders in smokers. (See Table 72-1.)

B. **Second-hand smoke** puts those individuals exposed at increased risk for respiratory infections, asthma, lung cancer, and coronary artery disease (CAD).

C. Health benefits are evident for individuals of any age who quit smoking.

D. Over the past 30 years, public awareness of the health benefits of stopping smoking has motivated smokers to quit. There has been a major decline in the prevalence of cigarette smoking.

E. Smoking prevention and cessation are still not given a major priority by medical practitioners or the health insurance industry.

F. About half of American smokers have now quit. Among those, the vast majority have stopped smoking on their own with multiple attempts of quitting "cold turkey," with or without tapering their nicotine consumption before quitting.

G. There is currently a much larger proportion of smokers who cannot quit, who continue to smoke heavily, and who are heavily addicted to nicotine. These individuals will probably need intensive interventions to quit smoking.

Table 72-1. Medical Effects of Cigarette Smoking

Cardiovascular disease	Cancers
Coronary artery disease	Lung
Cerebrovascular disease	Larynx
Peripheral vascular disease	Oral cavity
Aortic aneurysm	Esophagus
Chronic obstructive pulmonary disease	Bladder
Peptic ulcer disease	Kidney
Pregnancy complications—low birth weight	

II. Evaluation of Cigarette Smoking Cessation Methods

A. Although most smokers want to quit smoking and know that it is harmful for them to smoke, many quit-attempts fail within two weeks and two-thirds resume smoking within three months.

B. Effectiveness of smoking cessation programs can be evaluated by assessment of 1-year quit rates. **"State of the art" programs achieve 1-year quit rates in the 30–40% range.**

C. The two most common forms of smoking treatment are behavioral counseling therapy and nicotine replacement therapy, although adjunctive psychopharmacologic treatment is gaining in popularity.

    1. **Behavioral counseling therapy** is a cornerstone of treatment in specialized smoking cessation clinic settings. Behavioral therapy is a specific treatment technology that needs to be differentiated from didactic education about smoking because it is a far more effective tool than education alone. **Behavioral treatment involves education, training, support, and practice** in the following practices:

        a. Self-monitoring of cigarette smoking activity.

        b. Identifying the personally relevant emotional, cognitive, and behavioral cues, environmental settings, and external triggers for the urge to smoke.

        c. Anticipating triggers and using alternative strategies to avoid triggers, or if unavoidable, to handle the urges to smoke. Altering habits associated with cigarette use.

        d. Learning skills and techniques to deal with nicotine withdrawal and to prevent relapse after cessation.

        e. Evaluating prolonged or excessive symptomatology during preparation or quit attempts.

    2. **Nicotine replacement therapy** is commonly used for those individuals who demonstrate withdrawal symptoms or who are highly addicted. These agents can treat or minimize withdrawal symptoms. These therapies include use of the following:

        a. Nicotine chewing gum

        b. Transdermal nicotine skin patches

        c. Nicotine nasal spray

        d. Nicotine inhaler

    3. The use of nicotine chewing gum in medical settings is ineffective in improving quit rates. Nicotine chewing gum's use in smoking cessation clinics seems to be effective, owing to access to behavioral therapy, improved instruction about its use, or increased support and compliance. **The nicotine skin patch's use in general medical settings does improve quit rates.**

D. The most effective initial treatment for smoking cessation is the combination of both behavioral and nicotine replacement therapy, especially in those patients who are highly addicted to nicotine.

E. Wellbutrin is effective in smokers whose cravings are neither controlled by, or tolerated by, nicotine replacement and behavioral therapies. Other psychopharmacologic agents are also used to treat co-existent or emergent psychiatric symptoms while quitting smoking.

F. Acupuncture appears to be ineffective as a treatment for smoking cessation.

G. Hypnosis appears to be as effective as behavioral therapy alone.

III. Obstacles to Successful Smoking Cessation

The obstacles commonly observed in the process of smoking cessation include nicotine withdrawal symptoms, dependence on cigarettes to deal with stress and unpleasant feelings, weight gain, and the co-existence or development of co-morbid psychiatric symptoms or syndromes in the quitting process.

A. Nicotine is a powerfully addictive drug, capable of creating tolerance, physical dependence, and withdrawal symptoms.

1. **Withdrawal symptoms** include: craving, irritability, impatience, anger, anxiety, diminished concentration, increased appetite, and diminished sleep.

2. Nicotine withdrawal symptoms begin within an hour of cessation, persist strongly for several days, and still may be present for up to two to three weeks.

3. Nicotine withdrawal symptoms can be treated with nicotine replacement therapy, progressive taper of the number of cigarettes smoked, switching brands to one with a lower nicotine content, psychopharmacologic treatment, or a combination of the four.

4. Persistent or severe nicotine withdrawal symptoms have a broad overlap with psychiatric symptoms or syndromes and may well be better conceptualized and managed as such. This conceptualization is helpful especially if nicotine replacement therapy fails or the patient cannot withdraw after a prolonged period from nicotine replacement therapy without resumption of severe and persistent symptoms.

B. Dependency on cigarettes to cope with stress, anger, anxiety, and depressive feelings is common.

1. Cigarettes can become an automatic crutch to deal with various emotional states that prevents development of more adaptive skills (e.g., recognition of feelings and assertiveness to deal with these feelings).

2. Behavioral therapies designed to deal with ingrained patterns of coping are usually needed.

3. If behavioral therapies are unsuccessful, psychiatric evaluation and treatment, possibly including psychopharmacologic management, is indicated.

C. Weight gain

1. **Weight gain of 5 to 10 pounds is very common in smokers when they quit.**

2. Increased physical activity or an exercise program and attempts at limiting intake may provide some benefit. If there is persistent and large weight gain despite increased activity, psychiatric evaluation and treatment is warranted.

D. Co-morbid psychiatric disorders (mood, anxiety, and substance abuse) are exceedingly common in individuals who have difficulty quitting smoking. **Identification and treatment of these co-morbid psychiatric states have been shown to improve quit rates up to 50%.**

1. Many smokers who have difficulty quitting smoking have a history of depressive disorder or have current depressive symptoms or depressive disorder.

   a. It is typical for a person with a history of depressive disorder who stops smoking to develop a full-blown depressive disorder or depressive symptoms.

      i. **Failure in smoking cessation can be predicted in the first week after stopping by the presence of depressed mood, poor concentration, and persistent cravings.**

   b. **Antidepressant treatment in those smokers with depressive disorder has been shown to improve quit rates to the same level as those who are smoking and not depressed.**

2. Those patients with elevated anxiety or overt anxiety disorder (generalized anxiety disorder, panic disorder, or post-traumatic stress disorder) smoke at a higher rate than the general population. Those with anxiety disorders have a more difficult time quitting smoking when symptoms of their psychiatric condition are present at baseline or flare up during a quit attempt.

    a. Psychopharmacological treatment of anxiety disorders is indicated when highly anxious smokers cannot quit with standard smoking cessation techniques. Treatment may reduce the intensity of withdrawal symptoms.

    b. In smokers with elevated baseline anxiety, buspirone reduces withdrawal symptoms and improves quit rates with smoking cessation attempts.

3. Patients with attention-deficit disorder (ADD) frequently smoke. Nicotine reduces ADD symptoms, and it is common to see exacerbations in these symptoms with smoking cessation.

4. Manic-depressive or bipolar patients not infrequently become symptomatic, either manic or depressed, with smoking cessation.

    a. When working with smokers with bipolar disorder, advise patients to monitor their mood carefully. If prior quitting attempts have produced mood instability, recommend maximization of an anti-manic drug prophylactic regimen.

5. Substance abuse of other addictive drugs (e.g., alcohol, marijuana, stimulants, cocaine, or opiates) needs to be treated before attempting smoking cessation.

6. Patients with psychotic illnesses (e.g., schizophrenia) have great difficulty quitting smoking. Use of atypical antipsychotic drugs in the treatment of their psychotic symptoms has sometimes reduced the intensity of the smoking.

IV. Practical Treatment Strategies in the General Medical Setting

A. Ask all your patients if they smoke. Adopt a policy to determine smoking status at every patient encounter.

1. Besides routine outpatient visits, medical crises or inpatient hospitalizations may offer a "Golden Opportunity" to motivate quit attempts.

B. Advise your patients to stop smoking.

1. Personalize this concern based on your knowledge of the patient's life situation and health concerns and status. This approach will maximize the perception of overall benefits of smoking cessation to the patient.

C. Determine your patient's readiness to quit with Prochaska's stages of smoking cessation.

1. Precontemplation—no interest in cessation, denies impact of smoking
2. Contemplation—thinks about quitting, low confidence, has fears and concerns about quitting
3. Preparation—preparing to quit, is ready for smoking cessation intervention with little help
4. Action—has just recently quit smoking but can return to smoking fairly easily
5. Maintenance—has quit smoking quite some time ago and is not at major risk for relapse

D. Help your patients quit based on the individual patient's current stage of the quitting process.

1. Those precontemplators with little or no motivation or desire to quit and with denial of the impact of smoking on their health can usually be engaged non-judgmentally to

discuss the basis for their decision. This calm, evenhanded, but firm discussion can move some smokers to become contemplators. Those who persist in this mode, especially if it is pervasive in other areas of health behavior and life overall, warrant psychiatric consultation to look for frequently found underlying causes.

2. Contemplators usually have specific concerns or fears about quitting that stand in the way of quitting (see Obstacles to Successful Smoking Cessation). Detailed discussion of past quit attempts and the alternatives for dealing with these difficulties commonly move smokers to be ready to prepare to quit.

3. Preparation to quit involves several different pathways.

   a. Those smokers ready to try a quit attempt should be encouraged to set a quit date.

   b. Those smokers ready to try to quit with a history of relapse on prior quit attempts due to withdrawal symptoms in the first 3 weeks of the quit attempt should receive nicotine replacement therapy in addition to setting a quit date.

   c. **Those smokers who attempt to quit within the general medical setting should receive a follow-up appointment at whatever time they have relapsed historically when quitting or within the first two weeks after quitting, whichever is first.**

   d. Those smokers with low confidence in their abilities to quit, requesting specialized smoking cessation treatment, having symptoms after quitting that make relapse very likely, or making repeated unsuccessful attempts at quitting will benefit from a specialized smoking cessation program with behavioral group therapy and nicotine replacement therapy as needed.

   e. Those smokers who have failed all the preceding (a through d) steps or have current psychiatric symptomatology will benefit from psychiatric referral to treat cravings, severe withdrawal symptoms, low confidence, or overt co-morbid psychiatric disorders.

4. Those who have quit but are still at high risk for relapse in the first few months after stopping smoking benefit from follow-up to assess the development of treatable persistent symptoms (e.g., depressive symptoms, anxiety, irritability, or sleeplessness) whose improvement would reduce the risk of relapse.

V. Pharmacological Treatment Strategies

A. **Transdermal nicotine patches** can be used to relieve nicotine withdrawal symptoms.

   1. **Side effects**

      a. Skin irritation treated by rotation of patch sites.

      b. If the patient becomes allergic to the adhesive in the patch, switching patches to another adhesive system is advisable.

      c. Nicotine toxicity is rare but easily treated by removing the patch and using a lower-dose patch.

      d. If vivid nocturnal dreams, insomnia, and nervousness occur, they can be treated by removing the 24-hour patches (Habitrol, Nicoderm, Pro-Step) at bedtime or using the 16-hour patch (Nicotrol), which is removed before bedtime.

   2. **Initiation of therapy**

      a. The strongest-dose patch is begun at the time of smoking cessation, except for smokers who have stable CAD, weigh less than 120 pounds, or are not highly addicted to nicotine (smoke less than 12 cigarettes a day or less than a pack of low-nicotine cigarettes). These smokers begin on the medium- or intermediate-strength patch.

      b. Those smokers with unstable CAD should not use the patch. Smokers should not continue to smoke on the patch.

      c. The first strength of patch should be used typically for 4 to 8 weeks and the remaining lower-dose patches should be tapered every 2 to 4 weeks.

B. Nicotine chewing gum can also be used to relieve nicotine withdrawal symptoms.

   1. **Side effects**

      a. Nicotine toxicity can occur with inappropriate chewing technique. These symptoms include dyspepsia, hiccups, and dizziness.

      b. Nicotine chewing gum can cause jaw pain or loosen caps or other dental work.

   2. **Initiation of therapy**

      a. Patients need specific instruction on the use of nicotine chewing gum. With chewing of the gum, a peppery taste occurs, signifying nicotine release. At that point, the gum needs to be "parked" between the gums and the lips until the taste disappears and rechewed for up to 40 minutes per piece. Use of coffee or other acidic drinks may neutralize nicotine absorption.

      b. Nicotine chewing gum comes as Nicorette (2 mg per piece) or Nicorette DS (4 mg per piece). Double-strength gum is rarely used except for exceptionally addicted smokers. Nicorette is used initially at 8 to 12 pieces per day with a maximum of 20 pieces per day. It is used on a regular schedule (every half an hour) or as needed for cravings, depending on the intensity and frequency of the withdrawal symptoms and the ability of the smoker to anticipate the craving before smoking.

      c. In specialized treatment settings, nicotine chewing gum is being used in exceptionally addicted patients in conjunction with the transdermal nicotine patch.

      d. Nicotine chewing gum is tapered as feasible but used for periods up to 6 months. If tapering of nicotine chewing gum becomes difficult, consultation for behavioral therapy or psychopharmacological management is indicated.

C. Nicotine inhalers are very effective for highly addicted smokers. It appears that its progressively smaller peak inhalation dose when using an individual cartridge appears to subtly auto-taper those smokers most addicted to nicotine.

D. Nicotine nasal spray is highly effective for highly addicted smokers. After cessation is achieved, switch nicotine replacement to the nicotine inhaler, patch, or gum as tolerated.

E. Psychopharmacological treatments may be considered for those patients who have failed self-help, nicotine replacement, and behavioral therapy. They may also be indicated for those smokers who have certain symptoms or syndromes (anxiety, depression, sleep disturbance, or irritability) noted while smoking or during the cessation process. These interventions may be best begun after initial psychiatric consultation by those physicians with little or no experience using these agents.

   1. **Selective serotonin reuptake inhibitors** are antidepressants that are useful in those smokers who have baseline major depression or dysthymia, or who develop these symptoms with quit attempts. (See Chapter 14).

   2. **Buspirone,** a non-addictive serotonergic antianxiety agent, is useful in treating those smokers with anxiety, irritability, restlessness, and sadness while smoking or during withdrawal. Those smokers with elevated anxiety at baseline had significant improvement in quit rates with the addition of buspirone therapy.

      a. Initial dosages are 5 mg three times a day, and they can be raised weekly by 5 mg per dose up to 20 mg three times a day.

      b. Side effects include complaints of dizziness 30 minutes after a dose at the higher dosages. Taking the pill with food can usually eliminate this side effect.

      c. Buspirone is used for 6 months to a year after smoking cessation and then tapered in the same manner that it was started.

3. Bupropion (Wellbutrin XL) is a unique antidepressant that has recently been shown effective in helping intractable smokers who do not have a co-morbid psychiatric illness to quit smoking. It appears to help smokers who have had difficulties with excessive cravings.

   a. Side effects are sleep disturbance, agitation, drinking alcohol excessively, and an increased risk for seizure disorder. Those patients at increased risk for seizure or who have a seizure disorder should not take bupropion.

   b. Initiate therapy with Wellbutrin XL. It is available in two strengths, 150 mg and 300 mg, to allow for dosing flexibility. The usual target dose is 300 mg given once daily—initiated at 150 mg/day and then increased to 300 mg/day as early as day four, if adequately tolerated. The maximum total daily dose of Wellbutrin XL is 450 mg.

   c. Therapy should be continued for around 1 year.

Suggested Readings

Covey, L.S., Glassman, A.S., & Stetner, F. (1990). Depression and depressive symptoms in smoking cessation. *Comprehensive Psychiatry, 31,* 350–354.

Glassman, A.S. (1993). Cigarette smoking: Implications for psychiatric illness. *American Journal of Psychiatry, 150,* 546–553.

Littman, A. (1993). Review of psychosomatic aspects of cardiovascular disease. *Psychotherapy and Psychosomatics, 60,* 148–167.

Manley, M.W., Epps, R.P., & Glynn, T.J. (1992). The clinician's role in promoting smoking cessation among clinic patients. *Medical Clinics of North America, 76,* 477–494.

Prochaska, J.O., DiClemente, C.C., Norcross, I.C. (1992). In search of how people change: Applications to addictive behavior. *American Journal of Psychiatry, 47,* 1102–1114.

Rigotti, N., & Pasternak, R. (1996). Cigarette smoking and coronary heart disease—risks and management. *Cardiology Clinics, 14*(1), 51–68.

CHAPTER 73

Useful Exercise Programs and Strategies for Weight Loss

M. CORNELIA CREMENS AND PAUL M. COPELAND

I. Introduction

Only about **20% of Americans exercise at a level recommended for cardiorespiratory fitness, 40% exercise at a level less than that recommended for fitness, and the remaining 40% are sedentary.** Of those over the age of 65, 30% exercise; fewer than 10% of them exercise vigorously.

A reasonable question to ask is, What is the ideal or desirable weight for an individual patient? The average body weight for a given population has changed over time and it varies according to age and height, and from country to country. Although the problem of obesity and the need to lose weight differ within various cultures and societies, **obesity is and has been an ever-increasing problem in affluent Western societies; it carries with it increased medical consequences. Obesity increases the risk of coronary artery disease (CAD), cerebrovascular disease, diabetes, hypertension, degenerative arthritis, menstrual irregularities, infertility, gallbladder disease, sleep apnea, as well as cancers of the ovary, breast, endometrium, and prostate.**

II. Establishing the Ideal Weight for each Patient

Determining the ideal weight for each patient requires a complete physical evaluation of the patient and assessment of medical considerations for weight loss. (See Chapter 48: The Obese Patient.) In certain cases a full psychiatric evaluation may be indicated to eliminate any complicating psychiatric issues that may underlie the problem of obesity. Patients may assume they are overweight and request assistance in losing weight when actually they are well within the guidelines of the U.S. Department of Agriculture and the Department of Health and Human Services' new unisex weight guidelines (Table 73-1).

A. Recommended Weight Guidelines Using Body Mass Index
   Within these guidelines at each height the recommended weight translates into a body mass index (BMI) of about 19 to 25 (18.9 to 24.9) for all heights, sexes, and ages. BMI is computed by multiplying the weight in pounds by 700 and dividing the result by the square of the height in inches (Table 73-2). For example, the BMI for a person 5 feet 10 inches tall who weighs 150 pounds is calculated **as follows:**

$$150 \text{ lbs} \times 700 = 105,000$$
$$70 \text{ inches} \times 70 \text{ inches} = 4,900$$
$$105,000 \ / \ 4,900 = 21.4$$
$$21.4 = \text{BMI}$$

Table 73-1. Weight Guidelines of the U.S. Department of Agriculture and the Department of Health and Human Services

Height (without shoes)		Weight (in pounds without clothes)
Feet	Inches	
4	10	91–119
4	11	94–124
5	0	97–128
5	1	101–132
5	2	104–137
5	3	107–141
5	4	111–146
5	5	114–150
5	6	118–155
5	7	121–160
5	8	125–164
5	9	129–169
5	10	132–174
5	11	136–179
6	0	140–184

B. Extent of the Need to Lose Weight

Determining the ideal weight for a given patient requires calculation of the BMI and assessment of the patient so that an appropriate exercise program can be tailored. The BMI provides the patient and physician with clear guidelines for goals to be set and progress monitored. Recent revisions of the weight guidelines reveal that weights at the lower end of the scale are recommended for those with a low ratio of muscle and bone to fat; those at the upper end are for patients with more muscular physiques (Table 73-2). Therefore, individuals who are not well-conditioned athletes fall in the lower ratio of muscle and bone to fat category, and should aim for a weight at the lower end of the scale. **Current research suggests that health problems related to obesity climb when the BMI exceeds 25.** While health problems increase with a BMI greater than 25, **improvements in health status can be achieved with smaller reductions in**

Table 73-2. Calculation of Body Mass Index

$$\frac{\text{Weight in pounds} \times 700}{\text{Height in inches squared}} = \text{Body Mass Index (BMI)}$$

Body Mass Indexes of 18.9–24.9 are ideal.

overweight. The results of the Diabetes Prevention Program showed that a decrease of 7% in body weight, achieved through a combination of diet and exercise, significantly reduced risk of diabetes. Furthermore, exercise has been shown to improve diabetic control even without a demonstrable change in body mass index.

III. Assessment for Exercise Prescription

Adoption of a healthier lifestyle starts with a regular exercise program that the patient can live with for the rest of his or her life. A detailed assessment of prior habits and medical history should be established initially. It is best that one does not fixate on the numbers on the scales; use them as guidelines to encourage the patient to adopt an achievable lifestyle that improves his or her health over the long term. Increasing exercise and decreasing fat intake can lower the risk of poor health without leading to the loss of a single pound. Therefore, **incorporating a combination of exercise, diet, and behavioral modification is ideal.**

A. Prior Habits

A full inventory of the patient's prior physical activity, physical health, mental health, functional status, nutritional assessment, medications, and weight changes over the years should be established.

1. **Physical Activity Assessment**
   a. Consider the type of physical activity the patient has enjoyed in the past.
      i. **The exercise program must be compatible with the patient's lifestyle and capability.**
      ii. **Activity must be readily accessible in the beginning.**
   b. **Advocate walking at first** to build up stamina and avoid injury. Patients may begin walking in their neighborhood or at the local mall. Malls are environmentally controlled, thereby eliminating the frequent excuse of rain, snow, or uncomfortable temperatures (e.g., too hot or cold).

2. **Nutritional Assessment**
   Begin with a detailed evaluation of daily eating habits. This enables the physician to educate, counsel, and motivate the patient to make positive changes in lifestyle. Having the patient keep a log of his or her diet for at least 2 weeks and reviewing it briefly helps identify areas where change can be initiated.
   a. **Weight Changes**
      i. **Determine if obesity began in childhood or is adult in onset** (i.e., is this a chronic or recent problem?).
      ii. **Determine if weight has fluctuated** over the past months or years.
      iii. **Identify patterns of weight gain and weight loss.**
      iv. **Rule out underlying psychiatric illness that contributes to weight changes.**
   b. **Eating Habits**
      i. **Review the patient's dietary log,** which outlines current eating habits.
      ii. Encourage regular meals and a balanced diet, instead of sporadic bingeing after periods of abstinence.
      iii. Review nutritious choices and healthy eating patterns to eliminate patterns of eating when emotionally aroused (e.g., happy, sad, angry, anxious, or frustrated).

B. Medical History

Important aspects of any exercise or weight loss program begin with a thorough medical history and physical examination. Medical conditions, such as hypothyroidism, Cushing syndrome, or polycystic ovary syndrome, which can contribute to obesity, should be considered. Regular exercise, with the goal of attaining a physiological adaptation known as the training or conditioning effect, is safe and beneficial for most healthy patients and patients with significant medical problems (e.g., myocardial infarction). The basic principles of exercise training apply to both medically ill and healthy patients alike.

1. **Conduct a general physical examination** that includes preventative screening testing.
2. **Assess mental or cognitive status.**
   a. Psychiatric illness can interfere with diet, nutrition, and patterns of exercise. For example, weight loss and fatigue may be prominent with depression and limit one's ability to exercise. Bulimia nervosa may engender the use of physical exercise as a compensatory behavior for binge eating and should be recognized prior to giving an exercise prescription. Binge-eating disorder, likewise, should be directly addressed with a view toward specific treatment.
   b. Dementia, delirium, organic brain syndromes, history of head trauma, hypothalamic injury, and other disorders associated with cognitive impairments can lead to excessive weight gain or weight loss. The etiology of these weight variations are not well understood, but has been thought to involve the area of the brain, "the appestat," that inhibits the patient's ability to control eating habits or results in an apathetic response to a food stimulus.
3. **Assess functional status.**
   a. Outline barriers to physical exercise (e.g., chronic disabilities).
4. **Review the use of medications.**
   a. Review all medications, including over-the-counter medications, and medications that may compromise performance (by causing dehydration or reduced stamina) or promote weight gain, such as, olanzapine.
   b. Review the use of non-medicinal drugs and substances, such as caffeine, nicotine, alcohol, homeopathic remedies, and various recreational substances (e.g., marijuana, cocaine, and amphetamines).
   c. Caution patients about using large doses of supplements or megavitamins to enhance performance.
   d. Answer questions regarding the use of anabolic steroids; these should be discussed early in the treatment.
5. **Determine socioeconomic status and living arrangements.**
   a. Factor in the extent of time involved in a nutritional and exercise program so that compliance and motivation can be enhanced.
   b. Prescribe a form of exercise that considers the economic impact on the patient.

IV. Exercise Program

The amount of activity or exercise is more important than the type, duration, or intensity of exercise. Getting started is the most difficult phase of exercise training (refer to section on motivation). Initiation of a walking program is simple, inexpensive, and safe; all one needs to begin is a good pair of walking shoes. Reasonable goals should be established that will ensure the continuance of the activity.

A. **Gauging/Determining an Appropriate Level of Exercise**
   If the goal is to lose weight, the prescription is simple: burn more calories than you consume. Aerobic exercise provides the energy to burn calories. The following three methods measure aerobic capacity. Measurement of the target heart rate is the

most practical. Exercising at a lower intensity for a longer period of time is as beneficial as exercising at a higher intensity for a shorter period of time. In general, the former is better for most people because it is less likely to result in injury or discomfort.

1. **Target Heart Rate** (see Table 73-3)
   a. Calculation of a target heart rate (THR) is simple.

$$220 - age \times 0.6 = minimum\ THR$$
$$220 - age \times 0.9 = maximum\ THR$$

   These two calculations gauge where the heart rate should remain while exercising to ascertain if the patient is pushing the limits of exercising or not exercising hard enough. The range should be between the minimum THR and the maximum THR. If one is below the minimum THR the patient is not exercising hard enough, but if above the maximum THR the patient is exercising too hard. Neither too low nor too high a heart rate is beneficial. The impact of medications that affect heart rate, e.g., beta-blockers, needs to be taken into consideration.
   b. Balancing the THR in this mid-range allows for the maximum benefit from a workout session. The trick is to make the heart work hard enough but not too hard.
      i. For example, a 40-year-old patient's goal would be to maintain a heart rate of 108 to 162 beats per minute.
      ii. Measuring the heart rate does not disrupt the exercise routine. One stops exercising, immediately measures the pulse for 10 seconds, and multiplies by six.
2. **Metabolic Equivalents (METs)**
   One MET is the amount of oxygen consumed at rest by the body (3.5 mL/kg/min); 1 MET burns about 1 kcal/min. **Moderate physical activity is defined as any activity performed at an intensity of three to six METs.** Many tables are available that list the METs related to various activities or exercises.
3. **Maximal oxygen uptake** (VO_2 max) is the amount of oxygen used during maximal exercise. The higher the amount of oxygen used during exercise the greater the exercise capacity. Regular exercise may slow the rate of decline of many physiological parameters in addition to the VO_2 max. Studies have noted a greater decline in oxygen capacity in sedentary older people than in those who are physically active. Decreased oxygen delivery leads to anaerobic work, and anaerobic metabolism increases fatigue.

Table 73-3. Target Heart Rates

Age (years)	Heart Rates (beats/minute)	
	Minimum	Maximal
20–29	115–120	172–180
30–39	109–114	163–171
40–49	103–108	154–162
50–59	97–102	145–153
60–69	91–96	136–144
70–79	90–94	127–135
80+	84	126

V. Designing the Exercise Program

Recent adult fitness recommendations include incorporation of a balanced program of both endurance and strength-training exercises performed on a regular schedule (i.e., at least three times per week). Exercise should be interesting, fun, easily accessible, vigorous, and not painful if it is to become habitual.

A. Endurance Training (cardiovascular or aerobic)
1. Endurance training
   a. **Involves exercise of large muscle groups, with many repetitions, at a low level of resistance.**
   b. Varies the intensity; it should be monitored using the THR (refer to Table 73-4).
   c. Involves exercise 3 to 7 days per week, beginning slowly.
   d. Involves 20 to 60 minutes per session, ultimately.
      i. Start with 5- to 10-minute sessions to build stamina and avoid injury.
      ii. Progress slowly to avoid injury, but it is essential to increase and push to gain maximal benefit.

B. Resistance Training
1. **Strength training or weight-lifting involves the repetitive contraction of muscle groups against resistance.** One begins with a few repetitions against a limited resistance and increases slowly. The training effect is determined by the amount of resistance, not the type.

Table 73-4. Beginning an Exercise Program

1. **Medical examination** by primary care physician
2. **Review with a physician** the following:
   prescribed medications
   type of exercise
   frequency, intensity, and duration of exercise
3. **Reassess progress** with a physician and/or trainer.
4. Increase by 10% approximately every 3–6 months.
5. **Begin slowly.**
   warm–up for 5–10 minutes
   exercise (conditioning) for 20–60 minutes
   cool–down for 10 minutes
6. **Exercise at least three times per week**
   (there is no added benefit noted if one exercises > five times per week)
7. **Exercise for 20 minutes to start (usually) increase by increments of 10 minutes up to 60 minutes per session**
8. **Dress appropriately,** with supportive shoes and loose clothing.
9. **Increase fluids for rehydration** after physical activity.
10. **Maintain a healthy balanced diet** while exercising.

C. Exercise Prescription

An exercise prescription begins with the identified activity that best suits the individual. Walking programs, especially brisk walking, are of great overall benefit.

1. **Know the basics.** Encourage patients to warm up and cool down, and stretch each time they exercise. This promotes safer, more enjoyable exercise.
   a. **Warm-up exercises** increase blood flow to muscles and joints.
   b. **Cool down** maintains venous return and cardiac output, prevents hypotension, and reduces lactate accumulation, which can lead to muscle soreness and stiffness.
   c. **Nutritional balance** increases in importance owing to increased energy expenditure with increased activity. The impact of medications that affect heart rate, e.g., beta-blockers, needs to be taken into consideration.
   d. **Ensure an adequate diet** to maintain energy and fuel for increased activity.
   e. **Ensure that hydration is maintained** to minimize hypotension and increase the excretion of metabolic acids and waste products.
2. **Determine the type of exercise. A combination of endurance or aerobic exercise and resistance exercise is optimum,** balancing both within a weekly schedule. One should choose an initial aerobic exercise with low impact (e.g., walking, cycling, stair climbing, or dancing). With regard to resistance training, weight may consist of body weight initially, as the weight of an arm or leg, and then increase to include weights or resistance bands.
   a. **The exercise activity should be tailored to the individual patient.**
      i. Ask about prior enjoyable or interesting activities.
      ii. **Begin with reasonable goals and avoid overtaxing muscles.**
3. **Choose the intensity of the exercise activity.**
   a. The vigor with which an individual exercises is reflected in the heart rate, both maximal THR and resting heart rate.
   b. Set a level of exercise that requires more effort than normal activity (usually at 60–70% of predicted maximal oxygen uptake).
4. **Establish the duration** of time exercising so that it is inversely related to the intensity of the exercise. Begin slowly, at times only 5 minutes per day, and increase steadily up to 30 to 60 minutes per day.
5. **Assure that the frequency of the exercise program ranges from 3 to 7 days per week.**
   a. Begin with 3 days per week and increase slowly to enhance endurance.
   b. Perform resistance training less frequently, starting at 2 days per week per muscle group; training of the same muscle group should not take place 2 days in a row.
6. **Increase the exercise** (endurance and strength) **slowly,** but encourage the patient to push ahead consistently.
   a. **A training or conditioning effect** occurs when a lower rate of glycogen is consumed and fat is used as an energy source.
   b. Increasing the intensity of exercise too fast in patients beginning a new program will increase anaerobic metabolism and the concentration of blood and muscle lactate.

VI. Motivation

Motivation of patients to exercise and lose weight often begins with the primary care physician (PCP). Educating and encouraging the patient to begin a program of improved nutrition and increased activity sets the stage for success. It is important that goals be congruent with those needed to achieve improvement in medical co-morbidities and remain realistic for the patient. **Consistent follow-up and positive reinforcement engages the patient;** eventually the patient will recognize the benefits of exercise. However, this intellectual emphasis is rarely enough to mobilize the patient.

A. Underlying depression, dementia, or other psychiatric conditions can further impair interest in improved nutrition and in regular exercise programs.

    1. Aggressive treatment of psychiatric illness and reversible causes of dementia may be essential to activate a sedentary patient.

B. Group activities engage patients in a more social form of exercise, allowing patients to have more fun while exercising and to improve their diet.

    1. Group exercise often involves a greater commitment, with the added peer pressure of group members encouraging each other to maintain their goals.

        a. Groups assist patients to participate in regular exercise.

        b. Groups provide a format for reinforcement of behavioral modifications regarding diet and exercise.

    2. Meetings with peers and influential role models may enhance the incentive seeded by the PCP.

    3. A formal referral to a behavioral therapist may be indicated in patients more refractory to treatment.

C. Patients may request **medications to lose weight.** Often patients who feel they do not have either discipline or motivation request medications. However, although medications are not a first-line treatment for weight loss, they are indicated for patients with morbid obesity.

VII. Strategies to Encourage Participation

Strategies need to be developed to help patients initiate and maintain a regular program of exercise and dietary control. One should first schedule an appointment dedicated to an assessment of the issue to determine an appropriate type of exercise and diet suited to the individual patient. Patients who are having fun, performing well, and minimizing their risk of injury are likely to continue their program of exercise and remain active and fit.

Suggested Readings

American College of Sports Medicine. (1990). The recommended quantity and quality of exercise for developing and maintaining cardiorespiratory and muscular fitness in healthy adults. *Medical Science and Sports Exercise, 22,* 265–274.

Boule, N.G., Haddad, E., Kenny, G.P., et al. (2001). Effects of exercise on glycemic control and body mass in type 2 diabetes mellitus. A meta-analysis of controlled clinical trials. *Journal of the American Medical Association, 286,* 1218–1227.

Centers of Disease Control and Prevention. (1996). Prevalence of physical inactivity during leisure time among overweight persons. *Journal of the American Medical Association, 275,* 905.

Chakravarthy, M.V., Joyner, M.J., & Booth, F.W. (2002). An obligation for primary care physicians to prescribe physical activity to sedentary patients to reduce the risk of chronic health conditions. *Mayo Clinic Proceedings, 77,* 165–173.

Fiatarone, M.A., O'Neill, E.F., Ryan, N.D., et al. (1994). Exercise training and nutritional supplementation for physical frailty in very elderly people. *New England Journal of Medicine, 330,* 1769–1775.

Haennel, R.G., & Lemire, F. (2002). Physical activity to prevent cardiovascular disease. How much is enough? *Canadian Family Physician, 48,* 65–71.

Knowler, W.D., Barrett-Conner, E., Fowler, S.E., et al. (2002). Diabetes Prevention Program Research Group: Reduction in the incidence of type 2 diabetes with lifestyle intervention or metformin. *New England Journal of Medicine, 346,* 393–403.

Lee, I., Hsieh, C., & Paffenberger, R.S. (1995). Exercise intensity and longevity in men. *Journal of the American Medical Association, 273,* 1179–1184.

Manson, J.E., Willett, W.C., Stampfer, M.J., et al. (1995). Body weight and mortality among women. *New England Journal of Medicine, 333,* 677–685.

Whelton, S.P., Chin, A., Xin, X., & He, J. (2002). Effect of aerobic exercise on blood pressure: A meta-analysis of randomized, controlled trials. *Annals of Internal Medicine, 136,* 493–503.

SECTION VII

Physician-Assistance Strategies

CHAPTER 74

Enhancing Patient Compliance with Treatment Recommendations

CHRISTINE GALARDY AND JOHN B. HERMAN

"The first barrier to bioavailability is compliance"
Ross Baldessarini, M.D.

I. Introduction

A. Definition

1. **Throughout the history of medicine, compliance has generally been defined as the extent to which the patient's behavior coincides with medical or health advice.** Compliance has been a key element of the doctor-patient relationship.

2. To many practitioners, the term compliant has implied that the patient is passive in the treatment of his or her illness; any deviation from the recommendations of the treating members of the medical team has been perceived as negative.

3. The more recent trend, however, has been to appreciate that collaborative efforts between physician and the patient are essential to optimize health care; the ultimate decision-making powers lie in the hands of the patient.

4. **Efforts are ongoing to replace the word compliant with more accurate descriptors, such as adherent or concordant.** In this chapter we will primarily use the traditional term, compliant, and its correlate, compliance.

B. Poor Compliance is Common

1. The non-attendance rate for patients with scheduled medical appointments is approximately 19–28%.

2. Hospital re-admissions result from a deviation from medical recommendations 5–40% of the time.

3. Medication doses are delayed or omitted by 30–50% of patients.

4. Only 50% of patients with chronic diseases take their medications as prescribed.

5. Treatment for depression is completed by only two-thirds of patients.

6. Prescriptions go unfilled within 1 month of their issue by 20% of patients.

7. Up to 80% of patients can be expected to deviate from medical treatment regime.

C. Reasons for Reluctance are Understandable

1. **Often patients require more detailed information regarding the condition for which they are being treated** and their disease process; moreover, the treatment goals and their expectations for achieving them need to be explored.

2. Deviation from recommendations can be considered intentional when the patient's decision is a conscious, well-considered choice that incorporates not only the biology of the condition being treated, but also contributing psychosocial factors. Optimally, this choice is made after a dialogue with the clinician; therefore, the behavior is not literally "non-compliant."

3. **Non-compliance is often an act of independence to regain control** of a condition that can at times appear to be beyond one's control.

II. The Adverse Impact of Non-Compliance

A. Non-Compliance Hurts Patients
1. Sub-optimal doses of medications may lead to increased morbidity.
2. Persistent symptoms due to non-compliance often result in unnecessary diagnostic tests and procedures.
3. Frustration with a patient's condition or with the medical system increases as a patient continues to suffer from further diagnostic testing and from the illness itself.

B. Non-Compliance May Hurt The Clinician
1. Eager to heal the sick, **clinicians may feel let down or even betrayed by a patient who is not adhering to treatment recommendations.** Clinicians devote their heart, soul, and sweat in the interest of reducing a patient's suffering. Non-compliance can be experienced as a personal affront to the clinician, leading to feelings of devaluation, and under-appreciation.
2. **Managing a patient who, as a consequence of non-compliance, does not improve can leave the physician feeling helpless, ineffectual, and angry.**
   a. The physician's role is to recognize disease and then to educate and to collaborate with the individual who must then accept (or reject, or compromise with) treatment options.
   b. Experienced clinicians appreciate that, at best, compliance is generally relative. The clinician does best to heed **Osler's advice (i.e., to react with equanimity to a patient's report of non-adherence).** Expressions of sympathy for the unremitted illness can be accompanied by curiosity about why the treatment was difficult to endure.

C. Non-Compliance Hurts Society
1. Incomplete treatment of infectious processes contributes to the development of drug-resistant bacteria and results in the general population's increased risk of exposure to virulent organisms.
2. Already strained medical resources may be wasted by non-compliance.
   a. The financial burden upon the U.S. health care system has been estimated at approximately $100 billion each year.
3. Non-compliance may contribute to inaccuracies in clinical research.

III. The Discovery of Non-Compliance

A. Where to Start:
1. The ability of a physician to predict patient compliance may be no better than chance alone.
2. Although patients who improve may not be following doctors orders, when a patient is *not* responding as expected to treatment, after reconsidering the diagnosis and treatment, the physician should also supportively investigate adherence with treatment.
3. **Some patients deny or reject their diagnosis for cultural, intellectual, or psychologic reasons.**
4. **Compliance is a challenge for those who have cognitive difficulty.**
5. **Patients who are unwilling to entertain that they have a condition that will benefit from medical treatment are less likely to adhere to treatment recommendations.**

6. Individuals who are missing appointments, important tests, or evaluations on a regular basis are more likely to be non-adherent with other treatment recommendations.

B. Asking the Question May Be the Best Way to Get the Answer

1. Not surprisingly, **the most efficient way to assess whether or not a patient is deviating from treatment recommendations is simply to ask the patient,** *"How's it going with the [medicine]?"*

    a. **Asking an individual what medications they are taking, and how they are taking them allows the clinician to assess the patient's understanding of the treatment recommendations.**

    b. Patients who take less than 80% of their prescribed medications doses are four times more likely to report missing medication doses when they are asked.

    c. **It is helpful to inquire about adherence in a concerned, empathic, yet informative manner,** such as, "Sometimes it is difficult to remember to take medication. Have you ever noticed that you occasionally forget to take your pills?" or "Let me confirm that my records are accurate. What medications are you taking?" as opposed to "Have you taken all of your medication?" or "Are you taking your pills as prescribed?"

2. Individuals conceal non-compliance out of fear of the clinician's reaction, out of shame for the diagnosis, or from fear of the treatment itself.

3. **When addressed in a non-pejorative manner, however, the discussion can strengthen the patient-physician relationship.** Direct discussion is easier to employ than time-consuming, complex, and unreliable methods of assessing medication adherence.

4. Try to determine the specific behavior patterns involved in medication non-adherence; this allows for the information obtained to be incorporated into the individual's treatment plan.

    a. Missing an occasional pill is common. Is a single missed dose safe? Should the dose be skipped? Should the next dose be doubled?

    b. When an individual consistently takes a lower dose than recommended, it suggests bothersome side effects at the higher dose, or that the desired effect has been achieved at this lower dose.

    c. Independent of therapeutic benefits or side effects, some patients simply feel psychologically better taking a lower than prescribed dose.

    d. Sporadic consumption of medications may indicate an insufficient understanding or acceptance of the illness being treated, or the treatment's mechanism of action. In this situation, education and empathy are crucial ingredients.

    e. The inability to afford treatment is a sad but common explanation for non-compliance; "Poverty can be a side effect of some medications."

    f. Over-use of medication suggests that the individual's symptomatology is not being adequately managed, that the recommendations have been misunderstood, or that the patient is misusing or abusing the medication. Medications are often shared with family, or friends, or are even sold for a profit on the street.

C. Alternative Methods of Determining Compliance Have Mixed Benefits

1. **Daily diaries allow the physician to track the consumption of prescribed medications, and serve as a daily reminder for patients.** Moreover, review of the diary allows the clinician to praise and to positively reinforce adherence to treatment recommendations.

2. **Reviewing the frequency with which medications are being refilled** can also provide a general sense of medication utilization.

3. **Pill counting** can enable calculations and estimations of actual medication consumption. Having a patient bring in their pill bottles and counting medications that remain in the bottle can be demeaning and may damage the patient-physician relationship.

4. **Electronic medication monitoring** suggests a precise method of determining medication-taking behavior. However, this method can be quite expensive and subject to tampering; it is of no practical use.

5. **Direct measures of drug levels and their metabolites** are accurate but problematic when used to determine compliance.

   a. The procedures involved for direct measurements of serum levels are invasive and costly.

   b. Medication levels do not account for the difference among individuals with regard to pharmacokinetics and metabolism, and may demonstrate over or under-treatment that is not a result of any changes in the patient's behavior.

   c. Drug levels reflect cross-sectional assessments in time and may not accurately represent day-to-day or long-term behaviors.

IV. Why Don't Patients Comply?

Whether submitting to a surgical procedure, or to a trial of medication with unknown efficacy and side effects, trust in the clinician's competence positively predicts the quality of treatment.

A. Powerful factors affecting an individual's adherence to medical recommendations are the style of the individual taking the medication and the clinician's appreciation of, and reaction to, their patient.

1. **Patient's beliefs:**

   a. It is essential to understand and to listen to the patient's interpretation of their symptoms.

   b. A patient may attribute their condition to etiologies quite different from those who believe in the medical model; they hold alternative beliefs as to what is needed to treat it, and for that matter if it even needs to be treated at all. Identifying and discussing these differences are essential.

   c. Shame plays a central role in illness and its treatment; disease can be interpreted as a personal shortcoming, as a failure of will, or as something for which a patient feels guilty. Non-compliance can represent an effort to reduce shame.

   d. Cultural beliefs impact not only a patient's interpretation of illness, but also the presentation of the illness (e.g., how it is described), and the interaction between the patient and the physician.

2. **Emotional Maturity and the Ability to Cope with Illness and Its Treatment**

   a. An adolescent may interpret an illness as something that is embarrassing, and as something to be ashamed of; moreover, an adolescent may be lacking the life experiences to place the illness in perspective, along a continuum from minor to serious. A teenager may also pursue the fantastical and wishful (but understandable) belief that somehow not submitting to the *treatment* will mean that he or she can avoid the *illness*.

   b. A young person may be affected considerably by their condition, and believe that both short- and long-term opportunities in one's education, career, finances, and relationships will be impacted.

c. A middle-aged person may have concerns about how disclosure of an illness might impact work and family, or affect life and health insurance premiums.

d. An older adult may be confronted with a newfound fear and awareness of mortality, as the first manifestation of an endless series of illnesses. Independence may be threatened and concerns may grow about the health of their life-partner, and the impact of their own health on that relationship.

3. **Past Experiences Inform the Present**

a. A patient's experiences with the health care system may evoke both positive and negative reactions (e.g., unreasonable feelings of fear, anxiety, helplessness, hopelessness, and loss of control). However, a clinician may also enjoy the rewards of a patient's prior treatments and the good will toward the system of care. Experience, with the health care system, good or bad, will forever impact the present. The patient must be understood with that in mind.

b. Experience with side effects is likely to prompt worry, concern, and questions to the clinician.

B. Compliance Varies Among Illnesses and Their Treatments

1. **Major Depression Feels Bad**

a. Depressed mood or sadness is a universally-experienced emotion. However, clinical depression is often mistaken by patients and by clinicians for this minor, natural and non-pathological state. Shame, denial, and ignorance (by patients and their clinicians) are the most frequent barriers to treatment.

b. Depression is a biologic, genetically-influenced chemical imbalance characterized by persistent depressed mood, feelings of hopelessness, decreased energy, and concentration, and by the capacity to experience pleasure.

c. Patients with depression often fail to care for themselves; they don't follow medical recommendations, they fail to take medications, and they forego appointments.

d. Treatment of the underlying depression may enhance adherence to general medical treatment.

2. **Mania/Hypomania Feels Good**

a. The euphoric manic/hypomanic state of bipolar I and II disorders is associated with an elevated mood and with an energy level that most patients find to be a positive experience when they are in such a state. Medications and treatments can result in a feeling of being slowed down, and those with mania are likely to be less adherent with such medications.

b. Bipolar disease is a particularly difficult illness to manage, as insight and judgement can be limited with regard to matters of health and life, and patients may not believe they have an illness that requires treatment.

3. **Anxiety Disorders Make Patients Nervous**

a. The anxiety disorders (including panic disorder) are associated with hypervigilance for both internal (physical) and external (real life) stimuli.

b. Severe anxiety disorders may render an individual unable to travel outside of their home or neighborhood to visit a clinician.

c. Initially a patient treated for an anxiety disorder is likely to notice subtle physical symptoms and relate those symptoms to medication side effects.

d. While some psychologic interventions, particularly cognitive-behavioral therapy (CBT) have been effective in treatment of anxiety disorders, a patient who has benefited from pharmacologic treatment will be particularly reluctant to reduce their medications.

e. It remains the better part of wisdom to avoid a struggle and to maintain a patient on whatever effective treatment is embraced.

4. Obsessive-compulsive disorder (OCD)

a. The characteristic rituals and checking behaviors of obsessive-compulsive disorder (OCD) have a wide spectrum in patients, from repeatedly counting pills before taking them, to fears of contamination, to the hoarding of objects, to being so paralyzed by rituals that they are unable to leave the house.

b. As with all illnesses, OCD is frequently unrecognized; identification of symptoms is the first obstacle to dealing with difficulties involved in adherence to treatment.

c. Identification of the obsession (e.g., contamination) or ritual (e.g., pill counting) may aide in the creation of a treatment plan that minimizes the triggers of the obsession or compulsion.

5. Psychosis

a. Failure to adhere with treatment is particularly devastating to the patient who suffers from chronic psychosis. Consequent recurrence of psychotic symptoms, including delusions, paranoia, hallucinations, and disorganized thought, predicts a slippery slope that further jeopardizes medical adherence.

b. At times, an individual's perception of reality can be so bizarre, yet so real to them, that there is nothing anyone can do (without proper psychiatric medication) to encourage adherence. Often use of long-acting, parenterally administered treatments is the best option.

c. Medical illnesses can also be incorporated into an individual's delusional thinking.

6. Substance abuse

a. Active substance abuse complicates treatment of all medical and psychiatric illnesses and conditions.

b. Oftentimes, individuals become addicted to alcohol and to other substances as a consequence of their own efforts to reduce emotional or physical pain. While the devastating physical and social sequelae of substance abuse demands treatment, the underlying and primary disorder must not be ignored. Treatment of substance abuse may fail without recognition and treatment of the primary psychiatric problem.

7. Personality disorder

a. The mere presence of a personality disorder does not predict medication noncompliance.

b. Frequently, however, medications, appointments, and adherence to recommendations can become a central issue in the interpersonal struggles to which these individuals are predisposed.

8. General medical problems

a. Patients with numerous general medical problems are more likely to be on multiple medications, which even aside from side effects, can result in confusion regarding medication instructions.

b. Medical problems may contribute to misunderstandings, and to resistance to further recommendations.

c. Impairments in vision, manual dexterity, cognition, and memory can all significantly limit an individual's ability to follow recommendations for medical treatment.

C. Treatment Must Comply with a Patient's Social Environment

1. Family

a. Acceptance by family and friends of the diagnosis and support of the patient's treatment is an important factor in compliance.

b. Engaging the family and the support system in a patient's treatment can be extremely valuable in assisting with adherence to medical recommendations.

2. Religion
   a. An individual's religious beliefs can impact their interpretation of what is, and what is not, appropriate and acceptable treatment.
   b. Addressing elements of religious and spiritual faith in the context of illness can be rewarding not only for the patient, but also for the treating clinician.
   c. The patient's religious beliefs that can be incorporated into illness management can help comfort a patient, and consequently enhance their compliance.
3. Culture and Society
   a. How an individual with an illness interacts with the health care system, at what stage they access the health care system, and how concerns regarding treatment recommendations are managed are to a large degree culturally-based.
   b. In certain cultures, specific illnesses can result in shame, yet in others they can be openly shared.
   c. Consideration of the patient's cultural practices and attitudes towards illness and its treatment enhances understanding of the patient's limitations with regard to adherence.

V. Treatment Strategies: Walking the Path Together

A. The clinician-patient relationship is the single most important factor in predicting compliance.
1. **Effort invested in understanding the patient's view of their illness is rewarded many times over.**
2. **The treatment goals of the clinician and the patient must be the same** and must be made explicit.
3. **Supporting a patient's beliefs, family, religion, and culture** comforts both the clinician and the patient.
4. **Patients generally appreciate the time that the clinician invests in teaching.** An unexpected and unsolicited call or note that expresses interest and concern for a patient's well-being often works wonders.
5. **Tailor the patient's treatment plan and recommendations** to coincide with their schedule or lifestyle.
   a. **Develop cues to remind patients when to take medications** ("with meals" as opposed to "three times a day," or "when you take Spot out" instead of "in the morning") can be helpful.
6. Reliable and supportive collaborators in the patient's life can be enormously helpful.
   a. Encourage open communication between the patient, family, and friends with regard to the illness or condition (when appropriate).
   b. Ask the patient to bring a friend or loved one to an appointment.

B. Dealing with Resistance Outside the Clinician-Patient Consulting Room
1. Patients are often ambivalent regarding initiation of a course of medication. Anxious, inexperienced, and poorly qualified, they should not be put in the position to argue the case for a treatment trial to their family. Should the clinician learn that a spouse or a loved one (or especially another treating clinician!) has concerns or objections regarding treatment recommendations, the clinician should immediately initiate a discussion of these concerns directly with the objecting person. As with the patient himself or herself, one should engage the reluctant objector and invite them to "walk the treatment path" along with you and the patient.

C. The Difference Between a "Trial" and a "Course" of Treatment

1. **Once an illness has been diagnosed a clinician must present treatment options in an open and neutral fashion.** By including the possibility that "no treatment" is an acceptable choice, the clinician sends a powerful message. The patient is not being asked to surrender autonomy, control, or free will. Thus, the patient is alerted that the authority to decide (and to struggle) resides not with the clinician, but within him or herself.

2. The Trial. **Clinicians try to do no harm as they try to reduce the suffering of their patients. Treatment is chosen only because enduring, untreated illness is a worse option.** Treatments that do not help will be discontinued. Treatments that have intolerable side effects will be discontinued. The patient can be reassured that even treatments which both help and which are free of side effects can, nevertheless, be discontinued should the patient so choose. In a sort of paradox, sometimes the best way for a patient to decide on a course is to undertake a trial. To discontinue treatment after such a trial becomes the strongest basis for a truly informed decision.

D. Clear Communications Help

1. **Provide clear verbal and written instructions.**
   a. A significant number of patients do not recall accurately verbal instructions, even when optimally delivered.

2. **Open communication enables the treating physician to meet a patient's expectations, and to enhance a patient's adherence with recommendations and trust in the medical system.**

3. **Discuss the concept of deviation from medical recommendations and treatment adherence in advance.**
   a. With such an approach, a patient will feel more comfortable reporting their difficulty with adherence.
   b. This strategy removes the negative, demeaning, and at times scolding tone from the subject of the non-adherence.

E. Specific Situations

1. **Attention to the patient**
   a. **Phone calls or mail reminders** can initially improve attendance, as can decreasing the interval between appointments.
   b. **When a visit is missed, the patient should be telephoned, and a new appointment rescheduled.**
   c. **Respect a patient's time** and limit waiting time in the office whenever possible.
   d. **Follow-up appointments should be made prior to the patient leaving the office.**
   e. **Return phone calls and pages as quickly as possible.**

2. **Short-term regimens**
   a. Medication dosing **regimens should be as simple as possible.**
   b. **Instructions should be clear,** and be provided both verbally and in written form.

3. **Long-term regimens**
   a. **Adherence drops off considerably as the length of the treatment regimen increases.**
   b. Continued education and discussion regarding the condition or the disease process and the need for treatment can be helpful.
   c. Attention to, and acknowledgement of, the effect of lifestyle changes can enhance the patient-physician relationship and adherence to recommendations when the patient feels heard and understood.

    d. **Frequent follow-up appointments can improve adherence** and help the patient continue to feel involved in treatment decisions.

Suggested References

Conrad, P. (1985). The meaning of medications: Another look at compliance. *Journal of Science and Medicine, 20,* 29–37.

Cramer, J.A., & Spilker, B. (Eds.). (1991). *Patient compliance in medical practice and clinical trials.* New York: Raven Press.

DiMatteo, M.R., & DiNicola, D.D. (1982). *Achieving patient compliance: The psychology of the medical practitioners' role.* New York: Pergamon Press.

Eisenthal, S., Emery, R., Lazare, A., et al. (1979). "Adherence" and the negotiated approach to patienthood. *Archives of General Psychiatry, 36,* 393–398.

Gerber, K.E., & Nehemkis, A.M. (Eds.). (1986). *Compliance: The dilemma of the chronically ill.* New York: Springer.

Haynes, R.B. (1976). A critical review of the "determinants" of patient compliance with therapeutic regimens. In D.L. Sackett, & R.B. Haynes (Eds.), *Compliance with therapeutic regimens.* Baltimore: Johns Hopkins University Press.

Haynes, R.B., Taylor, D.W., & Sackett, D.L. (1979). *Compliance in health care.* Baltimore: Johns Hopkins University Press.

Meichenbaum, D., & Turk, D.C. (1987). *Facilitating treatment adherence: A practitioner's guidebook.* New York: Plenum Press.

Sackett, D.L., Haynes, R.B., & Tugwell, P. (1991). *Clinical epidemiology: A basic science for clinical medicine.* Philadelphia: Lippincott Williams & Wilkins.

CHAPTER 75
Breaking Bad News

PAUL HAMBURG

I. Introduction

A. **Bearing news regarding death and disease is an ancient burden and privilege of physicians.** Physicians may disclose news of cancer, HIV illness, diabetes, Alzheimer's disease, schizophrenia, or the death of a child. Whether the bad news relates to death or to the diagnosis of a disabling illness, **the physician must bear the consequence of being a messenger of ill tidings.** With a word, the lives of a patient and a family are unalterably transformed. These moments are difficult for every physician; they are unforgettable for patients and their families. Telling bad news embodies elements of power as well as powerlessness for the physician. At such times medical science seems especially potent to the patient and family even as the illness and prognosis fall beyond the ability of the physician to cure.

B. **While no approach to telling bad news can fully lighten the burden or change the unwelcome facts, compassionate and effective communication can make an enormous difference for patients and their families.** Their pain can be assuaged by the physician's tact, hopefulness, willingness to listen, and professional presence. It is not unusual for patients to recall these very painful encounters with gratitude toward a physician who helped them face one of life's worst calamities.

C. **The physician's primary mission is to relieve suffering.** This basic principle is especially relevant to the communication of bad news. Such encounters offer an invaluable opportunity to mitigate pain even as interpersonal skills are strained by the nature of the information conveyed and the intensity of the feelings generated. This chapter suggests ways to maximize the physician's effectiveness in relieving the suffering of patients and families that are receiving bad news.

II. General Principles

A. **The most basic recommendation for a physician who is about to tell a patient or family bad news is to sit down with them in a private setting.** Sitting indicates that there will be time to converse and that the physician's full attention will be available. Even if the duration of the encounter is limited by the urgency of the clinical setting or by other emergent care that calls the physician away, sitting for a short time with the patient and family allows for a more compassionate encounter. In fact, a series of brief conversations is often more effective than a single prolonged meeting, since patients and their families cannot absorb large quantities of information while in a state of shock and agitation.

B. **A second general principle to guide a physician in conveying bad news is to be succinct.** In this highly stressful situation, brevity and technical simplicity are essential for communication to be effective. A patient who has just learned of a cancer diagnosis may be unable to absorb a complex presentation of treatment options replete with statistical comparisons. It is better to assure the patient initially that a number of options are available and schedule a time to consider them further. In this way, the patient is not flooded with terms, concepts, and data while emotionally overwhelmed and there is more time to look at the initial impact of the diagnosis and to listen to the patient's concerns.

C. **Finding concise words** to convey information that may be technically complex or emotionally burdensome is undoubtedly important, but **the third principle to guide a physician conveying bad news is to concentrate as much on listening as on speaking.** Hearing the family's and patient's questions and concerns is a prerequisite to knowing how to respond. **It is helpful to ask about their most serious concern, fear, or worry.** Each patient and family will have its personal set of concerns, depending on the circumstances of the illness and their lives. In considering their concerns, it is important to bear in mind that what matters most is not answering them fully but being willing to hear them out.

1. **Sometimes the preeminent concern is fear of pain.** The physician may be able to offer reassurances that the patient's pain can and will be addressed throughout the course of an illness.

2. **At times the most pressing concern for the patient is how to tell someone else:** a spouse, child, parent, employer, or colleague. The physician may be of direct assistance in informing other family members or may counsel the patient regarding the timing and details of disclosure.

3. Faced with death, a patient may be especially concerned with surviving long enough to witness an important milestone: the marriage or graduation of a child, or the closing of a major business deal. Sometimes the physician can offer a reasonable expectation that this will be possible even while conveying the bad news about a fatal outcome.

4. **The patient and family may particularly fear the loss of dignity** that often is associated with terminal illness. The physician can help them begin to address these concerns and make appropriate plans regarding extreme interventions to prolong life or to determine the location of terminal care.

5. **A significant concern may pertain to finances.** The physician can discuss issues of disability, loss of earning capacity, and anticipated medical expenses.

6. **Sometimes the patient is burdened by secrets** that may have new and difficult implications in the face of a life-threatening illness. These secrets can involve interpersonal relationships, work, and finances. The physician may serve as a confidant or confessor with regard to secrets that might otherwise constitute an additional burden to a terminally ill patient and his or her family.

7. **Finally, the patient and family may be preoccupied with spiritual questions,** such as the nature of death and the injustice of illness. While the physician may feel out of his or her realm of expertise in discussing these questions, hearing such concerns and validating their importance often provide significant relief of mental suffering.

D. **Another general principle is honesty.** At no time is trust more important between a physician, a patient, and a family than in the presence of severe illness or death. While it is unnecessary (and often contraindicated) to burden a patient with excessive or morbid details regarding the impending course of a severe illness, the physician should be scrupulously honest in answering all the questions posed by the patient. If the physician cannot answer the patient's question, it is appropriate to indicate willingness to consult the relevant medical literature or another physician in search of further information. If the questions cannot be answered on the basis of current medical knowledge, this too should be communicated explicitly. **Shared uncertainty, although a source of discomfort for both patient and physician, is ultimately much more bearable than dissimulation.** An important role of the physician is to help the patient live through the anxiety caused by uncertainties of diagnosis and outcome.

E. The issue of hope is an especially difficult one. **It is inappropriate to offer false hope at any time; it compromises trust and ultimately leaves the patient more alone and confused.** However, even in the most desperate situations, once the physician understands the patient's specific concerns, an element of hope usually can be offered honestly. This may be the hope for a statistically unlikely recovery, the relief of pain and aloneness, or a dignified and timely end to the patient's and family's suffering. It is vital to leave as much room for hope as honesty permits.

III. The Physician's Predicament

A. **Bearing bad news evokes a host of intense feelings in the physician.** Understanding these responses can make a burdensome task less confusing.

B. **The physician may feel professionally helpless** in the face of inexorable disease or death. Most persons chose to become doctors out of a desire to make a difference and cure illness. Death and devastating illness may feel like a personal injury to the physician, an assault on the physician's sense of effectiveness. While some physicians may respond with equanimity to the limits of what they can do for their patients, helplessness often evokes despair or rage.

C. **Confronted by a fatal illness or a devastating diagnosis, a physician may experience a sense of guilt and excessive responsibility.** It is difficult to be helpful to a patient and family while feeling burdened by unwarranted self-blame.

D. **The physician may experience great personal anxiety** in response to death or a destructive illness.
   1. **A particular patient or illness may provoke a physician's anxiety about death and disease,** sometimes because of common features of age or life situation, or be a reminder of a painful event in a physician's life, such as the terminal illness of a parent. While most experienced physicians have learned to protect themselves from identifying excessively with a patient's fate, that protection may fail in the face of an especially poignant clinical situation or during a period of illness or personal crisis in the physician's life.
   2. **A physician may become anxious about the intensity of his or her own feelings of grief.** The loss of a patient after months or years of a professional relationship ruptures a significant attachment for the physician. It may be difficult to accept how personal the loss feels.

E. **A physician may experience an overwhelming sense of failure** in the presence of death and inexorable illness.
   1. Adverse outcomes challenge the physician's confidence and sense of competence. It may be difficult to tolerate intense feelings of powerlessness and ineffectiveness.
   2. Illness can be a profoundly humbling experience for a physician. It is common to feel a sense of uselessness and loss of confidence.

F. **A physician may fear that the patient and family will blame the messenger.**
   1. **Fear of vindictiveness or legal retribution** may make it difficult to help a rageful distraught family.

2. **Anger is a basic component of grief.** For some people anger is mobilized as soon as they learn the bad news and may initially be directed at the bearer of the news. It is natural to fear such anger even if the physician is aware that it actually pertains more to the adverse event than to the messenger.

IV. The Grief Response

A. **Understanding the wide range of normal grief responses helps demystify the task of communicating bad news.**

B. **Normal grief responses are enormously variable.**
   1. **The nature of a loss profoundly affects the pattern of grief.** Unexpected or catastrophic losses are more likely to be overwhelming. Anticipated loss is usually less traumatic because of the opportunity to prepare. Every loss ruptures a bond between persons and thus injures the self. The nature of the bond that is ruptured (loving, hateful, dependent, ambivalent) shapes the effect of the rupture. The meaning of the relationship informs the internal injury provoked by a loss.
   2. **Mourning varies with the emotional style of the individual,** ranging from stoicism to hysteria, from intense denial to catastrophic reaction, with each style posing different challenges for the physician.
   3. **Cultural and religious differences define different repertoires of normal grief.** Some cultures encourage the exuberant expression of rage and sadness, while others teach forbearance and introspection. The physician will benefit from some familiarity with the patient's cultural traditions regarding death and grief.

C. Despite enormous personal and cultural variation in grief responses, certain general principles can help patients face death and personal loss.
   1. **Denial is an unconscious shield against unbearable realities.** It plays a protective role in facing the unfaceable. While denial may delay a patient's acceptance of real circumstances, it also serves a useful purpose. Denial can postpone psychological pain, allowing an overwhelming reality to be absorbed in bearable increments. Unless denial disrupts necessary medical care, the physician should allow this process to evolve at its own pace rather than insist on the immediate acceptance of a diagnosis or prognosis.
   2. **Grief provokes intense feelings of sadness and rage.** It also may induce a numbing absence of feeling. Normal grief can involve many permutations of these experiences, which may occur in different sequences and be expressed in a variety of ways. Grief tends to begin with an overwhelming onrush of feeling or intense numbing. As the numbing fades, there may be further waves of overwhelming sadness and agitation. Over time grief becomes less acute and allows the individual respites from intense emotion.
   3. **The duration of grief varies greatly but grieving often lasts longer than people expect.** The process of reconciliation to severe loss takes a long time, and the acute grieving period generally is followed by a longer interval during which the pain is milder but ordinary life has not yet resumed. During this period there may be lingering waves of anger and sadness and a continuing need for support and reassurance that may be more difficult to obtain as the moment of loss recedes into the past.
   4. **Grief profoundly affects personal relationships.** Its cascades of emotion interrupt ordinary life and change the individual's ability to be emotionally involved with

others. A parent may have difficulty relating to a child. This may be especially problematic after the death of a parent, when the surviving parent must grieve while supporting a bereaved child. Besides being a personal crisis, grief is a relational crisis that affects marriages, friendships, and family connections. The anger which is part of mourning may become especially disruptive to intimate relationships.

D. Some situational and personal factors predict a complicated or prolonged course of mourning.

1. Facing severe illness or death is among the most challenging life experiences, drawing on every resource and strength: personal, spiritual, and relational. **Generally speaking, individuals who have psychological strength, coping skills, supportive relationships, a caring community, and spiritual reserves are far more likely to withstand grief than are individuals who lack these elements.** A vulnerable, psychologically unstable, alienated, lonely, or marginal individual may predictably be overwhelmed by loss.

2. **Although the death of a deeply loved person evokes intense and prolonged grief, it generally is easier to recover from such losses than from the loss of someone for whom one's feelings are conflicted.** A hated parent or estranged spouse may pose a special dilemma in regard to grief. Feelings of guilt, resentment, rage, and regret may complicate grief and predispose a person to depression or despair. In responding to personal illness or facing impending death, similar considerations may apply: As difficult as loss may be for someone who is at peace with life, it is even more problematic for an individual who is discontented.

3. **Certain losses are overwhelming per se: the death of children, the sudden death of an entire family, and the trauma of war, urban violence, and international genocide.** In catastrophic situations additional supportive measures are predictably necessary to aid the survivors.

V. Special Circumstances

A. Some situations place a special burden on a physician who is communicating bad news.

B. The death of a child violates a basic human expectation. We are to some degree prepared to outlive our elders and even our peers, but we are not ready to mourn for our offspring.

1. Perhaps the loss of a child is ultimately beyond grief; at the very least it leaves a deep scar on parents and marital relationships. A physician who must convey the news of a child's death or fatal illness has a special burden but also may be able to offer vital ongoing support for the parents as they grapple with their loss.

2. **Fetal and perinatal death** poses a special predicament. While the loss of a pregnancy is less devastating than the death of a living child, the intensity of attendant grief often surprises parents. It is important to realize the magnitude of the emotional investment parents make in a pregnancy, even early in its course. Parents may need permission to express their grief, especially in the absence of funerary rituals and customs that assist in the mourning process. The physician can help mitigate the impact of those who urge grieving parents to get over their loss quickly and minimize its significance.

C. Deaths that occur suddenly and without warning pose a special problem in regard to grief. The circumstances may be violent, there has been no opportunity to prepare for the loss, and there is no opportunity for reconciliation or a farewell.

D. Disaster situations, both human-made and natural, pose a special challenge for physicians. The volume of destruction and death is numbing for caregivers and rescue personnel, and the volume of grief may be overwhelming. There may be little time to console relatives, and compassion may be limited by exhaustion, personal traumatization, and self-protection. In these situations group support may be as important for the physician as it is for the survivors and their relatives. In the contemporary crisis of international terrorism, the impact of shared danger can both encourage empathy and overwhelm caregivers, who may fear for their own safety or worry about the fate of their own families and loved ones.

E. All too often, physicians (especially house staff, emergency room physicians, and *intensivists*) bring the message of death or a devastating diagnosis to a family they have never met before. The lack of ongoing trust, familiarity, and a pre-existing relationship makes such encounters especially difficult. If at all possible, it is mutually beneficial if the physician can take the time to ask about the family and the patient. By learning who the patient was in life and becoming even slightly acquainted with the family, the physician can temper the strangeness of the moment and feel more able to help.

F. Covering physicians. With current medicolegal and clinical concerns about physician fatigue and excessive working hours for house staff, it is ever more likely that patients who die in the hospital will do so at a time when a covering physician is on the scene. **Families may have difficulty hearing bad news from a stranger rather than the physician with whom they have communicated over the course of the illness.** The covering physician may also feel uncomfortable assuming this role with a family that he or she has never met. Providing timely access to more familiar members of the treatment team may help mitigate the difficulty of such encounters.

VI. Helpful Strategies

A. Several measures can be helpful for a physician who must communicate bad news to a patient and family.

B. During the initial encounter the impact of bad news may limit the quantity and scope of what can be addressed effectively. Large amounts of technical information regarding a disease or its treatment will not be absorbed in the presence of shock, denial, and emotional overload. **This time is often best used to provide rudimentary information, gauge its impact, address pressing questions, and schedule another visit.**

    1. Revisits aid in treatment planning and exploring in greater depth issues raised in an initial meeting with a patient who has just been diagnosed with a severe or life-threatening illness.

    2. **Revisits with the family are also very useful after the death of a patient.** Meeting after an interval of days or weeks can help answer lingering questions, address ongoing concerns, and provide an opportunity to ascertain how family members are coping with their grief. It may provide an opportunity to intervene if an individual shows early signs of pathologic grief or depression.

C. Support in the form of group or individual counseling may be useful for the patient or family.

    1. **Patients with life-threatening or debilitating illnesses often feel isolated and alone with their fate.** Groups that share an HIV diagnosis, cancer, arthritis, or

manic-depressive illness offer a chance for empathic understanding, mutual support, and education and permit the patient to feel useful to others.

2. **Grieving families also may benefit from time-limited groups** that share the loss of a child, the death of a relative by violence, or a traumatic experience in a war or catastrophe.

D. Support also may be useful for the physician.

1. While physicians learn to cope with the stress of their profession, including its particular burden regarding death and the communication of bad news, there may be occasions that prove unusually difficult.

2. At times the difficulty is specific to a particular situation: the loss of a patient to whom one was especially attached, a death that has evoked excessive feelings of guilt and responsibility, the death of a patient with whom one has identified strongly. At times it is the accumulation of many smaller burdens that proves excessive. Sometimes a previously tolerable burden becomes overwhelming because of coincident stressful events in the physician's life, such as personal or family illness.

3. Whatever the cause, when the toll of being a messenger of bad news causes depression, despair, self-doubt, insomnia, cynicism, or hopelessness in the physician, it is important to seek help from colleagues, family members, spiritual advisers, or a mental health professional.

VII. Conclusion

A. The physicians' ancient task of communicating bad news constitutes both a burden and an opportunity. By sitting and listening to patients and their families, taking into account both the physician's and the patient's emotional responses, it is possible to take full advantage of the chance to relieve suffering, which is the physician's most fundamental and compelling mission.

Suggested Readings

Cassem, N.H. (1978). Treating the person confronting death. In A.M. Nicholi (Ed.), *The Harvard guide to modern psychiatry.* Cambridge, Mass.: Belknap Press of Harvard University Press, pp. 579–606.

VandeKieft, G.K. (2001). Breaking bad news. *American Family Physician, 64*(12), 1975–1978.

CHAPTER 76

Maintaining Boundaries in the Doctor-Patient Relationship

RONALD SCHOUTEN

I. Introduction

A. At first glance the roles of doctor and patient are obvious, but there are multiple opportunities for those roles to be blurred and for both doctor and patient to step outside their respective roles. For the doctor-patient relationship to function optimally, it is important that those roles be filled consistently, honoring the appropriate **boundaries.** In this way, both parties have a set of rules which guide the relationship and allow the patient to trust the physician and know what to expect from the relationship.

1. The issue of **boundary crossings** (minor but potentially important blurring of the boundaries) and the more serious **boundary violations** (in which the boundaries are clearly transgressed) has been of great concern to mental health professionals. However, these concepts apply to all areas of medicine.

   a. **What constitutes a boundary crossing or violation is determined by both the nature of the action and the setting in which it occurs.** For example, in a rural area it may be appropriate for the family doctor to spend time with patients at a social gathering, while the same socializing in an urban practice may be considered a boundary crossing.

   b. Boundaries have been considered particularly important in psychiatry because of the uniquely personal nature of the problems treated, the feelings stirred up during psychiatric treatment, and the potential for the patient to develop a dependency on the doctor.

      i. **Transference and countertransference** (see Chapters 12 and 13) can lead to intense feelings between a doctor and a patient. These are feelings that are transposed from other relationships, including feelings that resemble "true love." Relationships and emotions, such as love, are common issues in psychiatric treatment; discussion of them increases the likelihood that such feelings will arise between doctor and patient. A physician who listens to a patient's personal problems, attempts to understand them, and accepts the patient for who he or she is may be the first person in the patient's life who has done this. This can result in the patient developing a deep, loving, and sometimes dependent attachment to the physician. When professional boundaries are honored, these feelings can be explored safely. When the boundaries are not honored, the patient can become confused and more damaged.

      ii. Transference and countertransference occur in all relationships, including the doctor-patient relationship in primary care. Primary care physicians (PCPs) must be aware of boundary rules which allow patients to feel safe and discuss personal matters with their doctors.

      iii. The nature of certain personality traits (e.g., dependency) and disorders (e.g., borderline personality disorder) may lead patients to actively challenge the boundaries of the relationship in a search for interpersonal fulfillment which they have not obtained outside the treatment setting.

2. The maintenance of professional boundaries has been the subject of both ethical and legal proscriptions. The basic principle of these limitations on physicians' behavior is that **physicians have a fiduciary duty to put the best interests of the patient ahead of the physician's interest.**

   a. The Hippocratic oath provides guidelines for physician behavior, including admonitions about appropriate boundaries, maintaining confidences, and avoiding sexual relations. **In 1989, the American Medical Association Council on Ethical and Judicial Affairs passed a rule which prohibits physician-patient sexual contact regardless of the physician's specialty.**

   b. Physician-patient sexual contact and other forms of physician exploitation of patients constitute the basis for discipline by physician registration authorities in all states.

   c. **The American Psychiatric Association has adopted a guideline that declares it unethical for a psychiatrist to have a sexual relationship with a former or current patient.**

   d. A number of states have enacted laws which make it a **criminal offense** for a physician to have a sexual relationship with a patient.

      i. Statutes vary in regard to whether they classify doctor-patient sexual contact as a misdemeanor or a felony. Some statutes distinguish between the first offense and repeated offenses.

      ii. While many statutes criminalize psychotherapist-patient sexual contact, the term *psychotherapy* is broadly defined in some statutes as "the professional treatment, assessment, or counseling of a mental or emotional illness, symptom, or condition." Thus, many of these statutes apply to PCPs who treat psychiatric illness.

      iii. Statutes also differ with regard to how they define the term *patient* and whether and when the prohibition applies.

B. Boundary issues are not limited to physicians. Increasing ethical, regulatory, and legislative attention has been paid to boundary issues concerning attorneys, clergy, and educators.

C. The emphasis on sexual contact in the literature on boundary violations should not detract from the importance of other boundary issues in the treatment of patients.

II. Selected Boundary Issues

A. Business Dealings between Doctor and Patient

1. The physician-patient relationship is fundamentally a business relationship. The terms of the contract state that the physician receives a fee in return for helping the patient with medical problems. The arm's-length nature of the relationship allows physicians to be objective in their dealings with patients.

2. **Involvement in other business dealings can detract from the distance, objectivity, and empathy necessary for the physician-patient relationship to succeed.**

   a. If Dr. A invests $200,000 in Mr. B's new business and the business fails, Dr. A will be hard pressed to deal objectively and compassionately with Mr. B's ensuing depression.

   b. If Dr. C buys a new car from his patient Mr. D, there is a strong likelihood that resentment and anger will develop when Dr. C learns that he could have purchased the car elsewhere for less money or if the car develops mechanical problems.

B. The Physical Examination

1. The physical examination is an extremely personal event which can involve the touching and observation of body parts in a way which ordinarily occurs only in the course of sexual activity.

   a. The use of overly familiar touching or language sends mixed signals to the patient which can invite further boundary violations or cause the patient great distress.

b. Some patients may be more sensitive than others to these issues. For example, patients who are victims of childhood abuse may be hypervigilant and extremely sensitive to any physical contact which could be interpreted as abusive. The physician is often unaware of the abuse history; failure to maintain appropriate professional boundaries and behavior with all patients may result in a considerable degree of unanticipated harm to the patient.

2. In addition to offending the patient and detracting from the patient's care, inappropriate behavior during a physical examination can lead to civil, and potentially criminal, litigation.

   a. Dr. A was sued for engaging in inappropriate sexual touching by Ms. B. Dr. A had become frustrated with Ms. B's frequent visits for vague physical complaints which he felt were psychosomatic in nature. In an effort to dissuade Ms. B from continuing this pattern, he performed a brusque and impersonal examination of her breasts and groin when she presented with a complaint of fatigue and swollen nodes. She experienced this examination as sexual and abusive, in part because it was reminiscent of events which had occurred during her childhood.

   b. Dr. C had to defend himself against a charge of battery (unpermitted touching without justification) after he forcibly conducted a physical examination of a resisting patient.

C. Social (Non-sexual) Relationships with Patients

1. In certain settings, such as small towns, social contact between physicians and patients is unavoidable. Confidentiality and cordiality without undue familiarity allow these treatment relationships to succeed.

2. Close friendships between a physician and a patient can compromise the physician's objectivity and lead to errors in judgment because of the physician's emotional involvement. The same principles apply here that apply in the context of physicians treating family members.

   a. Dr. D was the physician for his best friend, Mr. E. When Mr. E had a manic episode, Dr. D was unable to distance himself and commit Mr. E to the hospital.

   b. Dr. F saw her friend Ms. G for annual visits. This worked well until Ms. G began discussing her medical problems during social gatherings and calling Dr. F at home at all hours to ask advice about minor aches and pains. Dr. F was unable to set limits on those calls, as she would have done with other patients.

D. Gifts

1. Patients often give gifts to their physicians as a sign of appreciation, especially during the holiday season. Rejection of gifts can offend a patient, while accepting valuable gifts can compromise a physician's judgment.

   a. A patient may give expensive gifts in an effort to curry favor with the physician. The physician then may feel indebted to the patient and have his or her judgment influenced by this sense of indebtedness.

   b. **Highly personal gifts, such as intimate apparel, should serve as a warning that the boundaries of the relationship have been strained and perhaps violated.** In such circumstances, the meaning of the gift must be explored with the patient. When the gift is inappropriately personal, it may have to be returned after discussion with the patient.

2. Physicians on occasion give gifts to patients in honor of events such as weddings and the birth of children. This decision must be made carefully, keeping in mind how the act of gift giving may be interpreted by the patient and others. Such gifts should be modest and tasteful.

3. **Gift-giving and receiving in psychiatric practice can take on special significance because of the issues of transference and countertransference** discussed in

Chapters 12 and 13. Patients can attach great significance to both events. Some psychotherapists use small gifts as a therapeutic tool which indicate to patients that they are connected to the therapist and that the therapist is thinking of them outside the treatment setting. While this can provide comfort and a sense of stability to very disturbed patients, it can easily be misinterpreted as an indicator of personal feelings beyond those appropriate to the treatment. A physician who gives gifts in such a setting must be prepared to explain the meaning of the gift to the patient.

   a. When Dr. H went on vacation, she sent her patient Mr. I a postcard and brought him a small gift. Mr. I suffered from depression complicated by extreme sensitivity to abandonment, and he became distressed when Dr. H left town. Mr. I interpreted the card and gift as a signal that Dr. H thought about him constantly and romantically. He developed an infatuation with Dr. H that was unknown to her until Mr. I began stalking her.

   b. Ms. J gave her psychiatrist a gift to show appreciation for her help during an extended personal crisis. The gift was a day-long visit to an expensive spa, at which Ms. J said she would join Dr. K. Dr. K thanked Ms. J for the gift and commented on its very personal nature, which they then discussed as part of the treatment. She indicated that she could not accept the gift, and Ms. J instead made a contribution to a local charity.

E. Sex in the Treatment Relationship

1. As was indicated above, sexual relations with patients have received much attention in legal and ethical circles. The reasons why physicians get involved in these relationships vary. They include predatory sexual behavior by physicians seeking to take advantage of patients as well as infatuation on the part of physicians who are vulnerable because of their life circumstances. Some patients may be seductive or at least engage in behavior which may be interpreted by the physician as seductive. Nevertheless, **it is always the physician's responsibility to maintain appropriate boundaries. Failure to do so is always the fault of the physician.**

2. Sex with patients in the guise of treatment constitutes fraud and misrepresentation and may provide the basis for criminal prosecution in some states.

3. Sexual relationships with patients often result from the disparity in power and authority between doctor and patient. Such relationships are inherently coercive and lack consent.

4. Patients who have had sexual relationships with their physicians may suffer significant harm as a result. Such injury becomes a justifiable basis for a lawsuit against the physician.

   a. Dr. K, a PCP, engaged in a sexual relationship with Ms. L. She had come to see him for routine care but felt comfortable discussing the problems in her other relationships. Dr. K began extending her visits from 20 minutes to an hour, explaining that he was doing psychotherapy with her. He also began scheduling the visits during evening hours, when his staff had gone home. After the visits, they began having dinner together. This led to a sexual relationship. When Dr. K broke off the relationship, Ms. L became severely depressed and suicidal. After her hospitalization, she successfully brought a malpractice suit against Dr. K.

   b. Mr. M saw Dr. N, a PCP, for problems related to impotence. Dr. N saw Mr. and Mrs. M in counseling involving this issue. Dr. N encountered Mrs. M in a social setting, and a sexual relationship developed. Mr. M successfully sued Dr. N for malpractice and alienation of affections.

III. Handling Challenges to Boundaries

A. Be aware of the importance of boundaries in your practice and be clear with your patients about those boundaries.

B. When in doubt about boundary issues, consult a colleague or someone who has experience in this area. A good indicator that boundaries are being strained occurs when the physician begins doing things he or she would not do for other patients, such as changing appointments to the end of the day, allowing extended time, touching the patient affectionately, and giving the patient a ride home.

C. If boundary crossings occur, discuss them with the patient.

1. Let the patient know that such events are not a normal part of treatment and should not have occurred. For example, if a distressed physician tells a patient about his own marital difficulties, it should be made clear that this is an error on the physician's part. **Burdening the patient with concerns about the physician's well-being is always inappropriate and constitutes a breach of the fiduciary relationship.**

2. Ask the patient how he or she feels about the event. This can turn an error into a therapeutic event and serve as a warning to both parties.

D. If a boundary violation occurs, a consultant should be called in to see the patient and the physician so that the situation can be brought under control. The same is true for boundary crossings that cannot be addressed adequately by the physician alone. Keeping these events secret from colleagues and supervisors often leads to disaster.

1. For example, if a romantic relationship begins to develop between a physician and a patient, a consultant should be brought in to help the parties explore the clinical, ethical, and legal aspects of that relationship.

2. If the treatment relationship begins to take on erotic tones, a consultant or supervisor should be called for assistance.

3. Before a physician engages in any business activity with a patient, the boundary issues must be explored thoroughly. How will the treatment be affected if the business venture fails?

E. When in doubt, examine whether the activity is for the benefit of the patient or the physician.

Suggested Readings

Bisbing, S.B., Jorgenson, L.M., & Sutherland, P.K. (1996). *Sexual abuse by professionals: A legal guide.* Charlottesville, Va.: Michie.

Farber, N.J., Novack, D.H., Silverstein, J., et al. (2000). Physicians' experiences with patients who transgress boundaries. *Journal of General Internal Medicine, 15*(11), 770–775.

Gabbard, G.O. (Ed.). (1989). *Sexual exploitation in professional relationships.* Washington, DC: American Psychiatric Press.

Gabbard, G., & Nadelson, C. (1996). Professional boundaries in the physician-patient relationship. *Forum, 17*(2), 7–8.

Gutheil, T.G., & Gabbard, G.O. (1993). The concept of boundaries in clinical practice: Theoretical and risk-management dimensions. *American Journal of Psychiatry, 150,* 188–196.

Notman, N.T., & Nadelson, C.C. (1994). Psychotherapy with patients who have had sexual relations with a previous therapist. *Journal of Psychotherapy and Practice Research, 3,* 185–193.

Radden, J. (2001). Boundary violation ethics: Some conceptual clarifications. *Journal of the American Academy of Psychiatry & the Law, 29*(3), 319–326.

CHAPTER 77

Dealing with Psychiatric Issues in an Era of Managed/Capitated Care

Paul Summergrad and Michael S. Jellinek

I. Introduction

The development of managed care has changed not only primary care but psychiatric care as well. Primary care/psychiatric relationships were far from perfect before the advent of managed care. Communication was not always handled in an expeditious or clear fashion. However, primary care physicians (PCPs) had the choice and control to call a psychiatrist whom they trusted and be reasonably certain that their patient could be evaluated and treated without prior authorization. **The advent of managed care has included the following elements:**

- **Intrusive utilization review**
- **Mandated referral via 1-800 telephone numbers**
- **The carving out of mental health from general medical services**

PCPs no longer have the authority to refer patients directly for psychiatric or substance abuse services. They are not able to use known providers in a way that encourages communication and coordinated care. Furthermore, the carving out of mental health services often encourages the reduction of costs in the mental health sector without regard to the effect on primary care costs.

II. Prevalence of Psychiatric Disorders in the Population at Large

A. Large-scale, community-based epidemiologic surveys have estimated that in a single year:
   1. 17% of the population has an anxiety disorder
   2. 11% of the population has a substance abuse disorder
   3. 10% of the population has an affective disorder
   4. 3% of the population has a psychiatric disorder associated with severe impairment

B. **In primary care settings, patients who have a higher than expected use of care, or no definable medical condition, are likely to have a concurrent psychiatric or substance abuse disorder. In particular these cases include patients with:**
   1. **Fatigue**
   2. **Insomnia**
   3. **Headache**
      a. **Patients with these complaints and undiagnosed psychiatric disorders (including somatization) make increased use of primary care.**

III. Laws on Mental Health and Substance Abuse Treatment

In addition to findings demonstrating a high rate of mental health disorders in the general health care sector, studies done over the last 20 years have indicated repeatedly that there is a *de facto* mental health and substance abuse service system in the United States that relies heavily on the primary care sector—not mental health clinicians.

A. 10–20% of patients will have an active mental health disorder.

B. More than half of all ambulatory mental health services are provided in the general health care sector.

C. Many patients who are cared for in the general health care sector have unusual or atypical presentations of psychiatric illnesses. These cases include the following:

1. Illnesses that do not meet full diagnostic criteria for mental health or substance abuse services
2. Primary care patients with problem lists that contain an average of six problems. Psychiatric symptoms can modify or affect the presentation of these other disorders.

IV. Psychiatric Treatment in the Primary Care Setting

Psychiatric treatment (as is described in this volume) is more effective, based on randomized, controlled studies, than has ever been true before.

A. A wide range of effective psychopharmacologic agents are available to treat common affective syndromes (including depression, unipolar depression, and bipolar disorders) and a range of anxiety disorders (including panic disorder, obsessive-compulsive disorder, and chronic anxiety disorders).

B. Disorders that present in the general health care setting, for example, as major depression, dysthymia (minor depression), or panic disorder, are now treatable with success rates of more than 80% with standard, available psychopharmacologic agents.

C. The development of new psychopharmacologic agents, including the selective serotonin reuptake inhibitors, has changed primary care prescription practice.

1. Dosing of psychopharmacologic agents has become, in general, less complex.
2. These drugs often have fewer side effects and are safer in over-dosage, making them highly useful agents in the primary care setting.
3. Greater awareness and acceptance of psychopharmacology (in part due to direct consumer advertising) has increased the frequency of psychopharmacologic treatment.

V. Guidelines for Psychiatric Treatment in the Primary Care Setting

A. Become familiar with a few common problems in your primary care practice.

B. Include a few screening and rating instruments in your practice for case finding, and to monitor the outcome of treatment. These can include screening instruments such as the CAGE (see Chapter 52) for substance abuse or the SDDS-PC or PRIME MD (see Chapter 7).

C. Don't expect to manage or care for patients with rare, complex, or unusual psychiatric presentations. Such patients may need to be co-managed, however.

D. Become familiar with one or two drugs in a particular class. There is little need to know seven or eight tricyclic antidepressants or four or five of the newest selective serotonin reuptake inhibitors. Becoming familiar with one or two drugs, often those with slightly different side effects or half-life profiles, allows one to get a sense of patients' reactions to these agents and when reactions may be atypical.

VI. PCP–Psychiatrist Interactions

A. Under ordinary circumstances most physicians feel comfortable working with, and referring to, a relatively small number of specialists.

B. Define expectations for communication at the beginning: Primary care physicians should tell the psychiatrist by phone, letter, or e-mail an outline of the current problems facing the patient and the reasons for the consultation.

    1. **Helpful data includes the following:**

        a. **Intercurrent medical problems**

        b. **Past medical and psychiatric history**

        c. **Recent family losses or trauma**

        d. **Current medications that the patient has taken, including past trials of psychopharmacologic agents and reasons for their use**

C. Assess the feel of the doctor-patient interaction in the primary care setting. Many patients who most bedevil PCPs have multiple medical symptoms and psychiatric co-morbidities and are often the patients many PCPs most dread seeing. This is especially true of patients with somatization disorder or co-morbid personality disorders.

D. Expect and require a callback on the day of the consultation from the psychiatrist including the following information:

    1. **The overall view of the patient, diagnosis, needs, problems, and recommendations for immediate treatment**

    2. **A decision** (made either at the time of consultation or after evaluation) **regarding when or whether the psychiatrist will take over the care of the patient,** return the patient to the PCP, or co-manage the patient, and if so, for which aspects of care (i.e., psychopharmacologic or psychotherapeutic)

    3. **Determine whether the psychiatrist can refer the patient to another mental health clinician** if he or she needs specialized treatment (e.g., cognitive-behavioral, family, group, or individual psychotherapy). Psychiatrists need to communicate to PCPs after the consultation by letter in order to have a formal record of the consultation. Especially helpful are specific recommendations listed in the referral response, and guidelines for when to re-consult the psychiatrist. PCPs should expect promptness and reliability. Especially important is the ability of psychiatrists to work closely with physicians to accept referrals of an urgent nature in a timely fashion.

    4. A psychiatrist should be reachable in urgent or emergent situations. Psychiatrists who consult frequently with PCPs need to:

        a. Define for their staff and for the referring physicians when they can be interrupted

        b. Work with a team of consulting psychiatrists who are available at all hours

VII. Increasing Availability of Psychiatric Providers

Several other models are available for increasing availability of psychiatric providers. These models include:

A. The co-location of psychiatrists or other mental health clinicians in primary care settings

B. The hiring of mental health clinicians by primary care clinicians so they become their employees

C. Creation of psychiatric group practices in close proximity to primary care settings

D. The development of Psychiatry TeleConsultation Units. These units are staffed by psychiatrists and afford physicians direct phone access to a psychiatrist. This allows urgent and emergent problems to be triaged from the primary care setting, often while the patient is still there, directly to a senior psychiatric consultant. This model may allow for fewer formal psychiatric consultations, which may reduce expenses under capitation. Mechanisms to support teleconsult services under fee-for-service reimbursement systems have been difficult.

VIII. Interfacing with Psychotherapy

In an era of advanced psychopharmacologic treatment and greater diagnostic accuracy, PCPs should anticipate that for many patients psychotherapy may be a secondary or adjunctive treatment and that psychopharmacologic strategies may be tried first. This occurs for several reasons:

A. Psychopharmacologic treatment strategies are efficacious.

B. Patients often have such high levels of anxiety or depression that psychotherapy or cognitive-behavioral techniques are ineffective unless depression or anxiety is reduced.

C. Several models work in clinical practices.
  1. Current treatment models
     a. Patients may be seen back for psychopharmacologic management with a descending frequency of visits depending on the efficacy of treatment.
     b. This can often include frequent check-ins in addition to office-based visits, use of letters, phone, and unsecured terms (e.g., e-mail systems).
  2. For many disorders (e.g., major depression), studies show the best outcome with combined pharmacotherapy and psychotherapy.
  3. Some patients, especially those in the public eye or VIPs, may request "private" psychiatric or psychotherapy referrals.

IX. Health Care Economics

Significant data suggest that patients with intercurrent psychiatric and medical symptoms make more frequent use of medical evaluation and interventions. In particular, patients with depression, panic disorder, and somatization have increased utilization of general medical services.

A. This can occur when patients with undiagnosed disorders (e.g., panic disorder) make frequent emergency room visits.

B. Other situations occur in patients who have medical disorders (e.g., chronic obstructive pulmonary disease) who develop secondary panic in response to the breathlessness associated with their condition.

C. There are patients (e.g., those with somatization) who will rarely go outside of the general health care sector, but prefer to be treated by PCPs.
  1. These patients will need to be cared for predominately within the primary care sector using on-site psychiatric consultation or telephone consultation as appropriate.

2. Given the high frequency of patients presenting in primary care with non-specific complaints including fatigue and insomnia, frequent PCP evaluation or psychiatric consultation may be required.

D. Cost offset effects

1. In addition to the data suggesting the high frequency of medical use by patients with psychiatric disorders, there is evidence that the effective treatment, or at least management strategies of those psychiatric disorders, will likely reduce medical use.

2. In studies of somatizing patients, PCPs were instructed in standard care for somatizing patients including the following:

   a. Increased frequency of scheduled PCP-patient meetings

   b. Close attention to physical symptoms during the course of PCP visits

   c. Placement of limits on outside referrals

   d. Not defining the patients' problems as psychiatric

E. Patients treated in such a fashion had a reduced frequency of health care use in the two years following treatment.

X. Contracting for Mental Health and Substance Abuse Services

Because many mental health and substance abuse services are carved out of general health care contracts there may be a willingness on the part of many PCPs to move care from the primary sector to the mental health sector as soon as problems are diagnosed or become problematic. This often creates difficulties because the use of criteria by the managed care carve-out company may be different, or more restrictive, than that used by the PCP.

Additionally, because the incentives between the PCP and the mental health substance abuse carve-out company are not aligned, the managed care company may want to reduce mental health costs—even if a patient makes more primary care visits.

The mental health carve-out company may have little incentive to provide care for mental-health services that lower medical costs if it means increasing psychiatric treatment costs. In looking at contracts presented to primary care physician groups for evaluation, one needs to think carefully about the following issues:

A. Is the mental health substance abuse portion of the budget so low that it will cause care to be diverted into the general health care sector? For example, if the managed care company has agreed to a submarket capitation rate in order to "capture" new patients, it may be disinclined to allow referrals. Even if a contract is not globally capitated, are costs of psychopharmacologic agents borne by the PCP group or the mental health carve-out?

B. Does the company or the carve-out managed care organization have an interest and experience in dealing with issues that cross the medical-psychiatric interface? Patients with congestive heart failure do better when followed closely by behaviorally trained case managers who improve compliance. Will the mental health carve-out company support such care? Are the financial incentives and the clinical management systems aligned to support this?

C. Is there a group of psychiatrists from within one's own system that would be better positioned to care for patients in an integrated and complete way? Does the carve-out company use a network of providers and facilities separate from the rest of the medical system?

D. What would be most effective and acceptable to patients?

E. Would you prefer to go through a 1-800 number for referral of patients, or would you prefer care that is locally based and reliant on PCP and psychiatrist referral?

F. Are one's preferred specialists available through the carve-out company? How complex are the required authorization procedures? How intrusive or different are they from normal office procedure? Does the carve-out company have a full range of providers or a "shadow network" of providers who have limited access or who have left the network entirely?

G. Is there a way to increase and align the incentives between primary care and psychiatric care so that all groups are working closely for the optimal care of the patient in an integrated and non-carved-out fashion?

H. Can patients with co-morbid psychiatric and medical illness be hospitalized at the PCP's primary hospital?

I. Has mental health parity been fully implemented by the carve-out company or used as a rationalization to further limit care?

XI. When Should a PCP Strongly Consider a Referral or Consultation?

Although there are few published guidelines for specific disorders about when to consider a consultation, these general guidelines are helpful:

A. When a patient has new onset of psychotic illness, or has suicidal or homicidal ideation

B. When a patient has a marked change in personality or becomes fearful, agitated, and withdrawn, or will not communicate
  1. In all of these cases first consider the possible role of other neuropsychiatric or medical illnesses.

C. When a patient has a history of schizophrenia or manic-depressive illness.
Other conditions that often lead to referral are refractory childhood developmental conditions, complex behavioral disturbances (e.g., ADHD), and rare anxiety disorders (e.g., obsessive-compulsive disorder), and refractory illnesses of any kind.

D. If a patient has failed two courses of a standard antidepressant or antianxiety agent
  1. Under those circumstances, an evaluation should include the following considerations:
     a. The underlying psychosocial issues or alternative diagnoses
     b. The complex psychopharmacologic treatment regimens
     c. Other medical or neurologic disorders that are presenting psychiatrically
     d. Co-morbid psychiatric disorders (e.g., depression and substance abuse)

Mental health care is an indivisible element of primary care. Such care cannot be carved out; it can only be sub-optimized. Primary care physicians and psychiatrists working together must find a way to do better for the sake of their patients.

Suggested Readings

Chinman, G., Kelly, M., & Borus, J. (2002). Teaching residents the reality of current mental health care. *Harvard Review of Psychiatry, 10*(1), 56–58.

deGruy, F., III. (1996). Mental health care in the primary care setting. In *Primary care, America's health in a new era.* Washington, DC: Institute of Medicine, pp. D1–D19.

Kessler, R.C., McGonagle, K.A., Zhao, S., et al. (1994). Lifetime and 12-month prevalence of *DSM III-R* psychiatric disorders in the United States: results from the National Comorbidity Study. *Archives of General Psychiatry, 51,* 8–19.

Lin, E.H., VonKorff, M., Russo, J., et al. (2000). Can depression treatment in primary care reduce disability? A stepped care approach. *Archives of Family Medicine, 9*(10), 1052–1058.

Olfson, M., Marcus, S.C., Druss, B., et al. (2002). National trends in the outpatient treatment of depression. *Journal of the American Medical Association, 287*(2), 203–209.

Regier, D.A., Narrow, W.E., Rae, D.S., et al. (1993). The de facto U.S. mental health and addictive disorder service system. *Archives of General Psychiatry, 50,* 85–94.

Simon, G., Ormel, J., VonKorff, M., et al. (1995). Health care costs associated with depressive and anxiety disorders with primary care. *American Journal of Psychiatry, 152,* 352–357.

Simon, G.E., Katon, W.J., VonKorff, M., et al. (2002). Cost-effectiveness of a collaborative care program for primary care patients with persistent depression. *American Journal of Psychiatry, 158*(10), 1638–1644.

Simon, G.E., VonKorff, M., Rutter, C.M., & Peterson, D.A. (2001). Treatment process and outcomes for managed care patients receiving new antidepressant prescriptions from psychiatrists and primary care physicians. *Archives of General Psychiatry, 58*(4), 395–401.

Smith, G.R., Mort, K., & Karker, M. (1995). A trial of the effect of a standardized psychiatric consultation on health outcome and costs in somatizing patients. *Archives of General Psychiatry, 52,* 238–243.

CHAPTER 78

Coping with the Rigors of Medical Practice

BANDY X. LEE, HELEN KIM, AND EDWARD MESSNER

I. Overview

A. Introduction

Humanitarian ideals that once inspired the choice of a medical career can later lead to both professional success and stress. Certain psychological characteristics of physicians can be both adaptive and maladaptive: perfectionism, self-doubt, exaggerated sense of responsibility, and limited capacity for emotional expressiveness (Gabbard and Menninger, 1989). Medical training further encourages behaviors that contribute to burnout: long work hours with sleep deprivation, repression of feelings, and isolation from ordinary social situations.

When carried beyond residency and applied to their own personal lives, adaptive mechanisms that once sustained the physician through grueling training can leave him or her cynical, disillusioned, and unfulfilled at work and at home. Understanding the sources of stress and cultivating coping mechanisms can help physicians identify risks associated with medical practice and steer them toward preventive or ameliorating interventions.

B. Epidemiology

1. Despite the individual strengths of physicians, they commonly experience depression, substance abuse, and even suicide.
   a. In the United States, the number of physicians who kill themselves annually would fill an average-size medical school class.
   b. Female physicians on average die 10 years earlier than their male counterparts, the opposite of the sexual longevity ratio in the general population.
   c. Substance abuse often leads to physician impairment. Up to 12% of resident physicians reported increased use of substances compared with their use before training (Koran and Litt, 1988).
   d. Primary care physicians (PCPs) are particularly vulnerable to chemical dependence and psychiatric disorders associated with stress (Talbott, et al., 1987).

II. Etiologies for Physician Stress and Burnout

A. Dealing with Difficult Clinical Situations and Emotions

1. **Suffering**

   Physicians typically receive limited training in reassuring individuals who are uncomfortable, anxious, and suffering. The obligation to collect clinical information is superimposed on the anxiety of facing physical and emotional nakedness.

2. **Ethical conflicts**

   The patient's trust and reliance on the physician for information and advice raise numerous ethical issues. Within this setting, physicians often find themselves in the difficult position of trying to relieve pain as they inflict more through diagnostic procedures or drug side effects.

3. **Death and dying**

Death, dying, and suffering are all part of a physician's work experience. Physicians often counsel patients and families as they struggle with difficult issues (e.g., limiting treatment or withdrawing life support). The physician often assumes responsibility for prolonging life or facilitating inevitable death when confronted by these morally ambiguous predicaments.

4. **The perception of failure**

Finally, because death is often perceived as a failure of medical intervention by both the physician and the patient's relatives, physicians are ironically doomed to failure.

B. Responsibility without Authority

1. As medicine's front line, PCPs face the daunting task of keeping pace with a wide range of medical topics. Pervasive uncertainty about one's medical knowledge can be an enormously stressful aspect of practice. In addition, physicians must often make serious clinical decisions based on incomplete, conflicting, and untimely data. These stresses are compounded by other competing demands on physicians as they answer to institutions, insurers, patients, and families. Current health insurance reforms often establish standards of performance without physician involvement, which further undermines pride, morale, organizational commitment, and the physician's own efforts.

2. Medicine is still a field that attracts people who enter with a genuine desire to help others, often without the promise of recognition or reward. As one's perspective expands, however, this humanitarian impulse can lead to disillusionment, given that humanitarian values do not coincide well with market values, which govern much of the world and medicine today. Within their practices, physicians must deal with increasing restrictions in care, larger patient loads with less pay, and mounting paperwork. Outside their practices, they must exist within a society where industry keeps growing but where public health is deteriorating, both domestically and abroad.

C. Balancing Personal, Interpersonal, and Professional Roles

1. **Interpersonal Relationships**

Physicians often work in isolation and under adverse or competitive work conditions. We also tend to be staunchly self-reliant and reluctant to seek help with work or family life. This smoldering dissatisfaction often contributes to poor relationships with patients, relatives, and staff and leads to physician burnout.

2. **Conflicting Family and Professional Roles**

Traditional gender roles can also contribute to burnout and low job satisfaction. For instance, the pregnant physician must contend with not only the added demands of pregnancy, but also the historical prejudices of the wider medical culture. Within this work environment, maternity leaves are often characterized as extra entitlements that unfairly burden other colleagues rather than as rightful parts of an employee's benefit package. Female physicians often internalize this view and avoid asking for any accommodations in work schedule even if they are experiencing physical or emotional problems during or after pregnancy.

D. Cynicism and Discouragement

1. **Misanthropy**

   a. Instead of drawing out patients' feelings, physicians frequently find that patients evoke their own feelings of anxiety, defensiveness, and helplessness. Exposure to patients' suffering or hostility—in the form of manipulation, ingratitude, or even physical threats—can produce reactive misanthropy. In defense, one may not only lose warmth and concern for patients but can also develop crusty defensiveness or contempt.

   b. Misanthropic attitudes may evolve as a kind of self-protection in the face of the exhaustion and stressful experiences of medical practice. This kind of emotional isolation may carry over to all patients, so that one no longer recognizes patients who are appreciative, pleasant, and responsive to treatment.

2. **Expansion of antipathy**

   In its more malignant forms, the antipathy one develops toward patients may extend to other relationships, including those with fellow physicians, health care professionals, and even friends and family. It can color one's view of humanity as a whole, where one feels alone and develops a cynical evaluation of even those who might be a potential source of support. Such conflict with one's values and intentions can lead to self-punishment, guilt, and feelings of failure.

E. Legal Issues

1. In a litigious culture, the threat of malpractice suits can add to the tensions encountered in medical practice.

2. Even when not a defendant, a physician is sometimes required to testify as a witness in depositions or trials. This can be time-consuming as well as stressful.

III. When Coping Strategies Go Awry

A. How We See Ourselves

1. **Denial of vulnerability**

   As physicians, we wish to see ourselves as immune to impairments. One common way of coping with stress is to work harder and longer, which can ultimately cause even greater damage. Physicians often rely on defense mechanisms of repression, rationalization, denial, and reaction formation in the suppression and displacement of emotions. Over time, however, unexamined reactions to stressful situations can undermine relationships not only with patients but also with friends and family.

2. **Compromise of familial concerns**

   Marital or family concerns may be demeaned as not as important or urgent as saving lives and relieving pain. Too tired for empathic listening, reasonable conversation, or recreation, physicians often internalize their own concerns and become self-absorbed. For some, the demands of medical training, the rigors of establishing a practice, and the expectations of colleagues are used as excuses to postpone or avoid emotional intimacy in relationships.

3. **Deferment of referrals**

   Seeking help for personal or family problems is commonly misconstrued as an admission of weakness or personal failure. The stigma of a psychiatric diagnosis also keeps physicians from seeking appropriate care. Furthermore, to avoid public humiliation and disclosure to colleagues or licensing boards, many physicians feel unwilling or unable to ask for assistance. The stress of adopting an omnipotent, directive, and controlling stance can lead to god-like expectations and blame for human fallibility in oneself and others. This intolerance toward any personal vulnerability can undermine a physician's well-being as well as personal and work relationships.

B. How to Recognize Stress in Oneself

1. **Signs and symptoms**

Unmanageable stress can lead to clinical states of anxiety or depression that may have tragic consequences for clinicians, patients, and families if left untreated. Signals of psychic pain include feelings of overload and exhaustion, apathy, anhedonia, despair, headaches, gastrointestinal disturbances, and verbal incontinence. Other signs include longer and less efficient working hours; poor and irregular sleep and eating habits; disrupted family relationships; unaccustomed difficulties in memory, concentration, and problem-solving; and multiple suggestions by friends, relatives, or colleagues to seek help.

IV. Interventions

A. "Physician Heal Thyself"

As much as the health care profession requires the giving of oneself, it is necessary to recharge one's own emotional batteries. Each of us has a repertoire of methods for dealing with stressful situations that can be strengthened. Prevention of emotional overload can be achieved through anticipation of, and preparation for, difficulties, rather than through denial of them. Following are some examples of coping strategies:

1. **Make a systematic effort to process experiences** (e.g., by talking with a colleague or through introspection during a long commute). Dealing with the day's stresses can help one refrain from inflicting the emotional effects on family or other cherished relationships. Also, attempting to learn from and transform tragic events to growth-promoting ones can neutralize some of the misery that they inflict.

2. **Take your own history of responses to past stresses.** Physicians can apply this familiar skill to sort the useful strategies for coping from the counter-productive ones. Under stressful conditions, emotions often go unnoticed until they reach a painful level. Early signs might include unruffled competence at work followed by irritability or explosive anger at home. Clinicians who have not prepared for the stresses of practice may not even recognize the intensity of their needs or the desperation of their impulses.

3. **Make a list of methods that work.** Constructively channeled actions can discharge frustration and anger, such as through athletics and prudent sexual engagement. Readily available physical expressions include shouting into a bed pillow or running up stairs for release. Stretching or performing isometric exercises can also reduce muscle tension. A single episode of tearfulness does not indicate emotional instability but may in fact represent a restoration of balance.

4. **Maintain a healthy self-regard.** Caring for the mind and body and the appreciation of one's compassion, honesty, and perseverance can help individuals cope with stress. Also, the temptation during times of exhaustion to resort to poor eating habits can add weight, reduce fitness, and impair physical appearance, which can undermine attitudes about attractiveness and worth.

5. **Mentally rehearse potential problems or stressful situations and predict one's emotional reactions to them.** Imagining the expression of feelings can decompress intense surges of emotion, such as anger, sadness, or fear. Central to the usefulness of such expressive fantasies is the recognition that they are distinct from the corresponding actions; they need not, and usually should not, be enacted.

6. **Engage in directed fantasies** by imagining a scene that is affectively intense. A patient can be beaten up by thugs, or a superior might be hit in the face with a cream pie. The more uncivilized the fantasy, the more effective it can be in the management of pent-up emotion. In addition, the more unrealistic the fantasy, the easier it is to maintain the distinction between fantasy and the corresponding enactment.

7. **Dialogue with friends and family regarding anticipated unavailability.** This can help prepare them and sustain relationships. Lovers, spouses, and relatives may respond with anger or withdrawal, which may lead one to feel rejected or punished. On the other hand, as long as communication is maintained, adversity experienced together can lead to intimacy and mutual regard.

8. **Use humor and mutual support** with colleagues to magnify respites, triumphs, and the joy of learning while providing for a space to vent your rage and frustration.

9. **Relish mementos of happier times, recalling previous triumphs and rehearsing original goals.** Reassociation with familiar people, places, things, and activities can improve morale. Sustained by recollections of the pinnacles of one's life, the clinician will be in a better position to cope with daily stresses.

10. **Regard patients' behavior as a form of communication.** Collaborative relationships with patients seem to buffer against the worst effects of stress. Patients can evoke in the clinician feelings and attitudes comparable to those of others in the patients' past (complementary identification) and attitudes that the patient experiences (concurrent identification). Difficult behaviors may be a way of saying: "See! Now you know how I feel!" Understanding our own subjective reactions may be a source of clinical data about how to approach patients and recruit their individual strengths.

11. **Learn relaxation techniques and self-hypnosis to relieve stress.** Tension, sleep deprivation, over-stimulation, and the dread of returning to work without adequate rest may lure one to benzodiazepines, alcohol, or other sedating agents. Self-prescribed medications should signal caution at the first dose. As a safe and convenient alternative, self-hypnosis can induce sleep and reduce tension. Find a comfortable position and clear the mind of intrusive thoughts. Imagine yourself in pleasant surroundings and then picture your feet relaxing followed by relaxation of various segments of the body. Silent, sedating meditation can be brief depending on skill, practice, and extent of sleep deprivation.

12. **Temporarily suspend the requirement to be logical and relevant.** Observing the contents of one's mind and its spontaneous associations may lead to new insights. Mental experiences other than linear processes can evolve, connect, and merge into one another, and also interplay with our emotions and attitudes. Free association may lead one to ideas, feelings, and perceptions that were formerly outside of one's awareness, inducing delight in their complexity, generativity, and beauty. Poetry, abstract paintings, classical music, or other sources of mindfulness can further increase resiliency and connection with a deeper, stabler level of oneself.

13. With respect to gender issues, **physicians can greatly benefit from discussing dilemmas and decisions with colleagues and mentors** who have successfully confronted similar situations.

14. To cope well with legal issues, **the physician would do well to attend lectures and/or workshops on risk management.** When threats of litigation arise, it is in the physician's interest to seek the guidance of a professional liability insurance company and an attorney.

B. When to Consult

Professional consultation can add objectivity and expertise when a physician experiences overwhelming stress or burnout. An Athenian physician wrote in A.D. 2, "These are the duties of a physician: First . . . to heal his mind and to give help to himself before giving it to anyone else." Consider consultation for any of the following:

1. Depression (SIG: E CAPS) (see Chapter 14)
2. Suicidal ideation including wishes, intentions, plans, or actions (see Chapter 15)
3. Anxiety that interferes with personal or professional enjoyment (see Chapter 16)
4. Alcohol and drug abuse (see Chapter 52)
5. Rage and hatred expressed inappropriately
6. Interference with clinical skills or judgment
7. Impulsive or reckless behavior
8. Eating disorder symptoms

C. Types of Available Professional Help

1. **Psychotherapy** (see Chapter 2)

   Individual psychotherapy involves a commitment to meet with a psychiatrist for an initial evaluation in which both parties determine the appropriateness of therapy or medication. Individual therapy typically includes weekly meetings for short- or long-term therapy, ranging from months to years. Many physician-patients have found psychotherapy to be a powerful, life-enhancing experience.

2. **Psychopharmacology**

   If medications are indicated, these can be administered by a psychiatrist with or without ongoing psychotherapy. Some physicians may perceive needing medication as further admission of personal weakness. On the contrary, failing to treat biologically-based psychiatric conditions, such as major depression, is tantamount to denying insulin to the Type I diabetic; both omissions can produce fatal consequences.

3. **Couple and family therapy**

   Couple therapists and family therapists can be found at most mental health centers, psychiatric clinics, or private group practices. This support can help physician family relationships, which are paradoxically a major source of coping with the stress of medical practice and the first potential casualty of that stress.

4. **Autognosis or "self-knowledge" rounds**

   Autognosis rounds allow physicians to share their experiences as they identify their subjective reactions to clinical situations, use this information as diagnostic information, and learn how to minimize potential harmful effects of reactions to patients (e.g., managing anger toward a patient in a way that does not interfere with medical care). Autognostic techniques have proved useful to both medicine and psychiatry residents in groups conducted at the Massachusetts General Hospital.

5. **Support Groups**

V. Conclusion

At a Harvard Medical School commencement address, Dr. Ned Cassem charged the graduates with the following: "Fight down your grandiosity: learn to tolerate uncertainty and . . . remain more impressed by the mysteries and uniqueness of your patients than by your own expertise. Give yourself a break. Respect your own limits and vulnerabilities." More than warding off impairment and suffering, this makes more accessible the satisfactions and joys of medicine.

Selected References

Bennett, J., & O'Donovan, D. (2001). Substance misuse by doctors, nurses and other healthcare workers. *Current Opinion in Psychiatry, 14*(3), 195–199.

Boidaubin, E.V., & Levine, R.E. (2001). Identifying and assisting the impaired physician. *American Journal of the Medical Sciences, 322*(1), 31–36.

Cassem, E. (1979). Internship, liberty, death, and other choices. *Harvard Medical School Commencement Address.*

Firth-Cozens, J. (2001). Interventions to improve physicians' well-being and patient care. *Social Science and Medicine, 52*(2), 215–222.

Gabbard, G.O., & Menninger, R.W. (1989). The psychology of postponement in the medical marriage. *Journal of the American Medical Association, 261,* 2378–2381.

Gross, E.B. (1998). Gender differences in physician stress: Why the discrepant findings? *Women and Health, 26*(3), 1–14.

Hawton, K., Clements, A., Sakarovitch, C., et al. (2001). Suicide in doctors: A study of risk according to gender, seniority, and specialty in medical practitioners in England and Wales, 1979–1995. *Journal of Epidemiology and Community Health, 55*(5), 296–300.

Johnson, J.V., Hall, E.M., Ford, D.E., et al. (1995). The psychosocial work environment of physicians. The impact of demands and resources on job dissatisfaction and psychiatric distress in a longitudinal study of Johns Hopkins Medical School graduates. *Journal of Occupational Environmental Medicine, 37*(9), 1151–1159.

Koran, L., & Litt, I. (1988). House staff well-being. *Western Journal of Medicine, 148,* 97–101.

McGovern, M.P., Angres, D.H., Uziel-Miller, N.D., & Leon, S. (1998). Female physicians and substance abuse: Comparisons with male physicians presenting for assessment. *Journal of Substance Abuse Treatment, 15*(6), 525–533.

Messner, E. (1993). *Resilience enhancement for the resident physician.* Durant, Okla.: Essential Medical Information Systems, Inc.

Miller, N.M., & McGowen, R.K. (2000). The painful truth: Physicians are not invincible. *Southern Medical Journal, 93*(10), 966–973.

O'Connor, P.G., & Spickard, A. (1997). Physician impairment by substance abuse. *Medical Clinics of North America, 81*(4), 1037–1052.

Quill, T.E., & Williamson, P.R. (1990). Healthy approaches to physician stress. *Archives of Internal Medicine, 150,* 1857–1861.

Schear, W.A. (1990). Coping with the stress of malpractice litigation: CMIC Defendant Support Program. *Connecticut Medicine, 54*(10), 567–570.

Stern, T.A., Prager, L.M., & Cremens, M.C. (1993). Autognosis rounds for medical house staff. *Psychosomatics, 34*(1), 1–7.

Stewart, D.E., Ahmad, F., Cheung, A.M., et al. (2000). Women physicians and stress. *Journal of Women's Health and Gender-Based Medicine, 9*(2), 185–190.

Index

The letter *t* or *f* following a page number indicates that either a table or figure is being referenced.

AA (Alcoholics Anonymous), 508, 516
Abnormal Involuntary Movement Scale (AIMS), 58
Absence (petit mal) seizures, 227*t,* 232
Abstinence model, chronic opiate dependence, 517
Abuilia, 222
Abuse
   domestic violence. *See* Domestic violence, approach to
   victims, approach to patients who are, 108
Acamprosate, alcoholism treatment, 510
Acceptance, infertile patient, 413
Acetaminophen, tension headaches, 249
Activities of Daily Living (ADLs) Scale, 201, 471
Acupuncture for pain in HIV infection, treatment of, 378
Acute grief, approach to patient with, 153–156
   defining, 153
   duration, 155
   overview, 153
   pharmacological therapy, 155
      medication but not sedation, 155
   primary and secondary mourners, 153
   principles of managing, 155–156
   psychological interventions for, 154–155
   signs of, 153–154
Acute pain, approach to patient with, 314, 318–319; *see also* Pain
Acute stress disorder, approach to patient following, 535–536; *see also* Traumatic event
Acyclovir, neuropsychiatric side effects, 371*t*
ADD (Attention deficit disorder), 708
Addiction Severity Index (ASI), 57
Adjustment disorders
   obesity, 459
   pain, co-morbidity with, 314
ADLs (Activities of Daily Living Scale), 201, 471

Advance directives, terminally ill patients, 690–691; *see also* Treatment decisions at the end of life
Agnosia, 197
Agoraphobia, 77–78
   cognitive-behavioral therapy (CBT), 77–78
   panic disorder, 140
AHCPR Guideline on Depression in Primary Care, 27
AIDS, suicide risk and, approach to patient with, 130; *see also* HIV infection
AIMS (Abnormal Involuntary Movement Scale), 58
Akathisia, mimicking anxiety disorders, 361
Alcohol-abusing patient, 499–512
   alchohol abuse, definition of, 499*t*
   alchohol dependence, definition of, 499*t*
   benzodiazepine abuse risk, 149
   differential diagnosis, 505
   evaluation, 500–505
      interviewing the patient, 502, 505
      psychiatric and social problems associated with alcoholism, 500
      review of systems, 500
      screening tests, 501*t*–504*t*
   fatigue and, 333
   homeless patients, 596
   managing dual-diagnosis patients, 510–511
   overview, 499–500
   referral
      inpatient detoxification, 511
      specialized long-term alcoholism treatment, 511
   sexual dysfunction, 407*t*
   somatization disorder and, 273
   treatment, 509–510
      detoxification, 509
      long-term treatment, 509–510
      medications, 509–510

   treating associated symptoms, 510
   treatment strategies, 505–509
      action/active quitting begins, 508–509
      contemplation to preparation, moving patients from, 507
      maintenance, relapse prevention, 509
      motivational interviewing techniques, 507
      pre-contemplation to contemplation, moving patients from, 507
      preparation to action, moving patients from, 507–508
      stages of behavioral change, 506*t,* 506–507
   violent patient, 572
Alcohol dependence
   definition of, 499*t*
   suicide risk, 130
Alcoholics Anonymous (AA), 508, 516
Alcoholism, prevalence in heroin addicts, 518
Alcohol Use Disorders Identification Test (AUDIT), 501*t*–502*t*
Alcohol withdrawal, mimicking anxiety disorders, 362
Allergies. *See* Multiple environmental allergies, approach to patient with
Allodynia, 316
Almotriptan (Axert), migraine headache treatment, 247
Alosetron (Lotronex), irritable bowel syndrome (IBS) and, 354
Alpha-methyldopa, interaction with monoamine oxidase inhibitors, 617*t*
Alprazolam (Xanax)
   anxiety disorders, 148*t*
   anxiety in terminal illness, 495*t*
   nausea and vomiting, treatment for, 364
   premenstrual syndrome (PMS), 426
   sexual dysfunction, 396*t,* 407*t*
   violent patients, 573

Amantadine (Symmetrel)
  antidepressant-induced
    fatigue and sedation, 621*t*
    sexual dysfunction, 624*t*
  cocaine dependence, 516
American Academy of Neurology
    Criteria for HIV-1 associated
    cognitive/motor complex, 374*t*
American Medical Association
    (AMA), 744
American Psychiatric Association
    (APA), 744
Americans with Disabilities Act
    (ADA), 386, 589
Amitriptyline (Elavil)
  adverse effects, 614*t*
  analgesic use, 326*t*
  anxiety disorder, 147
  depression in terminal illness, 493*t*
  effects on heart and cardiovascular
    system, 634*t*
  GI side effects, 356*t*
  irritable bowel syndrome (IBS), 356*t*
  post-traumatic stress disorder
    (PTSD), 541
  seizures with, 228*t*
  weight gain, 619
Amoxapine (Asendin)
  analgesic use, 326*t*
  seizures with, 228*t*
Amphetamine (Dexedrine)
  attention-deficit/hyperactivity
    disorder (ADHD), 290*t*
  seizures with, 228*t*
Amphetamines, monoamine oxidase
    inhibitors, interaction with, 617*t*
Amphotericin B, neuropsychiatric side
    effects, 372*t*
Amprenavir, neuropsychiatric side
    effects, 371*t*
Amtihypertensives, sexual dysfunction,
    407*t*
Analgesic adjuvants, 325
Analgesic Ladder (WHO), 319*f*
Analgesics, interaction with monoamine
    oxidase inhibitors, 617*t*
Analgesic therapies for pain. *See* Pain,
    approach to patient with
Anastrazole, neuropsychiatric side
    effects, 362*t*, 363
Androgen replacement, 433
Anesthetics, seizures with, 228*t*
Aneurysms, headaches from, 245
Anger
  angry or demanding patients,
    approach to, 106–107; *see
    also* Personality disorders

chronic illness and, 305
infertile patient, 413
Anorexia nervosa, approach to patient
    with, 82, 171–180
  clinical picture, 172
  defining, 171
  diagnoses, 171
  diagnostic criteria, 176–177
  epidemiology, 172
  evaluation, 173–175, 174*t*–175*t*
  infertility and, 414
  medical complications, 174–175
  mortality and, 172
  overview, 171–172
  primary care physician's role, 171
  psychiatric differential diagnosis, 176
  risk factors, 172
  treatment strategies, 177–179
    cognitive-behavioral therapy
      (CBT), 82
Anorexigens, monoamine oxidase
    inhibitors, interaction with, 617*t*
Anorgasmia, antidepressant-induced side
    effect, 624
Anosognosia, 222
Antibacterials, neuropsychiatric side
    effects, 371*t*
Anticholinergic effects of antidepressants,
    management of, 118, 622–623;
    see also Antidepressant-induced
    side effects
Anticholinergics
  nausea and vomiting, post-chemo-
    therapy treatment for, 365
  sexual dysfunction, 407*t*
Anticonvulsants, 122
  depression, 122
  pain in HIV infection, 378
  sexual dysfunction, 396*t*
Antidepressant-induced side effects,
    management of, 613–627
  anticholinergic effects, 622–623
  cardiovascular effects, 615–618,
    629–644, 630*t*–637*t*
  central nervous system effects,
    619–622
  dermatologic side effects, 625–626
  discontinuation effects, 626
  excessive sweating, 626
  gastrointestinal effects, 618–619
  general principles of management,
    613–615, 614*t*
  hair loss, 626
  headache, 626
  overview, 613
  sexual side effects, 623–625
  weight gain, 619

Antidepressants
  anxiety associated with HIV
    infection, 376
  anxiety disorders, 145–147
  attention-deficit/hyperactivity
    disorder (ADHD), 294–297
  atypical, 118–120
  drug-drug interactions, 657, 658*t*–664*t*
  first choice: selective serotonin
    reuptake inhibitors (SSRIs),
    116–117
  generalized anxiety disorder (GAD),
    142
  glucocorticoid use, neuropsychiatric
    complications from, 527*t*
  insomnia, 257
  irritable bowel syndrome (IBS) and,
    355
  misconceptions in the use of, 122
  monoamine oxidase inhibitors
    (MAOIs), 120–121
    interaction with, 617*t*
  multiple environmental allergies, 346
  natural, 673–676
    essential fatty acids (EFAs), 675–676
    folic acid, 674–675
    inositol, 676
    S-adenosyl methionine (SAMe),
      637*t*, 644, 674
    St. John's wort (SJW), 673–674
    Vitamin B$_{12}$, 674–675
  organ transplant patients, 388
  panic disorder, 141
  postpartum depression, 449
  pregnancy, 437
  premenstrual syndrome (PMS), 425
  seizures with, 228*t*
  serotonin norepinephrine reuptake
    inhibitors (SNRIs), 117
  sexual dysfunction, 396*t*, 407*t*
  social phobia, 142
  switching, 123
  tricyclic antidepressants (TCAs),
    117–118, 294–295
Antiemetic treatments and their side
    effects, 364–365
Antiepileptic drugs, 234
Antifungals, neuropsychiatric side
    effects, 372*t*
Antihistamines
  anxiety in terminal illness, 495*t*
  insomnia, 257
    in HIV/AIDS patients, 377
Antimicrobials, seizures with, 228*t*
Antineoplastics, seizures with, 228*t*
Antiparasitics, neuropsychiatric side
    effects, 371*t*

Antipsychotic medications, 644–648,
    645*t*, 647*t*
  cardiovascular side effects, 644–648,
    645*t*, 647*t*
  drug-drug interactions, 665–666, 667*t*
  multiple environmental allergies, 346
  pregnancy, 437
  sexual dysfunction, 396*t*, 407*t*
  violent patients, 574
Antisocial personality disorder, commonly
    co-morbid with alcohol abuse,
    500
Antivirals, neuropsychiatric side effects,
    371*t*
Anxiety Disorder Interview Scale,
    Revised (ADIS-R), 55
Anxiety disorders
  alcoholism, 505, 510–511
    co-morbidity with, 510–511
    differentiating from, 505
  cancer patients, 359
  chronic illness and, 305
  differentiating from depression, 116
  dizziness and, 264
  glucocorticoid use, 523*t*
  homeless patients, 596
  infertility and, 417
  insomnia, 257
  menopause and, 429, 432
  multiple environmental allergies and,
    344
  non-compliance, 729
  obesity, 459, 464
  organ transplant patients, 389–390
  pain, co-morbidity with, 314
  pregnancy, 435, 438*t*
  premenstrual syndrome (PMS) and,
    423
  prevalence in primary care settings, 3
  referrals for, 29*t*
  screening tests for, 55
  sexual dysfunction, 409
  sexually assaulted patient, 549
  smoking cessation and, 707
  somatization disorder and, 273
  suicide risk, 130
  terminal illness, 494–495
Anxiolytic-hypnotics
  natural, 676–678
    kava, 677–678
    melatonin, 678
    valerian, 676–677
Anxiolytics
  cardiovascular side effects, 650
  drug-drug interactions, 666, 668
  organ transplant patients, 388
  sexual dysfunction, 396*t*, 407*t*

Anxious patient, approach to, 137–152;
    see also Anxiety disorders
  co-morbid depression, 143–144
  course of anxiety disorders, 139
  defining anxiety, 137
  differential diagnosis, 139–140
  epidemiology, 138
  etiology, 137–138
  impact of anxiety disorders on quality
    of life, 138
  panic, problems with diagnosing in
    primary care, 139
  populations of particular interest, 139
    cardiac patients, 139
    dyspneic patients, 139
    gastroenterology patients, 139
    patients with dizziness, 139
  primary psychiatric disorders, 140–143
  reactive or situational anxiety, 144
  treatment, general considerations, 144
  treatment, non-pharmacotherapy, 151
    cognitive-behavioral therapy
      (CBT), 151
    psychotherapies, 151
  treatment, pharmacotherapy,
    145*t*–151
    alternative agents, 150
    antidepressants, 145–147
    benzodiazepines, 148*t*–149
    buspirone, 149
    combining antidepressants and
      benzodiazepines, 150
    discontinuation, 150–151
Aphasia, 197, 221*t*
Apraxia, 197
Aripiprazole (Abilify)
  effects on heart and cardiovascular
    system, 634*t*, 644
  rehabilitation patients, 485*t*
Arousal phase disorders, sexual
    dysfunction, 398–399
Arrhythmias, cardiovascular side effects,
    618
Arteriovenous malformations (AVMs),
    headaches from, 245
ASI (Addiction Severity Index), 57
L-Asparaginase, neuropsychiatric side
    effects, 362*t*
Aspirin, headache, 248
Atenolol
  central nervous system side effects,
    619
  premenstrual syndrome (PMS), 426
Atomoxetine
  adverse effects, 291*t*
  attention-deficit/hyperactivity disor-
    der (ADHD), 291*t*, 296–297

Atrioventricular (AV), 618
Attention-deficit disorder (ADD), 279
  smoking cessation and, 708
Attention-deficit/hyperactivity disorder
    (ADHD), approach to patient
    with, 185, 282, 287–299
  alcoholism, co-morbidity with, 511
  overview, 287
  treatment, 289–298
    antidepressants, 294–297
    general principles, 289
    stimulants, 289, 292–293
    strategies, 297–298
  violent patients, 573
Atypical antidepressants, 118–120,
    119*t*
  depression, 123
  drug-drug interactions, 665
Atypical antipsychotics
  weight gain, 453*t*
AUDIT (Alcohol Use Disorders Identifi-
    cation Test), 501*t*–502*t*
Auditory hallucinations, 162
Auras, 229
Autonomy at the bedside, 687–689*t*; *see
    also* Treatment decisions at the
    end of life

Baclofen (Lioresal), seizures with,
    228*t*
Bad news, breaking, 735–741
  general principles, 735–737
  grief response, 738–739
  helpful strategies, 740–741
  overview, 735
  physician's predicament, 737–738
  special circumstances, 739–740
Barbiturates
  cardiovascular side effects, 650
  monoamine oxidase inhibitors, inter-
    action with, 617*t*
  seizures with, 228*t*
  sexual dysfunction, 407*t*
Battered women. *See* Domestic violence,
    approach to
Beck Depression Inventory (BDI),
    53–54, 474
Behavioral assignments, 72–73
Behavioral therapy, 13–14; *see also*
    Cognitive-behavioral therapy
    (CBT)
  chronic fatigue syndrome (CFS), 329
  erectile dysfunction, 411
  sexual dysfunction, 401–402
  smoking cessation, 706
  specific phobias, 143
Behavior modification, weight loss, 460

Behavior problems of children and adolescents, approach to, 279–286
  brief evaluation, 284
  clinical perspectives and decision making, 282–285
  innovative office models, 285
  overview, 279
  prevalence, 279
  primary care providers, 285
  recognition, 279–282
  referral, 285
  treatment strategies, 285
Benign positional vertigo, 265
Benzodiazepines
  alcohol detoxification, 509
  anxiety
    associated with HIV infection, 376
    disorders, 148t–149
    following a trauma, 539
    in terminal illness, 495t
  cardiovascular side effects, 650
  central nervous system side effects, 619
  cocaine-induced anxiety, 518
  delirium in terminal illness, 497t
  dementia, 210
  denial, managing, 586
  eating disorders, 178
  generalized anxiety disorder (GAD), 142
  insomnia, 148, 257
    in HIV/AIDS patients, 378
  multiple environmental allergies, 346
  panic disorder, 141
  postpartum psychosis, 449
  pregnancy, 438t, 440
  rehabilitation patients, 485t
  seizures, 228t
  sexually assaulted patient, 549
  side effects, 149
  social phobia, 142
  treatment refusal, approach to, 579
  violent patients, 573, 574
  withdrawal, mimicking anxiety disorders, 362
Benztropine (Cogentin)
  violent patients, 572
Beta-blockers
  anxiety disorders, 150
  dementia, 210
  seizures with, 228t
Bethanechol (Urecholine)
  antidepressant-induced sexual dysfunction, 624t
Binge-eating disorder (BED), 452, 458
Biologic agents, neuropsychiatric side effects, 362t, 364

Bipolar disorder, approach to patient with, expansive, or irritable mood, 115, 181; see also Elevated
  alcoholism, co-morbidity with, 511
  chronic fatigue syndrome, co-morbidity with, 337
  cognitive-behavioral therapy (CBT), 76–77
  course of illness, 181–182
  diagnosis, 181
  fatigue and, 333
  homeless patients, 596
  morbidity and mortality, 181
  prevalence of, 181
  sexual dysfunction, 398
  smoking cessation and, 708
Black cohosh (Cimicifuga racemosa), 678–679
  adverse effects, 679
  natural medication for PMS symptoms, 678–679
Blessed Dementia Scale (BDS), 56
Blurred vision, antidepressant-induced side effect, 622
Body dysmorphic disorder (BDD), 165, 167
  diagnostic criteria, 167
Body mass index (BMI), 451, 713–715
  calculation of, 714t
  recommended weight guidelines using, 713–715, 714t
Boundaries in doctor-patient relationship, maintaining, 743–747
  business dealings, 744
  gifts, 745–746
  handling boundary challenges, 747
  overview, 743–744
  physical examination, 744–745
  sexual relationships, 746
  social (nonsexual) relationships, 745
Brain failure, 199
Breast-feeding, 450
  presence of psychotropics in breast milk, 450
Brief Psychiatric Scale (BPRS), 55–56
Bright Futures: Mental Health, 280
Bromocriptine (Parlodel)
  cocaine dependence, 516
  premenstrual syndrome (PMS), 426
Bulimia nervosa, approach to patient with, 82, 171–180
  clinical picture, 172
  defining, 171
  diagnoses, 171
  diagnostic criteria, 176–177
  epidemiology, 172

  evaluation, 173–175
  infertility and, 414
  inositol, 676
  medical complications, 174–175
  premenstrual syndrome (PMS) and, 424
  primary care physician's role, 171
  psychiatric differential diagnosis, 176
  risk factors, 172
  treatment strategies, 177–179
    cognitive-behavioral therapy (CBT), 82
Buprenorphine (Buprenex)
  acute pain, 322t
  cardiovascular side effects, 651
  heroin dependence, 517
Bupropion (Wellbutrin), 119, 294
  adverse effects, 291t, 614t
  analgesic use, 326t
  antidepressant-induced
    fatigue and sedation, 621t
    sexual dysfunction, 624t
  attention-deficit/hyperactivity disorder (ADHD), 291t
  bulimia nervosa, contraindicated in patients with, 464
  cardiovascular side effects, 617, 618, 630t–633t, 639
  dementia, 210
  depression, 119
    in terminal illness, 493t
  effects on heart and cardiovascular system, 634t
  HIV/AIDS patients, treating depression, 373
  monoamine oxidase inhibitors, interaction with, 617t
  obesity, 461–462
  organ transplant patients, 388
  rehabilitation patients, 485t
  seizures with, 228t
  side effects, 119, 294
  smoking cessation, 711
  weight gain, 619
Buspirone (Buspar)
  antidepressant-induced sexual dysfunction, 624t
  anxiety disorders, 149
    associated with alcoholism, 510
  anxiety in terminal illness, 495t
  cardiovascular side effects, 650
  dementia, 210
  effects on heart and cardiovascular system, 634t
  generalized anxiety disorder (GAD), 142

obsessive-compulsive disorder
(OCD), 168, 169
premenstrual syndrome (PMS), 426
smoking cessation, 710
violent patients, 574
Busulfan, seizures with, 228t
Butorphanol (Stadol), acute pain, 322t

Cafergot, migraine headaches, 248
CAGE Questionnaire, 57, 501t
Calcium channel blockers
drug-drug interactions, 664t
migraine headaches, 248
Cancer, approach to patient with, 359–366
adaptive versus maladaptive psychological responses, 360–361
antiemetic treatment and side effects,
364–365
chemotherapy treatment, 363–364
evaluation, 359–360
overview, 359
psychiatric symptoms with medical
etiologies, 361–363
psychosocial interventions, 365–366
treatment strategies, 365
Carbamazepine (Tegretol)
cardiovascular side effects, 649
chronic pain, 319, 323t
dementia, 211
drug-drug interactions, 657, 661t
in HIV/AIDS patients, 380
effects on heart and cardiovascular
system, 634t
elevated, expansive, or irritable mood,
187
pain in HIV infection, 378
post-traumatic stress disorder (PTSD),
541
pregnancy, 438t, 440
seizures, treatment of, 232, 233t
violent patients, 574
Cardiac failure, organ transplant patients,
387
Cardiac patients, panic disorder, 139
Cardiopulmonary disease, suicide risk
and, 131
Cardiovascular side effects of antidepressants, 615–618
Cardiovascular side effects of psychotropic agents, 629–652
Celebrity patient, approach to, 603–610
celebrity, impact of, 604–605
criminals, 608–609
family members, 608
medical celebrity, 608
non-medical concerns, 606–607

overview, 603
physician considerations, 607–608
publicity, impact of, 603
ten commandments for a VIP's
doctor, 609–610
timing and place, 605
Centers for Disease Control and
Prevention (CDC), 368
classification system for HIV
infection, 368t
Central conduction of nociception, 311
Central nervous system (CNS), side
effects of antidepressants,
619–622
anticholinergic toxicity, 622–623
fatigue/sedation, 620
high-frequency tremor, 619–620
hypomania or mania, 622
jitteriness/increased anxiety, 620
myoclonus, 621
sleep disturbance, 620–621t
suicidal ideation, 622
Central sleep apnea, 258
Character disorders, insomnia and, 257
Chaste tree berry (CTB), natural medication for PMS symptoms,
678–679
Chemotherapeutic agents, neuropsychiatric side effects of, 362t,
363–364
Child Behavior Checklist (CBCL), 280,
284t
Childhood absence, 231
Childhood epilepsy, 231
Children's well-being: risk and protective factors, 283t
Chlorambucil (Leukeran), seizures with,
228t
Chlordiazepoxide (Librium)
alcohol detoxification, 509
anxiety disorders, 148t
anxiety in terminal illness, 495t
Chlorpromazine (Thorazine)
anxiety in terminal illness, 495t
delirium in terminal illness, 497t
effects on heart and cardiovascular
system, 634t
seizures with, 228t
violent patients, 574
Chronic alcohol use, 206
Chronic fatigue syndrome (CFS), approach to patient with, approach
to patient with, 335–340; see
also Fatigue
defining, 335
evaluation, 336–337

overview, 335–336
prognosis, 339
psychiatric differential diagnosis,
337–338
treatment strategies, 338–339
Chronic lung disease, homeless patients,
597
Chronic medical illness, approach to
patient with, 301–310
caring, 309
chronic illness experience, 304–305
adjustment reactions, 305
defense mechanisms, 304–305
meaning of chronic illness, 304
crisis of medical illness, 301–303,
302f
medical supportive psychotherapy,
308–309
overview, 301
personality types, 305–308
Chronic pain, approach to patient with,
314–315; see also Pain
treatment, 319–320
Chronic renal failure, suicide risk and,
131
Cilansetron, irritable bowel syndrome
(IBS) and, 355
Cimetidine (Tagamet), sexual dysfunction, 396t
Circadian rhythm sleep disorders, approach to patient with, 252t; see
also Disordered sleep
Citalopram (Celexa)
adverse effects, 614t
anxiety disorder, 146
cardiovascular side effects, 630t–633t
depression in terminal illness, 493t
effects on heart and cardiovascular
system, 634t
irritable bowel syndrome (IBS), 356t
obsessive-compulsive disorder
(OCD), 168
pregnancy, data supporting safety, 437
rehabilitation patients, 485t
Civil commitment, approach to,
577–581; see also Treatment
refusal
legal restrictions on, 577
overview, 577–578
process, 578–579
Classification of sexual dysfunctions, 394t
Clingers, approach to patients who are,
107
Clinical disability evaluation, approach
to, 589–591; see also Patient
seeking disability benefits

Clinical Global Improvement (CGI) Scale, 53
Clinical Institute Withdrawal Assessment (CIWA-Ar), 509
Clofibrate (Atromid), sexual dysfunction, 396t
Clomipramine (Anafranil)
    adverse effects, 614t
    analgesic use, 326t
    depression in terminal illness, 493t
    effects on heart and cardiovascular system, 634t
    obsessive-compulsive disorder (OCD), 143, 167, 168
    premenstrual syndrome (PMS), 426
    seizures with, 228t
Clonazepam (Klonopin)
    antidepressant-induced side effect, 619
    anxiety disorders, 148t
    anxiety in terminal illness, 495t
    chronic pain, 319, 323t
    denial, managing, 586
    insomnia, 256t
    mania associated with HIV infection, 376
    obsessive-compulsive disorder (OCD), 168, 169
    pain in HIV infection, 378
    post-traumatic stress disorder (PTSD), 541
Clonidine (Catapres)
    adverse effects, 291t
    attention-deficit/hyperactivity disorder (ADHD), 291t
    post-traumatic stress disorder (PTSD), 541
    sexual dysfunction, 396t, 407t
    short-term adverse effect, 296
Clorazepate (Tranxene)
    anxiety disorders, 148t
    anxiety in terminal illness, 495t
Closed head injury. See Head injury (closed), approach to patient following
Clozapine (Clozaril)
    cardiovascular side effects, 645t
    drug-drug interaction in HIV/AIDS patients, 380
    effects on heart and cardiovascular system, 634t
    seizures with, 228t
Cluster headaches, approach to patient with, 244; see also Headache
    characteristics of pain, 244
    epidemiology, 243
    onset and duration, 245

precipitating and ameliorating factors, 246
    treatment, 249
Cocaine Anonymous, 516
Cocaine or opiate-abusing patient, approach to, 513–519
    concomitant substance abuse/ dependency, 518–519
    diagnostic criteria for psychoactive substance use syndromes, 514–515t
    evaluation, 513–514
    opiate abuse and dependence, 517–518
    overview, 513
    seizures with, 228t
    treatment strategies, 516–517
        disrupting binge cycle, 516
        management of acute cocaine intoxication, 516
        pharmacotherapy of craving and withdrawal, 516–517
        relapse prevention, 516
Codeine
    acute pain, 321t
    heroin dependence, 518t
Cognition-enhancing natural remedies, 679–680
    ginkgo biloba, 679–680
Cognitive-behavioral therapy (CBT), 14, 69–73, 75–84
    anxiety associated with HIV infection, 377
    anxiety disorders, 151
    basis of, 69–70
    binge-eating disorder (BED), 463
    bipolar disorder, 76–77
    bulimia nervosa, 463
    chronic fatigue syndrome (CFS), 329
    clinical rapport: motivation and compliance, 70–71
    common elements, 71–73
        behavioral assignments, 72–73
        cognitive interventions, 71–72
        contingency management, 73
        exposure interventions, 72
        informational interventions, 71
        outcome, definition and monitoring of, 71
        relapse prevention skills, 73
        self-monitoring, 71
        skill rehearsal, 72
    defining, 69
    depression, 75–76
    eating disorders, 82, 178
    effectiveness of, 69

generalized anxiety disorder (GAD), 79, 142
    hypochondriasis, 277
    and insight-oriented therapy, differences between, 69
    menopause patients, 433
    obsessive-compulsive disorder (OCD), 79–80, 143
    panic disorder, 77–78, 141
    personality disorders, 83
    post-traumatic stress disorder (PTSD), 80–81, 143, 541
    premenstrual syndrome (PMS), 425
    psychotic disorders, 83
    referral for, 83–84
    social phobia, 78–79
    specific phobia, 81–82
Cognitive dysfunction, screening tests for, 56
Cognitive interventions, 71–72
Collaborative treatment by primary care providers and psychiatrists, 3–11
    barriers to diagnosis and treatment of psychiatric disorders in primary settings, 4–5
    communication, 8–9
    outpatient primary care psychiatry models, 5t, 5–6
        alternative models, 7–8
    overview, 3
    successful, 9t–10
Co-morbid depression, 143–144
Co-morbid psychiatric disorders, 177
Complex partial seizures, 225t, 230
Compliance, enhancing
    etiologies, 728–731
    non-compliance, 726–728
        adverse impact of, 726
        discovery of, 726–728
        overview, 725–726
        treatment strategies, 731–733
Components of pain, 311
Compulsive behaviors, approach to patient with, 167; see also Obsessive-compulsive disorder (OCD)
Computed tomography (CT), use of, 61–62, 63t; see also Neuroimaging techniques
    acute management of seizures, 230
    indications, 64
    versus magnetic resonance imaging (MRI), 62, 63t
    MRI versus, 62–63, 63t
Concomitant substance abuse/ dependency, 518–519

Conduct disorder, commonly co-morbid
     with alcohol abuse, 500
Consent. *See* Informed consent
Constipation, gastrointestinal side effects
     of antidepressants, 619
Consultation, approach to making, 27;
     see also Referral
Contingency management, 73
Continuation therapy, 124
     depression, 124
Continuous pain in the terminally ill, 314
Continuous positive airway pressure
     (CPAP), 259
Contrast agents, seizures with, 228*t*
Conversion disorder, 273, 275
     somatization disorder and, 273
Convulsive status, 233–234
Coping with infertility, 419
Coronary artery disease (CAD), 713
Corticosteroids
     neuropsychiatric side effects, 362*t*, 363
     organ transplant patients, 390
     weight gain, 453*t*
Co-trimoxazole, neuropsychiatric side
     effects, 371*t*
Countertransference, 590–591, 743
Creutzfeldt-Jacob disease, 206
Crisis approach to medical illness,
     301–303, 302*f*
CT. *See* Computed tomography
Cuprolithiasis, 263
Cushing's disease, suicide risk and, 131
Cushing's syndrome, 456
Cyclic antidepressants, weight gain, 453*t*
Cyclosporine (CYA)
     organ transplant patients, 390
     seizures with, 228*t*
Cyclothymia, fatigue and, 333
Cypropheptadine (Periactin)
     antidepressant-induced sexual
          dysfunction, 624*t*
     diarrhea, 618*t*, 619
Cytarabine (Cytosar), neuropsychiatric
     side effects, 362*t*, 364
Cytochrome P450 isoenzymes
     drug-drug interactions, 657, 658*t*
Cytosine arabinoside, neuropsychiatric
     side effects, 372*t*

D-amphetamine (Dexedrine)
     attention-deficit/hyperactivity dis-
          order (ADHD), 289
Danger to self/others, criterion in civil
     commitment process, 578–579
Dapsone, neuropsychiatric side effects,
     371*t*

Decreased libido, antidepressant-induced
     side effects, 623
Dehydroepiandrosterone (DHEA), 122
     depression, 122
Delavirdine, neuropsychiatric side
     effects, 371*t*
Delayed orgasm, antidepressant-induced
     side effects, 624
Delirium
     dementia and, 206
     glucocorticoid use, 522, 523*t*
          neuropsychiatric complications
               from, 527*t*
     HIV dementia, 375
     medical and neurological causes, 363
     during rehabilitation, 479
     terminal illness, 495–497, 497*t*
Delusional disorders, approach to patient
     with, 166; *see also* Hallucina-
     tions and delusions
     during rehabilitation, 480
Dementia. *See* Memory problems or
     dementia, approach to patient
     with
     functional neuroimaging, 66
     during rehabilitation, 480
     steroid, 526
Dementia of the Alzheimer's type
     (DAT), 197, 199
Denial, 102
     chronic illness and defense
          mechanisms, 304
     infertile patient, 413
     management of, 583–587
          assessing denial, 584–585
          differential diagnosis, 584
          overview, 583–584
          strategies for managing, 585–587
L-Deprenyl (Eldepryl), 120
     depression, 120
Depression, approach to patient with,
     111–125
     antidepressants, frequent miscon-
          ceptions in use of, 122
     cancer patients, 359
     changing drug treatment, 123
     chronic illness and, 305
     co-morbid, 143–144
     continuation and maintenance
          therapies, 124
     dementia and, 115, 206
     dizziness and, 264
     dysthymic disorder. *See* Dysthymic
          disorder
     epidemiology, 112–113
     evaluation, 114–115

     factors limiting adequate dose,
          duration, and compliance,
          122–123
     folic acid, 674
     glucocorticoid use, 522, 523*t*
          neuropsychiatric complications
               from, 527*t*
     headaches and, 247
     homeless patients, 596
     infertility and, 417, 419
     inositol, 676
     major. *See* Major depressive disorder
          (MDD)
     non-compliance, 729
     organ transplant patients, 389–390
     overview, 111*t*–112
     pain, co-morbidity with, 314
     pregnancy, 435, 438*t*
     prevalence in primary care settings, 3
     psychiatric differential diagnosis,
          115–116
     referrals to a psychiatrist, 29*t*, 124
     during rehabilitation, 479
     screening tests for, 52–54
     sexual dysfunction, 398, 409
     sexually assaulted patient, 549
     smoking cessation and, 707
     St. John's wort (SJW), 643–644,
          673–674
     suicide risk, 76
     in terminal illness, 491–493
     treatment strategies, 116–122
          cognitive-behavioral therapy
               (CBT), 75–76
          combined psychotherapy and
               pharmacotherapy, 121
          electroconvulsive therapy (ECT),
               121
          light therapy, 122
          pharmacotherapy with anti-
               depressants, 116–121
          psychotherapy, 121
          vitamin B$_{12}$, 674
Depression after delivery (DAD), self-
     help group, 449
Dermatologic side effects of anti-
     depressants, 625–626
Desipramine (Norpramin)
     adverse effects, 290*t*, 614*t*
     analgesic use, 325, 326*t*
     anxiety disorder, 147
     attention-deficit/hyperactivity dis-
          order (ADHD), 290*t*
     bulimia nervosa, 464
     cocaine dependence, 516
     depression in terminal illness, 493*t*

Desipramine (Norpramin) *(continued)*
  effects on heart and cardiovascular system, 634*t*
  irritable bowel syndrome (IBS), 356*t*
  pregnancy, 438*t*
  premenstrual syndrome (PMS), 426
  seizures with, 228*t*
Desire phase disorders, sexual dysfunction, 398
Despondency, during rehabilitation, 479
Detecting disorders. *See* Screening tests used for detection of psychiatric disorders
Detoxification, alcohol, 509
Dexamethasone, nausea and vomiting, 364
Dexloxiglumide, irritable bowel syndrome (IBS) and, 355
Dextroamphetamine
  adverse effects, 290*t*
  attention-deficit/hyperactivity disorder (ADHD), 290*t*
  cardiovascular side effects, 650
  depression in terminal illness, 493*t*
  effects on heart and cardiovascular system, 634*t*
  HIV/AIDS patients, treating depression, 373
  HIV dementia, 375
  rehabilitation patients, 485*t*
Dextromethorphan
  cardiovascular side effects, 616
  monoamine oxidase inhibitors, interaction with, 617*t*
Diacetylmorphine, heroin dependence, 518*t*
Diarrhea, gastrointestinal side effects of antidepressants, 619
Diazepam (Valium)
  alcohol detoxification, 509
  anxiety disorders, 148*t*
  anxiety in terminal illness, 495*t*
  cocaine intoxication, 516
  sexual dysfunction, 396*t*, 407*t*
  sexually assaulted patient, 549
  violent patients, 573
Diclofenac (Voltaren), pain, 318*t*
Diet
  irritable bowel syndrome (IBS) and, 355
  weight loss, 460
Diethylpropion, obesity, 461–462
Difficult patients. *See* Personality disorders, approach to
Digoxin (Lanoxin)
  sexual dysfunction, 396*t*

Dilaudid (Hydromorphone)
  acute pain, 320*t*
Diphenhydramine (Benadryl)
  insomnia, 256*t*
Diphenoxylate hydrochloride (Lomotil)
  diarrhea, 618*t*, 619
Disability assessment, approach to, 593; *see also* Patient seeking disability benefits
Discomfort, during rehabilitation, 480
Discontinuation side effects of antidepressants, 626
Disordered sleep, approach to patient with, 251–261
  hypersomnia, 258–259
  insomnia, 254–258
  parasomnias, 260
  periodic leg movements of sleep, 260
  restless legs syndrome, 260
  sleep-wake schedule disorders, 260
  terminology and classification, 251*t*–253*t*, 251–254
Disorders of extreme stress not otherwise specified, 536–537
Displacement, chronic illness and defense mechanisms, 304
Disquiet, during rehabilitation, 480
Disruptive behavioral disorders
  during rehabilitation, 479
  violent patients, 573
Disulfiram (Antabuse)
  alcoholism treatment, 509–510
  cardiovascular side effects, 651
  drug-drug interactions, 668
  effects on heart and cardiovascular system, 634*t*
Divalproex sodium (Depakote)
  cardiovascular side effects, 630*t*–633*t*, 649
  effects on heart and cardiovascular system, 635*t*
  elevated, expansive, or irritable mood, 187
Dizziness, approach to patient with, 263–267
  diagnostic criteria, 265–266
  evaluation, 263–264
  overview, 263
  panic disorder, 139
  psychiatric differential diagnosis, 264
  treatment, 266
Doctor-patient relationship. *See* Boundaries in doctor-patient relationship, maintaining
Docussate sodium (Colace), constipation, 618*t*, 619

Domestic violence, approach to, 553–558
  diagnostic criteria, 557
  evaluation, 555–557
  overview, 553–555
  psychiatric differential diagnosis, 557
  treatment strategies, 557–558
Donepezil (Aricept)
  cognitive enhancement, 208
  effects on heart and cardiovascular system, 635*t*
L-Dopa, interaction with monoamine oxidase inhibitors, 617*t*
Dopamine
  cocaine dependence, 516
  monoamine oxidase inhibitors, interaction with, 617*t*
Dopaminergic agents, depression, 123
Doxepin (Adapin, Sinequan)
  adverse effects, 614*t*
  analgesic use, 326*t*
  anxiety disorder, 147
  depression in terminal illness, 493*t*
  effects on heart and cardiovascular system, 635*t*
  irritable bowel syndrome (IBS), 356*t*
  post-traumatic stress disorder (PTSD), 541
  seizures with, 228*t*
  weight gain, 619
Doxycycline, premenstrual syndrome (PMS), 426
Droperidol (Inapsine)
  effects on heart and cardiovascular system, 635*t*
  migraine headaches, 248
  nausea and vomiting, post-chemotherapy treatment for, 365
  violent patients, 574
Drug abuse. *See* Alcohol-abusing patient; Cocaine or opiate-abusing patient
Drug-drug interactions, 653–669
  antidepressants, 657, 658*t*–664*t*
  antipsychotics, 665–666, 667*t*
  anxiolytics, 666, 668
  classification, 654–657
  clinical decision making, 653–654
  involving cytochrome P450 isoenzymes, 657
  miscellaneous, 668
  mood stabilizers, 657
  overview, 653
Dry mouth
  antidepressant-induced side effect, 493*t*, 622

DSM-IV-PC (Diagnostic and Statistical Manual of Mental Disorders, 4th ed., Primary Care Version), 27, 45, 89
  criteria for anorexia nervosa, 176
  criteria for bulimia nervosa, 176–177
  criteria for major depressive disorder, 112*t*
  disorders based on presenting symptoms, 47
  disorders usually first diagnosed in infancy, childhood, or adulthood, 48
  elements that inhibit the recognition and treatment of psychiatric conditions, 43–44
  genesis of, 44
  guiding principles of, 44
  how to use, 45–46
  mental conditions or symptoms, other, 48
  psychosocial problems that are not formal diagnoses, 48
  screening test, 52
  sections of, 45
Duloxetine (Cymbalta)
  effects on heart and cardiovascular system, 635*t*
Dyspareunia, approach to patient with, 399–400; *see also* Sexual dysfunction
Dyspepsia, gastrointestinal side effects of antidepressants, 618–619
Dyspneic patients, panic disorder, 139
Dyssomnias, approach to patient with, 251*t*–252*t*; *see also* Disordered sleep
Dysthymic disorder, approach to patient with, 111–113; *see also* Depression
  alcoholism, differentiating from, 505
  DSM-IV criteria for, 113*t*
  epidemiology, 113
  sexual dysfunction, 398

Eating disorders. *See* Anorexia nervosa, approach to patient with; Bulimia nervosa, approach to patient with; Obese patient, approach to
  cognitive-behavioral therapy (CBT) for, 82
  referrals for, 29*t*
Eating disorders not otherwise specified (ED NOS), 459
Echopraxia, 222

Edinburgh Postnatal Depression Scale, 445*t*–447*t*
Efavirenz, neuropsychiatric side effects, 371*t*
Ejaculatory dysfunction, antidepressant-induced side effect, 623
Electroconvulsive therapy (ECT)
  brain injury, treatment of, 241
  cardiovascular side effects, 121, 644
  depression, 121
  glucocorticoid use, neuropsychiatric complications from, 526
  obsessive-compulsive disorder (OCD), 169
  postpartum psychosis, 449
  during pregnancy, 440
  rehabilitation patients, 484
Electroencephalogram (EEG), 229
Eletriptan (Relpax), migraine headaches, 247
Elevated, expansive, or irritable mood, approach to patient with, 181–196
  diagnostic criteria, 189–195
  evaluation, 182–184
  overview, 181–182
  psychiatric differential diagnosis, 184–185
  treatment strategies, 185–189, 190*t*–193*t*
Encouraging patients to live healthier lives. *See* Lifestyle changes
Endurance training, 718; *see also* Exercise programs and strategies for weight loss
Enflurane (Ethrane), seizures with, 228*t*
Entitlement, 101
Ephedrine, interaction with monoamine oxidase inhibitors, 617*t*
Epilepsia partialis continua, 230
Epilepsy, approach to patient with, 225; *see also* Seizures
  suicide risk, 131
  surgery, seizures, treatment of, 234–235
Epinephrine (adrenalin)
  monoamine oxidase inhibitors, interaction with, 617*t*
Erectile dysfunction, approach to patient with, 409; *see also* Impotence
  antidepressant-induced side effects, 623
Ergotamine tartarate, cluster headaches, 249
Erythematous maculopapular rashes, 625

Escitalopram (Lexapro)
  adverse effects, 614*t*
  anxiety disorder, 146
  depression in terminal illness, 493*t*
  effects on heart and cardiovascular system, 637*t*
  irritable bowel syndrome (IBS), 356*t*
  obsessive-compulsive disorder (OCD), 168
Essential fatty acids (EFAs), 675–676
Estazolam (ProSom), insomnia, 256*t*
Estrogen
  etiology of menopause, 430
  etiology of postpartum mood disorders, 444
  postpartum depression, 449
  sexual dysfunction, 396*t*
  weight gain, 453*t*
Ethanol, seizures with, 228*t*
Ethosuximide (Zarontin), seizures, treatment of, 232
Etodolac acid, pain, 318*t*
Etomidate, seizures with, 228*t*
Euthanasia, 691; *see also* Treatment decisions at the end of life
Excessive sweating, antidepressant-induced side effects, 626
Executive dysfunction, 197
Exercise, weight loss, 460
Exercise programs and strategies for weight loss, 713–721
  assessment for exercise prescription, 715–716
  encouraging participation, 720
  exercise program, 716–719
    designing, 718*t*–719
  ideal weight, establishing, 713–715, 714*t*
  motivation, 719–720
  overview, 713
Explicit threats, criterion in civil commitment process, 579
Exposure interventions, 72
Extrinsic sleep disorders, approach to patient with, 252*t*; *see also* Disordered sleep
Eye movement desentization and reprocessing (EMDR), 542

Family and Medical Leave Act, 589
Family in crisis, approach to, 559–565
  crisis meeting, 560–563
  overview, 559–560
  referral, 563–564
Family intervention, chronic illness and, 309

Family therapy
  eating disorders, 178
  for physician stress or burnout, 762
  violent patients, 574
Famotidine (Pepcid), nausea, 618t, 619
Fatigue
  antidepressant-induced side effect,
    620
  approach to patient with, 329–334
    examination of patient, 331–332
    interview, 330–331
    medical history, 329–330, 330t
    overview, 329
    psychiatric differential diagnosis,
      332–333
    treatment, 333–334
Fearful or paranoid patient, approach to,
    108–109; see also Personality
    disorders
Felbamate (Felbatol), seizures, treatment
    of, 233t
Female orgasmic disorder, 399
Female sexual arousal disorder, 398–399
Fenfluramine, premenstrual syndrome
    (PMS), 426
Fenoprofen (Nalfon), pain, 318t
Fibromyalgia, 336
Fiorinal, migraine headaches, 248
FK506 (Tacrolimus)
  organ transplant patients, 390
Flashback, response to traumatic stress,
    536
Flucytosine, neuropsychiatric side
    effects, 372t
Flumazenil (Romazicon)
  cardiovascular side effects, 651
5-Fluorouracil (Efudex), neuropsychi-
    atric side effects, 362t, 364
Fluoxetine (Prozac)
  adverse effects, 614t
  analgesic use, 326t
  anxiety disorder, 146
  binge-eating disorder (BED), 464
  bulimia nervosa, 178, 464
  cardiovascular side effects, 630t–633t
  depression in terminal illness, 493t
  eating disorders, 178
  effects on heart and cardiovascular
    system, 635t
  GI side effects, 356t
  irritable bowel syndrome (IBS), 356t
  obesity, 461
  obsessive-compulsive disorder
    (OCD), 168
  post-traumatic stress disorder
    (PTSD), 541

pregnancy, data supporting safety, 437
premenstrual syndrome (PMS), 425
rehabilitation patients, 485t
sexual dysfunction, 396t
Fluphenazine (Prolixin)
  effects on heart and cardiovascular
    system, 635t
Flurazepam (Dalmane)
  anxiety disorders, 148t
  insomnia, 256t
Flurbiprofen, pain, 318t
Fluvoxamine (Luvox)
  adverse effects, 614t
  anxiety disorder, 146
  binge-eating disorder (BED), 464
  depression in terminal illness, 493t
  effects on heart and cardiovascular
    system, 635t
  GI side effects, 356t
  irritable bowel syndrome (IBS), 356t
  obsessive-compulsive disorder
    (OCD), 168
  post-traumatic stress disorder
    (PTSD), 541
  rehabilitation patients, 485t
Folic acid, 674–675
  natural antidepressants, 674–675
Frontal intermittent rhythmic delta
    activity (FIRDA), 239
Frontal lobe seizures, 230
Frovatriptan (Frova)
  migraine headaches, treatment of, 247
Functional Dementia Scale (FDS), 475,
    476t

Gabapentin (Neurontin)
  anxiety disorders, 150
  chronic pain, 319
  migraine headaches, 249
  seizures, treatment of, 233t
Galantamine (Reminyl)
  cognitive enhancement, 208
Gamete intrafallopian transfer (GIFT),
    415
Ganciclovir, neuropsychiatric side
    effects, 371t
Gastric bypass, weight-loss surgery, 463
Gastroenterology patients, panic dis-
    order, 139
Gastrointestinal side effects of antide-
    pressants, 618t, 618–619
  constipation, 619
  diarrhea, 619
  nausea and dyspepsia, 618t–619
Gemcitabine, neuropsychiatric side
    effects, 362t, 364

Gender identity disorder, sexual
    dysfunction, 398
Generalized anxiety disorder (GAD),
    approach to, 141–142; see also
    Anxious patient
  alcoholism, co-morbidity with,
    510–511
  cognitive-behavioral therapy (CBT),
    79
  defining, 141–142
  infertility and, 419
  kava (Piper methysticum), 677–678
  multiple environmental allergies,
    344
  sexual dysfunction, 398
Geriatric Depression Scale, 473t, 474
Geriatric patient, approach to, 469–477
  diagnostic criteria, 474
  evaluation, 469–474
    examination of patient, 472–474
    identification of presenting
      problem, 469–470
    interview, 472
    medical history, 470–472
    geriatric syndromes, 470t
    overview, 469
    scales and questionnaires to evaluate,
      474–475
Gingko biloba, 208, 679–680
  adverse effects, 680
  cognition-enhancing natural remedy,
    679–680
Global Assessment of Functioning Scale
    (GAF), 57
Glucocorticoids, approach to patient re-
    ceiving, 521t; see also Steroids
  adverse effects, 523t
  preparations, 522t
  selected indications for use, 521t
Gonadotropin-releasing hormone agonist
    (GnRH)
  premenstrual syndrome (PMS), 425
Granisetron
  nausea and vomiting, treatment for
    post-chemotherapy, 364
Gravely disabled criterion, criterion in
    civil commitment process, 579
Grief, approach to patient with,
    153–156; see also Acute grief
  fatigue and, 333
  infertile patient, 413
  response, breaking, 738–739; see also
    Bad news
Group therapy
  description of, 15–16
  eating disorders, 178

Guanfacine (Tenex)
  adverse effects, 291*t*
  attention-deficit/hyperactivity
      disorder (ADHD), 291*t*
Guanfacine (Tenex)
  post-traumatic stress disorder (PTSD),
      541
Guilt/self-blame, infertile patient, 413

Hair loss, antidepressant-induced side
    effect, 626
Hallucinations and delusions, approach
    to patient with, 157*t*–158*t*,
    157–164
  evaluation, 158–161, 159*t*
    complete physical examination, 161
    general recommendations, 158
    interview, 160–161
    medical history, 160
  overview, 157*t*–158*t*
  postpartum depression, 448
Hallucinogens, violent patients, 572
Haloperidol (Haldol)
  anxiety in terminal illness, 495*t*
  delirium in terminal illness, 497*t*
  effects on heart and cardiovascular
      system, 635*t*
  nausea and vomiting, post-chemo-
      therapy treatment for, 365
  obsessive-compulsive disorder
      (OCD), 168
  pregnancy, 438*t*
  rehabilitation patients, 485*t*
  seizures with, 228*t*
  sexual dysfunction, 396*t*
  violent patients, 574
Hamilton Rating Scale for Anxiety
    (HAM-A), 55
Hamilton Rating Scale for Depression
    (HAM-D), 52–53
The Harvard Department of Psychiatry
    National Depression Screening
    Day Scale (HANDS), 54
Headache, antidepressant-induced side
    effect, 626
Headache, approach to patient with,
    243–249; *see also* Cluster
    headaches; Migraine headaches;
    Organic headaches; Psychogenic
    headaches; Tension headaches
  characteristics of headaches, 244–245
  epidemiology, 243–244
  evaluation, 243–247
  overview, 243
  psychiatric differential diagnosis, 247
  treatment strategies, 247–249

Head injury (closed), approach to patient
    following, 237–242
  diagnostic criteria, 240
  evaluation, 237–239
  overview, 237
  psychiatric differential diagnosis,
      239–240
  symptoms, 240
  treatment strategies, 240–241
    psychopharmacology, 241
    rehabilitation, 240–241
Head trauma, suicide risk and, 130
Health Care for the Homeless (HCH)
    programs, 601
Healthier lives. *See* Lifestyle changes
Hepatic failure, organ transplant patients,
    387
Hepatotoxicity, 677
Heroin overdose, 517
Highly active antiretroviral therapy
    (HAART), 368
HIV-associated dementia, 373
HIV infection, approach to patient with,
    367–383
  clinical evaluation, 369–379
    anxiety and difficulty coping with
        illness, 376–377
    general approach, 369, 372
    HIV dementia, 373–375
    insomnia, 377–378
    major depression, 372–373
    mania, 375–376
    pain, 378
    substance abuse and dependence,
        378–379
    suicide, 379
  epidemiology, 368*t*, 368–369
  homeless patients and, 597
  interaction between HIV/AIDS and
      psychiatric illness, 369,
      370*t*–373*t*
  overview, 367
  treatment, 380
    pharmacotherapy, 380
Homeless patient, approach to,
    595–602
  assessment, 598–600
  definitions of homelessness, 595
  medical overview, 597
  overview, 595*t*–596
    demographics of homelessness,
        596
    prevalence of homelessness, 596
  prevalence of psychiatric diagnoses
      among the homeless,
      596–597

primary care practice, implications of
    homelessness for, 598
  treatment strategies, 600–601
Homeopathy, 680–681
Hopkins Symptom Checklist-90
    (SCL-90), 350
Hormonal therapy, postpartum
    depression, 449
Hormone replacement therapy (HRT),
    approach to patient entering,
    432–433; *see also* Menopause
  weight gain, 452*t*
Hormones
  neuropsychiatric side effects, 362*t*, 363
  sexual dysfunction, 407*t*
Hospice, 488–490
Huntington's chorea, suicide risk and,
    131
Huntington's disease, 199
Hydromorphone (Dilaudid)
  acute pain, 319, 321*t*
  heroin dependence, 518*t*
Hydroxyzine (Atarax)
  anxiety in terminal illness, 495*t*
Hyperalgesia, 316
Hypercalcemia, mimicking depression,
    363
Hyperpathia, 316
Hypersomnia, approach to patient with,
    254; *see also* Disordered sleep
  narcolepsy, 259–260
  obesity, 459
  postpartum depression, 448
  sleep apnea, 258–259
Hypertension, 616–617
Hyperventilation, 264
Hypervigilant patient, response to
    traumatic stress, 535
Hypoactive sexual desire disorder, 398
Hypochondriasis, approach to patient
    with, 166; *see also* Obsessive-
    compulsive disorder (OCD)
  chronic fatigue syndrome, 338
Hypomania
  antidepressant-induced side effect,
      622
  noncompliance, 729
Hypomanic episode
  DSM-IV criteria for, 194
Hypothyroidism, mimicking depression,
    363

Ibuprofen
  migraine headaches, 248
  pain, 318*t*
  tension headaches, 249

Idiopathic chronic fatigue, 335
Idiopathic environmental intolerance.
        See Multiple environmental al-
        lergies, approach to patient with
Idiopathic pain, 317
Ifosfamide, neuropsychiatric side effects,
        362t, 364
Illicit drugs, seizures with, 228t
Illness behavior, 308
Illness Behavior Questionnaire, 350
Imipenem-cilastatin, seizures with, 228t
Imipramine (Tofranil)
    adverse effects, 290t, 614t
    analgesic use, 325, 326t
    anxiety disorders, 147
        associated with alcoholism, 510
    attention-deficit/hyperactivity
            disorder (ADHD), 290t
    bulimia nervosa, 464
    depression in terminal illness, 493t
    effects on heart and cardiovascular
            system, 635t
    GI side effects, 356t
    irritable bowel syndrome (IBS), 356t
    premenstrual syndrome (PMS), 426
    seizures with, 228t
    sexual dysfunction, 396t
    weight gain, 619
Implied threats, criterion in civil
        commitment process, 579
Impotence, approach to patient with, ap-
        proach to patient with, 405–412;
        see also Sexual dysfunction
    diagnostic criteria, 409
    evaluation, 405–409, 406t–407t
    overview, 405
    psychiatric differential diagnosis,
            409
    treatment strategies, 409–411
        organically based erectile
                dysfunction, 409–410
        psychologically based erectile
                dysfunction, 411
Inattentive patient, response to traumatic
        stress, 535
Independent disability evaluation, ap-
        proach to, 591; *see also* Patient
        seeking disability benefits
Indinavir, neuropsychiatric side effects,
        371t
Indomethacin
    cluster headaches, 249
    pain, 318t
Infantile spasms, 231
Infertility, approach to patient with,
        413–420

causes, treaments, costs, and success
        rates, 416t
defining infertility, 413
evaluation and treatment, 414–416
impact of infertility on the couple,
        413–414
management, 418–419
overview, 413
pregnancy in an infertile couple,
        417–418
psychiatric consequences of infertility
        treatment, 416–417
Inflammatory bowel disease (IBD), 351t
    symptoms, 352
Informational interventions, 71
Informed consent, 35–39
    elements of, 36–38
        competency, 36–38
        information, 38
        voluntary, 38
    obtaining, 38–39
    overview, 35–36
Inositol, 676
    adverse effects, 676
    natural antidepressant, 676
Insomnia, approach to patient with,
        254–258, 255t; *see also*
        Disordered sleep
    diagnosis, 254
    glucocorticoid use, 523t
    HIV infection, 375, 377
    postpartum depression, 448
    primary, 258
    secondary to medical conditions, 257
    secondary to psychiatric problems, 257
    secondary to sleep apnea or central
            aveolar hypoventilation, 258
    secondary to substance abuse, 257
    treatment, 256–257
    types of, 255–256
Instrumental Activities of Daily Living
        Scale, 201, 471
Insulin
    seizures with, 228t
    weight gain, 453t
Integrative psychotherapy, 15
Intellectualization, chronic illness and
        defense mechanisms, 304
Interferon, neuropsychiatric side effects,
        362t, 364
Interleukin-2, neuropsychiatric side
        effects, 362t, 364
Intermittent explosive disorder, violent
        patients, 573
International Classification of Sleep
        Disorders (ICSD), 251

Interpersonal psychotherapy, 14
Interpersonal therapy, postpartum
        depression, 449
Interviewing. *See* Psychiatric interview-
        ing, approach to
Intractable seizures, 234
Intracytoplasmic sperm injection (ICSI),
        415
Intrauterine insemination (IUI), 415
Introjection, chronic illness and defense
        mechanisms, 304–305
Investigatory agents, cardiovascular side
        effects, 642–644
In vitro fertilization (IVF), 415
Involuntary civil commitment, 577
Irritability, glucocorticoid use, 523t
Irritable bowel syndrome (IBS), ap-
        proach to patient with, 349–358
    defining, 349
    evaluation, 350–353
    overview, 349t, 349–350
    psychiatric differential diagnosis,
            353–354
    treatment strategies, 354–358
Isocarboxazid (Marplan), 120
    analgesic use, 326t
    depression, 120
Isolation, infertile patient, 413
Isoniazid
    neuropsychiatric side effects, 371t
    seizures with, 228t
Isoproteronol, monoamine oxidase
        inhibitors, interaction with, 617t

Jitteriness, antidepressant-induced side
        effect, 620

Kava (*Piper methysticum*), 677–678
    adverse effects, 677
Ketoconazole, neuropsychiatric side
        effects, 372t
Ketorolac, pain, 318t

Labile mood, response to traumatic
        stress, 535
Lactobacillus acidophilus, diarrhea,
        618t, 619
Lamotrigine (Lamictal)
    cardiovascular side effects, 649
    effects on heart and cardiovascular
            system, 635t
    elevated, expansive, or irritable mood,
            187–188
    seizures, treatment of, 232, 233t
Letrozole, neuropsychiatric side effects,
        363

Levorphanol (Levo-Dromoran)
    acute pain, 321*t*
Levtiracetam, seizures, treatment of,
    232, 233*t*
Lidocaine (Xylocaine)
    chronic pain, 319
    pain in HIV infection, 378
    seizures with, 228*t*
Lifestyle changes, 699–703
    factors associated with, 699–702
    overview, 699
    physician's role in risk-factor
        reduction, 702–703
    strategies
        eating disorders. *See* Anorexia
            nervosa, Bulimia nervosa,
            Obese patient, approach to
        exercise. *See* Exercise programs
            and strategies for weight
            loss
        hypertension, 702
        smoking. *See* Smoking cessation
            strategies
        stress reduction. *See* Stress
            management
Light therapy, 122
    depression, 122
    side effects, 122
Limbic system surgery
    obsessive-compulsive disorder
        (OCD), 169
Lithium carbonate
    cluster headaches, 249
Lithium (Eskalith, Lithobid, Lithonate),
    123
    cardiovascular side effects, 649
    dementia, 211
    depression, 123
    drug-drug interactions, 657, 660*t*
    effects on heart and cardiovascular
        system, 635*t*
    elevated, expansive, or irritable mood,
        185, 186*f*
    glucocorticoid use, neuropsychiatric
        complications from, 527*t*
    obsessive-compulsive disorder
        (OCD), 168
    pregnancy, 438*t,* 439
    premenstrual syndrome (PMS),
        426
    prophylactic, for postpartum
        depression, 449
    seizures with, 228*t*
    sexual dysfunction, 396*t,* 407*t*
    violent patients, 574
    weight gain, 453*t*

Loneliness, chronic fatigue syndrome
    and, 338
Long-suffering, depressed, help-rejecting
    patient, approach to, 109; *see
    also* Personality disorders
Loperamide (Imodium A-D)
    diarrhea, 618*t,* 619
Lopinavir, neuropsychiatric side effects,
    371*t*
Lorazepam (Ativan), 148*t*
    alcohol detoxification, 509
    antidepressant-induced fatigue and
        sedation, 621*t*
    anxiety disorders, 148*t*
    anxiety in terminal illness, 495*t*
    central nervous system side effects,
        619
    delirium in terminal illness, 497*t*
    eating disorders, 178
    insomnia, 256*t*
    nausea and vomiting, treatment for,
        364
    post-traumatic stress disorder (PTSD),
        541
    rehabilitation patients, 485*t*
    sexually assaulted patient, 549
    violent patients, 573
Loxapine (Loxitane)
    effects on heart and cardiovascular
        system, 635*t*

Magnesium pemoline (Cylert)
    adverse effects, 290*t*
    attention-deficit/hyperactivity
        disorder (ADHD), 289, 290*t*
Magnetic resonance imaging (MRI), use
        of, 62, 64–65*t; see also*
        Neuroimaging techniques
    versus CT, 62–63*t*
    indications, 64–65
Maintenance of Wakefulness Test, 258
Maintenance therapy for depression, 124
Major depressive disorder (MDD),
        approach to patient with,
        111–113; *see also* Depression
    alcoholism
        co-morbidity with, 511
        differentiating from, 505
    chronic fatigue syndrome, co-morbidity
        with, 337
    DSM-IV criteria for, 112*t*
    epidemiology, 112–113
    fatigue and, 333
    HIV/AIDS patients, 372–373
    homeless patients, 596
    homeopathy, 680–681

infertility and, 417, 419
irritable bowel syndrome (IBS) and,
        353
multiple environmental allergies, 343
non-compliance, 729
obesity, 459
pregnancy, 435
sexual dysfunction, 398
somatization disorder and, 273
Maladaptive defenses of difficult
        patients, 100
Male erectile disorder, 399
Male orgasmic disorder, 399
Malingering, 231
Managed/capitated care era, dealing
        with, 749–755
    contracting for mental health and
        substance abuse services,
        753–754
    health care economics, 752–753
    increasing availability of psychiatric
        providers, 751–752
    laws on mental health and substance
        abuse treatment, 750
    overview, 749
    prevalence of psychiatric disorders,
        749
    primary care physician interactions
        with psychiatrist, 751
    psychiatric treatment in primary care
        setting, 750–751
    psychotherapy, interfacing with, 752
    referrals and consultations, when to
        consider, 754
Management of patient with infertility,
        418–419
Mania, approach to patient with,
        expansive, or irritable mood,
        184; *see also* Elevated
    antidepressant-induced side effect,
        622
    common co-morbid with alcohol
        abuse, 500
    glucocorticoid use, 522, 523*t*
        neuropsychiatric complications
            from, 527*t*
    HIV infection, 375–376
    noncompliance, 729
    pregnancy, 438*t*
    screening tests for, 55
    violent patients, 572–573
Manic-depressive disorder
    smoking cessation and, 708
Manic State Rating Scale (MSRS), 55
Manipulativeness, approach to, 105–106;
        see also Personality disorders

Maprotiline (Ludiomil)
analgesic use, 325, 326t
seizures with, 228t
Marital discord
infertility and, 417
Maximal oxygen uptake, 717
McGill Pain Questionnaire, 317
Meclofenamic acid
pain, 318t
Medical and surgical conditions causing
sexual dysfunctions, 395t
Medical conditions, insomnia secondary
to, 257
Medical illnesses, suicide risk and, 130
Medical supportive psychotherapy,
308–309
Mefanamic acid
pain, 318t
premenstrual syndrome (PMS), 426
Melatonin, 678
Memory problems or dementia, approach
to patient with, 197–212
dementia of the Alzheimer's type
(DAT), 197
diagnosis, 205–206
differential diagnosis, 206–207
epidemiology, 199
evaluation, 199–204, 200f, 202t
overview, 197, 198t
patient care, 207–211
terminology, 197
Meniere's syndrome, 265
Menopause, approach to patient
entering, 429–434
definitions, 429
epidemiology, 429–430
etiology, 430
evaluation, 430–432
examination, 432
overview, 429
physical and psychological
symptoms, 431t
psychiatric differential diagnosis, 432
treatment strategies, 432–434
patient education, 433–434
pharmacologic, 432–433
psychotherapeutic options, 433
Mental retardation
obesity and, 459
Meperidine
acute pain, 320t
cardiovascular side effects, 616
monoamine oxidase inhibitors,
interaction with, 617t
Meperidine (Demerol)
acute pain, 321t

drug-drug interactions, 665
heroin dependence, 518t
seizures with, 228t
Metabolic equivalents (METs), 717
Metamucil
constipation, 618t, 619
Metaraminol
monoamine oxidase inhibitors,
interaction with, 617t
Methadone (Dolophine)
acute pain, 321t
dosing, 517
heroin dependence, 517, 518t
Methantheline bromide
sexual dysfunction, 396t
Methotrexate, neuropsychiatric side
effects, 362t, 364
Methotrimeprazine
anxiety in terminal illness, 495t
Methyldopa
sexual dysfunction, 396t, 407t
Methylphenidate (Ritalin)
antidepressant-induced fatigue and
sedation, 621t
antidepressant-induced sexual
dysfunction, 624t
attention-deficit/hyperactivity
disorder (ADHD), 289, 290t
cardiovascular side effects, 650
depression in terminal illness, 493t
effects on heart and cardiovascular
system, 635t
HIV/AIDS patients, treating
depression, 373
HIV dementia, 375
monoamine oxidase inhibitors,
interaction with, 617t
rehabilitation patients, 485t
Methylsergide
migraine headaches, 248
Metoclopramide (Reglan)
nausea, 618t, 619
nausea and vomiting, post-chemotherapy treatment for, 365
Metronidazole, neuropsychiatric side
effects, 371t
Mexilitine
chronic pain, 319
Michigan Alcoholism Screening Test
(MAST), 57, 502, 503t–504t
Midazolam
anxiety in terminal illness, 495t
delirium in terminal illness, 497t
Migraine headaches
characteristics, 244
epidemiology, 243

onset and duration, 245
precipitating and ameliorating factors,
245–246
prevention, 248
prodrome, 246
treatment, 247–248
Mild euphoria, glucocorticoid use, 522
Milk of magnesia
constipation, 618t, 619
Mini-Mental State Examination
(MMSE), 56, 115, 203,
218t–220t, 360, 474
Minnesota Multiphasic Personality
Inventory (MMPI), 350
Mirtazapine
depression in terminal illness, 493t
Mirtazapine (Remeron), 119
adverse effects, 614t
antidepressant-induced sexual
dysfunction, 624t
anxiety disorders, 146, 257
cardiovascular side effects, 639
depression, 119
eating disorders, 178
effects on heart and cardiovascular
system, 636t
monoamine oxidase inhibitors,
interaction with, 617t
rehabilitation patients, 485t
side effects, 119
Miscellaneous drugs, seizures with,
228t
Moclobemide, 120
Modafinil (Provigil)
antidepressant-induced fatigue and
sedation, 621t
antidepressant-induced sexual
dysfunction, 624t
cardiovascular side effects, 651
Molindone (Moban)
effects on heart and cardiovascular
system, 636t
Monoamine oxidase inhibitors (MAOIs),
120t–121
adverse effects, 147, 614t
anxiety disorders, 147
attention-deficit/hyperactivity
disorder (ADHD), 293, 295
cardiovascular side effects, 616,
641–642
dementia, 210
depression, 120–121
dietary restrictions, 295
drug-drug interactions, 293, 664–665
drugs and foods contraindicated
during therapeutic use, 643t

obsessive-compulsive disorder
(OCD), 169
risk of lethal hypertensive crisis, 120
sexual dysfunction, 121, 146
social phobia, 142
weight gain, 121, 147, 453*t*
Mood disorders. *See* Elevated, expansive,
or irritable mood, approach to
patient with
DSM-IV definition of, 195
menopause and, 429
obesity, 459
pain, co-morbidity with, 314
postpartum, 443–450
pregnancy, 435
sexually assaulted patient, 549
violent patients, 572–573
Mood stabilizers, 210
cardiovascular side effects, 648–650
drug-drug interactions, 657
organ transplant patients, 388
postpartum psychosis, 449
Morphine
acute pain, 319, 320*t*–321*t*
heroin dependence, 518*t*
MRI. *See* Magnetic resonance imaging
Multiple environmental allergies, approach to patient with, 341–348
diagnostic criteria, 344
evaluation, 342–343
overview, 341
psychiatric differential diagnosis,
343–344
treatment strategies, 344–347
Multiple gestations, 418
Multiple physical complaints, approach
to patient with, 269–278
diagnostic criteria, 275–276
evaluation of the somatizing patient,
270–273
overview, 269–270
psychiatric differential diagnosis,
273–275
treatment strategies, 276–278,
277*t*–278*t*
Multiple sclerosis, 266
suicide risk and, 131
Multiple Sleep Latency Test, 258
Myocardial infarction (MI), 618
Myocarditis, 645
Myoclonus, 621
antidepressant-induced side effect,
621

Nabumetone
pain, 318*t*

Nalbuphine (Nubain)
acute pain, 322*t*
Naloxone (Narcan)
cardiovascular side effects, 651
heroin overdose, 517
Naltrexone (ReVia)
alcoholism treatment, 509
cardiovascular side effects, 651
effects on heart and cardiovascular
system, 636*t*
premenstrual syndrome (PMS), 426
Naproxen
pain, 318*t*
Naratriptan (Amerge)
migraine headaches, treatment of, 247
Narcissism, celebrities and, 604
Narcissistic personality disorder, 604
Narcolepsy, approach to patient with,
259–260; *see also* Disordered
sleep
diagnosis, 259
etiology, 259
prevalence, 259
treatment, 259–260
Narcotics, seizures with, 228*t*
Narcotics Anonymous, 516
National Co-morbidity Survey, 500
National Domestic Violence Hotline,
557
National Institute of Health (NIH), 671
Natural medications, 671–685
defining natural medications, 671
overview, 671–672
problems associated with use, 672–673
cost issues, 672–673
effectiveness issues, 672
safety issues, 672
recommendations for practitioners,
681–682
types of, 673–681
cognition-enhancing remedies,
679–680
homeopathy, 680–681
medications for premenstrual
syndrome, 678–679
natural antidepressants, 673–676
natural anxiolytic-hypnotics,
676–678
Nausea, gastrointestinal side effects of
antidepressants, 618–619
Nausea and vomiting, treatments for,
364–365
Nefazodone
adverse effects, 614*t*
cardiovascular side effects, 618
depression in terminal illness, 493*t*

eating disorders, 178
GI side effects, 356*t*
irritable bowel syndrome (IBS), 356*t*
monoamine oxidase inhibitors,
interaction with, 617*t*
premenstrual syndrome (PMS), 426
rehabilitation patients, 485*t*
weight gain, 619
Nefazodone (Serzone), 119–120
antidepressant-induced sexual
dysfunction, 624*t*
anxiety disorder, 146
depression, 119–120
effects on heart and cardiovascular
system, 636*t*
post-traumatic stress disorder (PTSD),
541
side effects, 119
Nelfinavir, neuropsychiatric side effects,
371*t*
Neurasthenia, chronic fatigue syndrome
and, 338
Neuroimaging techniques, use of, 61–66
indications, 64–66
computed tomography (CT), 64
dementia, 66
general guidelines, 65
magnetic resonance imaging
(MRI), 64–65, 65*t*
pre-electroconvulsive therapy
neuroimaging, 65
seizures, 66
modalities, 61–64
computed tomography (CT),
61–62, 63*t*
magnetic resonance imaging
(MRI), 62, 63*t*
positron emission tomography
(PET), 63, 64*t*
single photon emission computed
tomography (SPECT),
63–64, 64*t*
overview, 61
Neuroleptic
postpartum psychosis, 449
rehabilitation patients, 485*t*
Neuroleptics
anxiety in terminal illness, 495*t*
cardiovascular side effects, 630*t*–633*t*
delirium in terminal illness, 497*t*
dementia, 210
eating disorders, 178
glucocorticoid use, neuropsychiatric
complications from, 526, 527*t*
obsessive-compulsive disorder
(OCD), 168

Neuroleptics *(continued)*
  organ transplant patients, 388
  pregnancy, 438*t*
  seizures with, 228*t*
  violent patients, 574
Neuropathic pain, 315–316
Neuropsychiatric complications from
    steriod use, 522–526
  risk factors, 524–526
Neuropsychiatric dysfunction, approach
    to patient with, 213–223
  evaluation, 213–222
    behavioral, 216–222
    general, 213–216, 215*t*–216*t*
  overview, 213
Nevirapine, neuropsychiatric side
    effects, 371*t*
Nicotine chewing gum, 710
Nicotine replacement therapy
  smoking cessation, 706
Nightmares, response to traumatic stress,
    536
Nociception, 311–312
  central conduction of, 312
  peripheral conduction of, 311
Nocturnal myoclonus, approach to
    patient with, 260; *see also*
    Disordered sleep
Nocturnal penile tumescense (NPT), 408
Noncompliance, enhancing, 726–728;
    see also Compliance
  adverse impact of, 726
  discovery of, 726–728
Nonepileptic seizures, 231
Nonsteroidal anti-inflammatory agents
    (NSAIDs), 311, 318*t*, 325
Norepinephrine
  monoamine oxidase inhibitors,
    interaction with, 617*t*
Nortriptyline (Pamelor), 257
  adverse effects, 290*t*, 614*t*
  analgesic use, 325, 326*t*
  anxiety disorders, 147, 257
  attention-deficit/hyperactivity
    disorder (ADHD), 290*t*
  depression in terminal illness, 493*t*
  effects on heart and cardiovascular
    system, 636*t*
  pregnancy, 438*t*
  premenstrual syndrome (PMS), 426
  seizures with, 228*t*
Nucleoside antiretrovirals, HIV
    dementia, 375

Obese patient, approach to, 451–467
  etiology, 451
  evaluation, 451–457

examination of patient, 456–457*t*
  general recommendations, 451–452
  interview, 455–456
  medical and psychiatric history,
    452–454, 453*t*
  psychiatric differential diagnosis,
    458–459
  treatment strategies complicated by
    psychological factors or psy-
    chiatric illness, 459–465
  treatments for obesity, 460–463
  treatments for psychiatric illness
    and psychological factors,
    463–465
Obsessive-compulsive disorder (OCD)
  irritable bowel syndrome (IBS) and,
    354
  non-compliance, 730
  sexual dysfunction, 398
  somatization disorder and, 273
Obsessive-compulsive disorder (OCD),
    approach to patient with,
    approach to, 143, 165–170;
    see also Anxious patient
  cognitive-behavioral therapy (CBT),
    79–80
  definition of OCD, 143, 165
  diagnostic criteria, 167
  evaluation, 165–166
  onset and course, 143
  psychiatric differential diagnosis,
    166–167
  support groups, 170
  treatments, 143
  treatment strategies, 167–170
    electroconvulsive therapy (ECT),
      169
    first-line behavioral therapy: expo-
      sure and response preven-
      tion, 169
    first-line pharmacotherapy: SRIs,
      167–168
    limbic system surgery, 169
    second-line pharmacotherapy: SRI
      augmentation and alterna-
      tive monotherapies,
      168–169
Obsessive-Compulsive Foundation,
    170
Obsessive-compulsive personality disor-
    der (OCPD), 167
Obstructive sleep apnea, 258
OKT3, organ transplant patients, 390
Olanzapine (Zyprexa)
  anxiety in terminal illness, 495*t*
  cardiovascular side effects, 630*t*–633*t*,
    645*t*, 646

delirium in terminal illness, 497*t*
dementia, 209
  effects on heart and cardiovascular
    system, 636*t*
  elevated, expansive, or irritable mood,
    187
  nausea and vomiting, post-chemo-
    therapy treatment for, 365
  rehabilitation patients, 485*t*
  violent patients, 574
Ondansetron
  alcoholism treatment, 510
  nausea and vomiting, treatment for
    post-chemotherapy, 364
Opiates
  abuse. *See* Cocaine or opiate-abusing
    patient, approach to
  pain in HIV infection, 378
  sexual dysfunction, 396*t*, 407*t*
  violent patients, 572
Opioids, 320–325, 321*t*–322*t*
  adverse effects, 320, 323–324
  monoamine oxidase inhibitors,
    interaction with, 617*t*
Oral hypoglycemics
  monoamine oxidase inhibitors,
    interaction with, 617*t*
Organic brain syndromes
  homeless patients, 596
  organ transplant patients, 389
Organic headaches
  characteristics, 244
  onset and duration, 245
  precipitating and ameliorating factors,
    246
Organ malformation, risk of during
    pregnancy, 436
Organ Procurement and Transplant
    Network (OPTN), 386
Organ transplantation, approach to
    patient undergoing, 385–392
  evaluation of patient, 386–391
    post-transplant patient, care of,
      389–391
    pre-transplant psychiatric
      evaluation, 386–391
  overview, 385–386
    psychological evaluation of
      potential donors, 385
    recipient selection, ethical/
      medicolegal
      considerations, 386
Orgasm phase disorders, sexual
    dysfunction, 399
Orlistat
  obesity, 461–462
Orthostasis, 615

Orthostatic hypotension, 615, 645
Outpatient primary care psychiatry
        models, 5–6
    alternative models, 7–8
Oxaprozin
    pain, 318*t*
Oxazepam (Serax)
    anxiety disorders, 148*t*
    anxiety in terminal illness, 495*t*
    rehabilitation patients, 485*t*
Oxcarbazepine (Trileptal)
    cardiovascular side effects, 649
    elevated, expansive, or irritable mood,
        187
Oxycodone (Percodan, Roxicodone)
    acute pain, 322*t*
    heroin dependence, 518*t*
Oxymorphone (Numorphan)
    acute pain, 322*t*

Paclitaxel, neuropsychiatric side effects,
        362*t*
Pain, approach to patient with,
        311–328
    analgesic therapies, 317–327
        acute pain treatment, 318–319
        analgesic adjuvants, 325
        chronic pain treatment, 319–320
        multi-disciplinary approach, 327
        non-pharmacological approaches,
            318, 325–327
        opioids, 320–325, 321*t*–322*t*
        pharmacological approaches, 317
    classes of, 314–317
        acute pain, 314
        chronic pain, 314–315
        continuous pain in the terminally
            ill, 314
        idiopathic pain, 317
        neuropathic pain, 315–316
        reflex sympathetic dystrophy
            (RSD), 316–317
    overview, 311–314
Pain, HIV infection and, 378
Pain, verbal analog scale, 317
Palliative care, approach to patient
        receiving, 487–498
    general approach to, 490–491
    neuropsychiatric complications of
        terminal illness, 491–497
        anxiety, 494–495
        confusion and delirium,
            495–497*t*
        depression, 491, 492*t*–493*t*
    overview, 487–488
    practical problems in entering patients
        into, 488–490

Panic attacks
    in pregnancy, 435
Panic disorder, approach to, 77–78,
        140–141*t*; *see also* Anxious
        patient
    alcoholism, co-morbidity with, 510
    chronic fatigue syndrome, co-morbidity
        with, 337
    cognitive-behavioral therapy (CBT),
        77–78
    defining, 140
    demographics and course, 141
    fatigue and, 333
    homeopathy, 680–681
    infertility and, 419
    inositol, 676
    irritable bowel syndrome (IBS) and,
        353
    limited-symptom attacks, 141
    multiple environmental allergies, 344
    nature of, 77
    sexual dysfunction, 398
    treatments, 141
Papaverine
    erectile dysfunction, 410
Paraphilias
    sexual dysfunction, 398
Parasomnias, approach to patient with,
        252*t*–253*t*, 260; *see also*
        Disordered sleep
Paregoric
    heroin dependence, 518*t*
Paresthesias
    antidepressant-induced side effect,
        621
Parkinson's disease, 205
Paroxetine (Paxil)
    adverse effects, 614*t*
    anxiety disorders, 146, 257
        associated with alcoholism, 510
    bulimia nervosa, 178
    cardiovascular side effects,
        630*t*–633*t*
    depression in terminal illness, 493*t*
    effects on heart and cardiovascular
        system, 636*t*
    GI side effects, 356*t*
    irritable bowel syndrome (IBS), 356*t*
    obsessive-compulsive disorder
        (OCD), 168
    post-traumatic stress disorder (PTSD),
        541
    rehabilitation patients, 485*t*
Passive-aggressive disorder
    sexual dysfunction, 398
Patient compliance. *See* Compliance,
    enhancing

Patient seeking disability benefits,
        approach to, 589–594
    disability assessment, 593
    overview, 589*t*–591
    psychiatric disability evaluation,
        591–593
Pediatric Symptom Checklist (PSC),
        280, 281*t*, 284*t*
Pemoline (Cylert)
    cardiovascular side effects, 650
    depression in terminal illness, 493*t*
    effects on heart and cardiovascular
        system, 636*t*
Penicillins, seizures with, 228*t*
Pentamidine, neuropsychiatric side
        effects, 371*t*
Pentazocine (Talwin)
    acute pain, 322*t*
Peptic ulcer disease, suicide risk and, 131
Pergolide (Permax)
    antidepressant-induced fatigue and
        sedation, 621*t*
    antidepressant-induced sexual
        dysfunction, 624*t*
Periaqueductal gray (PAG), 312
Perilymph fistula, 263
Perimenopause, definition, 429
Perinatal toxicity, risk of during
        pregnancy, 436
Periodic leg movements of sleep,
        approach to patient with, 260;
        see also Disordered sleep
Peripheral conduction of nociception,
        311
Perphenazine (Trilafon)
    effects on heart and cardiovascular
        system, 636*t*
    nausea and vomiting, post-chemo-
        therapy treatment for, 365
    seizures with, 228*t*
    violent patients, 574
Persistent insomnia, 256
Personality Disorder Examination
        (PDE), 57
Personality disorders
    pain, co-morbidity with, 314
    premenstrual syndrome (PMS) and, 424
    screening tests used for, 57
    sexual dysfunction, 398
    somatization disorder and, 273
    suicide risk, 130
    violent patients, 573
Personality disorders, approach to,
        97–103, 105–110
    clinical presentations, 99–102
        angry or demanding patient,
            106–107

Personality disorders, approach to
clinical presentations (continued)
dependency, 99
fearful or paranoid patient,
108–109
long-suffering, depressed, help-
rejecting patient, 109
maladaptive defenses, 100
manipulativeness, 105–106
projections onto the doctor,
99–100
seductive or dramatic patient,
107–108
withdrawn, unsociable, or remote
patient, 108
etiology of personality disorders,
97–99, 98f
non-compliance, 730
scope of problem, 97
Personality types and chronic illness,
305–308
Phencyclidine, seizures with, 228t
Phenelzine (Nardil), 120
adverse effects, 614t
analgesic use, 326t
anxiety disorders, 147
cardiovascular side effects, 616
depression, 120
effects on heart and cardiovascular
system, 636t
premenstrual syndrome (PMS), 426
sexual dysfunction, 396t
weight gain, 619
Phenobarbital
seizures, treatment of, 232, 233t
Phentermine
monoamine oxidase inhibitors,
interaction with, 617t
obesity, 461–462
Phentolamine
erectile dysfunction, 410
Phenylbutazone
pain, 318t
Phenylephrine
monoamine oxidase inhibitors,
interaction with, 617t
Phenylpropanolamine
monoamine oxidase inhibitors,
interaction with, 617t
Phenytoin (Dilantin)
chronic pain, 319, 323t
migraine headaches, 248
seizures, treatment of, 232, 233t
Physician-assisted suicide and euthanasia,
691; see also Treatment
decisions at the end of life

Physician's role in risk-factor reduction,
702–703; see also Lifestyle
changes
Physician stress and burnout, coping
with, 757–759; see also Rigors
of medical practice
etiologies for, 757–759
Pick's disease, 205
Pimozide (Orap)
effects on heart and cardiovascular
system, 636t
obsessive-compulsive disorder
(OCD), 168
Piroxicam
pain, 318t
Pizotifen
migraine headaches, 248
Polysomnography, 254
Polysubstance abuse, 511
Positive and Negative Symptoms Scale
(PANSS), 56
Positron emission tomography (PET),
use of, 63, 64t, 230; see also
Neuroimaging techniques
Post-concussive syndrome, approach to
patient following, 238t; see also
Head injury (closed)
Postpartum mood disorders, approach to
patient with, 443–450
breast-feeding, 450
classification of disorders, 443
postpartum "blues," 443
postpartum depression, 443
puerperal psychosis, 443
diagnostic criteria, 448
etiology, 444
overview, 443
predictors of disorders, 444
prophylyaxis, 449–450
screening for, 444–447
treatment, 448–449
Post-transplant patient, care of, 389–391
long-term follow-up, 389–390
short-term care, 389
treatment, 390–391
Post-traumatic seizures, 230
Post-traumatic stress disorder (PTSD),
approach to patient following,
approach to; Traumatic event,
143; see also Anxious patient
alcoholism, co-morbidity with, 500,
511
cognitive-behavioral therapy (CBT),
80–81
defining, 143
epidemiology, 537

homeless patients, 596
irritable bowel syndrome (IBS) and,
353
multiple environmental allergies, 344
nature of, 80
onset and course, 143
organ transplant patients, 389
sexual dysfunction, 398
sexually assaulted patient, 549
treatment, 143
Post-traumatic vertigo, 265
Pre-electroconvulsive therapy neuroimaging, use of, 65; see also
Neuroimaging techniques
Pregnancy
in an infertile couple, 417–418
loss, impact of, 418
seizure treatment and, 234
Pregnant patient, approach to, 435–441
course of psychiatric disorder during
pregnancy, 435–436
electroconvulsive therapy (ECT)
during pregnancy, 440
overview, 435
pharmacologic intervention versus
risk of untreated psychiatric
disorder, 436
psychotropic drugs in pregnancy,
437–440, 438t
risk of untreated maternal psychiatric
disorders, 437
screening for psychiatric illness
during pregnancy, 440
Premature ejaculation, 399
Premature requests for limiting life-
sustaining treatment, 691; see
also Treatment decisions at the
end of life
Premenstrual dysphoric disorder, 422
differentiating from depression, 116
Premenstrual syndrome (PMS), approach
to patient with, 421–428
DSM-IV research criteria for, 422t
epidemiology, 422–423
evaluation, 423–424
overview, 421–422
physical and psychological symptoms, 421t
psychiatric differential diagnosis, 424
treatment strategies, 424–426, 427t
Premenstrual syndrome (PMS)/
menopausal symptoms
natural medications, 678–679
black cohosh (Cimicifuga
racemosa), 678–679
chaste tree berry (CTB), 679

Pre-transplant psychiatric evaluation,
  386–391
  diagnosis, 387
  factors which complicate, 387
  objectives, 386–387
  treatment, 388
*Primary Care Evaluation of Mental
  Disorders* (PRIME-MD), 27
Primary mourners, approach to patient
  with, 153; *see also* Acute grief
Primidone
  seizures, treatment of, 232, 233*t*
Procaine, seizures with, 228*t*
Procarbazine, neuropsychiatric side
  effects, 362*t*, 363
Progesterone
  etiology of postpartum mood
    disorders, 444
  postpartum depression, 449
  sexual dysfunction, 396*t*
Projection, chronic illness and defense
  mechanisms, 304
Projective identification, 100–101
  chronic illness and defense
    mechanisms, 304
Project Match, 505
Prolonged sleep latency
Propanolol
  migraine headaches, 248
Prophylaxis
  postpartum depression, 449–450
  pregnancy, 438*t*
Propoxyphene (Darvon)
  heroin dependence, 518*t*
Propranolol (Inderal)
  central nervous system side effects, 619
  post-traumatic stress disorder (PTSD),
    541
  seizures with, 228*t*
  sexual dysfunction, 396*t*, 407*t*
  violent patients, 574
Prostaglandin E1 (Alprostadil, Caverject)
  erectile dysfunction, 410
Protease inhibitors
  HIV dementia, 375
  neuropsychiatric side effects, 371*t*
Protriptyline (Vivactil)
  adverse effects, 614*t*
  analgesic use, 326*t*
  effects on heart and cardiovascular
    system, 636*t*
Pseudoephedrine
  monoamine oxidase inhibitors,
    interaction with, 617*t*
Pseudoseizure, 231
  versus seizure, 231*t*

Psychiatric disability evaluation, approach
  to, 591–593; *see also* Patient
    seeking disability benefits
Psychiatric disorders
  suicide risk, 129
Psychiatric interviewing
  approach to, 19–26
    common errors in interviewing, 25
    conceptualizing psychiatric
      conditions, 19–20
    creating an atmosphere conducive
      to self-revelation and
      mutual treatment planning,
      20–21
    data gathering, 22–23
    interviewing difficulties, 23–24
    negotiation and treatment planning,
      24–25
    overview, 19
  rehabilitation patients, 481*t*, 482
Psychiatric problems
  insomnia secondary to, 257
Psychiatry, natural medications in,
  671–685
Psychoanalytic psychotherapy, 13
Psychodynamic therapy
  eating disorders, 178
Psychoeducational therapy, 14–15
  anxiety associated with HIV
    infection, 377
Psychogenic headaches
  characteristics, 244
  onset and duration, 245
  treatment, 249
Psychopharmacology
  for physician stress or burnout, 762
Psychosis
  glucocorticoid use, 522, 523*t*
    neuropsychiatric complications
      from, 527*t*
  non-compliance, 730
  pregnancy, 438*t*
  steroid, 522
  suicide risk, 130
Psychostimulants, 122
  adverse effects, 493*t*
  brain-injury, treatment of, 241
  cardiovascular side effects, 650–651
  dementia, 210
  depression, 122, 123
  depression in terminal illness, 493*t*
  violent patients, 572, 574
Psychotherapy, 13–17
  anxiety disorders, 151
  depression, 121
  group therapy, 15–16

irritable bowel syndrome (IBS), 355,
  357
medical supportive, 308–309
menopause patients, 433
organ transplant patients, 391
for physician stress or burnout, 762
premenstrual syndrome (PMS), 425
psychotherapist, what to ask before
  referring to, 16
types of, 13–15
  behavior therapy, 13–14
  cognitive therapy, 14
  integrative psychotherapy, 15
  interpersonal, 14
  psychoanalytic psychotherapy, 13
  psychoeducational therapy, 14–15
  supportive therapy, 15
Psychotropic agents, cardiovascular side
  effects, 629–652
  antidepressants, 629–644, 630*t*–637*t*
    investigatory agents, 642–644
    monoamine oxidase inhibitors
      (MAOIs), 641–642
    second-choice antidepressants, 639
    selective serotonin reuptake
      inhibitors (SSRIs), 629,
      638–639
    tricyclic antidepressants (TCAs),
      639–641
  antipsychotics, 644–648, 645*t*, 647*t*
  anxiolytics and sedative-hypnotic
    agents, 650
  mood stabilizers, 648–650
  overview, 629
  psychostimulants, 650–651
  substance abuse, agents used to treat,
    651
Psychotropics
  in pregnancy, 437–440
  presence of, in breast milk, 450
  rehabilitation patients, 485*t*
  seizures with, 228*t*
  sexual dysfunction, 396*t*, 407*t*
Psychotropics, approach to patient
  receiving, 529–533
  diagnosis, 530
  education, 530
  family involvement, 531
  medications, 529
  negotiating medication changes,
    531–532
  overview, 529
  tracking
    compliance, 530–531
    relevant medical parameters, 532
    side effects, 530–531

Psychotropics
  tracking (continued)
    stressors, 531
    target symptoms, 530
Puerperal psychosis, 443
Pulmonary emboli, mimicking anxiety
    disorders, 362
Pulmonary failure
  organ transplant patients, 387
Purified protein derivative (PPD), 597

Quazepam (Doral)
  insomnia, 256t
Quetiapine (Seroquel)
  anxiety in terminal illness, 495t
  cardiovascular side effects, 630t–633t,
    645t, 646
  delirium in terminal illness, 497t
  dementia, 209
  effects on heart and cardiovascular
    system, 636t
  rehabilitation patients, 485t
Quinolones, seizures with, 228t

Rantidine (Zantac)
  nausea, 618t, 619
Rape. See Sexually assaulted patient,
    approach to
Rational Recovery, 516
Reactive anxiety, 144
Reduplicative paramnesia, 222
Referral, approach to making, 27–34
  for alcoholism
    inpatient detoxification, 511
    specialized long-term treatment, 511
  clinical situation or treatments that
    warrant, 29t
  collaborative care or referral, 33t, 33–34
  consultation or referral, 27
  for family therapy, 563–564
  making, how to, 31–32
  overview, 27
  patient non-acceptance, 32–33
  practitioner to refer to, 29, 30t
  presenting recommendation to
    patient, 29–31, 30t
  psychiatric diagnoses that warrant a
    referral, 28, 28t
Reflex sympathetic dystrophy (RSD),
    316–317
Regression, chronic illness and defense
    mechanisms, 304
Regressive dependency
  chronic illness and, 305
Rehabilitation, approach to patient
    requiring, 479–486
  evaluation, 481t, 481–483

overview, 479
range of problems that may be experi-
    enced during rehabilitation,
    479–481, 480t
treatment, 484–485
  pharmacological, 484–485
  psychiatric, 484
  psychological, 484
Relapse prevention, 509
Relapse prevention skills, 73
Renal failure
  organ transplant patients, 387
Reserpine
  sexual dysfunction, 407t
Resistance training, 718; see also Exercise
    programs and strategies for
    weight loss
Respiratory index, 259
Restless legs syndrome, approach to
    patient with, 260; see also
    Disordered sleep
Rheumatoid arthritis, 525
  suicide risk and, 131
Right to refuse treatment, 577–578
Rigors of medical practice, coping with,
    757–763
  etiologies for physician stress and
    burnout, 757–759
  interventions, 760–763
  overview, 757
  when coping strategies go awry,
    759–760
Risperidone (Risperdal)
  anxiety in terminal illness, 495t
  cardiovascular side effects, 630t–633t,
    645t, 646
  delirium in terminal illness, 497t
  dementia, 209
  effects on heart and cardiovascular
    system, 636t
  elevated, expansive, or irritable mood,
    187
  obsessive-compulsive disorder
    (OCD), 168
  post-traumatic stress disorder
    (PTSD), 541
  rehabilitation patients, 485t
  violent patients, 574
Ritonavir, neuropsychiatric side effects,
    371t
Rivastigmine (Exelon)
  cognitive enhancement, 208
Rizatriptan (Maxalt)
  migraine headaches, treatment of, 247
Rome Criteria, 350
Ruminations, 166
Russell's sign, 456

S-adenosyl methionine (SAMe), 122,
    637t, 644, 674
  depression, 122
  natural antidepressant, 674
  side effects, 674
Safety, approach to violent patient, 567
Saquinavir, neuropsychiatric side effects,
    371t
Schizoaffective disorder
  bipolar disorder, 185
Schizophrenia
  alcoholism
    co-morbidity with, 511
    differentiating from, 505
  bipolar disorder, 185
  chronic fatigue syndrome, 338
  common co-morbid with alcohol
    abuse, 500
  homeless patients, 596
  referrals for, 754
  screening tests used for, 55–56
  sexual dysfunction, 398
  smoking cessation and, 708
  violent patients, 572
Screening for psychiatric illness during
    pregnancy, 440
Screening tests used for detection of
    psychiatric disorders, 51–60
  alcohol, 501–504
    Alcohol Use Disorders
      Identification Test
      (AUDIT), 501t–502t
    CAGE Questionnaire, 501t
    Michigan Alcoholism Screening Test
      (MAST), 502, 503t–504t
  anxiety, 55
    Anxiety Disorder Interview Scale,
      Revised (ADIS-R), 55
    Hamilton Rating Scale for Anxiety
      (HAM-A), 55
    Yale-Brown Obsessive-Compulsive
      Scale (Y-BOCS), 55
  cognitive dysfunction, 56
    Blessed Dementia Scale (BDS), 56
    Functional Dementia Scale (FDS),
      475
    Mini-Mental State Examination
      (MMSE), 56, 474, 475t
  depression, 52–54
    Beck Depression Inventory (BDI),
      53–54, 474
    Clinical Global Improvement
      (CGI) Scale, 53
    Edinburgh Postnatal Depression
      Scale, 445t–447t
    Geriatric Depression Scale (GDS),
      473t, 474

Hamilton Rating Scale for Depression (HAM-D), 52–53

The Harvard Department of Psychiatry National Depression Screening Day Scale (HANDS), 54

Zung Self-Rating Depression Scale (SDS), 54

drug side effects, 58

Abnormal Involuntary Movement Scale (AIMS), 58

mania, 55

Manic State Rating Scale (MSRS), 55

Young Mania Rating Scale (Y-MRS), 55

personality disorders, 56–57

Personality Disorder Examination (PDE), 57

Structured Clinical Interview for *DSM-III-R* Personality Disorders (SCID-II), 56–57

schizophrenia, 55–56

Brief Psychiatric Scale (BPRS), 55–56

Positive and Negative Symptoms Scale (PANSS), 56

social functioning, 57–58

Global Assessment of Functioning Scale (GAF), 57

Self Adjustment Scale (SAS), 58

Structured Clinical Interview for *DSM-IV* (SCID), 52

substance abuse, 57

Addiction Severity Index (ASI), 57

CAGE Questionnaire, 57

Michigan Alcoholism Screening test (MAST), 57

Seasonal affective disorder (SAD), 122

Secondary mourners, approach to patient with, 153; *see also* Acute grief

Sedation

antidepressant-induced side effect, 620

Sedative-hypnotics

multiple environmental allergies, 346

Sedatives

sexual dysfunction, 396*t*, 407*t*

valerian, 676–677

Seductive or dramatic patient, approach to, 107–108; *see also* Personality disorders

Seizures, approach to patient with, 225–236

diagnostic strategies, 232

differential diagnosis, 230–232

evaluation, 225*t*–228*t*, 225–230

functional neuroimaging, 66

overview, 225

treatment strategies, 232–235

epilepsy surgery, 234–235

pharmacologic, 232–234

Selective serotonin reuptake inhibitors (SSRIs), 116*t*, 116–117

adverse effects, 146, 493*t*, 614*t*

anxiety disorder, 145

cardiovascular side effects, 616, 629, 638–639

dementia, 210

depression in terminal illness, 493*t*

dizziness, 266

drug-drug interactions, 657, 662, 663*t*

eating disorders, 178

first choice in antidepressants, 116*t*

HIV/AIDS patients, treating depression, 373

monoamine oxidase inhibitors, interaction with, 617*t*

obesity, 462

obsessive-compulsive disorder (OCD), 143, 167

organ transplant patients, 388

post-traumatic stress disorder (PTSD), 143, 541

premenstrual syndrome (PMS), 425

rehabilitation patients, 485*t*

side effects, 117

smoking cessation, 710

social phobia, 142

weight gain, 453*t*, 619

Self Adjustment Scale (SAS), 58

Self-help groups, postpartum depression, 449

Self-monitoring, 71

Serotonergic agents

insomnia in HIV/AIDS patients, 377

Serotonergic syndromes, 120

Serotonin norepinephrine reuptake inhibitors (SNRIs), 117*t*

anxiety disorder, 145

depression, 117

side effects, 117

Serotonin reuptake inhibitors (SRIs), 178

bulimia nervosa, 178

Sertraline

adverse effects, 614*t*

binge-eating disorder (BED), 464

bulimia nervosa, 178

cardiovascular side effects, 630*t*–633*t*

depression in terminal illness, 493*t*

GI side effects, 356*t*

irritable bowel syndrome (IBS), 356*t*

obesity, 461

obsessive-compulsive disorder (OCD), 168

premenstrual syndrome (PMS), 426

rehabilitation patients, 485*t*

sexual dysfunction, 396*t*

Sertraline (Zoloft)

analgesic use, 326*t*

anxiety disorder, 146

effects on heart and cardiovascular system, 637*t*

post-traumatic stress disorder (PTSD), 541

Sexual and gender identity disorders

referrals for, 29*t*

Sexual assault

homeless patients, 596

Sexual aversion disorder, 398

Sexual dysfunction

infertility and, 417

Sexual dysfunction, approach to patient with, 393–403

antidepressant-induced side effects, 116–121, 118, 623–625

diagnostic criteria, 398–400

evaluation, 393–397, 394*t*–397*t*

not otherwise specified, 400

overview, 393

psychiatric differential diagnosis, 398

treatment strategies, 400–402

organically based disorders, 400–401

psychologically based disorders, 401–402

Sexually assaulted patient, approach to, 545–551

epidemiology, 545

etiology, 545–546

evolutionary theory, 545

neurophysiologic theories, 546

personality theories, 546

evaluation, 546

examination of the patient, 547–549

overview, 545

psychiatric differential diagnosis, 549

treatment strategies, 550–551

legal, 550–551

medical, 550

pharmacotherapy, 551

psychological, 550

Sexually transmitted disease, 550

Sexual pain disorders, 399–400

Sexual relationships, boundary violations and, 746

Sexual side effects of antidepressants, 623–625

Short, Portable, Mental Status Questionnaire (SPMSQ), 475

Silbutramine
binge-eating disorder (BED), 464
monoamine oxidase inhibitors, interaction with, 617t
obesity, 461–462

Sildenafil (Viagra)
antidepressant-induced sexual dysfunction, 624t
erectile dysfunction, 409–410

Simple partial seizure, 225t

Single photon emission computed tomography (SPECT), use of, 63–64, 64t; see also Neuro-imaging techniques

Sinoatrial (SA), 618

Sinus headaches, characteristics of, 245

Sinus tachycardia
cardiovascular side effects, 617

Situational anxiety, 144

Skill rehearsal, 72

Skin diseases, homeless patients, 597

Sleep apnea, approach to patient with, 258–259; see also Disordered sleep
diagnosis, 258–259
insomnia secondary to, 258
treatment, 259

Sleep apnea, fatigue and, 333

Sleep-wake schedule disorders, approach to patient with, 254; see also Disordered sleep

Smoking cessation strategies, 705–711
evaluation of methods, 706
obstacles, 707–708
overview, 705t
pharmacological treatment strategies, 709–711
practical treatment strategies, 708–709

Social functioning, 57–58
screening tests, 57–58

Social phobia, approach to, 78–79, 142; see also Anxious patient
cognitive-behavioral therapy (CBT), 78–79
defining, 142
homeopathy, 680–681
onset and course, 142
treatments, 142

Sodium valproate
migraine headaches, 249

Somatization disorder, 274–275, 275t
chronic fatigue syndrome, co-morbidity with, 337
irritable bowel syndrome (IBS) and, 353–354
multiple environmental allergies, 343

Somatizing patients. See Multiple physical complaints, approach to patient with

Somatoform disorders
pain, co-morbidity with, 314
premenstrual syndrome (PMS) and, 424

Specific phobias, approach to, 142–143; see also Anxious patient
cognitive-behavioral therapy (CBT), 81–82
defining, 142
onset, 142
treatments, 143

SPECT (single photon emission computed tomography), 230

Spinal cord injuries, suicide risk and, 131

Spironolactone
sexual dysfunction, 407t

St. John's wort (Hypericum perforatum; SJW), 643–644, 673–674
adverse effects, 673
depression, 122
drug-drug interactions, 673–674
natural antidepressant, 673–674

Status epilepticus, 233

Steriod-suppressing agents, 122
depression, 122

Steroid
dementia, 526
dependence, 526
psychosis, 522
withdrawal syndrome, 526

Steroids, approach to patient receiving, 521–528
neuropsychiatric complications from steriod use, 522–526
management of, 526–527t
risk factors, 524t, 524–526
related neuropsychiatric syndromes from steriod use, 526
steroid use and complications, 521t–522

Steroids, neuropsychiatric side effects, 372t

Stevens-Johnson syndrome, 187

Stimulants
attention-deficit/hyperactivity disorder (ADHD), 289–293
organ transplant patients, 388

Stress
infertility and, 414
smoking cessation and, 707

Stress management, 85–93
chronic stress and psychiatric disorders, 89–90
evaluation, 88–89
overview, 85t, 85–86
primary sources of stress, 86–88
daily hassles, 86
economic difficulties, 88
environmental, 88
organizational changes, 87
personality influences, 87
physical ailments, 86
psychiatric disorders, 87
self-doubt, 86
social relationships, 87
treatment strategies, 90–92, 91t
non-pharmacologic interventions, 90–92, 91t
pharmacologic interventions, 90

Structured Clinical Interview for DSM-III-R Personality Disorders (SCID-II), 56–57

Subarachnoid hemorrhage, headaches from, 245

Substance abuse
agents used to treat, cardiovascular side effects, 651
bipolar disorder, 185
counseling, treatment for organ transplant patients, 389
insomnia secondary to, 257
non-compliance, 730
organ transplant patients, 390
pain, co-morbidity with, 314
premenstrual syndrome (PMS) and, 424
screening tests for, 57
smoking cessation and, 707

Substance abuse and dependence
HIV patient, 378–379

Substance-related disorders
referrals for, 29t

Suicidal ideation
antidepressant-induced side effect, 622

Suicidal patient, approach to, 127–135
current suicidal tendencies, evaluation of, 127t–129
approach to patient at potential risk, 128
corroboration with family and friends, 129
examination of mental status, 129

hopelessness, 129
patients, 127
possible precipitants, 129
social supports, 129
suicidal ideation and intent, 128
suicidal plans, 128
difficulties in assessing suicide risk,
133–134
clinician factors, 134
evaluation itself, 134
patient factors, 133–134
overview, 127
prevalence in primary care settings, 3
risk factors, examination of, 129–131,
130t
demographic factors, 129
familial factors, 131
medical illnesses, 130–131
past/present suicidal tendencies,
131
psychiatric disorders, 130, 129
social influences, 131
treatment of suicide risk, 132–133
disposition, 133
initiation, 132
medical conditions, stabilization
of, 132
self-harm, protection from, 132
serial assessments of mental status,
132
Suicide
HIV/AIDS patient, 379
Suicide risk, approach to patient with, 76,
129–134; see also Depression
depressed patients, 76
Sulfonylureas
weight gain, 453t
Sulindac
pain, 318t
Sumatriptan (Imitrex)
migraine headaches, treatment of, 247
monoamine oxidase inhibitors,
interaction with, 617t
Supportive therapy, 15
Sympathomimetics
rehabilitation patients, 485t
Syncope, 231
Systemic lupus erythematosus (SLE),
525

Tachycardia, 645
Tacrine (Cognex)
cognitive enhancement, 208
drug-drug interactions, 668
Tamoxifen, neuropsychiatric side effects,
362t, 363

Target heart rate, 717t
Tegaserod (Zelnorm)
irritable bowel syndrome (IBS) and,
354
Temazepam (Restoril)
insomnia, 256t
rehabilitation patients, 485t
Tenofovir, neuropsychiatric side effects,
371t
Tension headaches
characteristics, 244
onset and duration, 245
precipitating and ameliorating factors,
246
treatment, 249
Teratogenic risk, 436
Theophylline, seizures with, 228t
Therapeutic donor insemination (TDI),
415
Thiabendazole, neuropsychiatric side
effects, 371t
Thiazide diuretics
sexual dysfunction, 396t
Thiazides
sexual dysfunction, 407t
Thiazolidinediones
weight gain, 453t
Thioridazine (Mellaril)
anxiety in terminal illness, 495t
delirium in terminal illness, 497t
effects on heart and cardiovascular
system, 637t
sexual dysfunction, 396t
Thiothixene (Navane)
effects on heart and cardiovascular
system, 637t
pregnancy, 438t
seizures with, 228t
Thyroid
depression, 123
Tolmetin
pain, 318t
Tonic-clonic (grand mal) seizures, 230,
232
Topiramate (Topamax)
binge-eating disorder (BED), 464
cardiovascular side effects, 649
effects on heart and cardiovascular
system, 637t
elevated, expansive, or irritable mood,
187
migraine headaches, 249
obesity, 461–462
seizures, treatment of, 232, 233t
Topotecan, neuropsychiatric side effects,
362t, 364

Tracheostomy, 259
Transcutaneous electrical nerve
stimulation (TENS), 312, 378
Transdermal nicotine patches, 709
Transference, 590–591, 743
Transient insomnia, 255
Tranylcypromine (Parnate), 120
adverse effects, 614t
analgesic use, 326t
anxiety disorders, 147
cardiovascular side effects, 616
depression, 120
effects on heart and cardiovascular
system, 637t
obsessive-compulsive disorder
(OCD), 169
Traumatic event, approach to patient
following, 535–543
defining a traumatic event, 535
immediately following, 537–539
evaluation, 537–538
treatment, 538–539
months to years following, 542
overview, 535
responses to traumatic stress,
535–537
weeks to months following, 539–542
evaluation, 539–540
treatment, 540–542
Trazodone (Desyrel), 120
adverse effects, 614t
analgesic use, 326t
antidepressant-induced fatigue and
sedation, 621t
anxiety disorders, 150, 257
dementia, 210
depression, 120
depression in terminal illness, 493t
effects on heart and cardiovascular
system, 637t
GI side effects, 356t
irritable bowel syndrome (IBS),
356t
post-traumatic stress disorder (PTSD),
541
sexual dysfunction, 396t
side effects, 120
Treatment decisions at the end of life,
687–695
advance directives, 690–691
autonomy at the bedside, 687–689t
definitions, 687
forgoing life-sustaining treatment,
resolving conflicts about,
693–694t
overview, 687

Treatment decisions at the end of life,
    (*continued*)
  palliative care, approach to patient
      receiving, 693; *see also*
      Palliative care
  physician-assisted suicide and
      euthanasia, 691, 693
  premature requests for limiting
      life-sustaining treatment,
      691
Treatment non-compliance
  chronic illness and, 305
Treatment recommendations, enhancing
    patient compliance with. *See*
    Compliance, enhancing
Treatment refusal, approach to, approach
    to, 577–581; *see also* Civil
    commitment
  approach to, 579–580
  overview, 577–578
  process, 578–579
Triazolam (Halcion)
  insomnia, 256t
Tricyclic antidepressants (TCAs),
    117–118t, 294–295
  adverse effects, 147, 295, 493t, 614t
  anxiety associated with HIV
      infection, 376
  anxiety disorder, 147
  cardiovascular side effects, 617,
      639–641, 640t
  central nervous system side effects,
      619–620
  chronic pain, 319
  cocaine dependence, 516
  depression, 117–118
  depression in terminal illness, 493t
  drug-drug interactions, 662t–663t
  HIV/AIDS patients, treating
      depression, 373
  insomnia in HIV/AIDS patients,
      377
  migraine headaches, 248
  monoamine oxidase inhibitors,
      interaction with, 617t
  obsessive-compulsive disorder
      (OCD), 143, 167
  pain in HIV infection, 378
  pregnancy, 437, 438t
  sexual dysfunction, 396t
  side effects, 117–118
  social phobia, 142
  weight gain, 619
Trihexyphenidyl (Artane)
  violent patients, 572

Triiodothyronine
  antidepressant-induced fatigue and
      sedation, 621t
Trimethoprim-sulfamethoxazole,
      neuropsychiatric side effects,
      371t
Trimipramine (Surmontil)
  analgesic use, 326t
Triptans
  contraindications and warnings, 248
  migraine headaches, treatment of,
      247
  potential interactions, 248
Tuberculosis, homeless patients, 596

Unilateral neglect, 220, 222
Unipolar depressive disorder, 111t, 113
United Network for Organ Sharing
    (UNOS), 385
Urinary hesitancy and retention
  antidepressant-induced side effects,
      622–623

Vaginismus, approach to patient with,
    400; *see also* Sexual dysfunction
Valerian, 676–677
  adverse effects, 677
Valproate
  mania associated with HIV infection,
      376
Valproic acid
  dementia, 211
  drug-drug interactions, 657, 660t
  glucocorticoid use, neuropsychiatric
      complications from, 527
  pregnancy, 438t, 439
  seizures, treatment of, 232, 233t
Valproic acid (Depakote)
  chronic pain, 323t
  post-traumatic stress disorder
      (PTSD), 541
  weight gain, 453t
Vascular dementia, 205
Venlafaxine (Effexor)
  adverse effects, 291t, 614t
  anxiety disorder, 146
  attention-deficit/hyperactivity
      disorder (ADHD), 291t
  cardiovascular side effects, 616, 617,
      618, 639
  depression in terminal illness, 493t
  effects on heart and cardiovascular
      system, 637t
  GI side effects, 356t
  irritable bowel syndrome (IBS), 356t

monoamine oxidase inhibitors,
      interaction with, 617t
  rehabilitation patients, 485t
  weight gain, 619
Venlafaxine (Effexor XR)
  post-traumatic stress disorder
      (PTSD), 541
Verapamil
  migraine headaches, 248
Vertical banded gastroplasty, weight-loss
    surgery, 463
Vertigo, approach to patient with, 263,
    265–266; *see also* Dizziness
Very low calorie diets (VLCDs), 460
Vinblastine, neuropsychiatric side
      effects, 362t, 364
Vincristine, neuropsychiatric side
      effects, 362t, 364
Vinorelbine, neuropsychiatric side
      effects, 362t, 364
Violence. *See* Domestic violence,
    approach to; Violent patient,
    approach to
Violent patient, approach to, 567–575
  evaluation, 567–571, 568t–569t
  general recommendation, 567
  overview, 567
  psychiatric differential diagnosis,
      572–573
  treatment strategies, 573–575
Visual hallucinations, 162
Vitamin B$_6$
  premenstrual syndrome (PMS),
      424
Vitamin B$_{12}$, 674–675
  natural antidepressants, 674–675
Vitamin E, 208

Warfarin
  drug-drug interactions, 664t
Weight gain
  antidepressant-induced side effect,
      619
  smoking cessation and, 707
Weight loss (when not dieting) or gain
  postpartum depression, 448
Withdrawal, infertile patient, 413
Withdrawal symptoms, smoking
    cessation and, 707
Withdrawn, unsociable, or remote
    patient, approach to, 108; *see
    also* Personality disorders

Yale-Brown Obsessive-Compulsive
    Scale (Y-BOCS), 55

Yohimbine (Yocon)
    antidepressant-induced sexual
        dysfunction, 624*t*
    erectile dysfunction, 409
Young Mania Rating Scale (Y-MRS), 55

Zaleplon (Sonata)
    insomnia, 256*t*

Ziprasidone (Geodon)
    cardiovascular side effects, 645*t*, 646
    effects on heart and cardiovascular
        system, 637*t*
    rehabilitation patients, 485*t*
    violent patients, 574
Zolmitriptan (Zomig)
    migraine headaches, treatment of, 247

Zolpidem (Ambien)
    antidepressant-induced fatigue and
        sedation, 621*t*
    drug-drug interactions, 668
    insomnia, 256*t*
Zung Self-Rating Depression Scale
    (SDS), 54